Foundations for Excellence:

75 Years of Duke Medicine

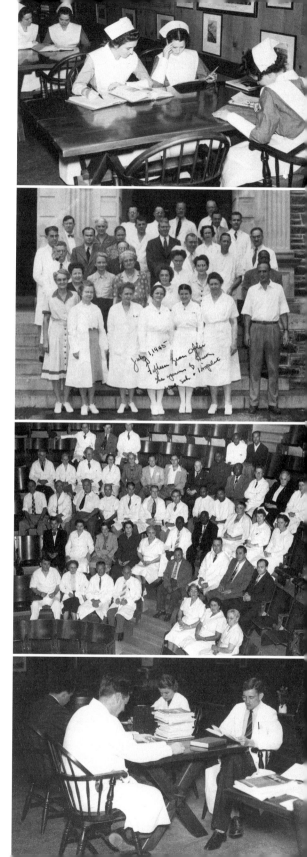

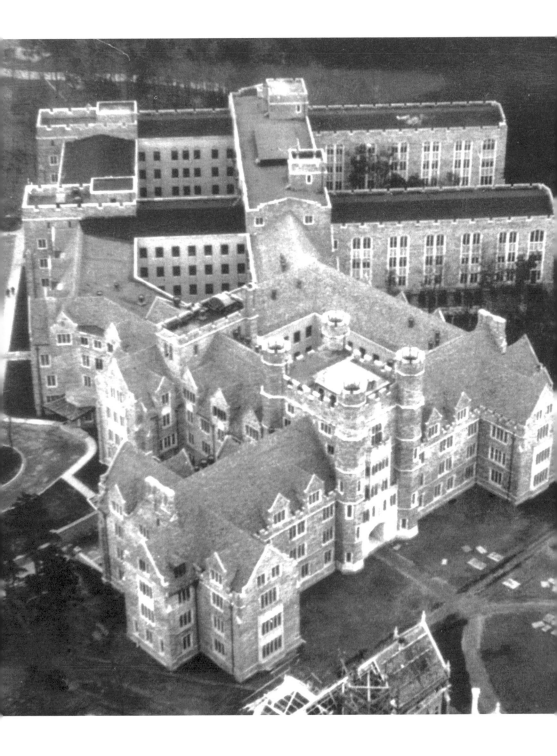

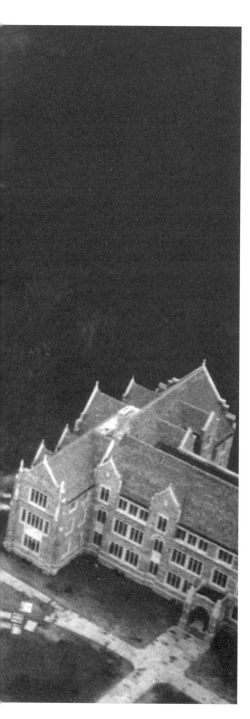

FOUNDATIONS

FOR EXCELLENCE:

75 YEARS OF

DUKE MEDICINE

By Walter E. Campbell

EDITED BY MAURA HIGH

DUKE
MEDICINE
75
EST. 1930

Duke University Medical Center Library

Durham, North Carolina

© 2006 Duke University
All rights reserved

Library of Congress Control Number: 2006928768
ISBN 0-9672946-4-9

Design and typesetting by Molly Renda
Printed by The Stinehour Press

Published by Duke University Medical Center Library
Durham, North Carolina

5   4   3   2   1

Photographs in the front pages are from the Duke University Medical Center Archives and show views of the hospital, library, staff, and patients taken between 1930 and 1945.

PAGE I, School of Medicine Library, 1940s; Members of the original School of Medicine staff, 1945; Duke University School of Medicine faculty and Duke Hospital staff in Duke Hospital amphitheater, 1950; School of Medicine Library, ca. 1945. PAGE II–III, Duke University Medical Center campus, including the School of Medicine and Duke Hospital, ca. 1930. PAGE XVII, Patrons in the reading room of the School of Medicine Library, 1937; Pediatric patients and their families waiting for treatment in the pediatrics ward of Duke Hospital, 1940s; Operation under Sterilamp using ultraviolet light, 1937; Division of Educational Media Services, Medical Illustration, undated.

For Mary Lee

On the twenty-first anniversary of her life in Duke Medicine

CONTENTS

IX   LIST OF ILLUSTRATIONS

XIII   FOREWORD BY MARY D. B. T. SEMANS

XV   ACKNOWLEDGMENTS

I   INTRODUCTION

18   CHAPTER 1: Duke Medicine and the Foundations of Health Care Reform in the American South

28   CHAPTER 2: The Corporate Hand and Duke Medicine: Research and Leadership

64   CHAPTER 3: Between Two Worlds: Duke Medicine from 1938 to 1940

100   CHAPTER 4: World War II and Duke Medicine

146   CHAPTER 5: After the War: The Politics of Duke Medicine, 1946–1950

204   CHAPTER 6: Duke Medicine at the Crossroads, 1950–1960

262   CHAPTER 7: Race, Place, and the Mission of Duke Medicine, 1960–1980

312   CHAPTER 8: Duke Medicine and the Concept of Oneness, 1980–1989

346   CHAPTER 9: Duke Medicine and the Health Care Business, 1989–2004

394   EPILOGUE: A Compassionate Global Business

399   APPENDIX 1: List of Departments and Chairs

405   APPENDIX 2: List of Fellows and Honorees

407   NOTES

435   BIBLIOGRAPHY

447   INDEX

LIST OF ILLUSTRATIONS

F.1 Osler ivy ceremony

1.1 The second Watts Hospital building
1.2 The first Lincoln Hospital building
1.3 Replanting of the Osler ivy

1.1 View of the West Campus quadrangle, 1931
1.2 The trustees of The Duke Endowment, 1925
1.3 Duke Hospital and medical school faculty, 1932
1.4 School of Nursing staff, nurses, and students, 1931
1.5 Dr. Wilburt C. Davison

2.1 Rear view of the Davison Building
2.2 Dr. Joseph W. Beard
2.3 Dr. David T. Smith
2.4 Dr. J. Deryl Hart and a team of surgeons
2.5 Duke University School of Medicine, viewed from the campus quadrangle
2.6 George G. Allen
2.7 Dr. J. Deryl Hart
2.8 Dr. Frederic M. Hanes
2.9 Dr. Robert A. Lambert

3.1 Aerial view of Duke University campus and PDC building, ca. 1940
3.2 Dean Wilburt C. Davison with Joseph and Dorothy Beard

3.3 African American pediatric patients and their families
3.4 Highland Hall
3.5 Dr. Richard S. Lyman
3.6 The "colored" registration area of Duke Hospital
3.7 An annual hospital picnic, with Stan Lordeaux and Dr. F. Bayard Carter
3.8 The waiting room of the 1940 addition to the Private Diagnostic Clinic
3.9 Drs. Richard S. Lyman, Wilburt C. Davison, Robert L. Flowers, Adolf Meyer, Robert S. Carroll, and Frederic M. Hanes

4.1 Cadet nurses on the steps of the Hanes Annex
4.2 Dr. Walter Kempner
4.3 Number of inpatients and outpatients at Duke University Medical Center, 1940–46
4.4 Technicians at work in the laboratory of Dr. Walter Kempner
4.5 The Bell Research Building under construction, 1945–47
4.6 Dr. Maurice H. Greenhill confers with the head nurse in Psychiatry
4.7 Dr. Hans Lowenbach observes a patient's reaction to electroshock therapy
4.8 Conscientious objectors working on Meyer Ward

4.9 Operating room of the 65th General Hospital

4.10 Physician with a patient at the Duke Hospital Blood Bank

4.11 Dr. Wilburt C. Davison, Doris Duke, and Dean William H. Wannamaker at the Jones Construction Company shipyard, Brunswick, Georgia

5.1 The Hanes Annex

5.2 Map of Duke University and Duke Medical Center, 1956

5.3 Circulation desk and patrons in the Duke University Medical School Library

5.4 Duke Hospital's nurses using portable x-ray equipment

5.5 Clementine Amey and Harriett Amey

5.6 Customers waiting in line at the cashier's window

5.7 Medical alumni reunion, April 27, 1950

5.8 Oscar Ross Ewing, Harold J. Gallagher, and Willis Smith

5.9 Drs. Jack D. Myers, Walter H. Cargill, John B. Hickam, and Eugene A. Stead Jr.

5.10 A nurse examines a child in a community clinic

5.11 The Department of Social Services at Duke Hospital

5.12 Judith Farrar, Mary Duke Biddle Trent, and Mildred P. Farrar

6.1 The Private Diagnostic Clinic under construction, 1955

6.2 Campaign postcard for Willis Smith

6.3 Rice dieters enjoy a meal together

6.4 Dr. H. Grant Taylor responding to a question from Eleanor Roosevelt

6.5 Dr. Paul M. Gross and Dr. A. Hollis Edens with Gordon Dean

6.6 Dr. Barnes Woodhall

6.7 Dr. Leslie B. Hohman and Irene Cherhavy with a young patient

6.8 University of North Carolina president Gordon Gray and Duke University president A. Hollis Edens

6.9 The Duke Out-Patient Clinic

6.10 The Surgical Instrument Shop

6.11 The Durham Veterans Administration Hospital

6.12 Dr. Ewald W. Busse

6.13 Dr. D. Gordon Sharp using an electron microscope

6.14 Faculty and students in the laboratory of the Research Training Program

7.1 New main entrance to the medical center and adjacent buildings, 1970

7.2 Drs. J. Deryl Hart and Douglas M. Knight, at the dedication of the Deryl Hart Pavilion

7.3 Dr. William G. Anlyan

7.4 Dr. Philip Handler

7.5 Dr. James B. Wyngaarden

7.6 Thelma Ingles with Virginia Arnold of the Rockefeller Foundation

7.7 Dr. Eugene A. Stead Jr. examining a patient

7.8 Dr. David C. Sabiston Jr.

7.9 The board of trustees of The Duke Endowment, 1961

7.10 North Division of Duke Hospital under construction in the late 1970s

7.11 Dr. E. Harvey Estes Jr.

7.12 Major figures in the history of Duke Medicine

8.1 North Division of Duke Hospital and the Bell Building, ca. 1980

8.2 The Department of Psychiatry at Duke University Medical Center

8.3 Duke University president Terry Sanford reading the medical center's in-house publication

8.4 Dr. Dani P. Bolognesi

8.5 John A. McMahon

8.6 The PRT (personal rapid transit) system

8.7 Drs. Ewald W. Busse, Thomas D. Kinney, William G. Anlyan, Barnes Woodhall, and J. Deryl Hart
8.8 Dr. Robert J. Lefkowitz

9.1 Levine Science Research Center
9.2 Dr. Robert M. Califf
9.3 Dr. Ernest Mario
9.4 Dr. Charles Johnson
9.5 Dr. Jean G. Spaulding
9.6 MaryAnn E. Black
9.7 Ruby L. Wilson
9.8 Mary T. Champagne
9.9 Drs. Arthur C. Christakos, Dan G. Blazer, Ewald W. Busse, William G. Anlyan, Ralph Snyderman, Charles E. Putman, and Doyle G. Graham
9.10 Dr. Charles E. Putman and a model of the Levine Science Research Center
9.11 Dr. H. Keith H. Brodie with Douglas M. Knight and Terry Sanford
9.12 Dr. H. Keith H. Brodie, Philip "Jack" Baugh, Dr. William G. Anlyan, and Dr. Ralph Snyderman
9.13 Dr. Ralph Snyderman and Nannerl O. Keohane

E.1 The Ralph Snyderman, M.D. Genome Sciences Research Building
E.2 Richard H. Brodhead and Dr. Victor J. Dzau

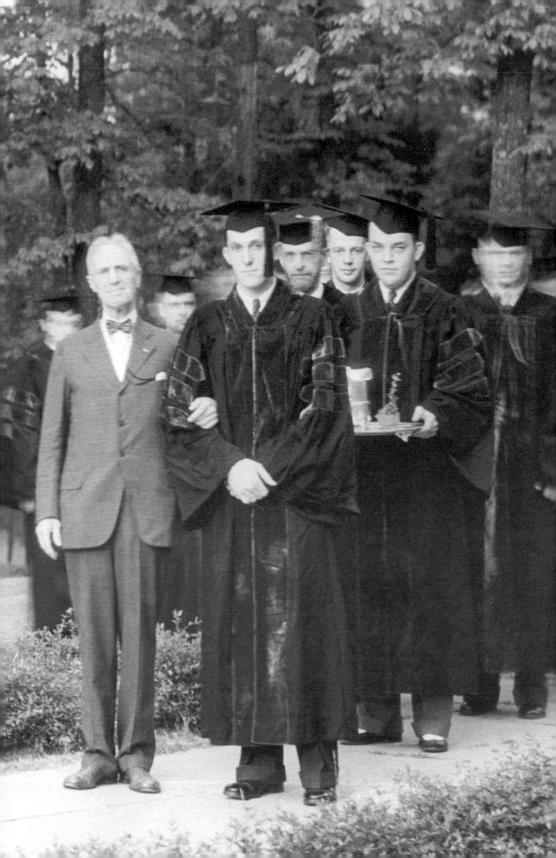

FOREWORD

On his second visit to the Johns Hopkins Medical School, William Preston Few, who had just been appointed president of the new Duke University, sent for Dr. Wilburt C. Davison, a staff member there who had been recommended by the great Dr. William H. Welch for the deanship of the future school of medicine at Duke. As Davison arrived in Dr. Welch's office, Dr. Few asked, "I have come for you. Are you ready?" Dr. Davison replied, "Yes, sir."[1] With those few words a great new medical institution began. That simple answer illustrates the firm resolve typical of Duke Medical School from its beginning.

Davison's determined response also reflects the inspiration of James Buchanan Duke, who, from the beginning of his philanthropic planning, felt that a hospital and medical school should be a major part of the new university he had envisioned. He established The Duke Endowment to provide for building Duke University and, a short time later, the medical center, with provisions for continuing support of both.[2] He was convinced that such a medical institution was an indispensable one.[3]

Mr. Duke invited Dr. Watson Smith Rankin, one of the country's outstanding health officers, to organize and administer the hospital section of The Duke Endowment. Subsequently, together, Dr. Rankin and Dean Davison, who shared similar views about medical education, hospitals, and preventive medicine, became a passionate force for medicine in the South.

F.1 Ivy planting ceremony in memory of Sir William Osler by the first graduating class of the Duke University School of Medicine, June 7, 1932. Dr. William S. Thayer of Johns Hopkins is escorted by class president, George William Joyner. *Duke University Medical Center Archives.*

Dr. Davison's deep respect for Sir William Osler's emphasis on bedside training had a profound influence on the new Duke Hospital's insistence on excellence in clinical care. Dr. Davison did not follow blindly the arrangements of other medical schools and felt that medical students should play a role in planning their course of study. He remembered the words of Sir William Osler: "How can we make the work of the student in the third and fourth year as practical as it is in his first and second? . . . The answer is take him from the lecture-room, take him from the amphitheatre,—put him in the out-patient department—put him in the wards."[4] Duke became known as a "hands-on" medical school.

It is refreshing to review the extraordinary history of the Duke Medical Center. Dr. J. Deryl Hart, founding chief of Surgery, has written, "One of our great assets was having Dave as our Dean for over thirty years."[5] The key to the medical center's rapid success was that Dean Davison brought a team of young physicians, the majority of whom were from Johns Hopkins, to open Duke's doors. They knew each other. They had worked together. They brought with them to Duke the high demands for quality expected of them at Johns Hopkins and they transferred these demands to their new school. "Each was told that if he could not work in harmony with those already appointed, he should not accept."[6]

This history is a tribute to the fervent dedication to their unusual teamwork and to their lifetime investments in one institution. It is a tribute to the joy of working together on a great mission.

Those founding physicians had a powerful conviction that their pulling together for greatness would produce success. The dean had said that he aimed to make Duke the best medical institution in the country, and his medical staff clamored for the same goal. They invested in the school. They poured their lives into the school. Very few left for greener pastures along the way because they felt that there weren't any. They stayed until they retired and finished their lives here, passing this flaming dedication on to the next generation.

Dr. Davison's reply to President Few rings in our ears, "I am ready."

Mary Duke Biddle Trent Semans

ACKNOWLEDGMENTS

As the author of this history, I cannot claim to be a neutral recorder. My ties, and those of my family, to Durham, to Duke University, and to Duke Medicine in particular, are close and go back a long way. We extend our gratitude to the many wonderful individuals we have met in the course of our lives and work here. There is little in the pages that follow about the legions of Duke Medicine employees who perform the kind of hospital work that I did and that my wife, Mary Lee, now does. Nor is mention made of the vast majority of service workers, physicians, staff, faculty members, and others who have made Duke Medicine what it is today. Their story awaits another time and another teller. What this anniversary history does provide is a story that combines my specific interests as a professional historian with the nature of the sources consulted and the important suggestions made by the book committee members with whom I worked.

I am indebted to many librarians and archivists for their generous assistance, especially Barbara Busse, Emily Glenn, Russell Koonts, Jessica Roseberry, Charles Rutt, and Mira Waller at the Duke University Medical Center Library and Archives; Tom Harkins, Tim Pyatt, and Nancy Thacker at the Duke University Archives; Elizabeth Steinberg at the Doris Duke Charitable Foundation Archives; and Beth Jaffe at the Rockefeller Archive Center. Eugene Lofton, Derrick Vines, and Sally Wardell were indispensable in meeting my many computer and networking needs at Duke, while the project's constant administrative tasks were handled patiently and ably by Michael Davidson, Tanika Hayes, Wilma Morris, Rick Peterson, and Vanessa Sellars.

The committee that oversaw this project shared with me their knowledge and interest in the history of Duke Medicine, as well as the insight, wisdom, and understanding they have gained from living and studying that history. Much of what is good herein was made better by their assistance and by the skilled and careful editing of Maura High, whose critical and engaged reading of the manuscript also helped transform it. The members of the 75th anniversary book committee were Edward Halperin, Margaret Humphreys, Ellen Luken, Frank Neelon, Suzanne Porter, Vicki Saito, Pat Thibodeau, and Robert Wilkins. I am thankful in particular to Pat Thibodeau, associate dean for library services, and Suzanne Porter, curator of the History of Medicine Collections at Duke, for their constant encouragement and support. In a time like our own, when the whole concept of libraries and knowledge are being revolutionized, their leadership will help guarantee Duke a central place in defining the new global order of information.

Foundations for Excellence:

75 Years of Duke Medicine

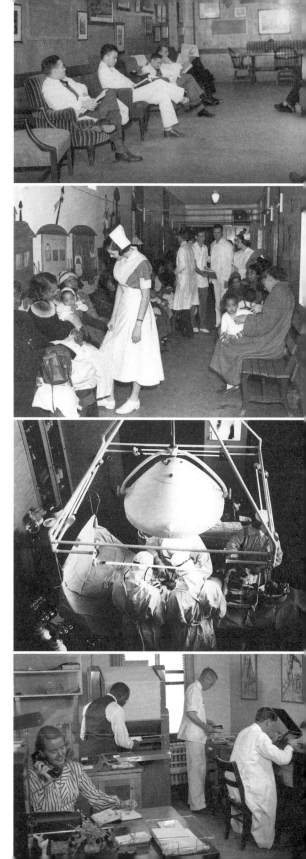

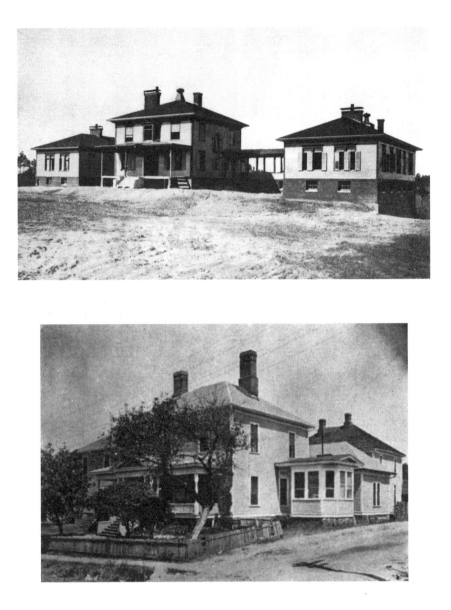

TOP: 1.1 The second Watts Hospital building, constructed 1909. *Duke University Archives.*

BOTTOM: 1.2 The first Lincoln Hospital building, constructed 1901. *Duke University Archives.*

Early in January of 1921, Dr. William Preston Few, the president of Trinity College, a small Methodist school in Durham, North Carolina, visited the offices of the Rockefeller General Education Board in New York. Few wanted some advice from Dr. Abraham Flexner, the board's director of medical education, who was then the world's leading authority on the topic.

Flexner was away in Europe, however, so Few spoke with E. C. Sage and together they drafted a memo to Flexner. "President Few of Trinity College called at the office January 7, 1921," they wrote. "He is desirous of conferring with Dr. Flexner in regard to the possible building of a Medical College in connection with Trinity College. Already a wealthy resident of Durham, Mr. George W. Watts, has made possible the building near to the college of a Hospital, known as Watts Hospital, for which there is already $1,225,000. Mr. Watts has indicated to President Few his willingness to complete the hospital and provide for it adequately and also erect a building for a Medical School. President Few is of the opinion that an opportunity is presenting itself now to create here in Durham a public health center for both white and colored people. He has assurances that a hospital for colored people also will be built."[1]

Few hoped to further Durham's cause by linking the proposed medical school to the new university that he and Trinity's major benefactor, the tobacco and electric utility magnate James Buchanan Duke, were planning. The General Education Board had given Vanderbilt University $4 million to reorganize its medical school in 1919, and Few believed a similar amount could be matched by the university being planned by Duke in Durham. "Of course, definite plans have not yet matured," the memo continued, "but President

Few is of the opinion that if the General Education Board could duplicate its gift made to Vanderbilt, he could secure a like amount for the University, not all of which, perhaps, going to the Medical School, for details have not yet been worked out. Just what proportion of the $4,000,000 might be available for the Medical School he is not yet prepared to say. This proposition involves, therefore, practically a $10,000,000 undertaking. In view of the precarious condition of the health of Mr. Watts, President Few is desirous of consummating plans at the earliest practicable date."

Few renewed his plea after returning to Durham, writing to Sage, "When you and I made the memorandum for Dr. Flexner concerning the possibility of making Durham a hospital, medical, and public health centre, I spoke to you of Mr. George W. Watts as being a wealthy man here much interested in the cause, but in precarious state of health. I now have to inform you that surgeons in Baltimore have operated on Mr. Watts and found cancer of the stomach in aggravated form. His life is, of course, a matter now of weeks or possibly months. You will therefore understand the urgency in getting the subject to Dr. Flexner's attention as soon as he returns from Europe and has opportunity to take it up."[2]

Founding of the City of Medicine

Watts died March 7, 1921, but "the cause" continued to grow and evolve in Durham, beginning not with a university medical center but with the development of Durham as a "city of medicine." New additions were soon made to Watts Hospital (the city's white hospital), and in 1924, through gifts and matching funds from James B. ("Buck") Duke, his brother, Benjamin N. ("Ben") Duke, and the city's black community, a new Lincoln Hospital was completed for Durham's African Americans. Shortly thereafter, Ben Duke also funded, in memory of his son, Angier Buchanan Duke, the construction of a nurses' home near Lincoln Hospital. These gifts reinforced an established collaboration of the Dukes and their father, Washington Duke (who had joined them in supporting the first Lincoln Hospital in 1901), with the city's black leaders, who pointed to the new facilities as "a striking example of what can be accomplished in a community when both races work together with a common objective."[3]

It was also in 1924 that Trinity College became Duke University through the provisions of Buck Duke's indenture creating The Duke Endowment. Only in 1930, however, five years after his death, did the dreams for Duke Medicine[4] finally emerge. By then Flexner had left the General Education Board, the board had ceased making large endowments for medical schools, and the university had used $4 million from Duke's estate to build a school of medicine and a 400-bed teaching hospital for blacks and whites. Not until the last minute did the General Education Board contribute to the cause: its $300,000 grant enabled Duke's school of medicine to open in 1930 as a four-year medical school—the first in North Carolina—rather than as a two-year school.

Since that time, the Duke University Medical Center (DUMC) has become one of the nation's leading academic medical centers and the primary catalyst for expanding Durham's reputation and service as a hospital, medical, and public health center. In 1950, the North Carolina Cerebral Palsy Hospital opened on Erwin Road, not far from Duke Hospital, and three years later the Veterans Administration opened a large hospital directly across Erwin Road from the expanding medical center. By the late 1960s, both the old Watts and Lincoln hospitals faced increasing deficits and outmoded facilities, and in 1976, after years of political and racial wrangling, a new hospital, Durham County General Hospital, was opened for all. As a result, Watts Hospital was closed and Lincoln began providing primary health services as the Lincoln Health Center. By 1998, Durham County General was known as Durham Regional Hospital and had become part of the new and expanding Duke University Health System. Today, Duke University is the fourth largest private employer in the state of North Carolina and the largest employer in Durham—the self-proclaimed "City of Medicine." DUMC also continues to rank among the top ten medical centers in the United States and is playing a leading role in attempting to transform the existing health care system through innovative developments in genomics, integrative medicine, and prospective health care.

DUMC has thus evolved since 1930 from an isolated medical outpost in the American South to a world-renowned institution with a global reach. How did it come so far so fast? Part of the answer is that original "cause." Duke's leaders have always been dedicated to Durham and to nurturing individuals and institutions that collaborate across the lines of race, sex, and class in support of education, health care, and leadership. At the same time, DUMC has always had access to the best of everything, from buildings, machines, and funding sources to ideas, information, and individuals. The monopoly capitalists who conceived the medical center in the 1920s linked it with established networks of trade, health care, finance, and research, and from the day it opened in 1930, DUMC's faculty and state-of-the-art facilities have dominated cutting-edge health and medical care in the southeastern United States.

Yet having the best of everything is no guarantee of success: DUMC has also depended on the ability of its leaders to adjust to changes in the environment and to shape the institution's future in creative ways. Much of Duke Medicine's continued success can be attributed, in fact, to the skill of its leaders in progressively expanding the institution's capacity and seizing every opportunity that emerged, piling advantage upon advantage.

The Mission and the Missionaries

The chapters that follow focus on the individuals and groups who shaped Duke Medicine's relationship with the private and public institutions dedicated to improving the nation's health and medical care. More specifically, the narrative describes the evolution and interplay of Duke Medicine with The Duke Endowment, Duke University, the Duke family, and James B. Duke's corporate interests; with the nation's largest foundations, particularly the Rockefeller Foundation and its related philanthropies; with the Private Diagnostic Clinic at Duke; with the state of North Carolina; and with the United States Public Health Service, especially the National Institutes of Health.

The Duke Endowment established the most important foundation for Duke Medicine's future excellence. The Endowment not only defined DUMC's mission and relationship to the state of North Carolina; its leaders also closely controlled the course of Duke University for the next 40 years: first, through the power accorded them in Buck Duke's indenture, and second, through the presence of three Endowment trustees on the seven-member executive committee of university trustees. The 1924 indenture gave the Endowment's trustees the power to fund a number of "schools" within the new Duke University, noting that "a Medical School" was among those that might "eventually" be included.

The Duke Endowment can aptly be described as a regional economic development plan that supported health care and education in North Carolina and South Carolina for men and women, blacks and whites, rich and poor. The Endowment embodied Buck Duke's personal experience and convictions as well as the programs of the Rockefeller Foundation and the Rockefeller General Education Board that had made North Carolina a laboratory for progressive health and educational reform in the early 20th-century American South. Unlike the Rockefeller philanthropies, however, the Endowment was directly intertwined with a for-profit business. Duke's Southern Power System (the Duke Power Company and its subsidiary companies) provided electrical power to the Piedmont Carolinas. As described by Duke in his indenture, "For many years I have been engaged in the development of water powers in certain sections of the States of North Carolina and South Carolina. . . . My ambition is that the revenues of such developments shall administer to the social welfare, as the operation of such developments is administering to the economic welfare, of the communities which they serve."[5]

Buck Duke established his private charitable foundation with $40 million in securities and then vastly increased that amount by the terms of his will. The common stock of his utility company, Duke Power, became the economic engine of the Endowment; indeed, the 1924 indenture creating the Endowment specifically designated both Duke Power securities and certain kinds of government bonds as the only financial instruments in which the 15 trustees could invest the foundation's funds.[6] Thus Duke Medicine emerged and developed as part of a larger ensemble of interests that linked the income of a nonprofit charity to a corporate, for-profit enterprise. As one close observer has written, "Not only had Duke attempted to make sure that the Endowment would always be there to help Duke Power meet its constant need for capital. He had also, in effect, given the virtual ownership and control of Duke Power to the Duke Endowment, as represented by its trustees."[7]

Buck Duke's indenture says nothing specific, of course, about the mission of Duke Medicine. The indenture simply mentions the possibility of establishing a medical school at Duke. The general purpose of the Endowment, as established in the indenture, is "to make provision in some measure for the needs of mankind along physical, mental and spiritual lines." The indenture charges the Endowment's trustees with distributing to certain institutions and programs the annual income of the foundation after the trustees themselves are compensated, and after additions are made to the original corpus (principal) of the trust. Duke University is the major beneficiary of the trust (receiving 32 percent of the income), and there are three other educational institutions named as beneficiaries: Davidson College in Davidson, North Carolina (5 percent); Johnson C. Smith University in Charlotte, North Carolina (4 percent); and Furman University in Greenville, South Carolina (5 percent). Another 32 percent of the distributed income goes to nonprofit hospitals in the Carolinas to help pay for the care of indigent patients, for building nonprofit community hospitals for both blacks and whites, and for converting existing for-profit hospitals into nonprofit community hospitals for all. The Endowment also gives 10 percent of its distributed income to orphanages for both races and 12 percent to certain specified beneficiaries of the Methodist Church in North Carolina.[8]

Funds for building and equipping the new university's medical center came from part of Buck Duke's holdings in one the world's great monopolies, the Aluminum Company of America. Duke acquired a one-ninth interest in Alcoa in the summer of 1925, and on October 10 of that year, just nine days before he died, Duke signed a codicil to his will providing $10 million to The Duke Endowment for building and equipping a medical school, teaching hospital, and dormitory for nurses at Duke University. Duke's executors apparently fulfilled this legacy by selling shares of 6 percent Alcoa preferred stock, which were separate from the larger group of Alcoa common stocks in his estate. Only $4 million was spent for the medical center projects, however, leaving $6 million in Alcoa preferred stock claimed by DUMC as medical center endowment and by the university as endowment for the larger institution.[9] The matter was not insignificant; although Duke Power stocks accounted for 80 percent of the Endowment's entire investment for the next four decades, over 95 percent of the foundation's remaining common stocks were in stocks connected with Alcoa's aluminum companies. And between 1960 and 1971, the value of those Alcoa stocks dropped from $110 million to $40 million.[10]

Duke Medicine was also staffed with the best physicians corporate America could recruit. DUMC got almost all of its original teaching faculty from the nation's leading academic medical school, the Johns Hopkins School of Medicine in Baltimore. Those who made DUMC a "little Hopkins" included Dr. Wiley D. Forbus, the founding chairman of Duke's Pathology Department, who wrote in 1952, in the first history of Duke Medicine, that the university's school of medicine had maintained from its beginning several "major objectives: (a) the cultivation and teaching of medicine on a strictly scientific basis; (b) the correlation of medical research with medical teaching at all levels of instruction, and (c) the continuous search for and experimentation with new or improved methods of teaching scientific medicine." Significantly, Forbus mentions nothing about actually *doing* research, for he wrote at a time when the role of research and specialization in Duke Medicine's future was being opposed by the medical center's most famous Hopkins transplant, Dr. Wilburt C. Davison, the founding dean of Duke's school of medicine. "From its beginning in 1930," Davison wrote in the same 1952 history, "Duke has been committed to and actively engaged in a program of training young men and women for academic and scientific careers, as well as for the practice of medicine, requiring exceptional clinical and preclinical preparation."[11]

The 1950s debate over the purpose of Duke Medicine reflected the clash between The Duke Endowment's original hospital mission and the explosion of research and specialization that followed World War II. Between 1927, when he was chosen to lead the new medical school, and his death in 1972, Wilburt Davison devoted himself to the Endowment's original mission. Davison considered it the duty of Duke Medicine to produce well-trained general practitioners as quickly as possible, with as many North Carolinians and southerners among them as practicable, and with the hope that some of these Duke-trained general practitioners would staff the well-equipped, nonprofit community hospitals being supported by the Endowment in the rural Carolinas. He and Dr. Watson Smith Rankin (who created the Endowment's hospital plan), joined the United States surgeon general, Dr. Thomas Parran Jr., on the latter's mission to study the Endowment's operations. Parran then used the information gleaned from that study to help design one of the most important pieces of health care legislation in American history, the 1946 Hospital Survey and Construction Act (widely known as the Hill-Burton Act).[12]

A New Mission: Research and the Training of Physician-Scientists

Research became a significant part of Duke Medicine in 1937 through the help of a private corporation. It took on added substance with public funding during World War II and assumed its current state of cutting-edge innovation in the late 1950s with the expansion of the National Institutes of Health. The 1937 effort involved Lederle Laboratories, a pharmaceutical company owned by one of the largest, most-diversified chemical companies in the world, American Cyanamid. Buck Duke had gained control of Cyanamid during World War I, and by the time DUMC opened in 1930, the company's three largest stockholder-officers were all trustees of the Duke Endowment. When Dr. Joseph W. Beard was hired as an assistant professor of experimental surgery at Duke, Lederle funded a laboratory for his cancer and virus research there. Within months of Beard's arrival at DUMC, he had created a profitable vaccine for equine encephalomyelitis and introduced Duke to issues of corporate-funded research that still confront university faculty today: who controls the data, who profits from them, and how. Four years later, on the eve of World War II, Cyanamid gave Duke an electron microscope—one of the nation's first—for use in Beard's laboratory at DUMC. Indeed, Beard's important wartime collaboration with the Rockefeller Foundation and the United States military on infectious diseases laid the foundation for Duke's reputation for excellence in medical research.[13]

Beard also embodied DUMC's close ties to the Rockefeller Foundation and to the network of personal and professional connections on which Duke Medicine was built. Beard's friend and mentor in surgery at Vanderbilt, Dr. Alfred Blalock, had studied at Johns Hopkins with Dr. J. Deryl Hart, the founding chairman of Duke's Department of Surgery. Blalock not only recommended Beard for the position at Duke; he later became department head and chief of surgery at Hopkins, where in 1964, his second in command, Dr. David C. Sabiston Jr., accepted the chairmanship of the Department of Surgery at Duke. As for Beard, after leaving Vanderbilt in the early 1930s, he did pioneering research in the New York and Princeton laboratories of the Rockefeller Institute under two of the nation's leading experts on viruses and cancer, Drs. Richard Shope and Peyton Rous. By the time he arrived at Duke, the Rockefeller Foundation was funding pellagra research at DUMC under Dr. David T. Smith, chairman of the Department of Bacteriology. Smith was focusing on a dietary disease that was common in the South, pellagra, which results from a deficiency of nicotinic acid.

Lederle supplemented funding for Smith's pellagra research in 1937, along with support for Beard, and over the next decade or so, Lederle and the Rockefeller Foundation supported research at DUMC on vitamins, nutrition, nicotinic acid, and the biochemical properties of proteins, especially serum proteins. This early foundation of corporate and philanthropic funding proved particularly effective in stimulating DUMC's excellence in the fields of immunology, biochemistry, and protein research, fields that defined much of molecular medicine in the last half of the 20th century. DUMC's best-known biochemists were Dr. Hans Neurath and Dr. Philip Handler, both Ph.D.'s. Neurath was brought to Duke in 1938 to do special protein research with Dr. William A. Perlzweig, the founding chairman of Duke's Department of Biochemistry. In the mid-1970s, together with Dr. James B. Wyngaarden, who was then chairman of the Department of Medicine, Neurath sat on the five-member advisory board that "hand-picked promising young clinical researchers" as Howard Hughes medical investigators.[14]

Phil Handler arrived at Duke in 1939, a year after Neurath. He succeeded Perlzweig as chairman of Biochemistry in 1950, and he remained active in research at DUMC until his election as president of the National Academy of Sciences in 1969. Handler was also a liberal political activist who considered basic research an extension of the Duke Endowment's irreversible mission in primary care. Handler's initial research at Duke, on the metabolism of nicotinic acid, helped elucidate one of the major principles of biochemistry: "that major metabolic pathways are essentially irreversible and that the interconversion of two metabolites usually proceeds by different metabolic pathways."[15] Between 1948 and 1949, moreover, Handler worked with the Atomic Energy Commission to make Duke one of four national centers for training postdoctoral fellows in the use of radioisotopes in medical research. The AEC funded the research program at Duke, as it did a radioisotope laboratory in Handler's department, and the program included courses "in nuclear physics, mathematics, statistics, genetics, biological effects of radiation, genetic effects of radiation, human genetics, biophysics and the medical application of tracer technic, and laboratory course in electronics, radioisotopes and tracers."[16]

Phil Handler also understood the significance of the famous "double helix" letter published in *Nature* in 1953 by James Watson and Francis Crick, and in the late 1950s, he mobilized a cross-campus alliance with the physical sciences to create the Research Training Program at Duke. Funded by Duke University, the Commonwealth Fund, and the National Institutes of Health, the RTP was started in 1959 under Dr. James B. Wyngaarden and made "specific provision for the training of students both as investigators and as clinicians." The RTP also served as a spur to Handler and others to embark upon a major revision of the medical school curriculum in 1961. The new curriculum was introduced in 1966 along with the Medical Scientist Training Program, an NIH-funded initiative that superseded the RTP. Indeed, Jim Wyngaarden was a member of the NIH committee that established the new training program, and he would serve as chairman of the Department of Medicine at Duke from 1967 until his appointment as director of the National Institutes of Health in 1982.

The Great Foundations, Psychiatry, and the Duke Family

The arrival of Beard, Neurath, and Handler in the late 1930s also co-incided with the efforts of Dean Davison and the then chairman of Medicine, Dr. Frederic M. Hanes, to have the Rockefeller Foundation fund a department of psychiatry at Duke. In January of 1940, after years of studying North Carolina's mental health needs, the Rockefeller Foundation granted $25,000 a year for seven years to establish what was then called the Department of Neuropsychiatry at Duke. The new department quickly became involved in health and welfare programs at every level of government, for blacks and whites, while its facility in Asheville, North Carolina, Highland Hospital (which had been given to the department in anticipation of its creation), extended the department's reach to the western part of the state.

By 1950, the Department of Neuropsychiatry was deeply involved in the care and training of World War II veterans and awaiting completion of the VA hospital being constructed on Duke's campus. But for various reasons the department fell apart in 1951, and was not put back together again until 1953, when, through the collaboration of the Rockefeller Foundation, the Commonwealth Fund, and the Josiah Macy Foundation, it was renamed the Department of Psychiatry. The department's new chairman, Dr. Ewald W. ("Bud") Busse, began focusing on issues related to child development, aging, and mental retardation, and once again the department flourished—at least until the mid-1960s, when it suffered a series of financial setbacks. Following the arrival in 1974 of Busse's successor, Dr. H. Keith H. Brodie, the department began to expand once again, and by the time Brodie became president of Duke University in 1985, Psychiatry was the third largest department at DUMC. Yet when Brodie himself returned to the department in 1993, after stepping down from the presidency, Psychiatry's inpatient bed count had been almost entirely eliminated as a result of the cost-cutting medical plans adopted by health maintenance organizations and insurance companies.

The Department of Psychiatry illustrates several developments in the history of Duke Medicine. DUMC has always been a laboratory for testing new approaches in teaching, research, and patient care, and the various individuals, institutions, and organizations funding these experiments—from the Duke family, The Duke Endowment, and the Rockefeller Foundation to the Commonwealth Fund and NIH—have had a stake in seeing that DUMC succeeds. Among those who wanted psychiatry to succeed at Duke were Alan

Gregg, the director of the Rockefeller Foundation's medical division; Frederic Moir Hanes, the second chairman of Duke's Department of Medicine; Mary Duke Biddle, the niece of Buck Duke; and Mrs. Biddle's daughter, Mary Duke Biddle (Trent Semans). Alan Gregg chose Duke University as one of five Rockefeller-funded centers for the study and promotion of psychosomatic (or whole-person) medicine in the United States. Hanes envisioned psychiatry as a way to advance his own deep interests in neurology. And the Biddle women were thankful for the psychiatric help Hanes secured for Mrs. Biddle during her mental illness in the early 1930s.

Buck Duke's daughter, Doris Duke, was likewise interested in the development of psychiatry at Duke. She began funding child guidance services at the university in the late 1930s, and in 1937 she supported the creation of the Department of Social Services at Duke Hospital. Three years later the department became an important link for the new Department of Neuropsychiatry to the other departments and to social and welfare agencies at all levels of government. The Department of Social Services also facilitated the Rockefeller Foundation's program in psychosomatic medicine at DUMC, providing help for what the first chairman of Neuropsychiatry, Dr. Richard S. Lyman, described as the "slow diffusion" of psychiatry into Duke's Department of Medicine. This flow was indeed slow under Hanes, who wanted Lyman to diagnose patients rather than treat them. Only in 1946, with Hanes's death, did Lyman get somebody he could work with as head of Medicine: Dr. Eugene A. Stead Jr. The Department of Psychiatry is unusual because it faltered, despite its excellent foundations. More than any other department at Duke, it remained a laboratory rather than the transformative institution that some of its earlier supporters had anticipated. Nevertheless, the story of the Psychiatry Department reflects the changing political and moral tone of the eras in which Duke Medicine has evolved. For DUMC was conceived in the tradition of private charity but matured and flourished in the "modern" era of the federal government's increasing responsibility for health care. And over the last two decades, the corporate-charity vision that had shaped much of DUMC's development has been transformed, by the political and moral ethos of the Reagan Revolution, by globalization and health maintenance organizations, by the largest business merger movement in American history, and by the simultaneous revolutions in biotechnology and genomics.

The PDC and the Business of Duke Medicine

To these personal, corporate, and philanthropic foundations of Duke Medicine, one must also add what is perhaps the most unique source of its excellence: the Private Diagnostic Clinic. The PDC is located in

Duke Hospital but it is not part of Duke University and it never has been. It is the private practice of the attending faculty of Duke's school of medicine. Attending faculty are M.D.'s who attend to patients; they are the physician-faculty of the medical school's clinical departments: Medicine, Pediatrics, Psychiatry, Surgery, Obstetrics-Gynecology, Ophthalmology, and so on. The PDC does not include, however, faculty appointed solely to the school's basic science departments, such as Anatomy, Pathology, Biochemistry, and Bacteriology; faculty in these departments usually are not M.D.'s (that is, are not physicians).

The PDC was formed in 1931, during the early years of the Great Depression, when Duke's first chief of surgery, Dr. Deryl Hart, negotiated a deal with the university that remained verbal until 1972. The deal required the PDC to set aside a certain portion of its collected fees in lieu of rent and other costs: "a percentage deduction was established to cover expenses (22.5 percent at first, with a subsequent drop to as low as 8 percent, and stabilizing at 10 or 11 percent)." The remaining funds collected by the practice were to be "distributed to the individual doctors concerned and to the hospital at a percentage based on services tendered." In other words, since 1931 the university has shared a financial interest with Duke Hospital and the medical school's clinical faculty in the PDC's bottom line.[17]

The PDC thus became, as it remains today, one of the great ironies and foundations of Duke Medicine. On a general level, it represents the very thing Abraham Flexner had tried to eliminate from medical education during his years at the Rockefeller General Education Board: moneymaking by medical school faculty. Flexner believed that medical faculty should not engage in private practice; that they should be paid for devoting themselves to teaching and research. The PDC's challenge to this charity tradition also raised warning flags within The Duke Endowment and Duke University itself. As Hart later explained the matter, "This was an undertaking of the doctors, not Duke University, which preferred not to be considered as engaged in the corporate practice of medicine. It was the opinion of the administration that if the name Duke was used in designating the private clinic, it might lead to the impression that Duke University was engaged in the private practice of medicine."[18]

Duke's administration was particularly worried about the impression the PDC might make on the North Carolina Medical Society, the state's white medical society. Not only did the society license physicians to practice in the state; it also wielded great power in the state legislature. More telling still, the society represented independent surgeons and general practitioners who engaged in single-physician practices and were strongly opposed to the growing trend of group practices like the PDC. According to the PDC, however, its group practice represented the efforts of Duke University to address both the concerns of the state medical society and the Depression-era needs of the medical school. "The University created this arrangement in part to make an appointment to the Medical School more attractive, by permitting faculty also to engage in private practice for profit; and in part to address North Carolina state law concerns arising from legal prohibitions against the corporate practice of medicine and the sharing of medical fees with non-physicians. The Private Diagnostic Clinic of physicians were self-governing and not subject to University direction."[19]

Duke Medicine, Duke University, and the State of North Carolina

The PDC's autonomy and income quickly made it a source of excellence and expansion as well as of friction within the medical center and beyond. The clinic split into medical and surgical divisions in 1937, at the request of Medicine's Fred Hanes, and though it described itself as self-governing, the PDC remained a benevolent dictatorship until the mid-1990s. It was controlled by the heads of its two divisions, each of whom held his position by virtue of his university chairmanship in the Departments of Medicine and Surgery, respectively. By 1960, the PDC was a powerful and successful business with tremendous potential for expansion and future growth. In addition to transferring significant amounts of money to Duke Hospital and the university, the PDC also paid its members good salaries and attracted promising new faculty by supplementing the university's token medical school salaries. At the same time, the PDC also used its newly established "departmental and development fund" to help finance the clinic and hospital additions of the 1950s; to create a number of referral clinics throughout central North Carolina; and to supplement funding from The Duke Endowment, the Rockefeller Foundation, and the Dorothy Beard Research Fund to construct the first building specifically built for the basic sciences at DUMC.

The PDC did more than fuel DUMC's postwar growth, however. It created additional political tension within the university, within The Duke Endowment, and within North Carolina. As salaries climbed at DUMC, they remained stagnant within the rest of Duke University, and in 1946, the newly elected chairman of Duke's board of trustees, Willis Smith, set out to curtail the power not only of the PDC and Duke Medicine but also of the Endowment trustees who tried to control the university. Smith made it his mission to prevent the Endowment from naming Dr. Wilburt C. Davison president of Duke University. The PDC and DUMC also found their postwar expansion plans subject to the wider political agendas of Willis Smith and university president A. Hollis Edens and to the planning agenda of the North Carolina Medical Care

Commission, the state body appointed to administer funds from the Hill-Burton Act.

The Medical Care Commission had more on its mind than Duke Medicine. In addition to the expansion plans for Duke Hospital, the commission's agenda included funding requests for the teaching hospital associated with Wake Forest College's new, private four-year medical school in Winston-Salem; for converting the University of North Carolina's state-supported two-year medical school into a four-year school; and for constructing a large teaching hospital in Chapel Hill to accompany the proposed four-year school.

The UNC proposal, in particular, posed a dilemma for the Endowment's trustees. The trustees had followed Buck Duke's wishes in creating Duke University and its medical center. The Endowment had pioneered in progressive health care reform, and its hospital program had become a model for the Hill-Burton Act, one of the most important pieces of federal health care legislation in the nation's history. And yet, for a variety of personal, political, and economic reasons, including the obvious competition with Duke Medicine, the Endowment would not support the UNC expansion proposal. The state legislature passed the proposal in 1947, however, despite vigorous opposition from the Endowment.

That politics proved tricky for the Duke interests illuminates a critical impulse at the heart of Duke Medicine's history. Buck Duke created the Endowment as a political and moral challenge to North Carolina Democrats like Josephus Daniels, the owner-editor of the Raleigh *News & Observer*, who had helped disfranchise black voters and many poor whites following the white supremacy campaigns of 1898 and 1900. Indeed, these racist campaigns had destroyed a revolutionary political alliance of blacks and whites, both Republicans and Populists, that the Republican Dukes had helped mobilize, elect, and hold power in North Carolina between 1895 and 1898. More specifically, Daniels and Duke were bitter personal and political enemies. Daniels had vilified Duke in the pages of the *News & Observer*, first, during the government's successful antitrust case against Duke's American Tobacco Company (1911) and later, during the early 1920s, when Buck Duke was seeking a rate increase for Duke Power from the state and Daniels was leading the movement to construct a "Memorial Hospital" at UNC.

Duke wanted his Endowment to perpetuate this political and moral challenge to the state's political leadership, and for the most part he succeeded. Duke Hospital opened in 1930 with black and white patients under the same roof—segregated, of course, by race, sex, and medical service, but also served all day and night by whites and blacks alike, from white nurses, students, and physicians to black service workers and housekeeping staff. Duke and DUMC also joined Doris Duke and Mary Duke Biddle Trent Semans in continuing the Duke family's support for Lincoln Hospital, Durham's all-black hospital, and for assisting (quietly) in the training and promotion of black professionals and technicians within Duke Hospital, especially in the Department of Social Services. Together with Duke University, moreover, both women also continued to support Durham's North Carolina College for Negroes (North Carolina Central University today).

The Endowment's opposition to the expansion of UNC's medical center thus fits an established pattern of personal, political, and institutional conflict that preceded the creation of Duke University in 1924. By opposing the 1947 measure, however, the Duke Endowment expanded the foundation of the rivalry and damaged what little collaboration had been fostered between the neighboring universities by the Rockefeller philanthropies in the 1930s. This institutional rivalry continued throughout the decades that followed, and became particularly intense during the health care crisis of the 1990s, when both universities created health systems to try to save their academic medical centers. Put simply, since World War II both Duke and UNC have become part of a larger political and economic matrix of sometimes cooperative but more often competitive federal, state, and corporate health interests, first with Hill-Burton, later with Medicare, Medicaid, and NIH funding, and today with biotech companies and drug research.

Fine-Tuning the Relationship

Amid this complicated and changing context, moreover, Duke's leaders have continued to expand and defend the economic engine that has driven Duke Medicine and much of the university since World War II: the PDC. The PDC's importance lies in its relationship with the university, the medical school, the hospital, and with competing medical interests such as those at UNC. Members of the PDC must be members of the medical school's faculty to join and participate in the practice; the PDC's physicians have priority on the beds at Duke Hospital; Duke Hospital is a part of the Duke Health System; and the PDC owns the community referral clinics that were established in the 1950s and expanded in the 1980s. By 1995 the PDC was transferring over to the medical school, the hospital, and the university more than $70 million a year. Protecting "the practice" became a principal strategy, in fact, pursued by Dr. Ralph Snyderman, Duke's chancellor for health affairs, and his colleagues, during the managed care crisis of the 1990s. In addition to revolutionizing the basic sciences at DUMC, Snyderman and his colleagues created the Duke Clinical Research Institute and forced the PDC to abandon its traditional power structure, facilitating thereby the democratization of "the practice" and aligning it more closely with the needs and goals of Duke University and its health system.

The close identification of Duke Medicine's success with that of Duke University has been likened at various times to "the tail wagging the dog." These part-to-whole tensions were obvious to at least one outsider during Duke Medicine's earliest days. In April 1931, in a cover story for *Time* magazine, a reporter noted the many distinguished visitors—"mostly medical educators"—who had attended the recent ribbon cutting for "the most prodigious new educational project in the land this century—Duke University, now nearly complete though little grass yet grows on its sandy campus, no ivy on its neo-Gothic walls of soft-colored fieldstone." According to the reporter, "The central ceremony of the day was the dedication of Duke's medical school and hospital. Apparently these instead of the University as a whole were selected for dedication because—though no Duke man would like to say so—the medical aspect seems bound to reach maturity and fame before the institution's other branches. Money can get results faster in medicine than in the less scientific fields of culture."[20]

Writing 65 years later, in his book *Keeping an Open Door: Passages in a University Presidency*, Dr. H. Keith H. Brodie recalled that when he became Duke's president in 1985, he aroused the "suspicion" of both medical and nonmedical faculty alike because of his eight years as head of Duke's Department of Psychiatry. His medical colleagues "wished they did not have to report to a university president who knew their business so well," while the faculty in the arts and sciences were even more skeptical. "Despite all I could say and do," Brodie recalled, "faculty outside the Medical Center feared that I would provide only token oversight of the physician-biomedical sciences coalition, allowing Duke's growth to emulate the Johns Hopkins model, where the arts, humanities, and social sciences play a subordinate role to medicine and medical research, and graduate studies receive a greater emphasis than undergraduate education. Duke history lent credence to their concerns, for our medical school had been founded with a core of Hopkins-trained physicians whose influence was still felt."[21]

Brodie's medical experience "impressed" the university's trustees, however, who believed in "the need for the president to understand the Medical Center." The trustees realized that the "complex relationship between a medical school, with its hospital and outpatient clinics, and the rest of the university presents an area of constant tension for chief executives of research universities." Brodie felt that "as president [he] could deal from a position of strength with the difficulties of uniting the medical and nonmedical components of the university": "I knew that Medical Center administrators had an understandable desire for autonomy based on the very different nature of their en-

1.3 Replanting of the Osler ivy, November 9, 1968, in honor of Dr. Wilburt C. Davison (with shovel). Dr. John P. McGovern (bending over) and Mrs. Mary D. B. T. Semans (far right) participate in the ceremony. *Duke University Archives.*

terprise. . . . Throughout my presidency I looked for ways to ameliorate this tendency of many of the medical staff to work without a sense of oneness with the institution."[22]

Duke's search for a sense of institutional oneness continued after Nannerl O. Keohane succeeded Keith Brodie as the president of Duke University in 1993. By then the medical center was at war with itself and the PDC was facing deep potential losses with the spread of managed care. Faced with the collapse of the nation's health care system, with its own bitter rivalries and internal disputes, and with the increasing dislocation of its supporting networks, DUMC turned to the university to help it create the Duke University Health System. Since then, Duke Medicine seems to have done more than survive. It now has a profitable health system and appears to have recognized the need for continued cooperation between the university's new president, Dr. Richard H. Brodhead, and the new chancellor for health affairs, Dr. Victor J. Dzau, who also serves as CEO of the Duke University Health System.

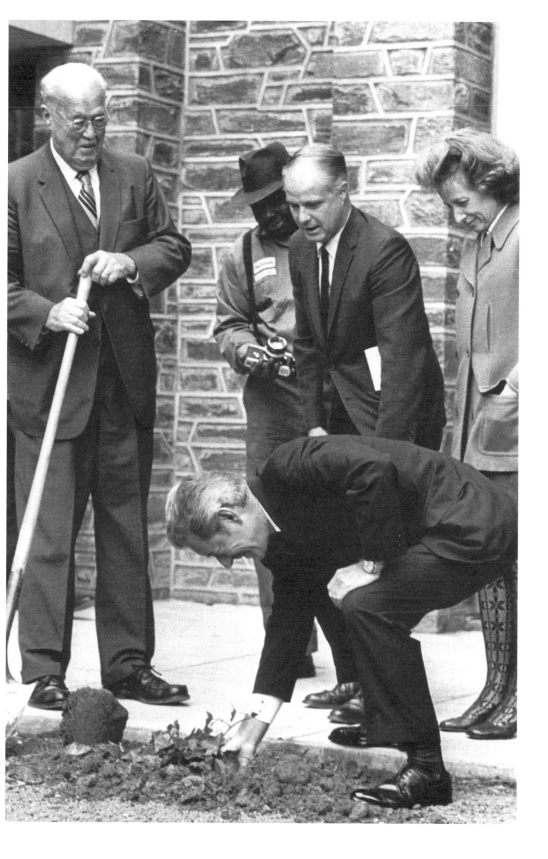

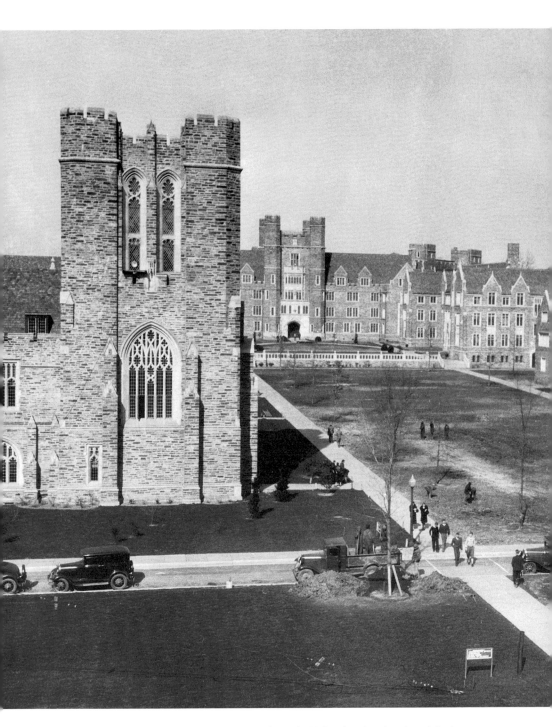

1.1 View of the West Campus quadrangle, Duke University, showing the original entrance to the school of medicine (Davison Building, center rear), 1931. *Duke University Medical Center Archives.*

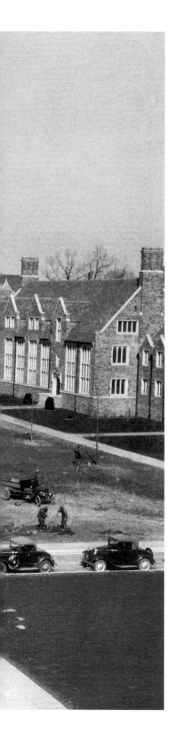

CHAPTER I:

Duke Medicine and the Foundations of Health Care Reform in the American South

The Duke University Medical Center opened in 1930, and for the next 30 years it depended heavily on the various personal, corporate, and philanthropic networks that connected it with James B. ("Buck") Duke and two great missionary enterprises, The Duke Endowment and the Rockefeller Foundation. Even before 1930 North Carolina had served as the laboratory for two major Rockefeller initiatives that lasted until the mid-20th century. One was the General Education Board, established in 1903 by John D. Rockefeller to aid education in the United States "without distinction of race, sex or creed."[1] The board placed particular emphasis on public education in the American South, especially for blacks, and it began its work in North Carolina because of the state's reputation for regional leadership in school reform. The board's programs lasted from 1903 to 1964.[2] The second was the Rockefeller Sanitary Commission for the Eradication of Hookworm Disease, which lasted from 1909 until 1914, and which was also funded by John D. Rockefeller. In 1914 the hookworm campaign was transferred to the Rockefeller Foundation's new International Health Board, where its programs included the control of yellow fever, malaria, and tuberculosis, as well as public health education, virus studies, and related research—programs that closely resembled the public health and research activities on which the Duke University Medical Center (DUMC) would initially focus. Although the International Health Board was disbanded in 1927 in a general restructuring of the Rockefeller Foundation, its work was continued in the foundation's new International Health Division. Finally, in 1951, the health division was merged with the foundation's medical sciences program and "public health activity was de-emphasized."[3]

Major Projects of the 1930s

Two of the central figures in the hookworm campaign, Dr. John Atkinson Ferrell and Dr. Watson Smith Rankin, became fast friends and important links in many of the networks of people and institutions that Duke Medicine inherited or created. Ferrell, a native of Clinton, North Carolina, graduated from the short-lived Raleigh medical branch of the University of North Carolina and worked as a teacher, public school administrator, and county health superintendent before becoming state director for the Rockefeller Sanitary Commission in 1909. Four years later the Rockefeller Foundation brought Ferrell to New York as associate director of the International Health Board, where he received national attention establishing county health departments as director of the foundation's public-health activities in North America. After retiring from the board in 1944, Ferrell served for two years as medical director of another philanthropy important to Duke Medicine, the John and Mary R. Markle Foundation. Ferrell eventually returned to North Carolina in 1946, where, for the next ten years, as executive secretary of the North Carolina Medical Commission, he oversaw the distribution of nearly $100 million in federal funds to more than 200 hospital projects throughout the state—including several projects at DUMC.[4]

Ferrell's colleague and frequent golfing partner, Dr. Watson Smith Rankin, was the key figure in linking Duke Medicine's public and private health networks. After earning his M.D. at the University of Maryland in 1901, Rankin, a native of Mooresville, North Carolina, did postgraduate work at the Johns Hopkins School of Medicine. He then returned to North Carolina as a professor of pathology at Wake Forest College, and between 1905 and 1909, as dean of Wake's two-year school of medicine, he investigated the prevalence of hookworm in the state. As a result of this work, Rankin was appointed secretary of the North Carolina State Board of Health (the state's first full-time health officer) in 1909, just as the Rockefeller commission started its hookworm campaign. The campaign brought Rankin widespread recognition, both within the state and beyond. He was elected to national offices in both

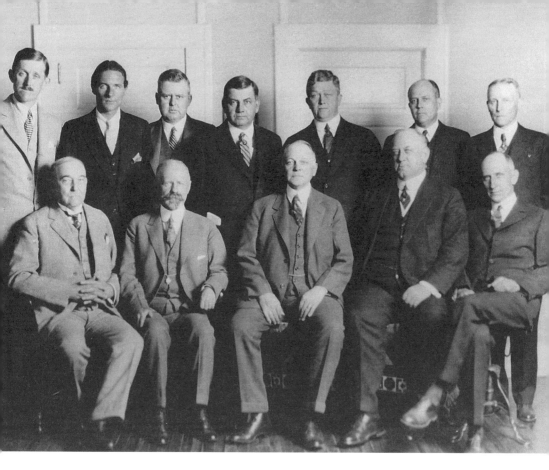

1.2 The trustees of The Duke Endowment, 1925. Seated, left to right: Jonathan E. Cox, William B. Bell, George G. Allen, William S. Lee, and Norman A. Cocke. Standing, left to right: Alexander H. Sands Jr., Anthony J. Drexel Biddle Jr., Walter C. Parker, Charles I. Burkholder, Edward C. Marshall, Watson S. Rankin, and Robert L. Flowers. *Photo courtesy of The Duke Endowment.*

the American Medical Association and the American Public Health Association, and in North Carolina, he later recalled, "the Legislature . . . were very good to me for sixteen years (I was a favored child)." Indeed, by the time he retired from the state board in 1925, North Carolina had more counties with full-time public health officers than any other state, and Rankin was "recognized as the nation's outstanding state public health officer."[5]

Rankin left state government to become head of the Hospital and Orphans Section of The Duke Endowment, where he remained as a trustee for the next 40 years. The hospital section was the most innovative and progressive aspect of the foundation's otherwise traditional approach to charity. On the most basic and immediate level, it provided nonprofit hospitals in North and South Carolina with a dollar a day for every bed occupied by a public (indigent) patient, regardless of race. On a more general level, Rankin devised a revolutionary plan for dealing with what many of his progressive colleagues considered a major source of escalating medical costs: the ownership and control of local hospitals by private individuals, usually physicians. At the time the Endowment began its work, for example, more than 50 percent of the hospitals in the Carolinas were privately owned, most by general practitioners. Believing that local hospitals would (and should) follow the same private-to-public ownership pattern as local schools, Rankin supervised the use of Endowment funds to assist in transferring the ownership and control of local hospitals from private individuals to community agencies.[6] [Figure 1.2]

Rankin was still in the early throes of developing the Endowment's hospital program when Duke University announced that it had selected Dr. Wilburt C. Davison of the Johns Hopkins School of Medicine to be dean of the school of medicine planned at Duke. "It is with great pleasure and encouragement that I have learned this morning of your appointment as Dean of the Medical Department of Duke University," Rankin wrote to Davison in January 1927. Although Rankin had agreed to Davison's appointment several months earlier, after meeting him at a medical conference, Rankin had yet to spend any time with the young pediatrician. But that was about to change. Rankin wrote: "I look forward to your coming to North Carolina with a great deal of interest and with very happy anticipations of the development in the very near future of a constructive program which will closely and advantageously relate the work of the Medical Department of the University with that of the Hospital Section of The Duke Endowment."[7]

THE COMMITTEE ON THE COSTS OF MEDICAL CARE

While Davison's appointment is frequently cited as perhaps the most important factor in Duke Medicine's initial success, Rankin's simultaneous involvement with the Committee on the Costs of Medical Care proved equally critical in shaping the early years of Duke's new hospital and medical school. Organized in 1927 by a small group of dissidents within the American Medical Association, the costs committee was a health services research group composed of health reformers and academics, including physicians, dentists, economists, public health officials, and hospital administrators. Funding for the committee came from several large philanthropic organizations, including the Rockefeller Foundation, the Carnegie Foundation, and the Twentieth Century Fund, and by the time it issued its final report in 1932, the committee had published more than 20 major reports on the costs and distribution of health services, 15 miscellaneous reports, and more than 30 reports authored in collaboration with other agencies.[8]

Watson Rankin was one of the 35 committee members who signed the group's final majority report, *Medical Care for the American People*, which was as controversial as it was revolutionary. The report was submitted along with several minority opinions to the National Conference on the Costs of Medical Care, which was held at the New York Academy of Medicine late in November of 1932. The commissioner of health for the state of New York, Dr. Thomas Parran Jr., opened the conference by reading a telegram from New York governor Franklin Delano Roosevelt, who had just been elected president of the United States. The telegram expressed Roosevelt's hope that the committee had "arrived at a practical policy for the present emergency."[9]

The associate director of the Committee on the Costs of Medical Care, Dr. Isadore Falk—who became director of research and statistics in Roosevelt's Social Security Administration—later summarized the majority's recommendations:

1. Comprehensive medical service should be provided largely by organized groups of practitioners, organized preferably around hospitals, encouraging high standards, and preserving personal relations.

2. All basic public health services should be extended to the entire population, requiring increased financial support, full-time trained health officers and staffs, with security of tenure.

3. Medical costs should be placed on a group payment basis through insurance, taxation, or both; individual fee-for-service should be available for those who prefer it; and cash benefits for wage loss should be kept separate.

4. State and local agencies should be formed to study, evaluate, and coordinate services, with special attention to urban-rural coordination.

5. Professional education should be improved for physicians, health officers, dentists, pharmacists, registered nurses, nursing aides, midwives, and hospital and clinic administrators.[10]

The *New York Times* gave front-page coverage to the committee's majority report under the headline "Socialized Medicine Urged in Survey." The AMA, too, detected a socialist bias in the majority report and preferred instead the blistering minority report signed by eight doctors who roundly condemned not only the idea of group practice but any departure at all from the traditional individual, fee-for-service practice. More flushed-face still was the editorial that appeared in the *Journal of the American Medical Association*. "The alignment is clear," JAMA proclaimed, "On one side the forces representing the great foundations, public health officialdom, social theory—even socialism and communism—inciting to revolution; on the other side, the organized medical profession of this country urging an orderly evolution guided by controlled experimentation."[11]

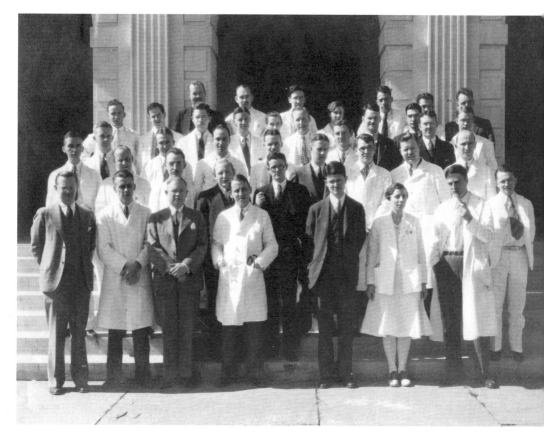

1.3 Duke Hospital and medical school faculty, 1932. *Duke University Medical Center Archives.*

By the time of the costs committee's "revolution," DUMC had already agreed with The Duke Endowment to adopt most of the committee's recommendations. In order to receive the Endowment's dollar-a-day charity, for example, DUMC, after opening its 400-bed hospital in 1930, worked closely with the state and local welfare agencies that sent it indigent patients and also paid for what the Endowment did not cover. As a result, the activities of DUMC increased in both scope and scale. [Figure 1.3] Between 1930 and 1932, the number of patients discharged from DUMC increased from 3,015 to 5,648, while the days of care it delivered increased from 14,887 to 67,672. Through the Duke Out-Patient Clinic, which opened in 1930, and the Private Diagnostic Clinic, which was established as a private group practice the following

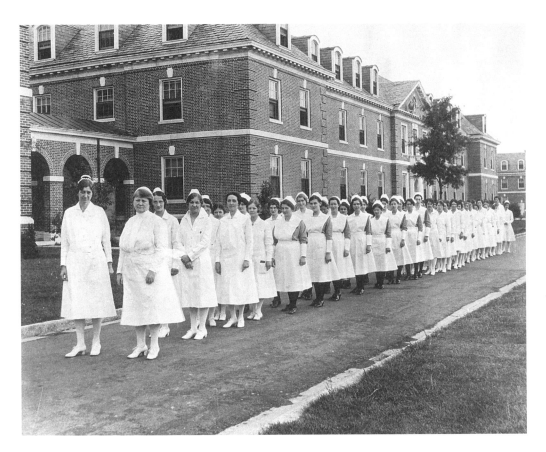

1.4 School of Nursing staff, Duke Hospital nurses, and students in the first class of the School of Nursing, 1931. *Duke University Medical Center Archives.*

year, the "entire population" received valuable diagnostic services. Although the outpatient clinic recorded only 2,988 diagnostic visits during its first six months of operation, that number jumped to 15,287 in 1931 and to 26,212 in 1932, as the clinic's diagnostic services "made it possible for physicians in general practice in this and surrounding states to obtain help in their medical problems not only for patients who could pay and who formerly were sent to Baltimore and Philadelphia, but also for the far greater number without financial means."[12]

By 1932, DUMC was also providing the professional education that the costs committee recommended. Duke's medical school accepted its first classes in the fall of 1930: 30 first-year students and 18 third-year students. It also acted on the advice of committee leader, Dr. Michael M. Davis, whose book,

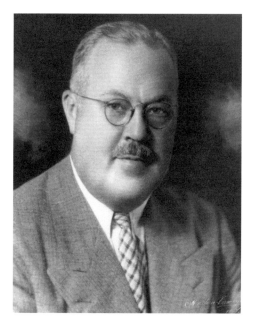

1.5 Dr. Wilburt C. Davison. *Duke University Archives.*

Hospital Administration: A Career, advocated internships at teaching hospitals for college graduates who wanted to train as hospital superintendents. Two administrative interns began at DUMC in 1930, and two years later they were appointed superintendent and assistant superintendent of Duke Hospital. What was more, DUMC's first class in the School of Nursing began in 1931, moved into a new nurses' home next to the hospital in 1932, and was graduated in 1933.[13] [Figure 1.4]

THE QUESTION OF INSURANCE

Rankin and Davison also gave close attention to one of the principal goals of the Committee on the Costs of Medical Care: group medical insurance. This involved their collaboration on some of the nation's first nonprofit Blue Cross plans. Their earliest effort, the Durham Hospital Association, nearly failed after its formation in 1929, only to be revived again in 1933 as the Hospital Care Association. "It was the first statewide hospital insurance plan in the world," Davison later claimed, "the first one to provide prepayment coverage for any group to *any* hospital, to enroll groups on waiver basis, and to give family dependents the same coverage as the employed certificate holder. It formed the pattern followed by all present Blue Cross Associations." Yet the plan also provoked suspicion among certain sectors of the state's medical community. "Many of the physicians in this and other states were suspicious that socialized medicine was back of the Hospital Care Association," Davison explained, "so Dr. Rankin, on the recommendations of Watts Hill and me, persuaded the Duke Endowment to appropriate $25,000 to enable Dr. Isaac H. Manning Jr., the President of the North Carolina Medical Society, and Graham L. Davis, Dr. Rankin's assistant, to go to England and study the British system. Dr. Manning, on his return, started the Hospital Savings Association with the blessing of the North Carolina Medical Society."[14] [Figure 1.5]

By 1937, however, the two Blue Cross associations were in "sharp" competition with each other, and many progressive observers were dismayed. One was Dr. C. Rufus Rorem, a member of the costs committee's research staff and director of the Committee on Hospital Service of the American Hospital Association. Rorem had been appointed to set up prepayment hospitalization plans with money from the Rosenwald Fund, one of the eight foundations that had originally supported the costs committee. "If there were one non-profit organization operating in the state (instead of two)," Rorem wrote to Rankin in May, "there could easily be a total of 150,000 subscribers in the state of North Carolina at the present time." Rorem had recently failed to get the two groups to consolidate, and he hoped that Rankin, as a trustee of both The Duke Endowment and the American Hospital Association, might have some suggestion. "My only reason for writing at all is because the eyes of the entire country are upon the North Carolina state-wide experiment, which, in my opinion, is being handicapped very definitely by what amounts to two separate state-wide non-profit corporations operating in the same area."[15]

It took another 30 years, however, to consolidate the two North Carolina "Blues," and during that time, despite the initial hostility, the Endowment's hospital program became the model for one of the most important federal health programs in American history, the Hospital Survey and Construction Act of 1946, commonly known as "Hill-Burton." In 1951, moreover, as the state's three medical centers—at Duke, the University of North Carolina, and Wake Forest College—competed for Hill-Burton funding, North Carolina was selected for a pilot study by the national Commission on Financing of Hospital Care—a body with close personal and programmatic connections to the Committee on the Costs of Medical Care. All of these developments were still years away in 1937, however, when the progressive elements of Duke Medicine became enmeshed with Duke's private research networks in corporate America.

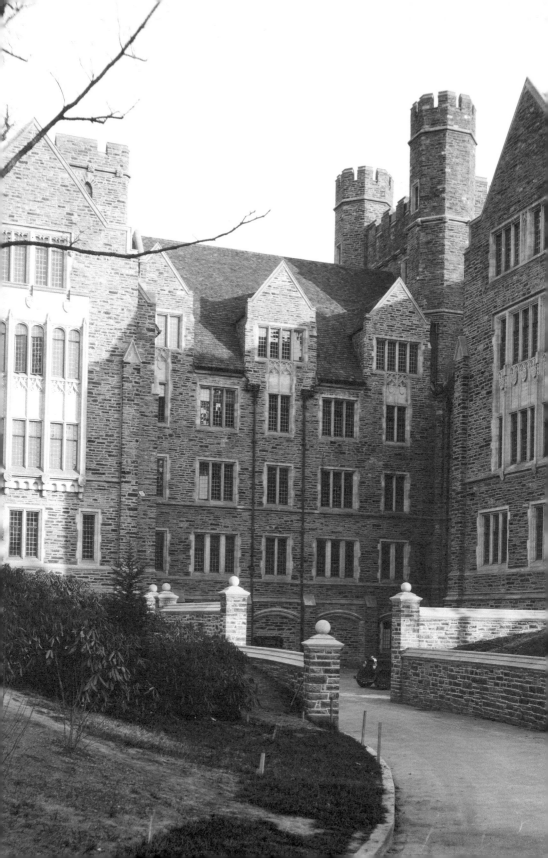

CHAPTER 2:

The Corporate Hand and Duke Medicine:
Research and Leadership

The foundations for Duke's modern academic medical center were laid in 1937, when the university's corporate and philanthropic partners helped Duke Medicine add large-scale research to The Duke Endowment's mission of subsidizing medical care for indigent patients and facilitating the growth of nonprofit community hospitals. The American Cyanamid Company joined the Rockefeller Foundation and The Duke Endowment in providing money, personnel, and equipment for research and teaching at DUMC. The Rockefeller Foundation also agreed to consider funding a psychiatry department at Duke, and the Private Diagnostic Clinic divided into the medical and surgical divisions that defined the practice for almost 60 years. The men who tried to sort all of this out within DUMC—Drs. Wilburt Davison, Frederic Hanes, and Deryl Hart— also depended upon decisions made outside of the medical center, especially in the board rooms of New York City.

Four loosely connected institutions—American Cyanamid, the Rockefeller philanthropies, The Duke Endowment, and the Doris Duke Trust—all had offices in the new RCA building at 30 Rockefeller Plaza in New York. The offices of the Rockefeller Foundation and other Rockefeller philanthropies, including the General Education Board and the Spelman Fund, occupied two contiguous floors of the building in 1937; a couple of floors up was the American Cyanamid Company and the office of one of its three controlling stockholders, 64-year-old George Garland Allen, who used his office there in his various roles as chairman of the board of The Duke Endowment, as a trustee of the Doris Duke Trust, as a member of the executive committee of Duke

---

2.1 Rear view of the Davison Building, originally the main entrance to the School of Medicine (right), and the rear of Duke Hospital (left). *Duke University Medical Center Archives.*

University trustees, and as president of the New Jersey–chartered Duke Power Company. The next three floors were also occupied by American Cyanamid, as was half of the next floor, where Cyanamid's 59-year-old president, William Brown Bell (another trustee of The Duke Endowment), had offices adjacent to those of Radio Corporation of America. A few floors farther up, near the top of the building, there were additional Rockefeller offices and a series of private dining rooms leased to six of the building's largest corporate tenants: Standard Oil, Shell Union Oil, the Rockefeller Foundation, American Cyanamid, Westinghouse, and RCA.[1]

Early Research Projects and Corporate and Foundation Support

One of the most important and peculiar stories of Duke Medicine involves Dr. Joseph Beard's discovery of a vaccine for equine encephalomyelitis in the fall of 1937, just months after his arrival at DUMC. Beard's discovery brought big money and big science to Duke. It also helped make Duke Medicine a key collaborator in government-sponsored research during World War II, and it facilitated DUMC's early connections with the National Institutes of Health. Beard's discovery also raises a number of intriguing and significant questions. Why was he working on an animal virus? How did he develop the vaccine so fast? Was his success simply chance and circumstance? Or was it a can't-miss deal, a combination of his research experience at the Rockefeller Institute and the money, men, and machines American Cyanamid put at his disposal? And what about the research and royalties from the vaccine? How were they to be controlled and divided? Who would benefit from them, in what ways, and for what purposes? Similar questions confront academic medical researchers today, and Beard's research served as valuable early experience for Duke in dealing with them.

Beard was working in the Princeton laboratories of the Rockefeller Institute when Duke hired him as assistant professor of experimental surgery in December of 1936. He and his colleague Dr. Ralph W. G. Wyckoff, a mechanical genius, were deep into research on the link between viruses and cancer. They were using the centrifuges Wyckoff had built to study the papilloma virus in rabbits. They were not very well liked by the rest of their colleagues, however. Although smart and talented scientists, they were also pushy and ambitious, and had little regard for the Rockefeller protocol of deferring to senior scientists in matters of shared discovery and publication.

Beard and Wyckoff hit it big in January of 1937, in the months before Beard took up his position at Duke. Beard explained the matter in a letter to his good friend Dr. Alfred Blalock, resident surgeon of the medical center at Vanderbilt University. "A few weeks ago I decided to make a final attempt to purify

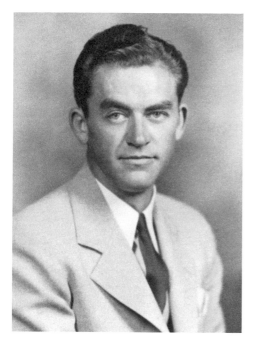

2.2 Dr. Joseph W. Beard. *Duke University Medical Center Archives.*

the virus responsible for the infectious papillomatosis in rabbits," Beard wrote early in February. "Some months ago Dr. Wyckoff moved to Princeton from the New York [Rockefeller] Institute and brought with him his ultracentrifuges. The program for the study of the virus included the using of these centrifuges. Much to our surprise and, as you can well believe, our gratification, we had obtained a heavy protein molecule from the growth within 48 hours." The next issue of *Science* magazine would include their description of the protein. "It is scarcely necessary for me to stress the importance of the purification of the protein which is associated with the infectiousness of an animal virus," Beard continued. "I have at best only five more months here in which I can participate in the work. It is very important that I derive as much benefit as possible from it."[2]

Among those who read the protein description in *Science* was Beard's mentor from the Rockefeller Institute in New York, Dr. Peyton Rous. Rous was one of the best of the outstanding scientists who worked at the institutes during this time, including Osvald T. Avery, whose 1944 discovery that DNA transmits hereditary information set the course of biological research during the rest of the century. Rous himself was awarded a Nobel Prize in Medicine in 1966 for his work on viruses and the origins of cancer. Indeed, it was under Rous in New York, between 1933 and 1935, that Beard had worked on what was then called the Shope papilloma virus—the virus from which Beard and Wyckoff had now purified (while working at the Rockefeller Institute in Princeton) the protein described in *Science*. Rous counseled Beard to follow Rockefeller protocol and do additional research before publishing something that claimed too much. "Do be very cautious, though," he wrote to Beard from New York, "and get the sanction of the powers that be before you come out in print. Best of luck to you and Wyckoff. I hope the virus crystallizes. Otherwise people will ask whether you have done more than merely concentrate it in association with a pathological protein."[3] [Figure 2.2]

In the meantime, Beard and Wyckoff turned their whirling centrifuges to the horse-brain virus and made considerable progress purifying it before being briefly interrupted by Beard's move to Durham. Once at Duke, Beard and his wife, Dorothy, began searching for funds to continue their virus research. Surgery's chairman, Dr. Deryl Hart, had told them that "research money was not exactly plentiful," and Beard later claimed he had offered to put up some of his "own salary to make the thing go. Inasmuch as I was making only $3,000 a year, however, I was somewhat loath to resort to such an extreme and distasteful measure without some exploration of other sources of funds beforehand. Dorothy and I then discussed the matter and decided that it might be possible to get some aid from Mr. Bell through Lederle Laboratories, a subsidiary of American Cyanamide [*sic*]. In a telephone conversation with him, he seemed sympathetic with our situation and suggested that I come to New York to discuss the problem with him."[4]

INITIAL CONNECTIONS WITH AMERICAN CYANAMID

Late in July of 1937, Cyanamid's president William B. Bell sent a telegram from New York to Dr. Wilburt Davison, the dean of Duke University's School of Medicine, saying he expected Davison and his party to meet him at 30 Rockefeller Plaza before taking a tour of Cyanamid's Lederle Laboratories in Pearl River, New York, and its Stamford Laboratories, in Stamford, Connecticut. Davison couldn't go, but he wired Bell to suggest that the new professor of experimental surgery, Dr. Joseph W. Beard, could come in his stead. In his reply, Bell invited DUMC's Dr. David T. Smith as well.[5]

Lederle Laboratories, the nation's leading producer of "veterinary biologicals," was located some 30 miles from Rockefeller Plaza. In their hour-long ride in the limousine, Bell, Beard, and Smith would have learned a little more about one another. Bell was a Quaker, an accomplished yachtsman, a trustee of The Duke Endowment, and president of American Cyanamid Company, one of the largest and most diversified chemical companies in the world. He was also an aggressive promoter of cancer research and an outspoken critic of President Franklin D. Roosevelt, having recently stepped down as chairman of the Republican Party's national Finance Committee.[6]

Dr. David Smith was an expert on tuberculosis and fungal and other infectious diseases, and as a victim of TB himself, he sometimes needed oxygen for support. Smith had directed the New York Hospital for Tuberculosis prior to coming to Duke in 1930, and he now held a dual appointment as chairman of the Department of Microbiology and as associate professor of medicine in the Department of Medicine. By 1937, Smith and his wife, Susan Gower, were the nucleus of a new Quaker meeting in Durham and were using grants from the Rockefeller Foundation for research involving fundamental biochemical and

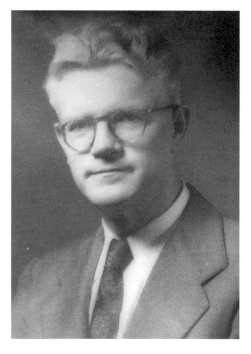

2.3 Dr. David T. Smith. *Duke University Medical Center Archives.*

analyses of pellagra.[7] As for the 35-year-old Beard, Bell probably knew as much about him as Smith did. He had heard Beard explain his research and had liked what he heard.[8] [Figure 2.3]

American Cyanamid had owned Lederle Laboratories since 1930, and since that time Bell had made it part of his own personal and corporate mission to eradicate animal and human diseases, especially cancer. Bell also wanted Cyanamid's companies to eliminate barriers between commercial and academic laboratories. That was the message, for example, of "The Commercial Laboratory," the lead editorial in Lederle's *Veterinary Bulletin* for July–August 1937. "Medicine, as a profession, has for years frowned upon commercialism," the editorial began; and medicine was still frowning on the commercialism of laboratories such as Lederle's, which produced "biologics and pharmaceutics . . . so vitally necessary to the practice of human and veterinary medicine." Bell wanted to end such prejudice and to do so through Cyanamid, which had reshaped and expanded Lederle since acquiring it. "No longer should the professor and, above all, the medico look down upon the hireling of the industrial laboratory as a money grubber," the editorial advised. "Ethical distinction between one and the other was based entirely on a false premise."[9]

The Lederle Laboratories were built in what another Lederle *Veterinary Bulletin* described as "a setting not unlike that of a typical American university. In fact many of the hundreds of visitors who tour the laboratories each year have remarked that a sort of academic atmosphere seems to pervade the premises. This is not a strange impression when one reviews the campus-like layout and the scholarly activities of a large portion of the personnel." Like universities, Lederle devoted separate buildings to the study of single or related subjects; and as in universities, too, many of Lederle's 1,100 employees held advanced degrees. What was more, "study for these specialists did not cease with the awarding of their college diplomas. They have chosen the mysteries of medicine as their life work: a life work that is dynamic, fascinating and challenging. Constant study is their lot, and they thrive on it."[10]

The conference room was full of Lederle specialists when Bell arrived with his guests from Duke. "Much to my surprise, he had arranged a formal round-table discussion," Beard later explained. "At this meeting of about 15 of us, we talked about all the possibilities of things that might be studied in virology in our laboratory [at Duke]."[11] Leading the discussion was Lederle's medical director, Dr. Arthur F. Coca. Founder and editor of the *Journal of Immunology*, Coca was one of the nation's leading allergists. He was also secretary-treasurer of the American Association of Immunologists, medical director of the Blood Transfusion Betterment Association, and clinical professor of medicine at New York Post Graduate Medical School. Coca had been Lederle's medical director since 1931, and through him, physicians at Cornell's Post Graduate Skin Clinic had received a concentrated form of "Lederle Tobacco Extract" for testing on patients in "the first opportunity for the analysis of tobacco in regard to the harmful sensitizing ingredients."[12] Coca had also started Lederle's *Veterinary Bulletin*, a slick, bimonthly publication that combined product promotion with summaries of the latest research done by government agencies and by Coca's professional colleagues in immunology at the Rockefeller Institute. More significant still, Coca had invested heavily at Lederle in the animals and equipment needed to develop a vaccine for equine encephalomyelitis (horse encephalitis), a disease that had threatened North America's horse population since the early 1930s.[13]

According to Beard, it was "Dr. A. A. Eichorn, a really grand old man of veterinary medicine," who turned the discussion toward the horse disease. "He suggested that one of the most pressing virology problems at the time was equine encephalomyelitis, which among farmers," Beard explained, "was known as 'blind staggers' of horses. The disease was affecting about 800,000 horses per year, many of which died, and many others were crippled and useless thereafter. This was a particularly critical matter, because of the implications with respect to very high-priced race horses, many of which had been lost from the disease."[14]

Eichorn may have suggested the horse encephalitis, but it was Lederle's search for a vaccine to fight it, and the belief that Beard could soon deliver one, that prompted the company to bring him to Pearl River in the first place. Beard had transferred to Duke the valuable how-to experience of his cancer research at the Rockefeller Institute in Princeton: how to isolate and purify the horse virus with a new research tool, the ultracentrifuge; how to grow large amounts of virus with a new technique involving chick embryos; and how to kill a virus and use its remains to develop a safe and efficient vaccine. To tie all of these together at Duke, however, Beard needed Lederle's support—but he needed more than money, he explained. He needed continued collaboration with his former colleague at the Rockefeller Institute in Princeton, Dr. Ralph W. G. Wyckoff. Wyckoff had not only built the ultracentrifuges in use at Rockefeller; he and Beard had also depended upon them for their own important horse virus research there. Wyckoff was a productive, experienced scientist, and a man of many talents. He had spent the last decade working at Rockefeller, in both its New York and Princeton branches, and during that time, he had helped himself and other scientists design, build, use, and fix—and then redesign, rebuild, and fix again—many of the machines and methods they needed in their research.[15]

After listening to Beard, the Lederle executives suggested something else that Duke might study: sulfanilamide. This new drug was proving particularly effective in treating serious infections in animals; indeed, Lederle itself had just released a report on it, "Sulfanilamide *Lederle*: A New Chemo-therapeutic Agent for Hemolytic Streptococcic Infections in Dogs." More intriguing still, while nearly all of the studies with sulfanilamide had involved only animals, the new drug was also proving beneficial in controlling certain streptococcal infections in humans. There were rumors, in fact, of the drug's success in treating other serious human infections. Some observers were even taken to hailing the introduction and use of sulfanilamide (and its allied "sulfa" drugs) as "epochal in the history of medicine." Cyanamid hoped they were right: sulfanilamide was manufactured by one of its largest subsidiaries, the Calco Chemical Company of Bound Brook, New Jersey.[16]

Bell took his Duke visitors to the animal-house side of the Lederle campus. The laboratories provided hutches, kennels, stables, and paddocks for the thousands of dogs, horses, guinea pigs, and rabbits that it studied. Many animals died in the course of the experiments. Horses were injected with the encephalitis virus, then killed and their brains were removed and studied, following a process recently developed at the U.S. Bureau of Animal Industry. The brain tissues were treated with formalin, and then the formalin-treated virus was used to create a vaccine. Unfortunately, the whole process was cumbersome, cruel, expensive, and very inefficient. The brains of injected horses contained such low concentrations of the virus that in order to produce even small quantities of vaccine, the company had to corral, care for, and dispose of large numbers of huge animals. All of which could be avoided, of course, if Beard could indeed produce a highly concentrated virus in chick embryos.[17]

The next day, Bell took his visitors to Cyanamid's new Stamford Laboratories, in Stamford, Connecticut. After a quick survey of the facility, the visitors listened to Dr. Bowling Barnes explain spectrophotometry and the company's infrared and ultraviolet spectroscopes. It was not immediately clear to anyone there how Duke might benefit from the spectroscopes; the scientists at Cyanamid's Calco Chemical Company were using the machines to standardize pigments and dye applications. Nevertheless, the visitors were impressed.[18]

After leaving Stamford, Bell returned to Rockefeller Plaza, while his guests went on to Brooklyn, where they visited the plant of Davis & Geck. Acquired by Cyanamid in 1930, Davis & Geck was the second largest manufacturer of surgical sutures in the world, eventually controlling some 70 percent of the domestic market. The company had profited handsomely from government contracts during World War I, much as Lederle had done, and like Lederle, Davis & Geck would do well during the war years ahead, providing 75 percent of the sutures required by the U.S. military. Smith and Beard were intrigued by Davis & Geck's filmmaking program. The company produced medical motion pictures to document new procedures and to assist in the training of doctors and nurses.[19]

As Smith and Beard headed back to Durham, Bell wrote to their dean about his "most interesting, stimulating and satisfactory visit" with them. "We spent Wednesday at the Laboratories in Pearl River," he explained to Davison. "As a result of our discussion,—and with particular thanks to Dr. Beard,—Lederle determined to go ahead with the installation of the super centrifuge at Pearl River and is in touch with Dr. Wyckoff whom they expect to retain when he goes to Pearl River on Monday or Tuesday of next week. We also hope to include his assistant and a helper." Bell also expressed his amazement at the spectroscopes at Stamford. "All I can say is that I never see this equipment or listen to our Dr. Barnes' explanation of it without having my imagination aroused and without feeling that through these facilities we should be able to see further into the structure of matter,—including pharmaceutical and bio-logical,—than man has seen heretofore. I believe that, on the conclusion of our visit, Dr. Smith and Dr. Beard to some extent shared this feeling."[20]

Davison was especially pleased that Bell proposed further collaboration between DUMC and American Cyanamid. Bell wrote to Davison, "I am very hopeful that, in some of the research work of the Medical School, you will find that these centrifuges will prove useful to you," as might the spectroscopes; "any light that it can throw on your research problems is at your disposal." Bell hoped Davison would visit Lederle and Stamford himself. "I trust that you recall having accepted my general invitation on this subject," he wrote, "and will follow it with something more specific as soon as I can work out some dates amongst which you may find one convenient to you." Finally, in a postscript, Bell wondered, "Do you suppose that Dr. [Walter M.] Nielsen of Duke University [Department of Physics] would be interested in a trip to our Stamford Laboratories? I would be most happy to have him make such a

2.4 Dr. J. Deryl Hart and a team of surgeons operating under the Westinghouse "Sterilamp," ca. 1936. *Duke University Medical Center Archives.*

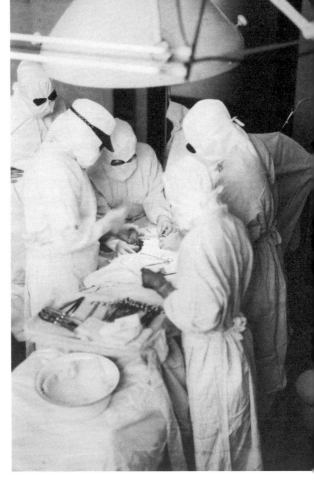

visit as my guest and I will, if you think it agreeable, make such a suggestion to him."[21]

Davison called the Physics Department and found that Nielsen "would like very much to visit the Stamford Laboratories." Davison also talked with Beard and Smith and found them "most enthusiastic over their trip." Smith seemed particularly pleased that Davis & Geck had asked him about the recent research in DUMC's operating rooms, where the head of Duke's Department of Surgery, Dr. Deryl Hart, had successfully used the Westinghouse ultraviolet "Sterilamp" to prevent airborne infections. As Davision explained it to Bell, "Dr. Smith told me that he discussed with the staff of the Davis & Geck plant the use of ultraviolet in the prevention of air infection, and they probably will install some of the lights as an additional precaution."[22] [Figure 2.4]

Less than a week later, Davison had lunch with Bell at Rockefeller Plaza and then visited the Stamford Laboratories in Connecticut. The dean was just as impressed as his colleagues had been. "Dr. Barnes, Dr. Jones and the others showed us everything and stimulated us in innumerable ways," he wrote thanking Bell. "Seeing the advance in other fields made us realize how much medicine needs to advance."[23] In a letter from Bell that crossed Davison's in the mail, the Cyanamid president expressed his delight with Davison's visit the day before. "My only regret is that I was unable to accompany you on your trip to Stamford. However, I trust that Dr. Jones and Dr. Barnes showed you the special pieces of equipment which I was most anxious to have you inspect, in the hope that they may contribute to those medical achievements which I am so anxious to see Duke University give to the world."[24]

Bell enclosed a pamphlet published by the *American Journal of Digestive Diseases and Nutrition* in his letter to Davison. "It contains a preliminary report on the treatment of cancer by a new principle extracted from nuclear material and called 'Anomin.'" The author of the report, Bell continued, was Dr. Beaumont S. Cornell, who had been "aided by the Duke Endowment in a study of certain aspects of pernicious anemia in the years before the medical school of Duke was organized." Cornell had abandoned his studies, however, after new liver treatments had decreased the threat of pernicious anemia, the disease from which James B. Duke was supposed to have died. Bell had heard nothing from Cornell in years, "until this report, unaccompanied by letter or otherwise, appeared in my mail today. I am passing it on to you," Bell explained to Davison, "for it may have some bearing on the subject which we were discussing."[25]

The "subject" they were discussing was a secret project that would require the coordination and collaboration of several Duke-related networks.[26] Physicians at the McLeod Infirmary in Florence, South Carolina, had been injecting extracts of the fungus *Aspergillus* into the tumors of advanced cancer patients; and to date, they reported, "some hundred advanced malignancies had received treatment, with consistent benefit subjectively and objectively, and with prolongation of life."[27] Encouraged by the results, the McLeod researchers had sought the advice of Dr. Watson Rankin, head of The Duke Endowment's Hospital and Orphans Section in Charlotte, North Carolina. Indeed, on the same day that Bell and Davison had discussed the secret project at Cyanamid's headquarters in New York, Rankin had been with the McLeod group at Pearl River, discussing with Coca and the other Lederle scientists how the two groups might collaborate on future *Aspergillus* research and product development.[28]

Lederle's response to the McLeod group, Bell explained to Davison, was "that what is needed now is a comprehensive plan, outlining a succession of steps including, in its proper place in the sequence, studies by a competent immunologist." While Lederle could analyze the data the immunologist collected, the latter "would probably have to do his work in the hospitals up to the point where it became a task of animal experimentation, in which case Lederle's facilities might be found advantageous. Whether this is true or not," Bell encouraged Davison, "I believe that you are the person to decide and, if it is true, to plan the project and assign the work. This kind of research can, I suppose, be handled effectively only by a well organized group, such as is rarely found outside of a faculty of a medical school. As I remarked to the trustees of the Endowment, the Medical School at Durham seems to me to possess, in an unusual degree, that open-mindedness, spirit and enthusiasm which are necessary to achieve results."[29]

Davison well understood the significance of the secret cancer project. Not only would it be the largest research program ever undertaken at DUMC; it also coincided with the signing by President Roosevelt of the National Cancer Institute Act, which provided $700,000 annually for cancer research and for better facilities for the diagnosis and treatment of cancer. Of more immediate importance to Davison, though, was the fact that the McLeod cancer project could reinforce the emerging collaboration between DUMC and American Cyanamid—a collaboration that now included more than just access to information and the latest technology. For Lederle had made a large grant to Beard in September to help him staff and stock a horse encephalitis research laboratory at Duke. As Beard later explained, "at that time, $6,500 was a considerable amount of money, and I was somewhat reluctant to take the responsibility for such an amount." But he did—under certain conditions. "We would have complete freedom to spend the money as fast as seemed necessary to carry on the work, but for a period of only three months. If, at the end of that time we had not made any progress, we would return the residual funds or continue as Lederle wished. They agreed to this plan, and we started the work."[30]

Davison was also well aware that the McLeod project was personally important to his close friend and mentor, Dr. Watson Rankin. Rankin had joined The Duke Endowment in 1925, after 16 years as head of the North Carolina State Board of Health, and it was Rankin who had designed the Endowment's hospital program for North and South Carolina. In addition to subsidizing indigent care in the region's nonprofit hospitals, the program provided grants for rural communities to build their own nonprofit hospitals and convert private, for-profit hospitals into locally owned and operated community hospitals. The McLeod Infirmary was one of the first for-profits to make the Endowment-funded conversion, and Rankin wanted to see what the McLeod researchers could do. Davison also considered Rankin the one person "to whom [he was] more indebted than anyone else."[31] Rankin had helped Davison plan and open DUMC in 1930 and had proved indispensable as an advisor to the young dean in the meantime. Significantly, too, Rankin was also a member of DUMC's faculty and had powerful connections with some of the nation's leading public health and medical officials. He was a close friend, for example, of Thomas Parran Jr., the new surgeon general of the United States. And his brother, Fred Rankin, a professor of surgery at the University of Louisville, was not only a son-in-law of Dr. Charles Mayo, a founder of the Mayo Clinic, but also a member of the American Medical Association's Council on Medical Education and Hospitals—the body that had recently rated Duke's medical school among the top 25 percent in the nation.[32]

Davison plunged into the planning with the spirit and enthusiasm that Bell had expected. He sent Smith to Pearl River to discuss the McLeod project and then joined Smith at The Duke Endowment offices in Charlotte to discuss the matter with Rankin and other foundation officials. Davison also asked several faculty members to evaluate the *Aspergillus* proposal. Dr. William A. Perlzweig, head of DUMC's Department of Biochemistry, counseled caution. "The biochemical excursions are phantastically wild and woolly, if not wholly, then for the greatest part. And yet they may contain a germ of a good idea. They ought to go on with their work on a modest scale," he advised. "If the preparations could be tested on rat or chicken tumors perhaps more ground could be covered in the preliminary work." A similar suggestion came from Dr. Robert J. Reeves, head of Radiology. "I would suggest study with laboratory and animal observations before going into the human element."[33]

But therein lay Davison's dilemma. The McLeod researchers saw no need for animal studies and had no use for Cyanamid's new equipment at the Stamford and Lederle Laboratories—at least, not yet. They believed they had already demonstrated the effectiveness of the *Aspergillus* extract in treating human tumors. What they needed now was "clinical material"—patients with certain conditions, most of them specific to women: "medullary forms of breast tumor with visible and palpable metastases; growths of the nature of the solid ovarian carcinomata, and those developing from the glandular epithelium of the uterus, together with certain intestinal cancers, would probably be the types most suited."[34]

Although human trials did not bother Davison, he soon discovered that Bell had a different approach in mind. In mid-September, the Cyanamid president notified McLeod that Lederle would not be contributing financially to their project. In the long run, Bell explained, "the general program can be best worked out by a completely rounded group of medical experts," experts, that is, like those at DUMC. "These experts should form a permanent group available each, some or all, for frequent and immediate consultation and advice. The probabilities of success will be greatly enhanced if most of the men in this group are accustomed to work together." As for what such a group would cost, Bell estimated "$25,000 a year for animals and material alone,—not to mention salaries, apparatus and buildings." But unless McLeod solicited "the aid and support of such a group as I have described," Bell would hesitate in making a contribution.[35]

By the end of September, the McLeod researchers had asked DUMC to direct their project and Davison had put a plan for it in Bell's hands. A committee of eight Duke physicians would control the project, Beard would chair the committee, and both Smith and Davison would serve on it. The *Aspergillus* extract would be administered to both animals and humans—in individual doses of

5,000 cc—and McLeod was to provide enough extract to test 300 mice, 300 rats, and 25 humans in "preliminary experiments." Duke would order the test animals from the Rockefeller Institute, and the human test subjects would be selected by Drs. Robert R. Jones Jr. and Roger D. Baker, the two physicians in charge of Duke's cancer clinic. If the animal tests proved negative, Duke would let McLeod know; if positive, the committee would send a report to McLeod and make no publication until after the South Carolinians published their "preliminary paper." The project would begin on December 3, with the injection of the selected Duke patients, and the animals would be tested once DUMC purchased and housed them.[36]

DUMC was already testing sulfanilamide by the time Davison submitted his plan for the McLeod cancer studies. Early in October 1937, Davison informed Bell that Duke's cancer clinic was "trying the effect of sulfanilamide in the shrinking of tumors in patients whose outlook is hopeless."[37] Interesting, Bell replied; and what if the results were favorable? "Would your next trial be with mice or rabbits in which the progress of the disease is not so far advanced? Or is it one of those instances where no harm could come to the patient and it is not necessary to restrict the experiment to hopeless cases?" Although Bell felt "no real warrant" in hoping for success, he knew that "the Calco Company, our subsidiary which manufactures sulfanilamide, is now receiving rumors of the trial of this material in all sorts of cases with the results reported favorable but not based on sufficient clinical experience to prove much of anything. Is Duke carrying on any experiments in other fields, with this material?" Bell asked.[38] Why, yes, Davison replied. Two of his own men in the Pediatrics Department. "Dr. Angus McBryde and Dr. Jerome Harris are now compiling our results of sulfanilamide therapy in miscellaneous conditions in children and Dr. Edwin P. Alyea is giving a paper at the Southern Medical Association Meeting in New Orleans on December 1st on his results of sulfanilamide therapy in gonorrhea in adults."[39]

RAISING CAPITAL

While the drug testing went forward at Duke, Cyanamid's three controlling stockholder-directors—Bell, George G. Allen, and longtime Duke attorney, William R. Perkins—set about raising capital to expand the company's research and development. They declared "a special dividend" of one dollar per share on the company's common stock and also approved their own "proposal to authorize 2,500,000 shares of new 5 per cent 10-par cumulative preferred stock, convertible into Class B common stock, and an increase in authorized Class B stock 3,000,000 to 3,600,000 shares." As the *New York Times* reported, "W. B. Bell, president, says in a letter to stockholders that the company requires a substantial part of its earnings for increased working capital and the expansion of its business."[40] Most of the special stock dividends went to Bell, Allen, and Perkins, of course, as would most of the new shares; but other individuals in the Duke-related networks also stood to benefit. Among the many members of the Duke and related families who held Cyanamid stock, for example, one of the largest blocks of nonvoting shares belonged to Walker P. Inman, the son of James B. Duke's widow by her first marriage. Several Duke Power executives also held Cyanamid shares, as did the director of The Duke Endowment's Hospital Section, Dr. Watson S. Rankin, who, from a peak of 1,300 shares in 1935, held close to 1,000 shares of Cyanamid in 1937.[41]

About a week before the Endowment's October board meeting, Davison sent Rankin a funding request from Duke University Hospital for $17,500. "We wish to apply, with the approval of the Administration of the University, to the Trustees of the Duke Endowment for assistance in enlarging and equipping the animal quarters of Duke Hospital." The funds were to be used for research and patient care: "The increasing routine diagnostic work of Duke Hospital, and the provision for research require each year greater expenditures for laboratory animals, and for their feeding and care. Every Wasserman reaction, virulence test for diphtheria, examination of spinal fluid for meningeal tuberculosis, and other daily problems in connection with the diagnosis and treatment of disease in patients require guinea pigs, rabbits, and rats. Pellagra, fungus diseases, and nutritional deficiencies, conditions which cause many deaths annually in North and South Carolina, can be studied only by the use of animals."[42] [Figure 2.5]

The Corporate Connection across Campus

Duke Medicine's plunge into corporate-sponsored cancer research coincided with several other significant developments on campus. By the late 1930s, Duke's Department of Chemistry was receiving $25,000 a year in research grants from one of Durham's largest industrial concerns, the Liggett & Myers Tobacco Company. Working under the direction of its chairman, Dr. Paul M. Gross, the Chemistry Department—which was the only department to occupy a building of its own on the university's new campus—conducted important research on the chemistry and diseases of tobacco, on nicotine and fertilizers, and on the cultivation of bright leaf strains of tobacco. Gross himself had developed two valuable cigarette patents, both of which he assigned to Liggett & Myers: one for a "Method of Manufacturing and Packaging Cigarettes" and the other for a "Method of Reducing the Nicotine Content of Tobacco." As the *New York Times* announced in December of 1936, "A 'tailor-made' process for reducing the nicotine content of tobacco was described yesterday by Dr. P. M. Gross, chairman of the Duke Univer-

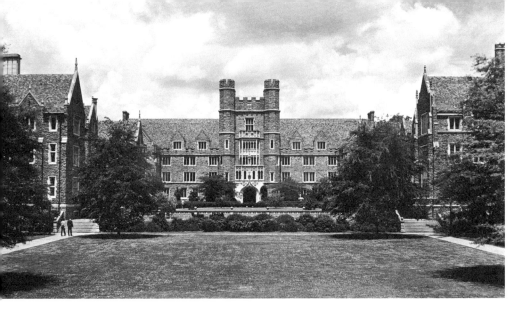

2.5 Duke University School of Medicine, viewed from the campus quadrangle. *Duke University Archives*.

sity Department of Chemistry, in an address at the University of Richmond. He said that ethylene oxide, first used successfully in a war on the injurious tobacco beetle, will reduce nicotine content to 1.1 per cent without seriously changing the aromatic qualities of the weed."[43]

Paul Gross was Duke Medicine's staunchest ally on campus for the next three decades. Gross, a graduate of Columbia University in New York, began teaching chemistry at Trinity College, Duke's predecessor, in 1919. His research progressed at Duke from tobacco soils and packaging cigarettes in the 1930s to radioactive fallout and the composition of tobacco smoke in the late 1940s and 1950s, and the general particulate composition of the environment from the late 1950s on. Gross became, in fact, one of the nation's foremost experts on the constituent particulates of environmental pollution. He also set the standard for corporate-sponsored scientific research at Duke in the early 1950s. From the tobacco companies that funded research in the chemistry department, Gross extracted the right to control and publish the data collected in such research, making it available to the companies only through publication. Gross also collaborated closely with Duke Medicine in bringing government-sponsored research to DUMC, first through the radioisotope programs sponsored by the Atomic Energy Commission in the late 1940s and then through the Research Training Program devised in the mid-1950s and implemented in 1959.

Yet it wasn't pathbreaking scientific research that most people thought about when they heard Duke University mentioned in the late 1930s. They thought about two things, both of which were making big news when the Endowment's trustees met in October 1937. One was the school's football team and its coach, Wallace Wade, whose recent winning ways had landed him on the cover of *Time* magazine for October 25. Duke's other well-known newsmaker was Dr. Joseph B. Rhine, head of the Parapsychology Laboratory in the university's Department of Psychology. Rhine's 1934 book, *Extra-Sensory Perception*, had drawn international attention, and early in 1937 the Duke University Press had printed the first issue of the *Journal of Parapsychology*. But neither of these publications had generated the popular buzz that now accompanied *New Frontiers of the Mind*, Rhine's story of clairvoyance experiments at Duke. Published on October 4, 1937, by Farrar & Rinehart, the book's release was coordinated with the simultaneous broadcast of a series of ESP experiments sponsored by the Zenith Radio Corporation. The book was also chosen as a Book of the Month Club main selection, and, in an advertising strategy not unlike that used earlier by James B. Duke at the American Tobacco Company, Farrar & Rinehart offered ESP cards to Zenith listeners and members of the book club.[44]

The Duke Endowment's Mission and Corporate Interests

In the same month as these stories were attracting wide media coverage, the trustees of The Duke Endowment were scheduled to meet. The October board meeting was one of 10 required each year under the terms of the Endowment's indenture, which also required "that at least at one meeting each year this Indenture be read to the assembled trustees." Most of the trustees had heard it many times. It delineated their duties and Buck Duke's reasons for establishing the Endowment. It also explained how the Endowment worked and the specific formulas for paying the trustees and figuring aid for the beneficiaries of the charitable trust—orphans, Methodist ministers and Methodist churches, nonprofit hospitals in the Carolinas, several private colleges in the region, and Duke University—which had been established under the terms of the indenture. The indenture also created the Endowment by weaving together an ensemble of for-profit and philanthropic networks in which the welfare of one part depended on the health of the others. The beneficiaries depended on the Endowment for funds, the Endowment depended largely on the stocks of the Duke Power Company, and Duke Power was controlled by the Endowment as the major stockholder. This interdependence of interests was expected to sustain the personal mission that Buck Duke had pursued during the last years of his life: to stimulate social, economic, and political development throughout—and beyond—the territory served by his various electric and water power properties in the Piedmont Carolinas. As

Duke himself put it in the indenture, his Endowment was a missionary enterprise: "From the foregoing it will be seen that I have endeavored to make provision in some measure for the needs of mankind along physical, mental and spiritual lines, largely confining the benefactions to those sections served by these water power developments."[45]

All of the trustees at the October meeting wanted to help the medical center, just as they also wanted to help the larger university of which it was part. But their interests, ideas, and goals varied, and they did not always agree on what "help" meant or how to distribute it effectively between the Endowment's two major beneficiaries, DUMC and Duke University. The board's only women, for example, the 24-year-old heiress Doris Duke Cromwell and her mother, Nanaline H. Duke, were estranged from each other. And there was no love lost between Doris Duke and the Endowment's two major figures, George G. Allen and William B. Bell, both of whom, as Endowment trustees, were also trustees of the Doris Duke Trust. While Doris Duke was a liberal Democrat, Allen and Bell were old-line conservative Republicans; while she supported Roosevelt with words, deeds, and money, they did everything possible to oppose the president; and while Doris Duke demanded greater control of her financial affairs, particularly with the trust fund her father had left her, Allen wanted to maintain the trustee structure controlling her trust and the investments underlying it.

At the same time, several of the Endowment's North Carolina trustees, including men who were also officers of the Duke Power Company in Charlotte, silently opposed the highly publicized fight that Allen, the company's president, had been waging since 1934 to prevent the federal government from funding a county-owned hydroelectric plant in South Carolina. Not only had the case generated bad publicity for Duke Power; the time and money spent fighting it had also further compounded financial problems for the company, the Endowment, and the university during the Depression. As an officer of the Rockefeller Foundation reported: "There is real concern over the Federal Gov't's loans for water power development in the Carolinas, which would affect the Duke interests. This would lessen the University income from endowment, over half of which is invested in Duke utilities." Only days before the trustees met, in fact, the United States Supreme Court agreed to hear arguments in the Duke Power case on December 3—the same day the McLeod cancer trials began.[46]

Despite their differences, however, the trustees shared a deep concern over another important question then before the Supreme Court: whether the Department of Justice could proceed with its antitrust suit against the Aluminum Company of America (Alcoa). The suit was the largest such antitrust action since 1911, when the Supreme Court had declared Standard Oil and

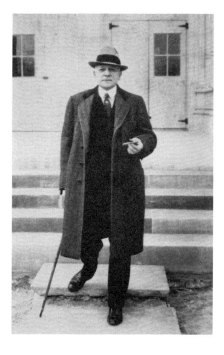

2.6 George G. Allen. *Duke University Archives.*

American Tobacco monopolies, and if the court allowed the government to proceed with its case against Alcoa, the Endowment's investment portfolio could be dramatically affected. James B. Duke had acquired a one-ninth interest in Alcoa in 1924, in a merger involving his Canadian water power properties, and in the years that followed Duke's death in 1925, his Alcoa stocks had become central to the building of the medical school and hospital. By the time the Department of Justice filed its suit in 1937, seven individuals and two groups (the trustees of The Duke Endowment and the trustees for Doris Duke) held almost 60 percent of the monopoly's common stock, as well as 63 percent of the common shares of its holding company, Aluminum Ltd., of Canada. Significantly, Alcoa securities represented more than 20 percent of the Endowment's portfolio of stocks and were the foundation's second largest investment after Duke Power.[47]

In addition to their concern over the Duke Power and Alcoa cases, several of the Endowment's most powerful trustees also shared a deep fear that the large number of horses they personally owned might become infected with the spreading epizootic of equine encephalomyelitis. Doris Duke and her husband, James H. R. Cromwell, maintained hundreds of horses at Duke Farms, their residence in Somerville, New Jersey; Cromwell's stepfather, Edward Stotesbury, owned some of the most valuable trotting horses in America; and the only American with a deeper investment than Stotesbury in blooded stock trotters was the nation's leading supporter of harness racing, William N. Reynolds of Winston-Salem, North Carolina. Reynolds, a brother of deceased tobacco magnate R. J. Reynolds, had recently retired as chairman of the R. J. Reynolds Tobacco Company. He had been a trustee of Duke University since 1927, an Endowment trustee since 1931, and a member of the executive committee of the Duke University trustees since 1933.

The motion to accept DUMC's funding request for equipping and expanding its animal facilities was made by George G. Allen, the Endowment's chairman. A short, balding man who smoked Cuban cigars and carried a cane, Allen was a native North Carolinian who was interested in the Methodist Church,

Duke University football, and extrasensory perception. He had started with Duke's American Tobacco in 1895, working in its bookkeeping department, and in 1922, Duke had asked Allen "to become associated with him in the handling of his personal affairs."[48] [Figure 2.6]

Since that time, Allen had been the most important financial nexus for the Duke-related networks. He was chairman of The Duke Endowment, president of Duke Power, a trustee of Duke University, and a director of American Cyanamid, Alcoa, the Texas Company (Texaco), the Guaranty Trust Company, and a number of other smaller enterprises. Between 1921 and 1935, moreover, Allen had also been vice chairman of the British-American Tobacco Company of London, where he would remain a director until 1950. Although he resigned from the Alcoa board when the government began its investigation, Allen would still be a director of Guaranty Trust when it merged with J. P. Morgan in 1959, and he would become a director and member of the executive committee of the merged Morgan Guaranty Trust. He would also continue on Cyanamid's board until 1957; serve on its executive committee; and act as chairman of its board for several years after Bell's death in 1950.[49]

Allen would also remain for the next two decades the most powerful decision maker within The Duke Endowment's ensemble of interests. He was Duke Power's president until 1949, when he would become the company's first chairman, a position he would hold until 1957. He would also continue as a trustee of Duke University, as a member of the university's executive trustee committee, and as chairman of the university's building committee until 1958. And he would still be chairman of the Endowment at the time of his death in 1960.[50]

Duke Medicine's Initiatives with the Rockefeller Foundation and the Duke Family

Duke Medicine's connections with the Rockefeller Foundation included more than Beard's hard science networks at the Rockefeller Institute. They also included the foundation's support for a department of psychiatry at Duke, a pursuit that affected not only Duke's institutional history but also the history of psychiatry in North Carolina.

DUMC's Rockefeller connections went back several decades to the shared business and political experiences of James B. Duke and John D. Rockefeller Sr. Rarely, if ever, seen together, and certainly not close friends, they nevertheless had much in common: both were Republicans and both had business enterprises that girdled the globe, including monopoly enterprises that were broken up by the United States Supreme Court in 1911: Standard Oil in Rockefeller's case, American Tobacco in Duke's. Paternalistic alike toward blacks and whites, both men were deeply religious and believed in the responsibility of great wealth to fund and direct the course of public health and social welfare in the United States. They were also deeply committed to developing the South and formed powerful enterprises for that purpose.

The Rockefeller Foundation was formed in 1913, more than a decade before The Duke Endowment, and was preceded by the Rockefeller Institute for Medical Research (1901) and by the Rockefeller Sanitary Commission for the Eradication of Hookworm Disease (1909–14). North Carolina had served as a leading laboratory both for the hookworm campaign and for the educational reforms promoted by the Rockefeller General Education Board. At the same time, one of the state's own public servants, Dr. John Ferrell, had become associate director of the Rockefeller Fund's International Health Board.[51]

It was also during these decades that Rockefeller philanthropy helped produce at Johns Hopkins the highly trained physicians who left there and opened DUMC in 1930. Chief among them was Wilburt C. Davison, the Hopkins-trained pediatrician who became DUMC's first dean. "Thanks to the foresight of the Rockefeller Foundation," Davison later wrote, "a number of long term fellowships and instructorships were established at the Hopkins so that those who wished to go into academic medicine had an opportunity for training." Funding for the Hopkins Pediatric Department alone had required "enough money to maintain twenty-five [physicians] at one time or another. . . . Practically all of that group became professors of pediatrics at one-third of the medical schools in this country, as well as in some of those abroad."[52] Likewise, all but a few of the original faculty at Duke's medical school had come directly from the Johns Hopkins medical school in Baltimore, and once they got to DUMC, they taught at a medical school underwritten with a grant from the Rockefeller General Education Board. This five-year, $300,000 grant had enabled DUMC to open in 1930 as a four-year medical school rather than as a two-year school.[53]

DUMC's opening had coincided, in fact, with a major reorganization at the Rockefeller Foundation involving both the retirement of its medical advisor, Dr. Abraham Flexner, and a reorientation in the foundation's programmatic emphasis to psychiatry. As the foundation's newly elected president, Max Mason, described the change, "it was not to be five programs, each represented by a division of the Foundation; it was essentially one program, directed toward the general problem of human behavior, with the aim of control through understanding."[54] According to the foundation's new director of medical sciences, Alan Gregg, the program would focus on psychiatry and psychobiology and give particular attention to neurology, for only through understanding and control of the nervous system could "physical pain and mental stress" be relieved.[55] In the widest sense, the foundation's psychiatric program was based on the general ideas of psychobiology and "psycho-somatic" medicine as advanced at Johns Hopkins University by psychiatrist Dr. Adolph Meyer. Meyer believed that no single factor explained illnesses in humans; rather, disease involved a multiplicity of intertwining psychological and physiological (somatic) factors as well as sociocultural forces.[56]

Between 1932 and the reorganization of Gregg's division in 1952, the Rockefeller Foundation would spend approximately $16 million on psychiatry, much of it for creating entirely new psychiatry departments in academic medical centers throughout the United States and Canada. During this time, the foundation also made large capital grants to existing departments for specific research and training programs.[57] In 1933, for example, the foundation funded a special psychiatry project at Harvard that deeply influenced the future chairman of Duke's Department of Medicine, Dr. Eugene Stead.[58] The mission of the Harvard program was to "'link psychiatry to the rest of medicine' by demonstrating that a teaching and research unit in psychiatry was an essential part of a general hospital." Likewise, the Harvard project was also expected to serve the foundation's larger goals for psychosomatic medicine: "to redefine existing disciplinary boundaries as to what constituted valid research, reinstate psychiatry's authority as a vital component of general medical and hospital practice, and extend the social role of the physician into the community." Put simply, Gregg and his colleagues believed that "the new science of man was not reductionist molecular biology but psychobiology and psychosomatic medicine—the holistic study of the entire organism, based on many disciplines ranging from anatomy to psychology and anthropology."[59]

DUMC had opened a psychiatric service in 1930, but staffing problems and inadequate funding had soon rendered it ineffective. It could not, for example, treat a member of the Duke family, Mrs. Mary Duke Biddle, for the severe depression she developed after her divorce in 1931 from Anthony J. Drexel Biddle Jr.[60]

Mrs. Biddle could not be treated at Duke because there was no psychiatric ward at that time in Duke Hospital. Fewer than 30 physicians in North Carolina were then interested in psychiatry, and it was not until March 1934, with the arrival of a Meyer-trained psychiatrist from Hopkins, Dr. Raymond S. Crispell, that psychiatry was truly practiced at DUMC—and only then within the Department of Medicine.[61] Fortunately for Mrs. Biddle, however, the chairman of Duke's Department of Medicine, Dr. Frederic Hanes, had worked as a neurologist at the National Hospital, Queen Square, London, and was able to refer her to his good friend, Dr. Robert F. Kennedy, a neurologist at Bellevue Hospital, who eventually helped her recover.

In the meantime, Drs. Davison, Hanes, and Crispell had worked out a political strategy to link Duke to improved mental health care in North Carolina. Their first step, drafting a resolution to the state legislature, was completed with the help of the Duke University law school in 1934, and early in 1935, Durham's state representative, Victor S. Bryant, offered the resolution to the North Carolina General Assembly. Adopted by the legislature on March 20, 1935, the resolution authorized the governor to appoint a commission to survey the state's mental health needs. The governor appointed Hanes, Crispell, Bryant, and two other men to the commission, and the Rockefeller Foundation funded the study. The appropriation was the "first of its kind made by the Foundation," the foundation reported, and "it was hoped that a practical result of the survey would be the establishment of a State Psychiatric Hospital at Durham with effective connections with Duke University."[62]

The study's importance to Rockefeller was made even clearer in the spring of 1936, as Hanes and his commission were completing their work. Gregg invited the entire commission to New York for dinner and discussions with some of that state's leading mental health officials. The meeting was held in the foundation's dining room in the RCA building at 30 Rockefeller Plaza. Gregg summarized the meeting in his diary: "I emphasized the importance of the Commission's work in our opinion as a control or model of such procedure in case as seems likely other states were prepared to follow the example of N.C." According to Gregg, the "principal issues in discussion were the question of centralization of state control and the possibility of increased economy or reduced expenditure in the present set-up." Also, "the advantage of a diagnostic hosp. of mental diseases in its relationship to the instruction of med. students emerged as a serious consideration and as part of the obvious desirability of extending public comprehension of the care of the defective and insane." Most of the participants at the New York meeting "favored a larger degree of centralization" but doubted that state costs could be reduced; indeed, they had described the need for at least two new mental hospitals in North Carolina.[63]

The commission's final report, introduced by Hanes and issued to the North Carolina legislature in January 1937, found it "humanly impossible" for the state's mental patients to obtain the care and attention they needed. Patient-doctor ratios were 528 to 1 and thus nowhere near the 150 to 1 recommended by the American Psychiatric Association. Patients at one state hospital were allocated 17 cents per day for food and only $1.10 a day for their total care. According to the Rockefeller Foundation, the North Carolina report established a unique and important precedent. "With the publication of this report something approaching adequate information on the state mental health service was, for the first time, made available. It is probably the best assemblage of information of its kind in the South and it is expected to serve as a valuable piece of evidence both immediately and in future."[64]

Hanes and his fellow commissioners made 16 recommendations, including "the development of Duke University as a center of psychiatric training" and "the development of the University of North Carolina as a training center for social workers and for clinical psychologists." Although the state's new governor, Clyde Hoey, initially ignored the report, Hanes and the foundation made progress in other directions. The report "had considerable effect upon the attitudes of state leaders (political, religious and educational) toward the subject of mental diseases," Rockefeller reported. "Among the more tangible effects of the survey are: increased appropriations by the legislature for enlarging state hospitals; the establishment of a Child Guidance clinic at Winston-Salem under excellent auspices and with strong community support; and the organization of a Society of Neurology and Psychiatry. The organization of local mental health societies was carried on by a member of the staff of the Commission utilizing Rockefeller Foundation funds."[65]

PSYCHIATRY AND SOCIAL SERVICES AT DUKE

In the meantime, Hanes asked the Rockefeller Foundation informally for help in establishing Duke Medicine's work in psychiatry. Early in September 1937, he and his wife, Betty, invited their friend Dr. Robert A. Lambert to their cottage in the mountains of western North Carolina. Lambert, the associate director of medical sciences at Rockefeller, was Alan Gregg's right-hand man, and after returning to New York, he summarized for Gregg his "Vacation in North Carolina with Dr. F. M. Hanes." According to Lambert, Hanes presented his "plans for further development of psychiatry at Duke" within the larger context of DUMC's growing need to expand its facilities. "There is a pressing need for additional beds for surgery and obstetrics as well as psychiatry which at present has no facilities for hospitalization of patients. It is expected that the Duke trustees will set aside some $600,000 for an addition to the hospital and that through this a 25 to 30 bed unit for psychiatry will be provided." Also, Lambert continued, "with a view to keeping psychiatry in close relation with internal medicine, it is H's idea that the psychiatric unit should be set up in the present building adjoining the medical ward." Hanes had also asked Lambert if the Rockefeller Foundation might endow a chair of psychiatry once the university had set up the proposed inpatient unit with beds, but was told that a "request for endowment would almost certainly be turned down; that there would be more hope for a grant over a limited period, assuming a strong case could be made."[66]

Lambert's discussions with Hanes occurred simultaneously with Lederle's funding of Beard's equine encephalomyelitis research and Doris Duke's support for both child psychiatry and a new division of social services at Duke.[67] The purpose of the division was to help coordinate and communicate information and services among the hospital, its patients, the medical school, and numerous community agencies. Division personnel, in addition to recognizing and explaining problems related to illness, organized lectures, courses, and roundtable discussions in order to demonstrate to medical students, nurses, and volunteer groups what medical social caseworkers could accomplish. Eventually staffed by progressive, professional medical caseworkers, the social services division was useful for DUMC both internally and externally. In addition to connecting DUMC's many services, the division cooperated with the University of North Carolina at Chapel Hill, providing three to six months of practical fieldwork training at Duke Hospital for graduate students in UNC's division of public welfare and social work. Through public and private agencies, moreover, and at every level of government throughout the state, DUMC's division of social services soon collaborated with "such community agencies as the Juvenile Court, churches, private family agencies, and various public welfare services, i.e., the Farm Security Administration, the State Department of Vocational Rehabilitation, the State Commission for the Blind, and the Child Welfare Services."[68]

While Doris Duke funded the new division, her private secretary, Marian Paschal, played a key role in helping Wilburt Davison establish and staff it. Paschal recruited some of America's best and brightest social workers to DUMC—women who had studied at the Simmons School of Social Work in Boston, at the University of Chicago School of Social Service, and at the New York School of Social Work (where Paschal herself had studied). As Davison later described her impact: "Miss Paschal, in collaboration with the State Welfare Authorities and under their supervision, investigated the social service needs in this area, and organized the Medical Social Service Division at Duke Hospital."[69] Paschal also proved important to DUMC as an officer and director of Independent Aid, Inc., the foundation chartered by Doris Duke in 1934. Between 1937 and her death a decade later, Paschal supported a variety of grants to DUMC from the foundation, including $15,000 to $30,000 annually for DUMC's division of social services.[70]

THE LARGER CONTEXT

These developments occurred against a background of movement for social change in the state. In the fall of 1937 Paschal also began working through Independent Aid with the North Carolina College for Negroes in Durham and, on a personal level, with the family of the school's business manager, Charles C. Amey. Although the Dukes had supported the black college for years—indeed, the chairman of its board of trustees was the vice president of Duke University, Dr. Robert L. Flowers—Doris Duke had had little or no contact with the school until Paschal and Amey met in mid-September during his fund-raising trip to New York. Surprised by the warmth and respect Paschal showed him, Amey wrote and thanked her after he returned to Durham. He also shared his experience with the college's long-time president, James E. Shepard, who immediately wrote Paschal that "Mr. C. C. Amey has told me about the very courteous interview you gave him, and of the deep interest you manifest in the success of this Institution. I cannot tell you how much I appreciate this."[71]

Shepard then recalled a similar experience of his own. "I shall never forget that way back in 1912 when I went to New York to see Messrs. J. B. and B. N. Duke and asked them for $1000, without any hesitancy they gave it. The Duke interest has not only followed this Institution, but they have shown an interest in everything for the uplift of the Negro. They inherited this interest from their father, Mr. Washington Duke, whom it was my privilege to call a friend." From that point on, Independent Aid became a regular contributor to the North Carolina College for Negroes and Paschal took a special interest in Amey's two daughters, one of whom would cross the color line at DUMC as a medical social worker in the Department of Social Services.[72]

Much of Independent Aid's expanded giving reflected the fact that Doris Duke received the second of three planned payments from her father's estate on November 22, 1937, her 25th birthday. She had received the first payment at age 21, and would get the final one when she turned 30. This time the payment was for some $18 million, and the media clamored for her to make a statement. Doris refused to discuss the matter, but her husband, James H. R. Cromwell, delivered a brief response on the radio. According to the *New York Times*, "Mr. Cromwell, who has been considered as a possible successor to [New Jersey] Governor-Elect A. Harry Moore as United States Senator, said in a radio speech last night that 'wealthy persons are no longer accumulating fortunes to leave monuments of themselves in the form of endowments to universities, but prefer to use the money and our best efforts to bring a greater measure of comfort, decency and security into the lives of our less fortunate fellow-citizens.'"[73]

Cromwell's comments reveal the delicate balance that Dean Wilburt Davison needed as he worked with Duke University's connections in the North. While Duke Medicine benefited from the dollars that Doris Duke dispensed, and while she practiced the progressive efforts her ambitious husband preached, the New Deal Cromwells were also challenging The Duke Endowment or, more specifically, its conservative Republican leaders, Allen and Bell. And Davison could not afford to alienate Allen and Bell, for, in addition to controlling DUMC's Endowment funds, the two powerful businessmen were using their extensive corporate connections to provide Duke Medicine with money, personnel, and machines. At the same time, DUMC's new psychiatric initiative required careful integration with the priorities of the Rockefeller Foundation's very liberal leader, Alan Gregg. Gregg and Allen saw each other regularly in New York, and they lived less than a mile apart in nearby Scarsdale, but they were worlds apart politically: Gregg was a leftist Democrat who usually voted socialist.[74] As for Wilburt Davison, he shared the prevailing liberal-leftism of both the Cromwells and Gregg, and he had little contact with the Endowment's Allen. Access to Allen, at least for university business, was controlled through the university's trustee on the Endowment, Duke's vice president, Dr. Robert L. Flowers.

Leadership and the Private Diagnostic Clinic

Wilburt Davison, Deryl Hart, and Fred Hanes constituted DUMC's core leadership during its first two decades of existence. All three men considered the medical center a special place, and each was dedicated, in his own way, to helping the medical center achieve the special goal set by James B. Duke for the entire university: "attaining and maintaining a place of real leadership in the educational world." Yet the three men also came from very different backgrounds, held different assumptions about the nature and extent of DUMC's growth and pursuit of research, and were connected to a variety of different webs and networks. The major source of conflict among them was the need for more space, particularly at the Private Diagnostic Clinic, and in choosing well or badly among policies and possibilities, they helped determine what ultimately became not only of themselves but also of their colleagues and Duke Medicine.

THE DEAN

Wilburt Davison was a patrician physician with the common touch. Standing over six feet tall and weighing more than 200 pounds, he was as comfortable lecturing to his professional colleagues as he was caring for children and drinking beer with his medical students. Davison was also a wonderful writer, with a keen sense of humor. As one long-time colleague described him, Davison "had a warm heart and a jovial disposition and he insisted on an informality that required everyone to call him 'Dave.'" [75]

Davison had grown up on Long Island Sound, the privately tutored son of a Methodist minister. After graduating cum laude from Princeton, he had attended Oxford on a Rhodes scholarship. There he had met the famous physician Sir William Osler, who became a friend and who, because Davison had asked to combine his two years of medical school into one, described him as "a new American colt who is wrecking a medical school tradition."[76] In between stints of medical service in wartime Europe, Davison had worked at the Rocke-feller Institute in New York, graduated from the Johns Hopkins School of Medicine, and married Atala Scudder, the daughter of Townsend Scudder, a former New York congressman and future state supreme court judge. Fol-lowing World War I, the young couple had moved to Baltimore, she to enter medical school at Johns Hopkins and he to take a pediatrics appointment at Hopkins. Davison was 34 years old and the assistant dean of Johns Hopkins Medical School when Duke president William P. Few hired him in 1927 to plan and launch Duke University's new school of medicine.

Since that time, Davison had learned several important lessons about Duke. One was that its financial means were not immune to wider economic forces; the Depression had demonstrated that, as had the antitrust litigation involv-ing Duke Power and Alcoa. Davison had also learned just how valuable the medical center was to public relations for Duke Power and The Duke Endow-ment when the Endowment promoted Duke Hospital's nonprofit good works to give Duke Power credit in its fight against government-funded electrical utilities. And in both of these lessons Davison was discovering yet another: that the trustees of the Endowment were more interested in the medical cen-ter than they were in the rest of the university. While the medical center had received the best of everything, the other departments gained little more than a grand façade of Gothic architecture. As one visitor from the General Edu-cation Board put in 1931, "The Univ. is quite an accomplishment as regards bldgs. And grounds; these are very striking and have many beautiful features. Unfortunately the whole endeavor was started with bldgs. Beautiful though they are, there is apparently no money for equipment and least of all for men. The new biology lab. has virtually no equipment and the small library is already overcrowded."[77]

Davison married, earned, and inherited money but practiced at DUMC a thriftiness that one Rockefeller officer attributed to "Dave's Scotch back-ground." Research was fine, in the young dean's mind, as long as gifts and grants supported it. But it always remained secondary to him, both person-ally and for the medical center. He focused instead on the medical school, on the clinical training of its students, and it was through them that he helped create what eventually became one of DUMC's most important and lasting net-works: the Duke Medical Alumni Association. At the same time, Davison was also developing a close personal relationship with Doris Duke—the closest she would have, in fact, with any other individual in the Duke-related net-works—and from 1947 until his death in 1972, he would serve as an officer and director of both her Independent Aid foundation and its successor, the Doris Duke Foundation.

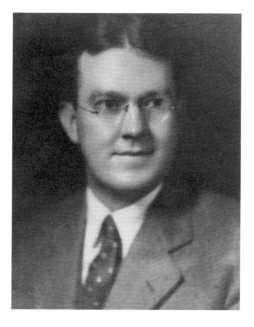

THE SURGEON

Davison had little in common with Deryl Hart, the head of Surgery, other than the fact that they were both over six feet tall and had worked at Hopkins at the same time. Two years younger than Davison, Hart had been raised on a farm in southwest Georgia and had been attending Emory when his father died. Needing the farm's income to continue his studies, Hart had maintained its operations while earning a bachelor's degree and then a master's degree in mathematics, his one true love in life. From Emory Hart had moved on to medical school at Johns Hopkins, where, after receiving his M.D. in 1921, he had completed a surgical internship with Dr. William S. Halsted. Hart had completed his residency at Hopkins, and was serving as a member of its faculty when Davison selected him as the first chairman of Duke's Department of Surgery. [Figure 2.7]

Hart was a reserved, formal man who spent much of his time in staff and student meetings performing calculations on his slide rule. He was more interested in research than Davison was, especially if it showed promise of saving money or producing revenue, but he embraced little of Davison's dedication to teaching and the medical students. "Dr. Hart was a superb surgeon who taught by precept," one chief resident from the 1930s recalled. "He did not like to talk while operating. We had to watch him very carefully and deduce for ourselves why he did this or that. He did not like to be questioned about why he did such-and-such, and he expected us to understand that."[78] One long-time colleague, fellow surgeon Clarence Gardner, later said of Hart: "Although he was a surgeon and educator by profession he was an architect and a financier by avocation."[79] Indeed, Hart was the architect of the most important for-profit business to emerge from Duke Medicine, the Private Diagnostic Clinic.

Beyond DUMC and the PDC, however, Hart's principal connection to the wider world was through his wife, Mary Elizabeth Johnson, a native of Raleigh. The couple had married in 1932, just months after the PDC was established, in a wedding described by the Raleigh *News & Observer* as "of widespread interest and outstanding in prominent social circles in the State." Mary was given away at the wedding by her uncle, John M. W. Hicks, the retired treasurer of the American Tobacco Company, while another uncle, Dr. J. Clyde Turner of Greensboro, the president of the Baptist State Convention of North Carolina, performed the ceremony.

Mary tried over the years to soften her husband's slide rule image by sending him to work with a boutonnière selected from the garden of their large, rambling house on the edge of campus. She was also the mother of his six children and a warm, generous matriarch to his students. "On the Wednesday night before each Thanksgiving," one former student recalled, "Dr. Hart and his wife, Mary, invited all the residents and interns in general and thoracic surgery for a turkey dinner at their beautiful home. Mary knew the backgrounds of the interns and their spouses, the names of all their children and what illnesses they had recently had. She and Deryl formed a team that served Duke well when he was chairman of the Department of Surgery and subsequently when he became president of Duke University from 1960 to 1963."[80]

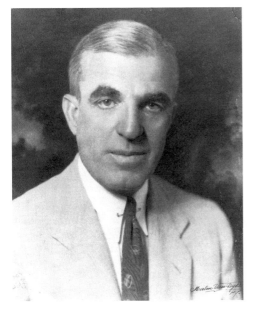

2.8 Dr. Frederic M. Hanes. *Duke University Medical Center Archives.*

THE PHYSICIAN-SCIENTIST

Though Davison and Hart were never close friends, they worked better with each other than they did with Fred Hanes, the chairman of the Department of Medicine. Unlike Hart in Surgery, Hanes had not been selected as Medicine's first chairman. Davison had chosen Harold L. Amoss, a graduate of Harvard Medical School, instead. But in 1933, in one of the more mysterious events in the early history of Duke Medicine, Amoss had resigned his position because of what Davison described to the Rockefeller Foundation's Alan Gregg as "financial difficulties." Davison also wrote later that Hanes "had been our professor of neurology from the beginning and would have been the original Duke Professor of Medicine if his friends hadn't told me that Fred would not be interested in the administration required of the chairman of the department. I was never so greatly misinformed."[81]

Actually, Davison probably had hoped to avoid giving Hanes such an important post. Born and raised in Winston-Salem, Hanes was a member of one of North Carolina's wealthiest and most prominent families. He had a sense of privilege and self-importance that reflected his position in a small, intertwined elite who saw their city as kind of a feudal manor. "These people were incredibly wealthy and wielded considerable influence on the local, state, and national level," one historian has noted. "They just assumed that they were the best men, and that they knew what was right for people."[82] Indeed, Hanes had access to a variety of powerful networks unmatched by anyone at DUMC or Duke University. He was also unmatched, it seems, at least among DUMC's faculty, in the depth of his racial prejudice and assumptions of privilege. [Figure 2.8]

Hanes had attended prep school at Woodberry Forest before graduating from the University of North Carolina in 1903. He received an M.A. from Harvard the following year, and then spent the next four years in medical school at Johns Hopkins. In 1908, Hanes moved to New York, serving as an assistant professor of pathology at Columbia University (along with Robert A. Lambert) and as a pathologist at Presbyterian Hospital. After a year of research at the Rockefeller Institute (1912–13), Hanes married a nurse, Elizabeth Peck, and served as an associate professor of medicine at Washington University Medical Department and then, briefly, as an assistant in neurology at the National Hospital in London. In 1914, he was professor of therapeutics at the Medical College of Virginia. Hanes returned to Europe again during the war, as a lieutenant colonel in the Medical Corps of the United States Army, commanding Base Hospital 65. (Coincidentally, Duke's hospital unit in World War II would be named the 65th General Hospital.)

Hanes spent much of the 1920s in private practice in Winston-Salem. He also established his own clinical laboratory, traveled with his wife, and busied himself with a number of lifelong hobbies. He collected paintings and books, particularly first editions of Boswell, Johnson, and their contemporaries. He also cultivated several original varieties of iris and would later play a major role in developing the Sarah P. Duke Gardens next to Duke Hospital. As late as 1925, at the age of 42, Hanes was playing polo with his brothers against the military teams that ponied up for matches at Fort Bragg.

As Davison had perhaps expected, Hanes complained about everything as chairman of the Department of Medicine. Sometimes it was in defense of DUMC, as when he wrote and criticized the local press for being unfair to Duke Hospital; other times it was simply cantankerousness, as when he asked the city to abolish the "barbaric" practice of blasting factory whistles so early in the morning. Inside DUMC, however, Hanes constantly found fault with the world around him—the linens used in the private rooms, emergency admissions, hospital rates, and equipment—and he fired off a continuous stream of grumbling memos and letters. Nor did the majority of medical students live up to Hanes's standards; those who were not completely "dumb" or "stupid" he might evaluate as "not a complete loss and may improve as time goes on."

By 1937, Hanes's most common complaint was the lack of space to expand, and in a letter to Davison in February of that year, Hanes complained that, while the wards of Duke Hospital were segregated by race and sex, the color line was not in place throughout the hospital. "When you come back I want you to study with us the question of getting the colored patients out of the present x-ray set-up," Hanes wrote to Davison. "As it is now we are mixing the colored and white indiscriminately which doesn't matter so much except in G. I. [gastrointestinal] work. Here both white and colored are compelled to use the same toilet facilities and this results in a very undesirable situation. Recently my mother went through a G. I. series and it was pretty bad. I have been thinking that we might find space in the basement where the x-ray equipment now being used could be set up for this purpose. This would make it convenient to the Medical Out Patient and would solve the question of fluoroscope for this division. The Equipment Committee has left untouched the amount earmarked for new x-ray equipment waiting your return. I strongly feel that we should modernize this part of the x-ray department, and if we could take some of the increasing load off by segregating the colored x-ray work I believe it would be a useful and feasible plan."[83] (This suggestion was in fact accepted.)

As insufferable as Hanes could be, he nevertheless championed the central importance of research to Duke Medicine and wielded significant influence within its powerful support networks. Late in 1936, for instance, Hanes had launched a $500,000 research fund at DUMC with a substantial contribution of his own. Named the Anna H. Hanes Research Fund in honor of his mother, the fund received additional donations from its namesake after she visited the hospital the following February. In Hanes's mind, research was the key to DUMC's future greatness. "We are going to stand or fall as an institution upon the scientific work done here," he believed. "It is not enough to sit like fat grub worms and merely treat disease. If Duke Medical School is to take top rank in the country it can only do so by the production of medical advances."[84] Hanes had already taken the first steps in launching Duke in that direction in 1934, when, through the Rockefeller Foundation's program to relocate refugee scholars from Europe, he had traveled to Germany and recruited Dr. Walter Kempner to DUMC. "I believe he will be a good man for us at Duke," Hanes had written the foundation after first meeting Kempner, "teaching some later on, and doing research from the start. I am very keen to get some real research going and this man is said to be original in his thinking."[85]

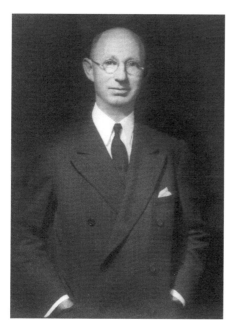

2.9 Dr. Robert A. Lambert. *Courtesy of the Rockefeller Archive Center.*

Through his family connections, moreover, Hanes also had the ear of the state's largest bankers and industrialists, the Duke University board of trustees, the Rockefeller Foundation, military leaders, insurance executives, members of the Duke and Biddle families, and members of the Roosevelt administration. In addition to the connections mentioned earlier, Hanes's family (the makers of "Hanes" knitted underwear) included several alumni and trustees of Trinity College, Duke's predecessor. Hanes's uncle, Pleasant Huber Hanes, was a Trinity graduate and a trustee of Duke University; in 1939 he would become chairman of the university's centennial fund-raising committee. Hanes's brother, Robert March Hanes, was president of North Carolina's largest bank, the Wachovia Bank and Trust Company, and from 1939 to 1940, he would serve as president of the American Bankers Association (the first North Carolinian to hold that office). Another of his brothers, John Wesley Hanes Jr., was a senior partner of Charles D. Barney & Company, a Wall Street investment firm; appointed to the Securities and Exchange Commission in 1937, John Hanes would be named assistant secretary of the Treasury in 1938. And then there was Hanes's brother-in-law, Robert Lassiter of Charlotte. Lassiter was chairman of the Federal Reserve bank in Richmond and served for years as vice president and then president of the largest corporate predecessor of Blue Cross and Blue Shield in the state, the Hospital Savings Association of North Carolina, Inc.[86]

Hanes's most important connection, at least for Duke Medicine, was his friendship with Dr. Robert A. Lambert of the Rockefeller Foundation. After working with Hanes in New York, Lambert, a native of Alabama, had served with the Army Medical Corps in Europe. He had then served as president of the American Near East Relief Committee in Syria, and on various Rockefeller assignments in Brazil, Central America, and Puerto Rico. Lambert made his first visit to Duke in 1930, before becoming Gregg's associate director, and he would visit it several times a year thereafter until his retirement in 1948. In his reports to the Rockefeller Foundation, Lambert frequently referred to Hanes as "my old friend and co-worker," and on one occasion he even described Hanes as "without a doubt one of those rare born-leaders, and withal a most excellent teacher."[87] Though his friendship with Hanes long preceded either's connections with Duke and the Rockefeller Foundation, Lambert's work with the medical sciences division elicited an initial response from Hanes that was both humorous and suggestive: "It must be grand to have Mr. Rockefeller's money to spend the way you do," Hanes wrote to Lambert. "I expect to see you in a loud checked suit with a brown derby hat when next you appear before our astonished gaze. Also should you find a million or two unexpended at any time please keep in mind poor little Duke Medical School which is struggling manfully to keep its head above the troubled waters."[88] [Figure 2.9]

THE CONFLICT BETWEEN SURGERY AND MEDICINE AND THE NEED FOR SPACE

By 1937, DUMC's troubled waters included a fierce struggle between Hanes and Hart over space, especially within the Private Diagnostic Clinic, where space meant money. Although the PDC was *in* Duke Hospital, it was not a part *of* Duke University. As Hart later explained, "The school and hospital were opened in 1930 during the depression; and over the following years, with the University income falling, we realized that securing an adequate clinical staff would be dependent largely on private practice, the development of which was slow in those years of financial hardships." Both immediate and cumulative benefits were expected from this private practice. Hart later noted that "in 1931, in order to render better service to the patients, to conserve the time of the teaching staff, to expand the income from private practice so that a part of it could be used for the development of an adequate staff, and to be able to compete for good teachers with institutions in large cities where a private practice might seem to the individual to be more certain of development, the Private Diagnostic Clinics were organized by the staff with the entire geographic full time group participating voluntarily."[89] Many in the group began practicing immediately, as cooperation from the university had been assured. "The officials of the school reasserted the rights of the staff to engage in private practice," Hart explained, "gave them permission to develop the clinics as a staff rather than University projects, and assured them that the institution would not use these organizations to restrict their rights in private practice or to delve into this part of their activities; an agreement that has never been broken or questioned by the University."

The PDC exceeded everyone's expectations. As new faculty were hired and more of the eligible clinicians practiced through the PDC, the number of private patients swelled, increasing the need for more hospital beds as well as for ambulatory patient services. Between 1932 and 1937, the number of patients discharged from Duke Hospital increased from 5,648 to 10,954, while the days of care they received jumped from 67,672 to 111,673. Yet the number of beds fell to approximately three per doctor, making it difficult for the faculty to generate the income promised them beyond the $2,000 to $3,000 salary the university paid them. In the meantime, the number of charity patients also continued to increase, as did the number of public (non-PDC) outpatients (from 26,212 in 1932 to 58,297 in 1937).

Hart described the need for more space in his 1971 book, *The First Forty Years at Duke in Surgery and the P.D.C.* "By 1937," he wrote, "expansion of the P. D. C. facilities became necessary, but space contiguous to the existing clinic was not available. As a result, two separate locations were used, with the cleavage falling naturally between the medical specialties (Pediatrics and Medicine, including Psychiatry) and the surgical specialties (Obstetrics-Gynecology and Surgery, including Ophthalmology)."[90]

The cleavage was nastier and much more disruptive than Hart intimated. Hanes's sister-in-law, Agnes Michel Hanes, had died two years earlier from an infection she had received following a radical mastectomy performed by Hart at Duke.[91] Early in August 1937, moreover, while Joseph Beard and David Smith were visiting Bell in New York, Hanes wrote to Hart: "All of us must recognize that the space available is extremely limited, and it will be necessary to use every available examining room in order to care for the private patient load." There were only two examining rooms available to the Department of Medicine, Hanes complained, while Surgery had six. "Obviously medicine is compelled to have more examining rooms at its disposal. In the nature of medical work more patients are seen than are seen by the surgical side. I don't know the exact figures but I should say the ratio would be about 5:1. This is not only the case of Duke Hospital but it is true of the practice of medicine and surgery in general."[92]

Hart continued his version of the story in his book, which was published almost 25 years after Hanes's death. "With the separation of the P.D.C. facilities, Dr. Hanes, Chairman of the Department of Medicine, expressed the wish that all of the medical specialties would function as a unit under his direction, and such an arrangement was considered desirable by all departments." And yet, as Hanes himself now reminded Hart, "I have pointed out to you before that, so far as I am aware, not one square inch of space has been given up by any clinical department for general hospital purposes except by the medical department. I repeat that the extension of the x-ray therapy department, the present blood chemistry laboratories and the recent separation of colored from white x-ray patients has all been done at the expense of medical space. We are now reduced to the point where we have not one foot of space available."[93]

Hart claimed in his book that it was the combination of the expanding PDC and Hanes's demands for separating the practice that led to its medical and surgery divisions. "As a result of this expansion and separation two divisions were organized—each bearing the original name 'Private Diagnostic Clinic'—and were designated 'Medical Division' and 'Surgical Division.' For the public image however, they operated as one." Hanes ended his 1937 letter to Hart by defending the Department of Medicine: "Finally, please let me say that there is a misapprehension current in regard to the attitude of the Medical Department, we have not the slightest desire to do anything unjust or unfair, or infringe in any way upon the rights of any department. What I do wish to make very plain is that any rearrangement of space must take into consideration the facts that I have mentioned above."[94]

By the fall of 1937, it was clear to everyone connected with Duke Medicine—patients, personnel, and philanthropists alike—that the center needed much more room than its seven-year-old facility could provide. Beard's research, the McLeod cancer project with *Aspergillus*, the division of social services, and the hoped-for expansion of psychiatry—all made the need to expand immediate and real. But how would this growth be financed, especially at the PDC, which was the most aggressive, expanding force within the medical center? "Duke," after all, was not part of the PDC's official title, and for a very good reason: the university believed that its name should not be associated with a private enterprise. The matter was a delicate one, both then and since. As Hart later noted, "Even though as presently operated the value of the P.D.C. activities has been recognized by most, others have advocated that the University take it over. At times this has become a problem for discussion."[95]

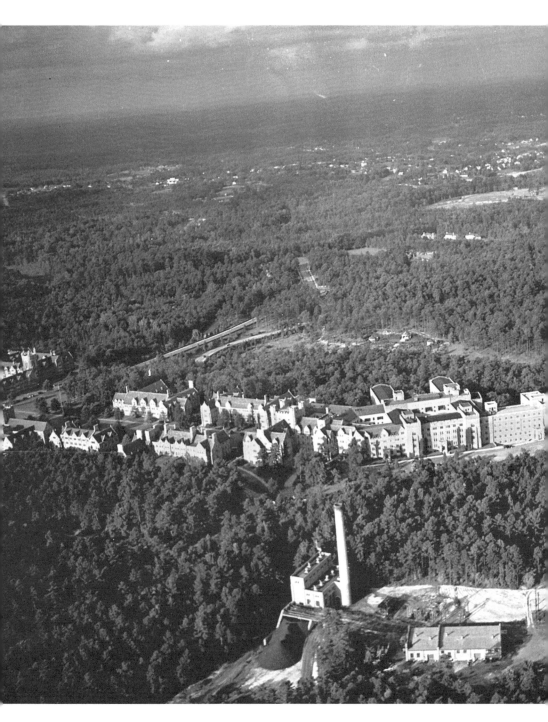

3.1 The Duke University campus (ca. 1940), showing the recently completed PDC building (white, right of center). *Duke University Medical Center Archives*.

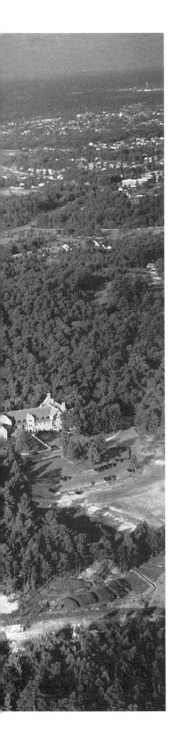

CHAPTER 3:

Between Two Worlds: Duke Medicine from 1938 to 1940

D uke University looked in two directions during its 1938 centennial celebration. The festivities looked back to the university's roots in rural North Carolina, to a private subscription school in Randolph County, and also looked forward through Duke Medicine, to a healthier state, region, and nation. The celebrations were a good example of what one historian has called the "nostalgic modernism" of American culture between the two world wars. "The crucial point is that the interwar decades were permeated by both modernism and nostalgia in a manner that may be best described as perversely symbiotic," Michael Kammen has written. "That is, each one flourished, in part, as a critical response to the other."[1]

Kammen's term also aptly describes the first decade and a half of Duke Medicine. The "nostalgic modernism" is there, for example, in Buck Duke's indenture, in the combination of his rural Methodist roots and his electric utilities. It is also there in his remarks on hospitals, science, and the importance of community. Hospitals, he wrote, "have become indispensable institutions, not only by way of ministering to the comfort of the sick but in increasing the efficiency of mankind and prolonging human life. The advance in the science of medicine growing out of discoveries, such as in the field of bacteriology, chemistry and physics, and growing out of inventions such as the X-ray apparatus, make hospital facilities essential for obtaining the best results in the practice of medicine and surgery." Duke, in providing funds for community hospitals, expected the communities themselves to share in the financial burden for indigent patients and building hospitals. "So worthy do I deem the cause and so great do I deem the need that I very much hope that the people will see to it that adequate and convenient hospitals are assured in their respective communities, with especial reference to those who are unable to defray such expenses on their own."[2]

Between 1938 and 1940 Duke Medicine remained enmeshed in the charity traditions of Buck Duke and his Endowment, even as it took on much of its modern shape: increased scientific research, the creation of a psychiatry department, a growing practice at the Private Diagnostic Clinic, and collaboration with the University of North Carolina on issues involving black health and education.

The Risks and Rewards of Research

In his experiments with the horse vaccine at Duke, Joe Beard faced many of the perils and profits of medical research, and through his work, both the university and its medical center gained early and important experience in dealing with academic medicine's modern mix of money, government, and culture. More specifically, Beard, Bell, and American Cyanamid expanded Duke Medicine's foundation as a laboratory for research, teaching, and patient care.

The secret cancer trials with the McLeod group proved particularly disappointing to everyone involved. None of the patients injected with the aspergillus extract showed any improvement, and early in January 1938, Duke abandoned its association with the project. Watson Rankin, the major link in the McLeod research, wrote to Davison from The Duke Endowment, "I think it is just as well that the relationship of both the University and the [Endowment] Trustees with the research work at the McLeod Infirmary terminate. We have one more payment to make on our appropriation, and they have already told me that they will not reapply for further assistance."[3]

Terminating the McLeod project did allow Joe Beard more time to focus on his horse virus research. His research was important for two closely related reasons. The virus annually threatened animals owned by small farmers and wealthy equestrians alike, in North America and South America, and, like the virus that caused the great flu pandemic of 1918, it might move to humans from its animal host. By the spring of 1938, Cyanamid's Lederle Laboratories had provided Beard with everything he had requested for his work, and the transfer of money, personnel, and equipment to Duke was paying off.[4] In addition to creating a vaccine that "was immeasurably cheaper and simpler to make than that produced with purified virus," Beard later recalled, he and his colleagues demonstrated for the first time "the efficacy of killed virus to induce active protection, whereas it had been previously thought that only live virus could be effective."[5]

Lederle's scientists had to see it to believe it. "They then made vaccine and tested it in both guinea pigs and horses," Beard later recalled. "Although they challenged their animals with about 50,000 infectious doses of virus given intracerebrally, every animal was solidly immune. Immediately after this demonstration, Lederle began producing the vaccine at a furious rate. They very shortly depleted the supply of fertile eggs in nearby places, and then began flying them in from long distances. At one time, they were using 40,000 eggs a day to prepare just equine encephalomyelitis vaccine."[6]

Despite repeated urgings from Bell and Lederle to apply for a patent, Beard initially demurred. "I was not much interested in being embroiled in such a matter myself, and Duke University was not about to be involved in any patent process."[7] On May 12, 1938, however, Beard applied for a patent, and Lederle, in announcing the new vaccine in the May-June issue of its *Veterinary Bulletin*, ran ads promoting the "new improved vaccine" along with a story that mentioned the work by Beard and Ralph W. G. Wyckoff. The price for the new vaccine—"sold only to veterinarians"—was $1.75 per treatment, with a five-treatment package offered at the reduced price of $7.00.[8] Lederle also began paying Beard a royalty of 5 cents for each dose of vaccine sold. "In the summer of 1938," Beard recalled, "I received a check of $1,110 which I spent for our own purposes." But his missionary impulse soon whispered back. "We began to worry then about possible increased income, and we thought we had better begin to make some arrangements to dispose of the royalties. . . . It seemed only reasonable to assign the royalties to Duke University, but at first the university seemed very warily reluctant to have anything to do with the patent."[9]

Up in New York, however, Bell and the Lederle group were so impressed with Beard's success that they brought him to Pearl River to discuss an expanded program of collaborative research. "Dr. Beard and his associates at Duke did a practically perfect job on equine encephalomyelitis," Bell wrote to Davison. "We believe that, while other diseases may present more complications, no one could approach them with more hope of success than he. It only remains for me to say that, while I know nothing of the details of these matters, I have a strong hunch that, with the new techniques now available, we are ready for the conquest of several of the great diseases. I believe that Dr. Beard,

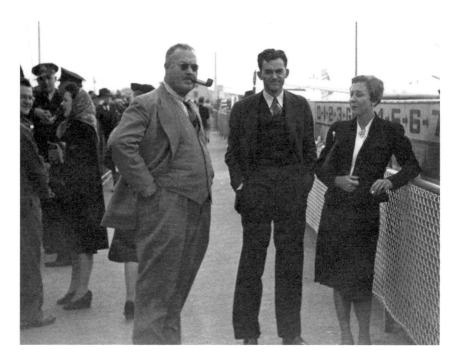

3.2 Dean Wilburt C. Davison, left, with Joseph and Dorothy Beard. *Duke University Medical Center Archives.*

with the backing of yourself and the group that surround you, are the people who can make this conquest. I need not tell you how delighted I shall be if the credit for these discoveries goes to the Medical School of Duke University."[10]

Beard's second royalty check made him gasp. It was "for more than $30,000," he recalled, "and, in consequence, we increased our efforts to get the University to do something about it." This time Duke cooperated; working closely with the Beards, the university established a research fund to accept the royalties. It also wrote the procedures to govern the fund, and gave the fund its name, the Dorothy Beard Research Fund. Unfortunately, physicians at Harvard Medical School were also seeing human patients infected with horse encephalitis, with over 30 cases soon reported. "The people at Lederle then became very frightened," Beard wrote, "because they had a rather large number of people engaged in making the vaccine. We debated some time the advisability of vaccinating everyone in contact with the agent. This was actually a most critical matter, because some people having had the disease either died or were mentally badly crippled afterward. . . . The fear was, of course, that the virus was not really entirely killed and that we would be taking the chance of infecting the people, or at least some of them, with live virus." And that included Beard and five or six of his co-workers at Duke.[11] [Figure 3.2]

Negotiating for Psychiatry

Late in April of 1938, as the virus experiments were peaking on the fourth floor of the medical school, Fred Hanes and Dave Davison were on the first floor, writing letters to Alan Gregg at the Rockefeller Foundation. Both men requested funds for a new department of psychiatry as part of the general expansion of the medical center, Hanes through a personal appeal and Davison as dean of the Duke University School of Medicine.

"The time has come when we feel that a determined effort must be made to establish an adequate Department of Psychiatry within the Department of Medicine," Hanes wrote to Gregg. "This cannot be done without the construction of a new building to provide not only for psychiatric beds, but neurological and neuro-surgical beds, housing for increased staff, etc. etc." The medical center was planning a new, million-dollar building, Hanes explained, "and we hope that the Trustees of the Duke Endowment will approve its construction as a capital item. Our medical school and hospital budget of $1,070,010 requires this year $510,157 from Endowment income, and the present set-up will call for a considerable yearly increase. The trustees are unwilling, therefore, to adopt a psychiatric program without some outside aid."[12]

Hanes then made his pitch. "If we could secure a seven year grant of $25,000, I believe the Trustees will approve our psychiatric program, and provide the needed space. Without this space I despair of seeing psychiatry adequately developed here, at least during my working time." Hanes then repeated his plan for developing psychiatry at Duke, referring to the program at the University of Rochester as "the same type of unit that I have in mind—a strong unit within the Department of Medicine. On Monday, May second, I shall be in New York, and will greatly appreciate an opportunity to discuss the matter with you and Lambert."

Davison said nothing in his letter about where psychiatry might fall within DUMC's departmental structure. He emphasized instead the progress DUMC was making, not only in fulfilling its original plans in psychiatry and other previously neglected fields but also in collaborating with other institutions and agencies. "When Duke University School of Medicine and Duke Hospital were opened in 1930," he wrote, "we could not provide adequately for neurology, preventive medicine, social service and psychiatry. We now have an active staff in neurology, neuro-surgery and neuro-anatomy, and hope for progress later in neuro-physiology. A Professor of Preventive Medicine and Public Health has been appointed, and arrangements have been made for cooperation in the field of teaching with the Division of Public Health of the University of North Carolina under Dr. M. J. Rosenau." In addition, Davison continued, a "Social Service Division has also been organized, which through the cooperation of Duke University and the University of North Carolina will form a part of a joint training school for medical social workers." Yet in psychiatry, he explained, "our facilities are still very inadequate. At present, we have an Assistant Professor and an Instructor in neuro-psychiatry, but we have no provision in Duke Hospital for psychiatric patients."[13]

Davison's pitch was similar to Hanes's. The plans for the new medical building included a psychiatric ward of 23 beds, but a Rockefeller grant of $25,000 per year for seven years was needed to pay for staff. "Duke University is appropriating $5,000. annually for this work," Davison wrote, "and will continue to do so, but we need the balance of $25,000 annually to complete the personnel." Davison ended his proposal with a list of potential benefits from such a grant. "The establishment of a clinic for psychiatry and mental hygiene at Duke, with the aid of the Social Service Division, the Legal Aid Clinic, the Family Service Association, the Juvenile Court and the Psychology Departments of Duke University and the University of North Carolina, would be very valuable, not only for the good that it could do individual patients, but for its educational value for the psychiatrists, pediatricians, and other members of the medical profession, social workers and the community at large." Beyond Durham and Chapel Hill, moreover, "clinics also could be held monthly in communities in North Carolina which have shown an interest in this work, which have sufficiently adequate medical and social facilities to carry on the work properly, and which would sponsor and help such clinics."[14]

There was a flurry of activity in the weeks that followed as Hanes shuttled between the Rockefeller Foundation in New York and the governor's mansion in Raleigh. Finally, early in June, Hanes asked Alan Gregg of the Rockefeller Foundation to visit Raleigh for a meeting with North Carolina governor Clyde Hoey. The governor was now "intensely interested in putting into practical application as soon as possible the suggestions" made by Hanes's commission the previous year.[15] "You may think that I am a bit insistent about your attendance at this meeting," Hanes explained to Gregg, "but the Governor especially requested that you be there if possible. This suggestion came directly from him that the Legislature, which meets this January, set up the proper organization for a Psychiatric Commission with the best Commissioner that we can obtain to direct and coordinate all the state[']s activities in mental work." The governor expected "considerable opposition from existing agencies" to the proposed changes, and he wanted Gregg's support in taking this step.[16]

Gregg agreed to meet with the governor but made it clear, either as a prod to further state action or as a way to dampen Duke's expectations, that his visit would not affect funding for a department of psychiatry at Duke. "In view of the indeterminate state of plans in North Carolina for the cure of insane and defectives," he wrote to Davison, "I am better able to record the suggestions in your letter of April 22 than to answer them. . . . Almost the only comment I could offer at present would be that I would doubt if our Board would be disposed to endow a department of psychiatry though it is at least possible that it would some time in the next three years consider a contribution to its development over a period of years."[17]

Hanes was in New York preparing to sail for a European vacation when Gregg arrived in Durham. Gregg spent most of the morning with Davison touring the home of Benjamin N. Duke. Duke's daughter, Mary Duke Biddle, was in town for the wedding of her daughter, Mary, to Dr. Josiah Charles Trent, and was considering giving the house to Duke University. "Davison raised the question of whether it would be satisfactory for psychiatric service," Gregg wrote of the mansion in his diary. "I thought it would be better as a convalescent hospital since it is too far away from the rest of the school, and psychiatry has suffered long enough from physical isolation from the rest of medicine."[18]

Gregg's meeting with the governor went better than he expected. "It is evident that N.C. is preparing to create a service unifying the present scattered mental hospitals," he noted. "Probability is that this service will be separate from Charities and Corrections and separate from Public Health work." It was also evident to Gregg "that North Carolina is willing to go outside the state for its first commissioner." These were just the kind of changes that the Rockefeller study had recommended.[19]

Poverty, Race, and Reform at Duke's Centennial Celebration

The reform of North Carolina's mental hospital system was just one of the many progressive efforts engaging Duke University at the time of its centennial celebration in 1938. There were also collaborative efforts under way between Duke and the University of North Carolina and between Duke Medicine and Durham's black hospital, Lincoln Hospital, in the fields of race relations and public health. Duke Medicine also made the centennial a public forum for the hotly debated question of the federal government's role in the nation's health care system.

The *New York Times* noted the university's celebration in a column headlined "Symposium To Mark Duke Centennial." "When Duke University lights 100 candles on her birthday cake this month," the newspaper explained, "alumni will send greetings from nearly every State in the Union and from thirty-one foreign countries. 'One Hundred Years of Southern Education in the Service of the Nation' will be the central theme."[20] Duke launched its centennial celebration late in October with a three-day symposium for 500 southern physicians. The symposium, both in its topics and its guests, reflected many of the medical and political currents then shaping DUMC's institutional journey. In addition to focusing on medical problems and diseases especially prevalent in the South, the program included discussions on the future of American medicine, featuring Dr. John Punnett Peters of Yale Medical School and Dr. Morris Fishbein, editor of the *Journal of the American Medical Association*.

In the widest sense, the symposium reflected Duke's position as a leading regional medical center dealing with the public health and medical problems of a poor, rural population in an undeveloped region. In a centennial pamphlet Davison noted the "special importance attached to Duke as a medical research center. The Duke University School of Medicine is the only clinical medical school in North Carolina," he wrote, "and Duke Hospital at present is serving a population of three million. The University thus has a unique opportunity to investigate diseases such as pellagra, sprue, nutritional deficiencies, fungus infections, and the formation of stones in the kidneys, which are found in much larger numbers here than in the Northern states in which most of the great medical centers are located."[21]

Two-thirds of North Carolina's 3.5 million inhabitants lived in rural areas during the 1930s, and African Americans comprised about one-third of the state's population. Birth and death rates were unusually high; 22.3 percent of children died under the age of 10, a rate almost twice the national average (11.8 percent); and midwives handled 65 percent of the black births in the state. The supply of hospital beds and physicians was also low; with 5.05 beds per 1,000 inhabitants, North Carolina ranked 45th of 48 states in 1939, while its ratio of 1 physician for every 1,346 inhabitants ranked it 46th among the states. And if the Duke, Watts, and Lincoln hospitals gave Durham County one of the highest physician-to-inhabitant ratios in the state, at 1 to 261, Tyrell County had a ratio of 1 physician to every 5,164 inhabitants.

Syphilis, tuberculosis, typhoid, diphtheria, brucellosis, sprue, erysipelas, and pellagra and other nutritional deficiencies—along with cancer, kidney disease, and heart disease—regularly challenged Duke's physicians and researchers. Hospital staff used more than 100 rooms on the first floor of the hospital to diagnose and treat an average of 400 outpatients a day at the Public Dispensary, usually without advance appointments. This outpatient service was especially important to the poor and others of limited means; the dispensary provided access to physicians in 18 different specialties at consultant fees that were lower than normal. First-time patients paid one to five dollars with return visits at 25 cents to one dollar, plus the full cost of x-rays and other materials used. By 1938, some 350,000 visits had been recorded at the dispensary, a number that would jump to more than a half million by World War II.

By the time of Duke's centennial, most of the medical center's research focused on nutritional studies related to the public health needs of the southern population. Dr. David T. Smith was one of DUMC's leading researchers; his primary focus was pellagra, and his principal funders were Lederle Laboratories and the Rockefeller Foundation, with additional funding provided by the Markle Foundation and Ciba Pharmaceutical Products. In the days that followed the centennial symposium, for example, Markle contributed $4,000 to sponsor Duke's professor of nutrition, Dr. William J. Dann, to conduct "nutritional studies on pellagra and related diseases."[22] And Markle made its grant within days of a presentation on pellagra by Smith and his wife at a meeting of the National Academy of Sciences. "Spectacular cures of the disease with the nicotine acid, a tasteless white crystalline substance resembling common table salt, were described at the meeting by Dr. David T. Smith and Susan Gower Smith of Duke University," the *New York Times* explained. "Their report was illustrated with colored motion pictures showing patients in the last stages of the dread poor man's diet disease, broken in mind and body, restored to life, health and well-being in the short period of ten days, a spectacle which the distinguished scientists present felt was one of the great modern miracles of science. Not only does nicotine acid offer the definite promise because of the cheapness and availability as a byproduct of tobacco, one of the South's principal products, it was pointed out; the elimination of the disease will also yield incalculable economic benefits to the Southern States in restoring the thousands of sufferers to a life of usefulness and productivity. The disease, even in its earlier stages, affects the mind as well as the body of the patient and greatly reduces his efficiency as a wage-earner."[23]

The centennial symposium also marked a transition in Duke Medicine's plans for a department of public health and preventive medicine. Davison had planned from the start to establish such a department, and in the fall of 1935, after refusing his repeated requests for funding, the Rockefeller Foundation had given him a grant to visit a number of university medical schools "for the purpose of conferring on methods and problems of teaching and research in preventive medicine."[24] The grant, part of a larger foundation initiative in the United States and Canada, sent Davison on what he called "my quest for knowledge of the teaching of public health and preventive medicine." Visits to Toronto University, Vanderbilt, Tulane, Louisiana State, and the universities of Cincinnati and Virginia had led him to an unexpected conclusion. "Although I realize that I am still too ignorant for a definite conclusion," he wrote to Rockefeller in April 1936, "I believe that for the next five years a separate department of public health and preventive medicine is not needed at Duke for the three following reasons: (1) All of the clinical and preclinical departments here are cooperating to permeate the curriculum with the preventive aspect of disease, (2) The courses at the other schools I visited, although more extensive, do not include much more than ours . . . and (3) the University of North Carolina, with which we are anxious to cooperate, has established a course headed by Dr. Milton J. Rosenau for the training of county health officers; our students have the privilege of attending lectures there and also Dr. Rosenau generously has offered to help with the teaching here."[25]

By the time of Duke's centennial, DUMC's division of social services was providing field training for UNC social workers, and the two universities were also sharing a new professor of preventive medicine. In September of 1937, Dr. Harold W. Brown, a former General Education Board fellow at Harvard, had joined the staff of Rosenau's division of public health in UNC's two-year medical school, and shortly thereafter, Davison had secured Brown's appointment to the medical school at Duke.[26]

Duke and UNC were also connected in several ongoing initiatives that, by the fall of 1938, involved their collaboration with private philanthropy and government agencies to improve race relations and black education in North Carolina. One such initiative had emerged in the early 1930s, in response to a proposal submitted to the Rockefeller General Education Board by North Carolina's director of Negro Education, Nathan Carter Newbold. Newbold had asked the Rockefeller philanthropy to fund a "Department of Studies, Information and Statistics on Negro Education and Life" at Duke, which would benefit from its proximity to the new School of Public Welfare at the University of North Carolina. "I am confident President [Frank Porter] Graham of the State University, and Dr. [Howard W.] Odum, Director of the School of Public Welfare, would readily and heartily agree to such a plan of cooperation."[27]

Newbold envisioned, moreover, that the new department would have the opportunity "for reaching and influencing leaders of thought in several major professions and occupations" through Duke's various graduate schools. Indeed, "many Duke faculty have already demonstrated keen interest in the problems of the Negro Race," Newbold explained, and his long list of interested faculty included such "new men" as Davison. Also, "in the very excellent Duke Hospital, which is part of the University, Negroes are cared for and nursed back to health on the same terms as are white people, and they are given equally comfortable accommodations."[28] [Figure 3.3]

At the urging of the General Education Board, Newbold had held conferences with all of the principals involved and each had expressed support for both the proposed department and the collaboration it would entail. Duke president William P. Few had appeared "glad" to set up the program, if he could get the money for it, and he also said he would "be most happy to cooperate fully and completely with our friends at the University of North Caro-

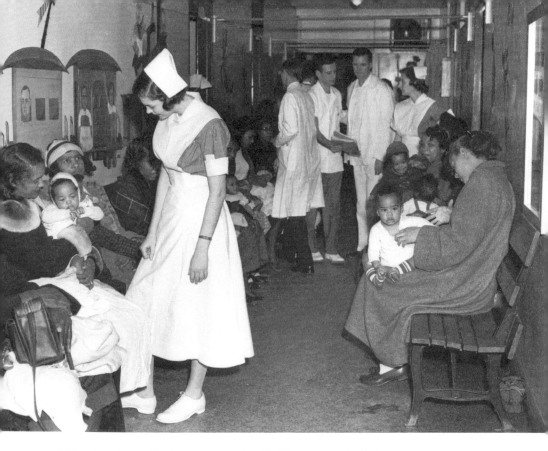

3.3 African American pediatric patients and their families at Duke Hospital. *Duke University Medical Center Archives.*

lina." Likewise, Newbold reported, all of the Chapel Hill group, including Odum and UNC's president Graham, "were interested. Dr. Odum stated that he believes Duke University is the proper place for beginning such a program and that so far as he is concerned he will take pleasure in working for the establishment of it there."[29]

Yet a more cautious response to the proposal had been offered in private by Odum and his faculty colleagues at UNC, all of whom were deeply involved in studies similar to those being proposed by Newbold for Duke. As Odum wrote to the General Education Board in April 1934, it was "our first reaction that such a program headed by Mr. Newbold would be an admirable thing for North Carolina and the South, and that we should like to join both in urging such a program and in the assurance of cooperation. There are, as I wrote you, a number of features that need maturing, and I should like very much to talk to you about some of the points in question."[30] Despite these efforts, nothing more was heard of a department of Negro studies at Duke. Rather, the two universities joined Newbold in 1934 in forming the Division of Cooperation in Education and Race Relations within the North Carolina Department of Public Instruction.

The division lasted more than a decade and marked a high point of collaboration between Duke and UNC. During that time the division worked with local, state, and federal agencies as well as with a variety of progressive foundations to support a number of initiatives aimed at improving race relations and black education in North Carolina. The division focused in particular on two closely related black institutions in Durham. One was Lincoln Hospital, a 100-bed hospital that derived over half of its income from two sources: the City of Durham (33 percent) and The Duke Endowment (21 percent). The other Durham institution was the North Carolina College for Negroes, one of the few state-supported liberal arts colleges for African Americans in the South. Both institutions were controlled (for the most part) by a small group of the city's black elite and were affiliated with a nursing school of 30 undergraduate students and eight graduate students.

THE DEVELOPMENT OF TWO BLACK INSTITUTIONS IN DURHAM

Newbold's Division of Cooperation in Education and Race Relations assisted Duke in establishing clinics at Lincoln Hospital during the hospital's reorganization in the mid-1930s. In 1934, Lincoln Hospital had been on the brink of failure. Thanks to the Duke family, its facilities were as modern as any of the region's best black hospitals, yet most African Americans who could afford to pay for their care went to Duke. That left Lincoln with the most indigent and desperately ill patients, as well as a group of equally desperate doctors who attempted surgeries that exceeded not only their own capabilities but also the strength of those they operated on. The result was a fatality rate twice that of the region's other black hospitals and then the embarrassing loss of accreditation by the American College of Surgeons. For Watson Rankin, head of The Duke Endowment's hospital section, these setbacks were particularly disturbing. Lincoln was as important to the Endowment as an exemplary black grantee as it was to the Duke family as a personal philanthropy. And yet, as Rankin had intimated to Lincoln's trustees, future foundation support for the hospital was contingent upon a reorganization of its affairs.[31]

Lincoln's trustees turned to Duke's Davison for advice, and though he gave it reluctantly, hoping to avoid involving the university in the matter, his collaboration with Rankin stimulated an initial reorganization at Lincoln that laced efficient white paternalism with local racial politics and in the process wounded black pride. The hospital's all-black staff resigned, and local white doctors (including one Duke physician) were put in charge of Lincoln's various services with black doctors as assistants. The change elicited bitter protest from many of Durham's black leaders, including the chairman of Lincoln's finance committee, C. C. Spaulding, and hospital trustee James E. Shepard, who was president of the North Carolina College for Negroes. Indeed, their intervention helped change the mechanism for reorganizing Lincoln Hospital, making it possible for black physicians to resume their positions as service chiefs once they proved their competence to a committee of white consultants.

The benefits of the reorganization had quickly become obvious. Mortality rates receded to normal levels, and new financial procedures combined with special funding from The Duke Endowment and the Rosenwald Fund had improved the hospital's economic prospects. By the time of Duke's centennial, several of Lincoln's physicians had resumed their head positions in the hospital's clinical services and Davison had helped Lincoln regain accreditation by the American College of Surgeons. By then, too, Newbold's Division of Cooperation had instituted a postgraduate clinic at Lincoln for black doctors in North Carolina, South Carolina, and Virginia. In addition, faculty from Duke, UNC, Watts Hospital, the North Carolina State Sanatorium, and the two-year medical school at Wake Forest College were conducting annual clinics at Lincoln "with the physicians receiving instruction from the bedside of the patients. These clinics last for a period of three days," Lincoln reported, "and at the end of the course held at Lincoln Hospital the doctors are invited to attend clinics being held at Duke University."[32]

As Duke prepared for the centennial symposium, Newbold and Shepard prepared a resolution requesting funds from the state legislature to establish, with the help of Duke and UNC, a graduate studies program at the North Carolina College for Negroes. According to the *New York Times*, Shepard expressed "the belief that Negroes trained in the professions can practice among members of their own race and find sufficient outlet for their talents. He envisions a graduate school that would be guided at the beginning by nearby Duke University and the University of North Carolina." Support for this training did come from the state, when the North Carolina General Assembly approved the graduate studies program for the black college.[33]

DEBATE OVER A NATIONAL HEALTH POLICY

Few of the physicians who attended Duke's centennial symposium were thinking about race relations and black education. Most wanted to hear the presentations by Peters, of Yale, and Fishbein, of the American Medical Association. The two men were locked in a furious debate over the future of American medicine; specifically, they were at odds over the question of a national health policy. Peters represented the Committee of Four Hundred, a group of "insurgent" physicians within the AMA who believed that "the health of the people is a direct concern of the government" and that a "national health policy directed toward all groups of the population should be formulated." Fishbein represented those who believed just the opposite, that the current system was just fine, that government should not concern itself with the health of individuals, and that it should, in fact, stay far, far away from formulating a national health policy. Where Fishbein feared a fatal dose of New Deal "socialized medicine," Peters prescribed more support from local, state, and federal governments for public health services, the "medically indigent," and medical research and education. Their debate was part of a larger one that continued for the next 20 years, and for which Duke Medicine continued to serve as a major forum.

There can be little doubt that the vast majority of Duke's doctors supported what Peters was preaching. His approach, after all, reflected the realities of most academic medical centers, where a physician's professional life was defined by research, teaching, and a group practice that served indigent and paying patients alike. In other words, Duke's physicians were not like Fishbein's supporters: independent, solo-practice doctors who depended upon private patients for their entire livelihood. Yet DUMC's leaders also prized the independence and autonomy they derived from private enterprise and the absence of government intervention. They agreed that the health system needed reforming, and that government at all levels was central to the process, but they also wanted to control the process to fit their own needs and goals.

Fred Hanes revealed a personal version of this mindset in the days that followed Fishbein's appearance at the symposium. In a Founder's Day speech to the Medical College of South Carolina, Hanes told his audience, "Only a few days ago I listened to a high official of the American Medical Association discuss the doctors' relation to the newer social trends, and I am firmly convinced that the attitude he adopted was so reactionary and non-cooperative that I shudder to think what capital the demagogues would make of it in Washington."[34]

The old order was changing, Hanes warned, "and whether we like it or not, medicine and medical practice are changing, too. Today the catch-word is 'socialized medicine,' and the term is used by many who have only the foggiest notion of its meaning. . . . The employment of physicians on salaries, to care for the indigent, was begun in Greece as early as 600 years B.C., and was quite general by 500 B.C." In fact, he argued, only in the past 50 years had individuals amassed private fortunes large enough to fund modern medical schools, medical research, and hospitals in the United States. "Rockefeller—Whitney—Harkness—Duke—you and I are witnessing the beginning of the end of these noble private philanthropies," Hanes predicted. In the future, taxation would prohibit the accumulation of great fortunes and "the government, state and national, alone will have funds to dispense for philanthropic purposes. . . . This immense and ever-increasing power of government is one that we physicians, if we are wise, will not try to resist, but will try to guide and direct. . . . My point is this: Should we not at once select the wisest and sanest heads among us to represent our interests in Washington, and seek by cooperation to influence and direct the trend of medical legislation which will surely be enacted by Congress very soon?"

Not coincidentally, perhaps, the major medical legislation then being considered in Washington at the time of Duke's centennial—the plan against which Fishbein was railing—was a plan based in part upon The Duke Endowment's community hospital system. Surgeon General Thomas H. Parran Jr., a leading AMA "insurgent," had studied the system the previous year for Roosevelt's Interdepartmental Committee on Health and Welfare Activities.[35]

Success and Controversy over the Horse Vaccine Study

Duke had hoped to feature Joe Beard's vaccine research at the university's centennial, but apparently baseless charges against his conduct of the research had cast a cloud over his accomplishment.

His research was, in fact, proving very successful. At the same time that the vaccine was saving hundreds of thousands of horses throughout the country, Beard was busy inoculating humans with it. The vaccination effort was one of the first examples, if not the first, of the long and fruitful relationship that continues today between Duke Medicine and the National Institutes of Health. As Lederle's *Veterinary Bulletin* explained, "After consultation with the National Institute of Health and Duke University, plans were made to protect all workers involved in handling the virus at these laboratories. Time was not taken to attempt to produce a more refined vaccine than that which had been found so satisfactory for horses. Approximately 130 members of the staff and technical group each received two intramuscular injections of the bivalent vaccine into the gluteal muscles at an interval of one week."[36]

Beard spent much of the fall of 1938 going back and forth "to Lederle every week by train, first to vaccinate the people and then to bleed them for the demonstration of antibodies." He eventually collapsed with exhaustion, however, and was forced to spend several days in Duke Hospital during the first part of December. Otherwise, he recalled, the process was both "a lot of fun" and "rather bizarre," given that 35 or 40 uninoculated humans eventually died in New England from equine encephalitis. Because it was mainly women who handled the virus at Lederle, most of the workers he vaccinated were women, and "the girls all knew about the cases in New England and the dangers of fooling with the virus. The result was many fainting fits, and girls were dropping all over the halls and restrooms. Fortunately, everything turned out well, and nobody at Lederle or at Duke showed any signs of the disease."[37]

Beard's discovery was a fundamental contribution not only to public health but also to Lederle Laboratories and to the future of Duke Medicine. In addition to demonstrating for the first time the efficacy of a killed virus to induce active protection, Beard's horse vaccine also provided protection against a disease that, like rabies, brucellosis, and tuberculosis, could spread from animals to humans. The vaccine saved many irreplaceable animals during the horse encephalitis epidemic of 1938–39, which was one of the most widespread in the history of the United States and Canada. As one prominent scientist wrote to Beard, "I believe that your development of the vaccine for horse encephalitis is one of the greatest contributions made by a scientist to the cause of the livestock industry for a long, long time—probably even as great as Dorset, Niles, and McBryde's development of the prophylactic measures for hog cholera."[38]

Certainly, too, the vaccine was profitable for Lederle both economically and for the prestige and publicity it generated. In 1938 alone Lederle sold over 1.3 million doses of the vaccine, and much to the delight of the veterinarians who administered it, as well as to those it helped, every animal that received the complete treatment survived. The profits generated by the vaccine enabled Lederle to recoup losses on unprofitable research, expand investments in other promising products, and promote the company's success in several huge exhibits at the 1939 New York World's Fair. Lederle mounted its exhibits in the Medicine and Public Health building as part of a space sponsored by the American Veterinary Medical Association and devoted to veterinary science and public health. A committee of "eminent specialists" controlled the exhibits and permitted "no advertising except a small incidental signature tablet on each, naming the sponsor." According to Lederle's *Veterinary Bulletin*, one of the company's exhibits dealt with the horse vaccine. "It relates pictorially the story of recent epizootics and the recently discovered relationship to encephalitis in children and supports public health efforts to control the next epizootic. Lederle also has a large exhibit on Pneumonia Serum therapy, and another on Allergy. In fact, the three exhibits make it the largest exhibitor in the building."[39]

The impact on Duke Medicine of Beard's success was also extensive. On the most basic economic level, he received almost $300,000 in royalties from his vaccine patent by the time it expired in 1958. The matter also prompted the university to establish procedures for dealing with such developments. In January of 1939, in an agreement with Duke, Beard assigned his royalties to the University and, more specifically, to the Dorothy Beard Research Fund, which was to receive "any and all sums accruing to or received by Duke University" under the terms of Beard's assignment. These sums were to be spent at the discretion of a committee consisting of Beard, Davison, and Hart, for "work done in the Division of Experimental Surgery, in the Department of Surgery, except that out of the first amount or amounts received by Duke University under this assignment" the committee was "empowered to expend an amount not exceeding 33 1/3% of the amount so received for purposes other than research or laboratory work, and that for each year thereafter during the life of this agreement said committee may expend a sum not in excess of 20% of the amount received during the preceding year for purposes other than research or laboratory work, provided that the funds so received were in excess of $5,000."[40]

The fund committee initially used Beard's royalty payments "rather generously" for research, chiefly for the salaries of additional staff, but additional grants soon covered all of those costs. Eventually the fund also "helped a considerable number of individuals with their personal financial problems," Beard recalled, and it also "bought houses and sold houses for members of our staff and others not in our laboratory." The fund became particularly important near the end of World War II, when it provided $51,516 of the $181,516 required to construct the Bell Building, the first DUMC building erected solely for medical research. The remaining funds for the Bell Building came from The Duke Endowment ($100,000), the Rockefeller Foundation ($10,000), and $10,000 each from the "departmental funds" of the medical and surgical divisions of the Private Diagnostic Clinic. By the time Beard retired in 1972, the fund still amounted to more than $150,000.[41]

Also important to Duke Medicine, both immediately and cumulatively, were the attention Beard received, the funding he attracted, and the reputation he established. Beard's initial success prompted Lederle to expand its collaboration with DUMC. The company not only provided funding for Beard's virus and cancer research; it also created a Lederle Fellowship in Biochemistry under the direction of Dr. William A. Perlzweig, chairman of DUMC's Department of Biochemistry. DUMC's first Lederle Fellow was Dr. Hans Neurath, a chemist who was later recognized as one of the founding fathers of modern protein science. Neurath and Perlzweig worked closely on "special projects" in protein chemistry funded by Lederle and the Rockefeller Foundation, and Neurath remained at DUMC until Perlzweig's death in 1950.[42]

Beard's success also brought DUMC an immediate increase in the size and number of grants it received. In 1939 alone it received research grants from private sources that totaled more than all of the grants from previous years combined. No new funders were involved, however; all of the grants came from DUMC's existing contributors and were made, with only a few exceptions, to the same researchers working on existing research problems. What the increased funding reflected in part was the perceived potential of a two-year grant from Lederle. The grant provided Beard and other researchers, including a physicist from Duke's Department of Physics, with access to an electron microscope built for American Cyanamid by the RCA Manufacturing Company. In fact, in 1941, at the end of the grant, American Cyanamid gave DUMC an electron microscope of its own. One of only 16 such instruments then in existence, the microscope was installed in Beard's division of experimental surgery.[43]

Beard's professional publications, moreover, as well as coverage of his work in the popular press, brought significant attention to Duke Medicine, helping it forge new links with federal agencies involved in health care and medical research. DUMC received its first grant from the National Cancer Institute in 1938—not for further encephalitis studies but for extending the cancer research Beard had brought with him from the Rockefeller Institute. Also important was Beard's collaboration with the National Institute of Health; his vaccine was a major advance in public health. Put simply, Beard quickly became one of nation's leading experts on the physical and chemical properties of viruses—a specialty almost unknown outside the Rockefeller Institutes. "With the beginning of the war," he later wrote, "we became involved with the Army, and I was an Associate Member of the Influenza Commission for many years. After the war, Mr. Bell continued to provide funds through Lederle Laboratories. We got money from the Influenza Commission, and, after 1950, the Public Health Service supported us very liberally with research."[44]

Beard's work was not without controversy, however, and a bitter one erupted just as he was allegedly being considered for the Nobel Prize. Early in 1939, his former adviser at the Rockefeller Institute in Princeton, Dr. Carl Ten Broeck, began making "every effort possible to prevent the granting of the patent" to Beard for the horse vaccine. At the same time, Ten Broeck charged Beard and Wyckoff with "unethical practices in their scientific relationships" and succeeded in having their membership applications rejected by the American Association of Immunologists.[45] The association's secretary, Dr. Arthur F. Coca, was also Lederle's medical director, and he was furious with the organization's actions. He immediately asked Beard and Wyckoff to write letters including anything that might help explain why their applications were rejected.

Both men assumed, correctly, that Ten Broeck was behind the matter, and in saying so to Coca they responded at considerable length to the unstated accusations that Ten Broeck *might* have made. According to Beard, Ten Broeck probably considered him as being "willful, disobedient and without the desirable spirit and loyalty expected of an employee of the Institute" and of having an "undesirable competitive attitude" in his cancer research. Beard also listed accusations of a more serious nature that might have been leveled at him: "I stole Dr. Ten Broeck's findings and ideas relative to work with the equine encephalomyelitis virus"; "I was apt to steal ideas from the young people at Princeton"; "the results of my work were placed in the hands of a commercial institution for the purpose of preventing proper distribution of a useful veterinary product"; and "I have unethically entered into a contract with a commercial institution for the purpose of obtaining a patent on a veterinary product by which it is charged that I have received unethical personal gain."[46]

With the letters from Beard and Wyckoff in hand, Coca pressed the association to form a "court" to decide the matter. "Some pressure has also come from Duke University," the association's president wrote. "I can guess that the Lederle interests are behind this effort, which seems to me to be very ill-advised." Most members of the association's governing council agreed; with the exception of Ten Broeck, they considered the problem best "cured by time."[47] They viewed the whole situation as a "mess" and had "no great desire to injure Beard and Wyckoff."[48] As far as Duke was concerned, maybe it was Ten Broeck who needed investigating. Davison suggested as much in his "Comments on the statements of Drs. Wyckoff and Beard." "The accusations against Dr. Wyckoff and Dr. Beard do not appear to be founded on facts, and are satisfactorily answered. . . . Is it possible that Dr. Ten Broeck has attempted to suppress scientific information, which was useful in preventing disease in animals and perhaps also in human beings?"[49]

Wise counsel from Dr. Peyton Rous quieted Coca's call to press the matter. Rous, a future Nobel Prize winner, had worked directly with everyone involved in the matter. "Beard and Wyckoff have been put in a hard position," Rous wrote to Coca, "and it speaks for their sincerity that they were willing to write their letters. Yet that does not mean that they were right in all that they did. Here the skein becomes so tangled that no court could unravel it. The net result of such a court would be to stigmatize even if it absolved them, to make a cause celebre from what might better be forgotten. The best validation of Beard and Wyckoff as worthy scientists will be what they now accomplish. Can scientific societies afford to exclude men who continue to do work of distinction? Do they not exist for such men?"[50]

A Core Academic Business: The Private Diagnostic Clinic

To this early foundation of corporate, philanthropic, and national attention, Duke Medicine also added a business that was controlled to a large extent by the physicians themselves, the Private Diagnostic Clinic. The PDC began driving Duke Medicine economically during World War II, and since that time it has been a principal source of university revenue outside of The Duke Endowment and alumni giving.

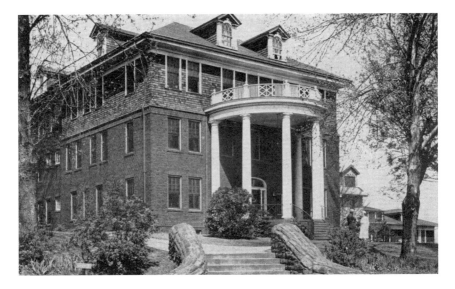

3.4 Highland Hall, part of the Highland Hospital complex in Asheville, North Carolina. *Duke University Medical Center Archives.*

The PDC's power was already in evidence in 1938 when it negotiated for its own five-story addition to Duke Hospital. The Endowment agreed to pay for the addition, and the university initially proposed that the PDC pay for rent, supplies, and secretaries in the new private addition. The proposed five-floor addition was, after all, about private patients. The three upper floors would add over 100 private beds to the hospital, while the bottom two floors were designed for the offices and examining rooms of the new PDC clinics. And it was this space—one floor each for the medical and surgical divisions of the practice—that concerned the university and the Endowment. Because the funds to build the PDC wing would come from monies otherwise earning interest as endowment, the trustees wanted a return on their investment from the private, for-profit group practice.

That was not an acceptable solution for some of the clinic's doctors, however. Having always received an office, supplies, and secretarial help as part of their compensation for teaching, they now considered the university's proposal a violation of their original agreement. They proposed instead to pay all of the clinic's operating expenses with the exception of rent; and in lieu of paying rent, they would *voluntarily* set aside into a "building and development fund for the Medical School and Hospital a percent of the income from private practice . . . to yield a sum greater in amount than the proposed annual rental."[51]

The deal was sealed with a nod and a handshake, and in mid-December 1938 the university and The Duke Endowment agreed to contribute $600,000 to build and equip the new five-floor addition. The deal proved to be almost as important to DUMC and Duke University as the formation of the PDC itself. When completed, the new PDC building generated substantial revenue for the practice and considerable power for the two men—Fred Hanes and Deryl Hart—who headed its two divisions and who held those positions because they chaired, respectively, the Departments of Medicine and Surgery in the School of Medicine at Duke University. The PDC's building and development fund proved particularly important, giving Hanes and Hart and their successors tremendous power in shaping Duke Medicine's future according to their own needs and visions. The result was an unusually high degree of departmental autonomy in which each clinical department acted as a separate unit with its own teaching and research programs. The system that emerged not only dispersed the centralized power formerly exercised by Davison and the Endowment; it also diminished the medical center's integration with the larger university.

Building a Department of Psychiatry at Duke

The new PDC building made room for the in-house psychiatric beds considered by the Rockefeller Foundation as a crucial prerequisite for funding a department of psychiatry at Duke. Fred Hanes visited the Rockefeller Foundation in New York to let Alan Gregg know that everything was falling into place. Gregg wrote in his diary that the Endowment trustees had approved construction that "would make possible 20–25 beds in psychiatry," and also that "the present proprietor of a mental hospital at Asheville . . . has signified his intention of leaving his property to Duke Univ. to be run as a mental hosp. or to be disposed of as the Duke Trustees may see fit." Gregg also pointed out in his notes on the meeting that "Hanes believes that the present prof. of psychiatry, Crispell, is not the man they want to head up psychiatry at Duke Med. Sch." At this early stage in the development of the department, issues were already arising that would cause difficulties in later years. Hanes believed that if the foundation supported psychiatry at Duke for five years at $25,000 a year, the university trustees "would assume formal responsibility for continuing to support the Dept." at the same level thereafter. Yet Gregg had to tell Hanes "that this could not come up for consideration during 1939 but that we would consider some such proposal sympathetically for 1940." Gregg also reflected in his diary, "Character of man they could secure would be important. . . . I should say that a definite and well established dept. of psychiatry with beds in the gen. hosp. is a very substantial improvement, immediate as well as cumulative, in contrast to the youngster under Hanes as a polyp in the dept. of med."[52]

The events that followed demonstrate the extent to which DUMC's psychiatry project, and as well as the development of psychiatry in North Carolina, shaped and were shaped by the goals of Alan Gregg's psychiatry program at the Rockefeller Foundation. By the time the state legislature met in 1939, Governor Clyde Hoey had acted on Gregg's earlier recommendations to reform the Division of Mental Hygiene within the State Board of Charities and Public Welfare. The new position of assistant director of the division was filled in June 1939, and in 1940, after close cooperation with the National Committee for Mental Hygiene, North Carolina went out of state—as Gregg had recommended earlier—to hire a psychiatrist as director.[53]

The Rockefeller Foundation handled DUMC's project with the care and collaboration it required. Securing beds in Duke Hospital had been easy enough, and Hanes appeared reconciled to the creation of a separate department of psychiatry. He even asked the foundation to "keep on the look-out for a Professor of Psychiatry for us and tell us his name when you find him." But finding the right person was as tricky as it was important. Hanes's ideas had to be considered, as did DUMC's needs and its plans for Highland Hospital, the hospital it was given in Asheville. As Hanes put it, "We are very anxious to get a good, common-sense administrator as well as a psychiatrist who has his feet planted on the ground. Eventually, if our present plans carry through we are going to have a very big psychiatric set-up here and in Asheville, and it will take a man of good administrative ability to organize properly such a program."[54] [Figure 3.4]

Hanes wanted that man to be a neurologist with training in psychiatry—someone who would complement the work of his former student, Dr. Robert W. Graves, now a professor of neurology at Duke, and Dr. Barnes Woodhall, a neurosurgeon who had recently come to Duke from Johns Hopkins. Early in 1939 DUMC sent Graves and Woodhall to Montreal, the center of Rockefeller psychiatry in Canada, where they became familiar with what Hanes called "the new brain wave instrument, which we have purchased"—the electroencephalograph. Adding the machine at Duke was just one example of how Hanes was "very anxious to help Graves and Woodhall in every way I can. I sincerely believe they are going to establish one of the foremost neurologic set-ups in the country," he wrote to Lambert. "There is nothing in the south of the nature of the organization which they are attempting, combining as it does excellent clinical material in abundance, neuro-pathologic technique . . . and an excellently equipped neurological examining room."[55]

No neurologists, however, were on the list of candidates suggested by Gregg and Lambert at the Rockefeller Foundation. Instead, they preferred a trained psychiatrist with an interest in biochemistry or neurophysiology. One of the foundation's top choices was Wendell S. Muncie, whom Lam-

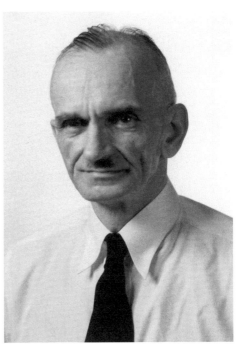

3.5 Dr. Richard S. Lyman. *Duke University Medical Center Archives.*

bert described as Adolf Meyer's "right-hand man in the teaching and administration of the Phipps Clinic" at Johns Hopkins. "At one time it was thought by some that Muncie would succeed Meyer but that now appears improbable," Lambert explained.[56]

Muncie was also the candidate preferred by Dr. Robert S. Carroll, founder of the Highland Hospital in Asheville. Carroll had established the hospital in 1904, and by the time he donated it to Duke in 1938, it was one of the leading centers of therapeutic psychiatry in America. Its most famous patient was Zelda Sayre Fitzgerald, wife of novelist F. Scott Fitzgerald. Fitzgerald had entered Carroll's care in 1936, after earlier treatments by Meyer and others had failed, and she would come and go at Highland until her tragic death there in a fire in 1948. Carroll accepted much of what Adolf Meyer taught about psychiatry and psychosomatic medicine, and Meyer considered Carroll "an excellent practical diagnostician and easily the best pragmatist in psychiatry in America."[57] Occupational therapy, especially being occupied outdoors, was Carroll's guiding principle. Work, eating right, exercise, and avoiding tobacco and alcohol—these ingredients, combined with religious faith and spirituality, were the keys, Carroll believed, to handling most nervous disorders. "The physical, mental and moral are intricately related even as the primary colors in the rainbow," he wrote in *Our Nervous Friends*. "Our nerves enter intimately into every feeling, thought, act of life, into every function of our bodies, into every aspiration of our souls. They determine our digestion and our destinies; they may even influence the destinies of others. . . . Can we ignore the omnipotence of the spiritual?"[58]

Carroll received Meyer's recommendation of Muncie for the Duke position in February 1939, just as Dr. Richard S. Lyman became Meyer's heir apparent at Johns Hopkins.[59] Lyman had just returned from China, where, since 1932, he had been a professor of neurology and psychiatry at the Rockefeller-supported Peking Union Medical College. Lyman had always had the drive and support to pursue his interests: he went from Yale and MIT to an American Red Cross camp in Serbia; he piloted airplanes in World War I and took an M.D. from Hopkins; served under Meyer as an associate in psychiatry and did postgraduate work at the National Hospital, in Queen Square, London; worked with Ivan Pavlov in Leningrad and became the first associate professor of medicine at the new, Rockefeller-funded medical school at the University of Rochester; served on the faculties of First National Medical School in Shanghai and Peking Union Medical College; and made films of his Chinese patients and used those films for teaching, diagnosis, and treatment evaluations. It was Lyman, not Muncie, that Meyer wanted to succeed him at Johns Hopkins.[60] [Figure 3.5]

Yet Alan Gregg also wanted Lyman at Duke, and in March he put Lyman's name at the top of the list in a discussion with Hanes. It was probable, Gregg wrote in his Rockefeller diary, "that Duke will be ready in 1940 for active work in psychiatry—they have taken on Asheville Hosp. for mental diseases . . . —23 beds will be provided for in the Duke Hosp. addition plus OPD [outpatient department] quarters. With the requirements at Asheville they might need as many as ten men—following discussed in about this order of precedence: Lyman, Gildea, Cameron at Albany, Finesinger, Muncie, Billings, Barrera, Watters, Rennie."[61]

Duke waited until the final centennial celebration in the spring of 1939 to announce Carroll's gift of Highland Hospital. It was a rewarding moment for the 70-year-old psychiatrist; having dedicated his life to the profession, he was now facilitating its expansion through the collaboration of Duke, Highland, and the Rockefeller Foundation. The occasion also seemed right for Carroll to promote his choice for the chair of psychiatry at Duke. "I spent an evening with Dr. Davison at Duke," he wrote to Muncie. "Three men are on the list for consideration. You are definitely Dr. Davison's choice, and in the course of time you will be asked to visit Duke."[62]

Muncie was indeed among the final three candidates for the position at Duke, but the medical school's selection committee interviewed only Lyman and Edwin Gildea, an associate professor of psychiatry at Yale. As Hanes explained the committee's deliberations to the Rockefeller Foundation, Duke could not facilitate Gildea's research interests in biochemistry. As for Lyman, Hanes found "his personal appearance a little disconcerting but on further acquaintance one realizes that he has an attractive personality and a keen mind." Several of the Duke men also knew Lyman from their days together at Hopkins, Hanes wrote, and "all like him very much." Hanes himself especially liked the fact that Lyman's "interests lie in the field of neuro-physiology and, in a way, duplicate somewhat the interests of Graves and Woodhall. He is very keen about the electro-encephalograph and seems to have done quite a little work with it." Lyman also told the search committee that he wanted the position at Duke.[63]

Hanes recommended Lyman to the Rockefeller Foundation as "the best man for the place," and the foundation agreed, giving Hanes the "go ahead with Lyman. As far as we can see there is no better available man for your job," Lambert wrote. This clinched the deal for Duke. "We decided unanimously to ask Lyman to take the tentative offer of professor of psychiatry," Hanes notified the foundation at the end of June. "He has been made thoroughly to understand that this position will depend entirely upon the carrying out of the plans we have made. I shall say no more myself in regard to the Rockefeller participation in these plans, since I feel now that it is a matter for the Dean entirely."[64]

What happened next is not exactly clear, but Carroll apparently offered to retain Muncie anyway, to head up a "Clinical Department" of psychiatry at Highland.[65] Carroll's plan called for Lyman to head the new department at Duke, where he would be responsible for research and theoretical work.[66] The arrangements seemed solid until Muncie declined the position in October. His reasons for doing so were both practical and prophetic: two men in charge was one too many, and the one in charge would face two sites separated not only by distance but by functions and allegiances that should be integrated.

At the same time, the Rockefeller Foundation heard from Lyman, who asked about future funding for psychiatry at Duke. "As the place grows more will be needed. Where will it come from?" he asked. Lyman wasn't hinting for future support from the foundation, Lambert explained; he was just wondering how Duke would do it. And the Rockefeller officer told him how: "I say the best evidence that Duke will take care of itself is found in the record of what the institution has done in its first ten years. The medical school finances have been admirably handled by Davison. I know of no other institution that has gone through the depression so well. Furthermore I point to the possibility of money coming to Duke from wealthy people in North Carolina, particularly the Hanes family."[67]

On January 19, 1940, the Rockefeller Foundation sent Davison and Hanes a telegram from New York: "Psychiatry grant approved twentyfive thousand yearly for seven years official letter follows in few days." The foundation, in summarizing the grant, noted its potential impact on the South: "Duke will be the first of the southeastern medical schools to establish a strong psychiatric unit with adequate clinical facilities and full-time staff. There is little doubt that the new department at Durham will influence similar developments already contemplated at Vanderbilt, the University of Tennessee, and the Medical College of Virginia, Richmond, and that it will stimulate efforts toward the better teaching of psychiatry at other southern medical schools."[68]

Patient Care and Teaching in the Prewar Years

By the time of DUMC's 10th anniversary in 1940, it had recently added a new psychiatry department, a new PDC building, a new head of the School of Nursing, a new Medical Alumni Association, a new war in Europe, and a new 65th General Hospital for the United States Army. It was time for moving forward and for looking back.

Duke's daily hospital census peaked at 433 inpatients on May 3, 1940—a month before the new building opened—and by its 10th anniversary in July, the hospital had given nearly a million days of care to more than 140,000 different inpatients. Fourteen percent of them came from within a 20-mile radius of the hospital; the rest journeyed from North Carolina's other 99 counties and 36 other states, and traveled an average distance of 70 miles.[69] By the end of 1940, 44,171 operations had been performed at Duke Hospital and 3,662 newborns delivered. The patients included both rich and poor and black and white, and they came because they wanted care or had no other choice.

The high number of charity cases caused concern and action. Duke Hospital "is more or less a dumping ground for the neglected and misfortunate patients in a large surrounding territory," one North Carolina physician wrote.[70] Many poor pregnant women also arrived at the hospital hoping for general assistance. As one medical social worker noted, "Many were still under the false impression that Duke Hospital served as a maternity home and child placing agency; and by coming here all responsibility for their problems would be assumed. When they discover that this is not the case many difficulties must be faced."[71]

From a charity rate that topped 90 percent in the early 1930s, Duke worked with its patients and county governments throughout the state to reduce the hospital's charity load. County welfare departments began paying part of the hospital costs, as did patients themselves and their support networks of churches, friends, and lodges. In 1940 Davison reported "seventy-two per cent of the patients still pay less than cost, but by having them contribute in accordance with their means, Duke Hospital, with the same amount of money, now is helping 13,000 patients to be treated annually instead of giving complete charity care to 4,000." The hospital had also adopted an inclusive or flat-rate plan in 1933, which was based upon a patient's ability to pay rather than on the actual costs. By replacing the usual room rate and other expenses with one single charge, the hospital "made it possible to estimate in advance the probable cost of hospitalization and to adjust the bill to the patient's resources. . . . The patient has been greatly benefited," Davison explained, "for there is no test or procedure needful to his medical care which is not given him."[72]

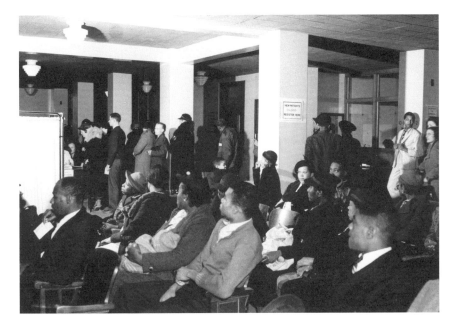

3.6 The "colored" registration area of Duke Hospital. 1940s. *Duke University Medical Center Archives.*

QUALITY OF CARE

Among the hospital's many satisfied patients were mill workers, politicians, and African Americans. Word of one grateful patient came from the president of a cotton mill in Roxboro, North Carolina. "Just a little story of human interest which pleased me very much indeed," the executive wrote to Duke's President Few, "and I believe will give you a few moments of pleasure. One of our employees had occasion to go to Duke Hospital and he has just returned. His appreciation of what was done for him at the hospital was very real, and one of the remarks that he made was 'They treated me just as nice as if I had been a millionaire.' I was very much pleased, and I am sure you will be too."[73]

North Carolina senator Josiah W. Bailey also felt grateful after his stay in Duke Hospital. "I have just returned from Duke Hospital where I received indescribable benefit," he wrote in the summer of 1938. "I very greatly enjoyed the stay in the hospital. When I got there, I was much worse off than I suspected, but after two weeks of rest and treatment, they tell me I am all right, but I must continue to rest for several weeks. . . . The hospital is a most unusual institution and it seems to me that it is conducted perfectly. I had really a good time there every moment. I like the doctors and the nurses and everybody else. I am very grateful that we have such an institution and am deeply attached to it. I shall be returning every six months and intend to do whatever they tell me to do."[74]

It's not clear how Jessie Perry felt about her stay in Duke Hospital, but her experience there reflected some of the basic realities of race and space at DUMC during its first decade. The 42-year-old African American woman arrived at Duke's outpatient clinic in January 1939 assisted by May McLelland, a white official at Peace College for women in Raleigh. "They gave her a pretty thorough going over but did not take any x-ray pictures," McLelland wrote to Watson Rankin at The Duke Endowment, "because they found her urine pretty clear but full of sugar. It seems her blood test also indicated a diabetic condition, so the first diagnosis centered around this condition. Knowing that she had been operated upon for a kidney stone condition, I insisted that the pictures be made, but it was then so late in the afternoon that I was advised to take Jessie back home and to bring here back on Tuesday morning, that being the day for the diabetic clinic."[75]

Bad weather and an early arrival on Tuesday enabled Perry and McLelland to be "among the first" to be seen in the diabetic clinic. "I think that it was fortunate for Jessie that she had a spell of kidney colic when we brought her in, and Dr. Stevens fell right to work to give her some relief, then to have the x-ray pictures made. When he found that she had kidney stones in addition to the other trouble, he made every effort to find a place for her in the hospital, and although it was three o'clock this afternoon before they could put her to bed, we were so thankful that they could find a place for her at all." Perry was expected to be in the hospital for at least a month. "We have raised enough money from gifts from our faculty and students to keep her there for thirty days," McLelland explained. "If Jessie gets well it will be due to the treatment that she will receive at Duke." For McLelland, the experience was an eye-opener. "The nurse in charge of the diabetic clinic told me that they have only fifty beds for colored people and that they need twice that number. She praised them as patients. Said they were so grateful and appreciative and always made good patients. I was most grateful for the consideration with which we were treated, and so I am all for adding the fifty beds. I hope that somehow it may be done." [Figure 3.6]

The physician who treated Perry was Dr. Joseph B. Stevens, a native of Greensboro, North Carolina. His career illustrates the scope and effectiveness of Duke's medical school. After graduating from Davidson College, Stevens had entered Duke's medical school in 1932 and had graduated in 1935 on the school's optional year-round, accelerated program. He had then interned at Duke and was in his residency there when he treated Perry as part of his instruction and experience. By the time Duke's Medical Alumni Association was formed in 1940, Stevens was one of the 374 graduates of the Duke University School of Medicine and one of 696 students (27 of them women) who had been accepted there during the decade—from 6,986 applicants. Stevens was also among the 25 percent of those selected who came from North Carolina; one of the 209 graduates who were still interns and residents at the time; and one of the 312 interns and residents who had spent between one and seven years at Duke Hospital. Eventually, Stevens served as an instructor in medicine before returning to Greensboro in 1946. In 1950, he became president of the Duke Medical Alumni Association.[76]

THE TEACHING OF MEDICINE

Duke's medical school offered a traditional four-year curriculum in addition to the more popular accelerated program that Stevens pursued. The four-year students spent their first two years in preclinical courses—anatomy, physiology, biochemistry, pathology, and microbiology—where they were taught basic science and laboratory work by faculty who also did laboratory research but did not see patients. Students then spent their last two years of medical school seeing patients in clinical courses—medicine, surgery, obstetrics, and pediatrics—where they were taught by faculty who also had privileges to practice in the PDC. By 1940, the Duke University School of Medicine included over 230 staff members involved in teaching, research, and patient care: 10 professors; 131 associate and assistant professors, associates, instructors, and assistants; 10 residents; 37 assistant residents; and 48 interns.[77]

The leading figures on the preclinical faculty were the founding heads of their respective departments, Dr. Wiley D. Forbus in Pathology and Dr. William A. Perlzweig ("Perly") in Biochemistry. Students from the graduating class of 1938 remembered that Forbus was "in the process of writing his book, *Reaction to Injury*, and continually lectured to us on this interpretation of pathology." Students considered Perlzweig's biochemistry course their most difficult, both for the subject matter and because Perly, a Russian native, spoke with "quite an accent." Davison was the most revered member of the clinical faculty and, indeed, of the entire medical center—with his tie askew, his collar unbuttoned, and his pipe alight, he offered a sense of humor and personal warmth unmatched among the other faculty. Hart and Hanes were considered very formal by comparison, but were memorable teachers nonetheless. One student recalled that Hanes "always wrote aphorisms on the blackboard at the start of each of his lectures; many of these were quotations from Hippocrates and other famous physicians or philosophers of the past." Another student remembered Hanes's saying, "'Blood means cancer until proven otherwise' exactly 5000 times during my career at Duke but it is still true."[78]

Most of Duke's students felt a "family-like" closeness during their years at the medical center. Rather than being greeted with the old medical axiom

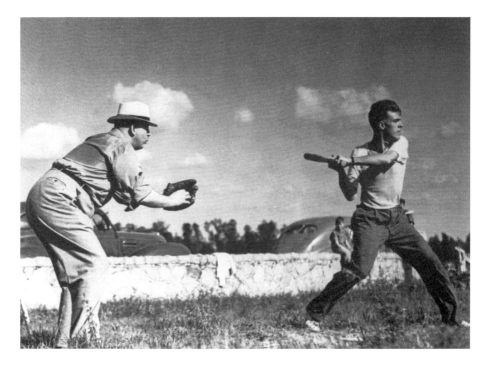

3.7 An annual hospital picnic, with Stan Lordeaux (M.D., Duke, 1940) at bat and Dr. F. Bayard Carter (chair of the Department of Obstetrics and Gynecology 1931–64) catching. *Duke University Medical Center Archives.*

that one of every three of them would fail, they were told from the start, one student reported, that they had been accepted as students because the school had faith in their ability to succeed. "This attitude amongst the faculty never changed and assured us that no matter what the difference in levels of intelligence, all of us had a chance to become physicians if we were diligent."[79] They also missed Duke after leaving it. At least that's what Hanes heard from one physician who was "permitted by the Rockefeller people to visit several clinics on his way down here. At all of the places he went he found some of our men serving as house officers and he says that in every way these men spoke with longing of their life at Duke Hospital. Their judgment is probably not too good," Hanes wrote, referring to their lack of experience, "but they insist they have seen nothing anywhere which is as good as they had here. I think we have a good spirit at this place based on an earnest desire to do well and a respect for the feelings and happiness of the men. I must say I think a great deal of our good feeling, as well as the feeling of those who left the house staff, is due to Mrs. Martin's culinary efforts. A satisfied stomach is very apt to produce a satisfied man. However, I hope their feelings are not based entirely upon this point!"[80] [Figure 3.7]

Among the nursing staff, however, and between the nurses and the men running Duke Medicine, feelings were not so "family-like" by 1940. Part of the problem was simply a long, disruptive transition in the original leadership at Duke's School of Nursing; it took more than a year to fill the position vacated by the school's first dean, Bessie Baker, who resigned in July of 1938 because of ill health. Yet it was also the nature of the transition, as well as the questions involved, that proved so disruptive. As Lambert noted in May of 1939, after a visit to Duke, Davison asked the Rockefeller Foundation for advice on a replacement for Baker. "Local feeling is against too academic a person and strongly in favor of some one who will emphasize the practical side," Lambert wrote. "In other words, a product of the Yale School is not wanted. . . . Miss Titus at Vanderbilt tried to make trouble at Duke by urging Miss Baker to insist on complete autonomy for the Nursing School. D[avison] thinks this would be impracticable and thoroughly inadvisable. . . . D. thinks the weakness in U.S. nursing education at the present time is on the practical side."[81]

Baker's successor, Margaret I. Pinkerton, was finally appointed on October 1, 1939. As dean of the School of Nursing, she served together with Davison and the hospital superintendent on a committee that handled the hospital's affairs. She also supervised two head nursing instructors (one for "theoretical" work and the other for "practical" work) and 12 instructors. Ultimately, moreover, she helped coordinate the school's 125 nursing students with the 130 graduate nurses and 12 ward supervisors who worked in Duke's 450-bed hospital. But what consumed Pinkerton's attention at Duke was a wider trend in which the "increasingly professional image of the nurse was leading, by the end of the decade, to a redefinition of nursing education that emphasized technical and professional competence more than training through primarily bedside apprenticeship."[82]

Duke's School of Nursing offered a three-year program leading to a "diploma of graduate nurse" or, with 60 additional hours of college work, a bachelor of science in nursing degree. Most of the school's first students were high school graduates with no college experience, but as the decade went on, more and more students arrived with some college preparation. By 1940, 20 percent of the school's graduates had earned the B.S.N. degree and the school's entrance requirements included at least one year of college. It was announced early in 1940, in fact, that beginning in 1941 completion of two years of college work would be required for entrance.[83]

In November of 1940, however, Duke reverted to the old definition of nursing education and abolished the B.S.N. option. It also withdrew from the Association of Collegiate Schools of Nursing. Duke's nursing school became

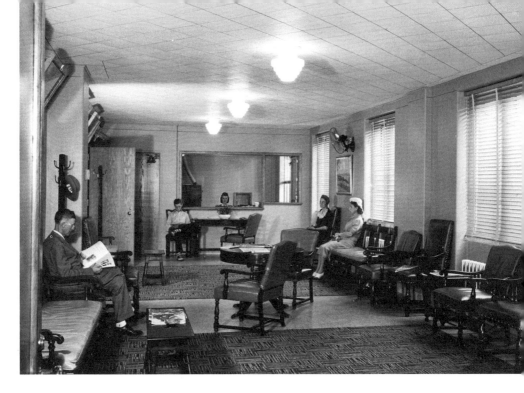

3.8 The waiting room of the 1940 addition to the Private Diagnostic Clinic. *Duke University Medical Center Archives.*

a hospital program within the School of Medicine, and nurses received their training directly from the departments in which they trained and from the small nursing faculty. Certainly, Davison pushed for the change; as noted above, he opposed, in principle, the swing of the "pendulum" away from practical nursing. The decision also reflected the strength and persistence of traditional gender roles in the medical profession; men, not women, were the profession's professionals. That was the way that many of Duke's physicians, apparently, wanted to keep it. "Most of the doctors had come from Hopkins," a former Duke nurse recalled, "and Hopkins doctors are pretty 'macho,' I guess is the present word for it. I like men and I like to be liked by men, but it was all pretty difficult because doctors did not want nurses to get a better education." Closely connected to these gender issues, moreover, were questions of economics. Nursing was the largest expense in the hospital's budget, and it cost more to hire degreed nurses than those holding only a diploma.[84] [Figure 3.8]

Yet the best explanation for Duke's decision to abolish the B.S.N. option is one that also accounts for timing. The decision coincided with the opening of the new PDC hospital wing and with Fred Hanes's plans for a new nurses' home. When the PDC wing opened on June 30, 1940, its 113 private and semi-private beds needed nurses, but since funds were not available to hire them, the hospital turned to students. Also at issue were the beds promised for the new Department of Neuropsychiatry; rather than locate them in the new building, as originally planned, they were placed, along with an 18-bed surgical nursery, in the former house staff dormitory on the third floor of the original hospital. The new psychiatric space became the Meyer Ward, in honor of Adolf Meyer, and the surgical nursery was named Matas Ward, after Rudolph Matas. As for the displaced house staff, some 75 in number, they found lodging where they could: in the hospital, in the basement of the nurses' home (Baker House), in dormitories and temporary cabins on campus, and in "cottages" nearby.[85]

Hanes offered to donate a new nurses' home in the days after the new wing opened. The existing facility, Baker House, provided housing for both student and graduate nurses, and though once separated from the original hospital, it now virtually embraced the new addition. Hanes wanted to use Baker House for the displaced, mostly male house staff, and in September 1940, he received word from Duke's president, Dr. William P. Few, that the university's Executive Committee had "voted to request the preparation of plans for the proposed Nurses Home and an estimate of the costs, these to be presented at the meeting late in November." Few died less than a month later, however, and Hanes's plans were put on hold.[86]

Changes under Way at the Outbreak of War

T he question of Few's successor was quickly answered. Duke's 70-year-old vice president, Robert L. Flowers, was made acting president in October, and early in 1941, he was elected as Duke University's second president. Other questions, however, could only be answered with time: How would the nursing staff adapt to the changes? Would the new wing deepen the hospital deficit and thus require even more money from the university's endowment? Would the clinical faculty become preoccupied with private patients in the new PDC and thus have less time, as some believed, for teaching and research? How would the new Department of Neuropsychiatry be coordinated with Highland Hospital and with Hanes's plans for neurology? And what about the war? The 65th General Hospital, a group of physicians at Duke, had already been recognized by the United States military, but would it be needed? If the United States entered the war what impact would it have on DUMC?

Many of these questions were on the minds of those who gathered at DUMC on November 29, 1940, for the dedication of the Department of Neuropsychiatry. The head of the new department, Dr. Richard S. Lyman, was especially preoccupied with questions of patriotism and professional obligation. Lyman had started at Duke in September, and early in November, he had requested a six-month leave of absence beginning in January. The army had asked him to join a group of physicians at the Aeromedical Laboratory at Wright Field in Dayton, Ohio. As he summed up his decision to Alan Gregg, "In the face of overwhelming needs for spontaneous willingness to 'lay to' and strengthen our position in this country, I feel that circumstances have made me unusually suited for one rôle (a physiologically-minded neuropsychiatrist interested in investigation and possessor of some past experience as a pilot) and so there is, to my mind, no choice."[87] Gregg had not been pleased, reminding Lyman that the Rockefeller Foundation's contribution to Duke had been "based upon the assumption that leadership in the new development in psychiatry would be prompt and close and that you would be in immediate charge of the undertaking."[88]

Lyman also managed to offend Dr. Adolf Meyer, the principal speaker at the dedication. As Hanes later explained to Gregg, Meyer "told Lyman that it was his intention to retire at the end of this year and asked Lyman if he would accept the professorship at Hopkins if it were offered to him. Lyman told him quite frankly that he would not, since he considered the opportunity here better than at Hopkins. This so upset Dr. Meyer that he went back to Baltimore in quite a huff. . . . This was all highly amusing to us here though I hope the rift is not a serious one."[89] [Figure 3.9]

Many of Duke Medicine's modern foundations were in place by the time the United States officially entered World War II. There was the "nostalgic modernism" of the Duke family toward its roots in Durham, and there was the Duke connection to some of the world's largest and most powerful corporations. There was the gargoyled Tudor Gothic of Duke's stone buildings and the study of proteins and viruses. There was a focus on practical medical education and the graduation of well-trained general practitioners. There was corporate-funded research, and there was research funded by philanthropy. There was the charity tradition of subsidized care for the indigent, and there was the for-profit group practice of the Private Diagnostic Clinic. And there was a growing base of medical school alumni. World War II would not eliminate the Duke family's hunger for wholeness in Durham. Nor would it cut the university's ties to corporate America, to the nation's great foundations, and to Duke's medical alumni. What the war did was stimulate unprecedented government support for biomedical research and for research in industries and at universities. The result for Duke Medicine was a struggle over the future direction of the medical center.

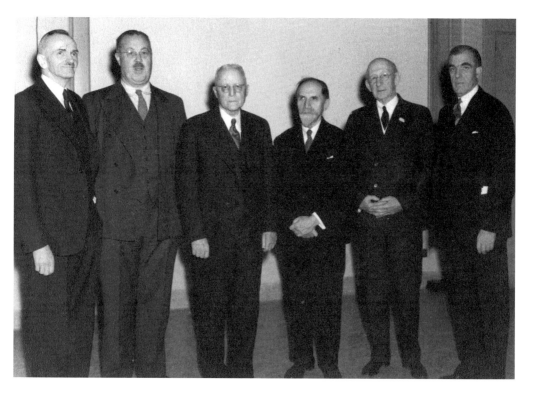

3.9 At the dedication of the Department of Neuropsychiatry, November 1940. Left to right, Drs. Richard S. Lyman, Wilburt C. Davison, Robert L. Flowers, Adolf Meyer, Robert S. Carroll, and Frederic M. Hanes. *Duke University Medical Center Archives.*

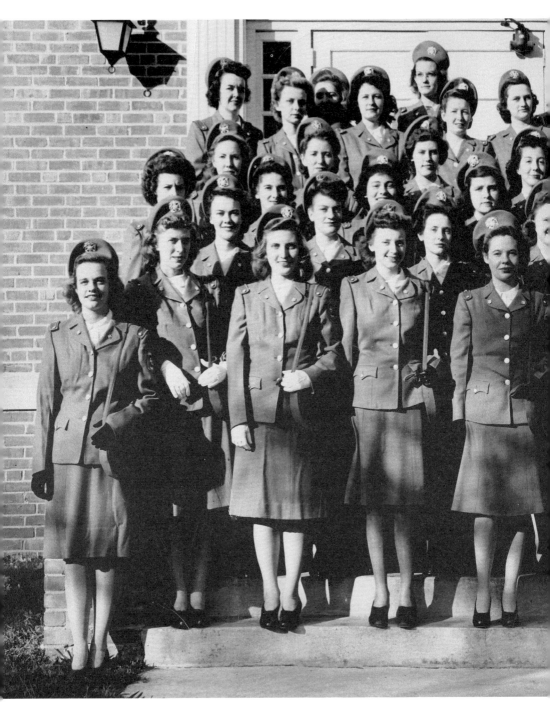

4.1 Cadet nurses on the steps of the Hanes Annex. *Duke University Medical Center Archives.*

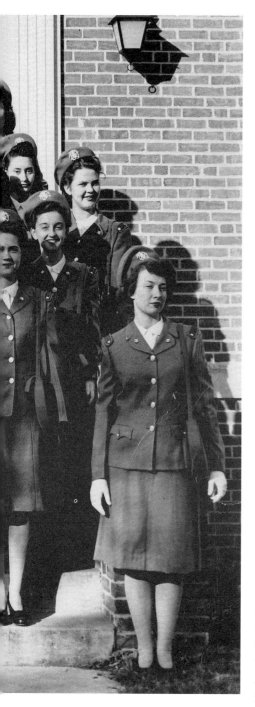

CHAPTER 4:

World War II and Duke Medicine

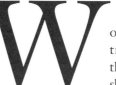orld War II transformed the relationship between money, government, and culture in the United States, and in the process, it not only expanded the foundations of Duke Medicine, through government-sponsored research and programs, it also challenged the charitable and general practitioner traditions developed by The Duke Endowment and Dean Wilburt C. Davison. Along with additional students, patients, research, and funding, the war brought the need for more space at DUMC and a vigorous debate over the purpose and future of the medical center. The war also marked the emergence of the Department of Neuropsychiatry as a catalyst for innovative research and collaboration, as well as for the care and training of returning veterans. What the new department failed to do, however, was sustain Highland Hospital in

the way that Davison and Hanes had planned: as a profitable enterprise capable of funding the department after the Rockefeller grant ran out. Instead, the Veterans Administration played that role, providing federal funds for treating returning veterans and making the Department of Neuropsychiatry one of biggest players in the PDC's private practice.

Serving the Military

D uke Medicine made its first contribution to the war effort after President Franklin D. Roosevelt signed the Selective Training and Service Act in September of 1940. In October DUMC organized the 65th General Hospital, an overseas army medical unit, as the first cohorts of men aged 21 to 36 registered for the draft. Not until July of 1942, however, did the 65th begin training and helping staff the large station hospitals at Fort Bragg in southeastern North Carolina, and only in the fall of 1943 was the 65th finally sent overseas.

Duke Medicine derived much of its pre- and postwar military work from the unique knowledge of its faculty and the medical center's location in close proximity to Fort Bragg and other military installations in North Carolina. By the time President and Mrs. Roosevelt visited Fort Bragg in March 1941, the base was on its way to becoming one of the largest military installations in the United States. From 5,400 troops in August of 1940, the base mushroomed to 67,000 troops in the summer of 1941 and to 160,000 at the height of the war.[1] To monitor the threat of infectious diseases at Fort Bragg, as well as throughout the military services and the public in general, the secretary of war created the Board for Investigation and Control of Influenza and Other Epidemic Diseases in January of 1941. Conceived with the flu pandemic of World War I in mind, the board initially planned a system of 12 commissions, each of which would be composed of active civilian researchers who were familiar with the needs of their specific areas and who would work side by side with their counterparts in the military. The commissions most closely associated with DUMC were the Commission on Epidemiological Survey, the Commission on Tropical Diseases, and two closely related commissions, the Commission on Influenza and the Commission on Acute Respiratory Diseases.[2]

The Commission on Epidemiological Survey created four investigative teams in February of 1941: one at Harvard, another at Stanford, a third at Duke, and the fourth at the Puerto Rico School of Tropical Medicine. Durham became the headquarters of the Fourth Corps Area of the commission, and its team was initially composed entirely of physicians from Duke. The team's director was Dr. David T. Smith, a bacteriologist, and its two professional staff members were Dr. Wiley D. Forbus, chairman of Duke's Pathology Department, and Dr. Daniel F. Milam, an associate in preventive medicine. Other Duke physicians who served as commission consultants to the secretary of war were Dr. Douglas H. Sprunt (influenza); Dr. Robert W. Graves (meningitis); Drs. Norman F. Conant and Julian M. Ruffin (tropical medicine and nutrition); and Dr. J. Lamar Callaway (syphilology and dermatology).[3] Of particular significance (as we shall see) were Dr. Joseph Beard's activities as a consultant for both the Commission on Influenza and the Commission on Acute Respiratory Diseases. Not only was the latter commission headquartered at Fort Bragg; its laboratory was also located in the Station Hospital there, and it received most of its financial support from four private foundations: the Rockefeller Foundation, the W. K. Kellogg Foundation, the Commonwealth Fund, and the John & Mary R. Markle Foundation. Much of DUMC's research during the war was directly related to the work of the commissions dealing with flu, respiratory diseases, tropical diseases, and nutrition, and was funded by a combination of grants from the Rockefeller and Markle Foundations, Lederle, and numerous other philanthropic and corporate interests.[4]

Among the initial concerns at Fort Bragg was the high prevalence of syphilis and other venereal diseases in North Carolina. Over 22,000 new cases of venereal disease were reported to the State Board of Health in 1940, with 36,000 active cases of syphilis under treatment in the state's public health clinics. Among the state's white population the prevalence of syphilis was 40 to 50 per 1,000, while the rate among the African American population was 150 to 180 per 1,000. To the president of the state's Medical Society, Dr. Hubert B. Haywood Jr., these figures boded ill for North Carolinians as well as for the young draftees coming to Fort Bragg. In his president's address to the society in May of 1941, Haywood pointed out that for every 1,000 black draft registrants from Harnett County (adjacent to Fort Bragg), 218 were found to have syphilis. "A problem of national importance is that of protecting men coming from the New England states," Haywood warned, "where the incidence of syphilis is low (80 per 1000) to army camps in a state like ours where the incidence of syphilis is high. The venereal disease rate in any army camp is a reflection of the conditions in the communities surrounding a camp."[5]

Similar concerns were also surfacing in Durham, where, in the summer of 1941, the War Department announced plans to build a large army camp 15 miles north of the city. Established the following February as Camp Butner, the 40,000-acre site was used by the Fourth Services Command of the Army Ground Forces for training and maneuvering combat troops. In addition to gasoline stations, grenade ranges, recreational facilities, and huge munitions storage facilities, Camp Butner eventually included one of the army's largest general and convalescent hospitals, a prisoner-of-war camp, and housing for 35,000 troops. One soldier stationed there later recalled, "The army ran a bus line into Durham. There was always long lines waiting for the buses and sometimes we stand in line for an hour in order to go to Durham. In Durham we went to the theaters, ate in the restaurants, and visited the U. S. O. clubs." In anticipation of their visits, the United States Public Health Service established a 200-bed Rapid Treatment Center for venereal disease in east Durham. Housed in a building formerly used for a National Youth Administration program, the Rapid Treatment Center was designed "to reclaim for the draft pool the large number rejected because of venereal disease and to remove and treat infected prostitutes from the city streets to safeguard the soldiers at the newly built Camp Butner."[6]

By the time the military announced its plans for Camp Butner, the Syphilis Clinic was one of the largest and most important outpatient clinics at Duke Hospital. Much of its activity reflected the high incidence of the disease in Durham, especially among the city's black population. As the head of DUMC's division of social services, Ruth (Elizabeth) Barker, pointed out in July of 1941, "Because of the problems created by syphilis, not only for the individual patient, but also for the community as a whole, we have spent considerable time this year with each new patient in relation to contacts and future treatments and in working out policies with the different local health departments, particularly the Durham County Department of Public Health." Also, Barker continued, "at the annual meeting of the North Carolina Medical Society at Pinehurst in May, Dr. J. L. Callaway, in charge of the Duke Hospital Syphilis Clinic, and the Social Service Department, presented an exhibit on 'The Role of the Medical Social Worker in the Control of Syphilis.'"[7]

DUMC's interest in the research and treatment of venereal disease also stemmed from the national syphilis control campaign of United States surgeon general, Dr. Thomas Parran Jr., and the development at American Cyanamid of a new line of sulfa drugs. Parran, in addition to authoring a well-received book on syphilis, *Shadow on the Land* (1937), had been instrumental in obtaining passage of the National Venereal Disease Control Act of 1938. The act made funds available for rapid treatment centers that employed the new sulfa drugs and, later, penicillin.

The act also gave American Cyanamid another reason to hire W. Harry Feinstone as its director of biological chemotherapy. "In 1939," Feinstone recalled, "I served on a committee of the U. S. Surgeon General to find agents to prevent infections in battle wounds. Most men dying on the battlefield were dying from wound infections. We introduced the use of dressings with sulfa powder and sulfa powder packets, which were included in each soldier's backpack. When injuries occurred on the field, a soldier or his buddy could apply the sulfa powder."[8] Between 1939 and 1944, Feinstone helped Cyanamid develop some of the most widely used sulfa drugs of the period. One was sulfadiazine, which Lederle Laboratories introduced in August 1941. According to the *New York Times*, the drug had been "used experimentally in a number of medical schools and hospitals against pneumonia and streptococcal and staphylococcal infections."[9] Feinstone also worked closely with Dr. Kenneth L. Pickrell, a future chief of Duke's division of plastic surgery, using Cyanamid's methyl cellulose-sulfadiazine films to wrap burns and other surgical wounds.[10] Although Duke experimented with several of Cyanamid's sulfa drugs, it appears not to have participated in the sulfadiazine trials. Among the physicians who subsequently used the drug for research, however, was the head of Duke's Syphilis Clinic, Dr. J. Lamar Callaway, who tested its effectiveness on several different types of venereal infections.[11]

Collaboration on a critical syphilis research problem—the search for a reliable serological test to detect the disease—illustrates one way in which private and public interests were woven together in Duke Medicine during the war. Working under a contract between Duke University and the federal government's Office of Scientific Research and Development, Beard, Callaway, and seven other researchers from three different departments at DUMC compared over 300 syphilitic and biological false-positive sera collected from military and private hospitals as well as from the clinics at Duke and the Rapid Treatment Center in Durham. Their results showed "that the antibodies of truly syphilitic sera, reactive with lipoidal antigen, differ from those of biologic false positive in certain chemical and immunological respects. The possibility of the application of these findings to the development of a practical method of differentiation is being explored."[12]

In addition to specialists in infectious disease, nurses were among the first personnel mobilized at Duke in preparation for the war. In July 1941, at the suggestion of the United States Public Health Service, Duke's School of Nursing increased its enrollment. It admitted 84 students for the October term instead of the usual 58. It also instituted an accelerated program, accepting between 54 and 121 students every nine months during the war. While the Public Health Service bore part of the costs of this program, the Kellogg Foundation also granted $4,000 to Duke for loans and scholarships in its School of Nursing.[13] [Figure 4.1]

Implications of the War Effort on Medical Education

Only after the attack on Pearl Harbor did the war begin to affect deeply the course of teaching, research, and patient care at DUMC. As one former medical student recalled, "On a Sunday morning, December 7, 1941, when we were fourth-year medical students, we were shaken by the radio reports of the disaster wrought by the sneak attack on Pearl Harbor. On the following morning, we huddled around a small radio in the Dope Shop [soda fountain] and heard Franklin Roosevelt declare war on Germany and Japan and utter those famous words about a day of infamy. Within one month, every member of our class had signed a commitment to join one or the other of our armed forces in service of our country."[14]

The country needed doctors. It needed them quickly. And it needed to help them finance their education. One major response was the "accelerated" program in medical education; students began attending medical school all year long and were graduated in three years rather than four. To help them pay for their education, private foundations provided grants to medical schools for scholarships and loans, and in 1943 the government subsidized students who entered the expedited medical training offered in the Army Specialized Training and Navy V-12 (S) Programs. Internships were also cut from a year to nine months, the length of residencies was shortened, and quotas were imposed for interns and residents so that nonteaching hospitals could have more interns. Medical schools also introduced new subjects, ranging from tropical medicine and gas warfare to trauma surgery, venereal disease, first aid, shock, and burn therapy. Making all of these measures difficult to implement was the fact the war absented many of those who taught medicine. The faculties left behind were often half their normal size and burdened with workloads even more demanding than the heavy ones they shouldered during peacetime.[15]

DUMC quickly adopted the accelerated program. "Ten days after Pearl Harbor," Davison later wrote, "Duke was the first medical school in this country to make the continuous 'four-quarter schedule' compulsory." The change was not a difficult one for Duke to make; the medical school simply made mandatory its previously optional year-round program. The medical school also increased the size of its entering class from 68 (in 1942) to 77 (in 1943) and admitted two classes of 75 students each in 1944, one in January and the other in October. To help these additional students finance their education, Duke's trustees voted a $6,000 supplement to the university's normal loan fund of $12,000, and the Kellogg Foundation provided a $10,000 grant for loans and scholarships. As for the number of interns and residents at DUMC, the total dropped from 48 interns and 77 residents in 1940 to 35 interns and 35 residents in 1945.[16]

MATERIAL SUPPORT FOR STUDENTS

A major difference between Duke and other medical schools became clear early in 1942 at a meeting in Chicago of the Congress on Medical Education and Licensure. While Davison arrived at the meeting with a loan fund that exceeded the financial needs of his students, most of his colleagues came from medical schools with meager resources and many students who, as a result of accelerated programs and the loss of summer employment, needed loans for their tuition and expenses. Much to Davison's dismay, the meeting voted to ask for $3 million a year in federal loans for students to meet the extra cost of summer study. Davison considered the request extravagant and, according to one report, stood up at the meeting and "suggested that students be charged 6 per cent in interest on any loan made to discourage unnecessary borrowing. He was booed for the suggestion. An ardent Newdealer from the Office of Education in Washington argued not only for no interest but for a discount of 20 percent in repayment—to encourage borrowing!"[17]

DUMC also differed from many other medical schools in the extent to which it participated in the Rockefeller Foundation's various wartime programs for foreign medical students and research fellows. Duke was among the 23 American medical schools (and only 3 in the South) that the foundation asked to take on one or two British medical students each year for their junior and senior clinical rotations. As Alan Gregg explained the program to Davison, "The air raids in London and elsewhere have imposed excessive demands upon all physicians and upon hospitals, whose structures have in several instances been partially destroyed. The conditions for deliberate, thorough, and adequate teaching in medicine are severely deranged. A considerable number of the teachers, furthermore, are called away from teaching to military or special civilian duties, and together with the profession as a whole, are exposed to injury and death in a measure that heightens the importance of adequate training for those who will be their successors." The British students paid for their own Atlantic crossings while the Rockefeller Foundation paid their tuition and living expenses. Duke's first two British students arrived in the fall of 1941, and though Davison offered them free tuition, the foundation paid approximately $1,200 per year in tuition and living expenses for each student. By 1944, Duke had hosted at least eight Rockefeller-sponsored British medical students, including several women.[18]

Beyond the additional funding, the British students brought talent and diversity to Duke and also contributed to the international flavor that characterized the medical center during and after the war. The first three British students were "in the upper third of their class," Davison reported in 1943, and the fourth, having just arrived, was doing "excellent" work. "All four of these students have entered into student activities and have made many friends. In addition to any benefit which they may have derived, they have been a real asset in broadening our medical horizons and in increasing Anglo-American friendship." Davison considered the four students "equal to the best students whom I have known during twenty-five years in American medical schools and three years at Oxford."[19] Another real asset was the wife of British student

Lawrence Liversedge. In the opinion of Dr. Henry I. Kohn, assistant professor of physiology and pharmacology, Mrs. Liversedge was "one of the best technicians at Duke. (She is a lawyer and knew nothing about laboratory work before coming to the U.S.) There is no charity in giving her a job at $75.00 a month. She should have a raise."[20]

DUMC's most diverse contingent of international students included a number of postgraduate fellows from Latin America who were sponsored by the Rockefeller Foundation and the United States government. The first Rockefeller fellows arrived at Duke in the fall of 1940 (one from Peru and one from Colombia) and were followed in larger numbers after the United States entered the war. "As its contribution toward better relations with Latin America," Lambert wrote in April 1942, "Duke is prepared to give board and lodging to any young doctor coming for postgraduate study whom we would sponsor. . . . I gather that dormitory facilities are ample for any reasonable number of South Americans." If the Latin Americans were more exotic than the British medical students, they also required more attention. The most common problem was language. "Foreigners with inadequate English take a lot of time," Davison explained in an interview with Rockefeller, and he offered as an example a doctor "from Mexico sent here under a grant from the Division of Cultural Relations of the State Department to study tropical medicine." The Mexican doctor tied up "half the time of a Puerto Rican resident who acts as his guide and mentor, as well as the attention of other staff members."[21]

The Rockefeller Foundation considered Duke an excellent option for its Latin American fellows, but it never insisted that they go there or that Duke take them. Lambert made DUMC's case, for example, in suggesting Duke as perhaps the best place for a young Mexican physician to train in surgery. "I would say that he should not go to the largest clinic or to the one with the most distinguished chief," Lambert wrote to a Mexican official, "but to a place where he would be reasonably certain to get the personal attention of an able surgeon-teacher and be given the opportunity to learn by practical experience as soon as he is qualified to participate in the work in wards and operating room." Lambert expressed great respect for the chiefs at Columbia Medical Center, Johns Hopkins, and the Mayo Clinic, but he also believed that the Mexican surgeon "might have a better opportunity at Tulane with Dr. E. W. A. Oschner or at Duke under Dr. Deryl Hart. Duke University Hospital (Durham, North Carolina) is outstanding among the hospitals of the South and the University has demonstrated in the past years a hospitality to our neighbors south of the Rio Grande." Lambert even went so far as to write a note to Davison in the margin of a copy of this letter: "Let me know if it is all right to make references to Duke in answering such letters." To which

Davison replied: "All of us here are greatly flattered and shall try to live up to the compliment."[22]

Rockefeller followed the same sort of diplomacy when asking Duke to take on "special" students from Latin America. After describing the "difficulties" of one such student (a young Colombian who had failed his comprehensive examinations at Yale Medical School), Lambert appealed to Davison on the student's behalf. "If there is a possibility of your letting him come to Duke on probation as a special student for one term, please give him a chance to present his case. Of course he will understand, as I shall, if you have to reply with a categorical 'No.'" DUMC answered with a qualified no; while Hanes and Davison wanted to give the student "another trial," they were unable, Davison claimed, "to convince the members of the admission committee, who feel that it would be letting down the bars for the future."[23] Somewhat later, the government of British Honduras asked for special assistance from Rockefeller's International Health Division in arranging laboratory training for a woman recently graduated from the Belize School of Nursing. In this case, there was no question of lower standards. The division contacted Davison at Lambert's suggestion, and Davison replied that DUMC would be "very happy" to accept her into its program in laboratory technique.[24]

The Rockefeller Connection

These cases reflect the Rockefeller Foundation's general approach to Duke Medicine between 1932 and 1956, the years in which the foundation's medical sciences division focused on the promotion of psychiatry and psychosomatic medicine. Through the patient benevolence of Lambert and Gregg, the foundation advised and assisted DUMC in any way it could and demanded in return only that Duke do what it promised to do. Which it always did—and then some. Particularly important to Duke was the fact that the foundation served as the world's largest and most important repository of information on the medical sciences and on the interests, performance, and personalities of physicians throughout the United States and around the world. The foundation proved indispensable, for example, in helping Duke find strong potential candidates for faculty positions, including Fred Hanes's successor, Dr. Eugene Stead, whose interest in and association with psychosomatic medicine was a major reason why Lambert later recommended him for the position. DUMC also shared a similar relationship with its other largest funders, The Duke Endowment and American Cyanamid, and for the most part, everyone concerned got what they wanted. DUMC got money, personnel, and equipment, Cyanamid got a group of talented collaborators, and the

Endowment got satisfaction and positive publicity from a medical center that excelled in patient care, teaching, and research. Put simply, it was as important to the Rockefeller Foundation that Duke's medical center succeed as it was to Bell at Cyanamid and to Allen and Bell at The Duke Endowment. And though each of these interests had somewhat different goals in mind, all placed collaboration with Duke Medicine above trying to command and control it.

Yet DUMC's inherited networks were also part of larger networks and systems that were likewise being affected by the war. World War II increased the momentum of two emerging forces at Duke, research and the Private Diagnostic Clinic, and the combination of the two provoked a struggle over expansion and governance within the medical center that eventually spread to the larger university itself. At the heart of these changes were Duke's connections with The Duke Endowment and American Cyanamid; with the largest Rockefeller philanthropies (the General Education Board and the Rockefeller Foundation, including its International Health Division); and with numerous federal agencies, including the National Research Council, the Office of Scientific Research and Development, the Office of the Coordinator of Inter-American Affairs, and the army commissions mentioned above.

THE GENERAL EDUCATION BOARD

As noted in earlier chapters, Duke's relationship with the Rockefeller General Education Board began early in the 20th century (with Trinity College, the university's predecessor) and included funding that had enabled DUMC to open as a four-year medical school in 1930. And yet, from the time of Duke's creation in 1924, the board had perceived several major "defects" in the university's relationship with The Duke Endowment. Put simply, the board worried about who would rule at Duke, in what ways, and for what purposes. As one board official noted in 1929, in discussing the proposed medical school grant:

(1) The Trustees of the Endowment Trust might at any time cut off the funds of the University, if the work of the University did not meet with their approval.

(2) Having this power, the Trustees would be strongly tempted to interfere with the freedom of the University, particularly in the field of Social Science.

(3) The Trustees of the Endowment Trust are not persons who understand clearly or sympathize deeply with the work of the University.

Overriding these supposed defects, however, and carrying the day for the 1930 medical school grant, was the General Education Board's desire to provide leverage to the men then leading Duke—"President Few, Mr. Flowers, Dean Davison"—in dealing with the potentially unsympathetic trustees at the Endowment. "A gift from the General Education Board would undoubtedly be interpreted as a recognition of confidence in their administration and would strengthen their hands."[25]

The 1930 grant to Duke had marked a turning point in the grant-making policies of both the General Education Board and the Rockefeller Foundation. Until that time the board, in addition to its focus on education in the South, and especially black education, had made multimillion-dollar grants to endow the creation of medical schools at a number of private universities throughout the United States. A major aim of these endowments, as formulated by the board's Dr. Abraham Flexner, was to eliminate moneymaking from academic medicine. Under the Flexner plan, medical school faculty were expected to eschew all private practice and concentrate instead on teaching and research. By 1930, however, Flexner had been forced to retire from the General Education Board, the Depression was on, the Rockefeller philanthropies faced diminished endowments of their own, and medical schools that lacked major endowments found it increasingly difficult not only to operate but also to attract and keep faculty without some sort of private practice. It was at this point, when the board had ceased making major endowments to medical schools, that the PDC was created at Duke and the board started coordinating its activities in medical education with the Rockefeller Foundation, which was reorganized simultaneously into five major divisions—Gregg's division of Medical Sciences being one of the most prominent. From that point on, the foundation practiced on a small scale, and in different ways, what the board had done with lump sum funding for entire medical schools. It made small, one- or two-year grants to individuals for teaching and research and only occasionally, as in the case of psychiatry, did it give larger multiyear grants to institutions.

Thereafter, the General Education Board focused on the social sciences at Duke, especially on projects with a regional emphasis, while the Rockefeller Foundation focused on the medical sciences at DUMC, also with a preference for regionalism. In 1935, for example, Duke had received a major grant from the board as part of a regional library partnership with the University of North Carolina, and late in 1939 the board began aggressively funding non-medical research projects at Duke: studies of industrial problems related to the economic development of the South, such as research on the cultivation of Turkish tobacco, forest ecology, and marine biology. The board renewed these grants during the war, and following the conflict, made similar new ones, which it then renewed after Dr. Hollis Edens, an associate director of the board, was elected Duke University's third president in 1948.[26]

*   *   *

Within months of the board's 1939 gift, the Rockefeller Foundation funded the centerpiece of its southern strategy in psychiatry—DUMC's Department of Neuropsychiatry—and made a three-year grant to Dr. Hertha Sponer, a German émigré in Duke's Department of Physics, for "researches in spectroscopy and applications to problems in experimental biology and medicine." Like the General Education Board, the foundation also made large grants to Duke for nonmedical research, specifically in the field of Latin American studies and economics.

Research, Researchers, and Their Funders

Underlying the nonmedical research at Duke was the collaboration of the Rockefeller Foundation and allied philanthropies with government agencies, especially the Office of Coordinator of Inter-American Affairs. Created by Roosevelt in July 1941, the Inter-American Affairs Office and its predecessor, the Office for Coordination of Commercial and Cultural Relations between the American Republics, brought Latin American fellows to DUMC and other American institutions with funding from the United States Public Health Service, the Rockefeller Foundation, and the Commonwealth Fund. More than 200 Latin American health professionals and scientists received fellowships between 1939 and 1943, and more than 250 fellows were appointed annually during the rest of the war and immediately thereafter. The fellowships were part of the Inter-American Affairs Office's mission to work closely with the Department of State to counteract growing Nazi influence in the Western hemisphere by providing "for the development of commercial and cultural relations between the American Republics." Its first director was Nelson Rockefeller.

One of DUMC's closest collaborations with both the federal government and the Rockefeller philanthropies occurred early in the war in the area of tropical diseases. Dean Wilburt Davison was the critical nexus. Davison was made a consultant to the newly formed Institute of Inter-American Affairs (a private corporation formed by Nelson Rockefeller in 1942). He also joined Dr. Lewis H. Weed, his "former chief" at Hopkins, on the National Research Council in Washington. Weed, as chairman of the NRC's Division of Medical Sciences, was a good example of how Davison and DUMC's connections with Johns Hopkins and Hopkins physicians became important contacts for DUMC during the war. Davison became Weed's assistant at the NRC's medical science division. "As Vice-Chairman of the Division during 1942 and 1943," Davison later wrote, "I left Durham every Monday evening and returned Friday or

Saturday morning, working an average of four days a week in Washington and doing my Duke dean's job on Saturdays and Sundays. I concentrated all of my week's teaching, ward rounds, and clinics on Mondays."[27]

Davison's work with Weed put him at the center of the war's emerging webs of military, medical, and industrial interests. In the spring of 1940, Weed, with the concurrence of the surgeons general of the army, navy, and U.S. Public Health Service, had made the National Research Council's Division of Medical Sciences the clearinghouse for creating advisory committees on medical problems related to the armed services. The first such committees—one on chemotherapeutics, the other on transfusions—had been formed that summer. The following June, moreover, with the creation by Roosevelt of the Office of Scientific Research and Development, Weed was appointed vice chairman of its Committee on Medical Research. The committee did not do research, however; it operated entirely by funding external contracts "with universities, hospitals, and other agencies conducting medical research." It also worked closely with the advisory committees of the National Research Council to "sponsor conferences on medical topics, submit reports and recommendations, and allocate research projects to investigators affiliated with various institutions."[28] Significantly, it was the success of the extramural programs of the Committee on Medical Research, and the eventual transfer of several of the committee's contracts to the U.S. Public Health Service, that undergirded the extramural research program adopted by the National Institutes of Health following the war.

TROPICAL DISEASES RESEARCH

Davison worked closely at the National Research Council with the Commission on Tropical Diseases, which focused on malaria, yellow fever, rickettsial diseases, and dysentery. Tropical diseases had long been a major concern of the Rockefeller philanthropies in Latin America, and Robert Lambert was a leading figure in the field. In 1926, for example, after five years with the Rockefeller interests in Brazil and Central America, Lambert had organized and become the first director of Columbia University's School of Tropical Medicine in Puerto Rico. The purpose of the school (which served, like Durham, as the headquarters for one of the four investigative teams of the Commission on Epidemiological Survey during World War II) was "to establish a great Pan American medical centre at Porto Rico for the cooperation between North and South America for the conquest of disease."[29] The Rockefeller connection, in fact, now included the army's Commission on Tropical Diseases. Not only was the commission headquartered at the Rockefeller Foundation in New York; its director was also the director of the foundation's International Health Division, Dr. Wilbur A. Sawyer; its laboratories were the laboratories of the Rockefeller Institutes in New York and Princeton; and its staff was composed almost entirely of scientists associated with those institutes.[30]

Davison's work with tropical diseases brought him into constant contact at the National Research Council with Sawyer and Archie S. Woods, vice president of the John and Mary R. Markle Foundation. "I have your letter of October 5," Sawyer wrote to Davison in 1942. "Mr. Archie S. Woods had talked with me about the plan for including some persons from Latin America among the lecturers giving instruction in your program. . . . Apparently Mr. Woods is very anxious to have this part of the program succeed. I shall make some inquiries before coming to Washington and I hope to have an opportunity to talk with you on October 15."[31]

Four months later, Davison journeyed to the jungles of Panama with Sawyer and Woods. The trip was arranged by the Commission on Tropical Diseases to investigate the "opportunities which might be developed for training medical officers in malaria and tropical disease at Panama and along the Pan-American Highway." According to one commission report, "Definite increases in opportunity, including the establishment of the Army School of Malariology, developed from this mission."[32] The mission also provided Davison with another opportunity. "One of my most interesting assignments during 1943 was trying to improve or rather to introduce the teaching of tropical medicine into the eighty-six medical schools because the danger of malaria, yaws and other diseases was greater than that from the Japanese and Germans. I spent two weeks in Central America, a week in Haiti and several weeks persuading our too few authorities on tropical medicine to give lectures at the medical schools. Harold W. Brown, who taught preventive medicine at Duke and Chapel Hill, gave more lectures on tropical diseases at more medical schools than anyone else."[33]

The government's work on tropical diseases, especially malaria, also affected research at Duke and established an important web of personal and professional relationships for Duke Medicine. Shortly before Davison left for Panama, Weed appointed Fred Hanes chairman of the National Research Council's committee on malarial research. "Dr. Weed has put me on some malarial research committees and I am dropping you a line in regard to one phase of this work," Hanes wrote to Davison. "I presume that the contribution we might make would be in the clinical testing of new drugs." Although DUMC saw too few malarial patients to depend on for such tests, Hanes noted that malaria could be induced in some of the center's syphilis patients—a procedure that was used to treat syphilis at the time. "If we use our general paretics and other types lues," he suggested, "we could have ideal experimental animals and at the same time be using the best therapy [the test drugs]." The central question for Hanes, however, was whether Duke could receive financial support for the hospitalization these tests would require: "I note in Dr. Weed's letter that he speaks of support for research objectives and I thought you might find out pretty exactly how this phase of the matter would work out." Davison politely pointed out to Hanes (who was soon appointed to the Committee on Medical Research of the Office of Scientific Research and Development) that the purpose of the National Research Council was to "see that drugs get tested rather than test them."[34]

Hanes visited the Rockefeller Foundation in New York shortly after Weed appointed him chairman of the council's malaria committee. There he lunched with Lambert and two of the scientists most closely associated with the nation's search for new and better antimalarial agents. One was Dr. George K. Strode, an associate director of Rockefeller's International Health Division, and the other was Dr. James A. Shannon, associate professor of medicine at New York University. Hanes was thoroughly briefed on the national antimalarial efforts that were then under way. Access to quinine, the most effective agent for treating malaria, had been cut off by the Japanese conquest of Southeast Asia, and treating the disease was critical to the expected U.S. invasion of the region, where malaria was endemic. Following the meeting, Hanes visited the International Health Division's malarial research facilities at the Rockefeller Institute and Shannon took him out to Welfare Island, where, under the auspices of both the National Research Council and the Office of Scientific Research and Development, and in the 100-bed New York University Research Service, Shannon was conducting clinical trials with the antimalarial drug Atabrine.

Back at Duke, Hanes asked his research assistant, Dr. Nancy Bowman Wise, if she would be interested in working with Shannon on the Atabrine project. For the previous two years, Wise, an M.D. from Yale, had been supervising research on brucellosis directed by Hanes and funded by the Rockefeller Foundation, the Anna M. Hanes Research Fund, and several private benefactors, including Hanes himself.[35] Hanes considered Wise an effective and exceptional physician: effective for having "done much to clear up a number of questions about the laboratory diagnosis of brucellosis," and exceptional because she was a woman who was dedicated to medicine. By 1943 Hanes had grown disappointed with a group of four or five women he had hired two years earlier in anticipation of losing his male staff members to the draft. The women were now leaving to get married or to take better jobs elsewhere, and, according to Lambert, Hanes considered the department "worse off than he would have been without them. Is more convinced than ever of the economic waste of giving women medical education."[36] With the exception, that is, of Bowman Wise, who was working closely on the brucellosis project with another exceptional young woman, Grace Kerby, a first-year medical student who in 1965 would become head of DUMC's division of rheumatic and genetic disease.

Hanes allowed Kerby to continue the brucellosis research after he "lent" Wise to Shannon for the Atabrine project at Welfare Island. The major result of this important project was the development of an Atabrine therapy that "enormously enhanced the capability of the U.S. military personnel to operate successfully in malaria-infested areas of Southeast Asia." Wise also continued to collaborate with her Atabrine colleagues following the war, and in 1948, shortly before Shannon began his long career at the National Institutes of Health, first as associate director of the National Heart Institute and then as the director of NIH (1955–68), Wise was one of the coauthors listed with him on a series of articles in the *Journal of Clinical Investigation*.[37]

NUTRITION RESEARCH

By the time Wise left for New York in April 1943, the laboratories at DUMC were jammed with people pursuing research projects funded by the federal government, as well as by Markle, the Rockefeller Foundation, other private foundations, Lederle Laboratories, and several different pharmaceutical companies. The most comprehensive program involved coordinated studies in nutrition associated with Dr. David T. Smith's work on pellagra and related vitamin deficiency states. In 1939, for example, DUMC collaborated with the North Carolina State Board of Health and Dr. John A. Ferrell of Rockefeller's International Health Division to organize a study of nutrition among mill workers at Bynum, North Carolina. To facilitate the study, DUMC became the state board's medical nutrition center and also appointed Dr. Daniel F. Milam, a Rockefeller fellow at the International Health Division, as an associate in preventive medicine at Duke. Milam directed the Bynum study; Duke's professor of nutrition, Dr. William J. Dann, did the laboratory work, which was funded by the Markle Foundation. Milam also served with Dr. David T. Smith on the army's Commission for Epidemiological Survey, and worked closely on other community nutrition studies with Dr. William J. Darby, a special fellow in nutrition with Rockefeller's International Health Division. Darby, a former fellow with the National Research Council, moved to Chapel Hill in 1943, where he served as assistant research professor of nutrition at UNC's School of Public Health while working at DUMC as both an instructor in preventive medicine and director of the state medical nutrition center.

The Markle Foundation was the single largest contributor to nutrition research at Duke between 1936 and the creation of its Markle Scholars-in-Medicine program in 1947. During that time, with only a few exceptions, Markle made numerous small grants through Davison, as dean of the School of Medicine, to the chairmen of several of Duke's preclinical departments—Smith (bacteriology), Perlzweig (biochemistry), and Forbus (pathology)—and also to Dann, the professor of nutrition. These grants were occasionally matched or supplemented by additional funds from the National Research Council, the Anna M. Hanes Research Fund, and other sources (including, on one occasion, Durham pharmacist C. T. Council, one of the creators of the "BC powder" headache remedy). Almost all of the projects Markle funded at DUMC dealt with nutrition studies related to the vitamin B complex, particularly nicotinic acid (B3) and riboflavin (B2).

VIROLOGY RESEARCH

In June of 1943, however, Markle made a grant to DUMC that was not directly related to nutrition research. The grant was made in the usual way—through Davison, to the medical school, and for the use of a member of DUMC's preclinical faculty—but it also had several unusual features. It was to be used by Dr. Douglas H. Sprunt, an original member of the army's Commission on Influenza; it required additional funds from Duke University; and the subject of the research was "the effects of amino acids and related compounds on viral resistance." So arcane was the subject, it seems, that when the grant was awarded to Duke, Markle's vice president, Archie S. Woods, wrote to Davison: "We should like to receive semi-annual reports briefly summarizing in words understandable to the layman, the progress of the study during the preceding six months' period."[38]

In addition to the increasing complexity of scientific research, the grant to Sprunt reflected Duke's connection to the wider, wartime collaboration between government and private industry. On a general level this encompassed Duke's relationship with American Cyanamid. Cyanamid and its subsidiaries made and processed some of the most harmful and healing products of the war: explosives, chemical weapons, and rubber additives, as well as albumin, blood plasma, sutures, and drugs. More specifically, the grant to Sprunt was part of a larger research effort connecting Cyanamid's Lederle with both the laboratory of Dr. Joseph W. Beard and the army's Commissions on Influenza and Acute Respiratory Diseases. In June of 1943 the Commission on Influenza was authorized by the surgeon general of the army to use students from specific units of the Army Specialized Training Program as test subjects for a vaccine being developed against the flu. Three months later, vaccine testing became compulsory for all units of the program—including a unit of some 50 to 60 medical students at Duke. The testing marked two years of research in which Lederle Laboratories and several other commercial companies had worked with the commission to develop a safe and effective flu vaccine.[39]

Joe Beard had one of the best virology laboratories in the nation by 1943.

He had an experienced staff, an electron microscope, and several ultracentrifuges and was perhaps the nation's leading authority on the size and shape of proteins and other large molecules. Grants from Lederle had expanded his virus research considerably, and he was also working with the Committee on Medical Research on contracts with the Office of Scientific Research and Development when he was appointed to the Commission on Acute Respiratory Diseases, headquartered at Fort Bragg.

In October 1943 Beard and his Duke colleagues joined Dr. John H. Dingle, head of respiratory diseases at Fort Bragg, and I. William McLean Jr., a fellow in virus research with the National Research Council, in publishing the "Isolation and Characterization of Influenza Virus B (Lee Strain)" in *Science*. The authors, in a note on their funding sources, listed what was in fact the core of supporters for research at DUMC during the war. "This work was aided by the Dorothy Beard Research Fund and by a grant to Duke University from Lederle Laboratories, Inc., Pearl River, N.Y. The investigation was also supported through the Commission on Acute Respiratory Diseases, Board for the Investigation and Control of Influenza and Other Epidemic Diseases in the Army, Preventive Medicine Service, Office of the Surgeon General, U. S. Army, and by grants from the Commonwealth Fund, the W. K. Kellogg Foundation, the John and Mary R. Markle Foundation and the International Health Division of the Rockefeller Foundation to the Board for the Investigation and Control of Influenza and Other Epidemic Diseases for the Commission on Acute Respiratory Diseases."[40]

By November of 1943 the army had developed a "highly but not completely, effective" vaccine for preventing influenza A and it wanted to begin vaccinating as soon as possible all army troops and other military personnel deployed overseas. It was at this point that Lederle made its largest grant yet to Beard, and it did so in a way that was becoming routine but also increasingly disturbing to Davison. It made the grant without consulting the dean, and it also made the grant directly to Duke rather than through him in the name of the medical school. As Lederle's laboratory director informed Davison, "Several days ago, in an informal discussion with Dr. Joseph W. Beard, we learned of his intent to undertake studies dealing with the porcine disease, hog cholera. He particularly emphasized researches to elucidate the fundamental nature of this etiologic agent, or virus, in the hope that the information gained would ultimately result in a better control of the disease." Lederle "intended" that up to 15 percent of the one-year grant "be used for providing of suitable animal and test quarters."[41]

Beard certainly needed the additional space. With a secretary, numerous technicians, and five full-time professionals working on virus research alone—not to mention the associated animals, cages, and laboratory equipment—

there was no room in his fourth-floor laboratory for anything else, much less for hogs. And it was critically important to have the hogs, for his cholera research had the potential for a double pay-off. In addition to the stated goal of the grant—to produce a better vaccine against hog cholera—the project was also designed to test on hogs the flu vaccine being developed for the army. In January 1944, Beard and Dr. Wendell Stanley of Princeton University met with the Commission on Influenza at the Rockefeller offices in New York and suggested that a purer, more stable vaccine could be created through the use of centrifuges. Within days, the commission recommended that the army collaborate with Beard and Stanley to produce a centrifuged vaccine that could then be tested on animals and humans and also be evaluated for the practicality of commercial mass production. Back in North Carolina, Beard built and stocked hog pens on his farm in Hillsborough, northwest of Durham, and began testing on swine the toxicity of the vaccines he was producing at Duke.[42]

Beard and his research team also became parties to an agreement made between Duke University and Lederle on March 6, 1944. Signed by Bell for Lederle and president Robert Flowers for Duke, the agreement gave the university some early and valuable experience with matters still confronting academic medical centers today. In its stipulations regarding corporate access to and control of the research data, as well as its method for distributing any profits that may be derived from the research, the agreement was almost exactly the opposite of the established protocol today. The agreement made Duke responsible for keeping all records associated with the study and for making those records "accessible to [Lederle's] authorized representatives." Duke was likewise obligated to keep Lederle "advised of the activities of the research and the results from time to time accomplished." Lederle was to own "any and all inventions" arising from the research; the Duke inventors (if any) were to apply for patents in the United States and other countries at the request and expense of Lederle; and Lederle would decide what to do with any patents granted. In return for these rights, Lederle agreed to pay Duke 5 percent of the net sales value of the invented products made and sold by the company after Lederle recovered the amount of the original and any subsequent grant. Beard and his wife, Dorothy, signed the agreement along with their colleagues, Drs. D. Gordon Sharp and A. R. Taylor.[43]

RESEARCH INTO KIDNEY DISEASE

Another foundation of Duke Medicine's excellence in research appeared in April 1944 with publication in the *North Carolina Medical Journal* of Dr. Walter Kempner's "Treatment of Kidney Disease and Hypertensive Disease with Rice Diet." Kempner had dedicated the past several years to collecting and

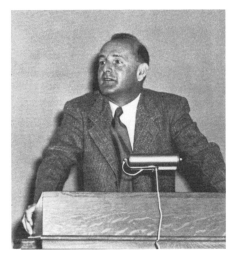

analyzing data on patients suffering with kidney disease, particularly nephritis, and hypertension. Working initially with severely ill patients on the public wards, Kempner, in an effort to ease the workload of their kidneys without compromising nutrition, tried them on a diet of rice, sugar, and fruit. His first major breakthrough had occurred in 1942 when a patient on the rice diet returned for a check-up after two months—rather than the prescribed two weeks. Her blood pressure was reduced, her eye-ground problems (retinal hemorrhaging) were resolved, and her heart had shrunk significantly in size. Kempner wasted no time in placing other patients on an extended rice diet therapy, and by 1943 Hanes was so impressed with the results that he insisted Kempner treat both private and ward patients. By 1944, Kempner had more than 200 case histories documenting success with the rice diet. [Figure 4.2]

But there were problems. Not with Kempner's research; it was impeccable. The trouble was getting people to recognize that. With the exception of Hanes, who was on the editorial board of the *North Carolina Medical Journal*, nobody believed Kempner's results. National journals rejected his articles before the *Journal* published them, and in June 1944, at a meeting of the American Medical Association in Chicago, he was greeted by derisive disbelief during a presentation of his spectacular results. Part of the problem was Kempner himself; he was a haughty Prussian aesthete who had been groomed from birth to be a scientist. He viewed most of his colleagues as dummkopfs, at least where art and research were concerned, and throughout the thirties he had longed to return to Germany. To most American physicians, a German Jew like Kempner—a man who was also a Germanophile at a young southern medical school—was not someone to be accorded immediate acceptance during World War II. And to make matters worse, Dean Wilburt Davison was one of Kempner's greatest skeptics. He disliked Kempner personally, he could not decipher his research, and he worried about Kempner's impact on the medical school and its faculty. By 1944, Kempner was generating more revenue than anyone else at the PDC, and many of the faculty—both clinical and preclinical alike—resented it.[44]

Shifts of Power and Focus

The research success of Beard and Kempner signaled the beginning of the end, in fact, of Davison's rule as dean of the medical school. As the PDC continued to flourish, and as the government eventually surpassed the private sector in funding research at DUMC—largely, at first, through Beard and Kempner's postwar grants from NIH—Davison's personal authority gradually declined. Eventually, he lost control of Duke Medicine's networks, both within the medical center and beyond, and his kingdom dissolved into a series of loosely affiliated fiefdoms, each ruled by an independent department chief. Medicine and Surgery continued as the largest and most powerful departments, and with their chairmen also at the head of the medical and surgical divisions of the PDC, they replaced Davison as the controlling authority at DUMC. Davison remained for years as the face of DUMC, representing it with the university and The Duke Endowment, and his emphasis on creating well-trained general practitioners also continued. But the heads of Medicine and Surgery became the primary power brokers within the institution and controlled many of its external connections with government and the private sector.[45]

By 1943, in fact, the rapid growth of the PDC and the research by Beard and Kempner were transforming Duke Medicine. Personnel shortages provoked some of the change; there were simply not enough faculty, staff, and nurses to cover teaching and private practice. At the same time, the creation of the Army Specialized Training and Navy V-12 (S) Programs brought in more than 100 fast-track medical students to Duke. So great was the need for teachers that several divisions were being taught exclusively by residents—with no backup. "If we are going to teach properly each division should have two men available," Hanes wrote to Davison in November, "otherwise sickness or necessary absence will result in no teaching at all." Medicine already had three divisions being taught by men "classed as Residents," Hanes explained, "which means they can and will be taken away for army service, leaving necessary teaching uncovered. These men should be classed as Instructors and placed on the list of *indispensable teachers*. We have been given a job to do for the *armed services* and we should demand the proper personnel to teach properly."[46]

TEACHING VERSUS PRIVATE PRACTICE

The following day Davison made and conveyed to Hanes several serious complaints against the Department of Medicine. Davison charged the department's senior medical staff with neglecting their duties as teaching consultants at the Outpatient Clinic in order to spend more time with private outpatients at the PDC. The dean also pointed out that the three residents Hanes wanted reclassi-

YEAR	INPATIENTS	OUTPATIENTS	
		PUBLIC	PDC
1940	12,517	98,627	
1941	12,766	104,056	
1942	12,936	86,629	
1943	14,086	84,601	25,600
1944	14,007	79,922	31,191
1945	14,000	78,541	47,500
1946	14,437	83,638	45,000

4.3 Number of inpatients and outpatients at Duke University Medical Center, 1940–46. *Wilburt C. Davison Papers.*

fied as instructors were actually spending more time with private patients than they were teaching, and that DUMC's senior medical students considered the department's teaching in the Outpatient Clinic as "inferior." Furious, Hanes ordered the PDC's business manager to prepare "a written report about this matter." He also asked his department faculty to chart in complete detail their own schedules, as well as those of the senior staff. And finally, Hanes posted a note at the Outpatient Clinic asking the senior medical students to respond anonymously to "rumors" regarding the quality of teaching they were receiving in the Department of Medicine.

The business manager was perplexed by Hanes's order. The PDC, he wrote, did not schedule appointments when its doctors were "assigned to OPC, ward rounds and other teaching duties. We never arrange appointments for those hours as we understand quite clearly that teaching comes first." Likewise, the faculty sent charts and letters to Hanes showing personnel schedules devoted overwhelmingly to teaching and research rather than to private practice. As for the fourth-year medical students, while they described as "good" or even "excellent" the department's teaching at the Outpatient Clinic, they couched their handwritten general comments with the discretion the forum deserved. Most said that they could use more time to work up their patients; that the teaching consultants might ask and answer more questions; and that having an occasional discussion with a specialist would be nice. At the same time, all of the responding students echoed one of Hanes's frequent refrains: the

Outpatient Clinic needed a neurologist. Hanes sent all of the documentation to Davison.[47]

Whether teaching actually suffered at DUMC because of increased attention to private patients is not clear. What is clear is that the number of public outpatient visits declined significantly at DUMC during the war while the number of PDC visits almost doubled. [Figure 4.3] These changes reflected to some extent the rationing realities of the war—the shortages of gas, oil, and tires that severely curtailed automobile travel, especially for the major population sector served by the Outpatient Clinic: the rural poor. After 1941, moreover, Duke Medicine faced competition in Winston-Salem from the combined facilities of the state's second four-year medical school, the Bowman Gray School of Medicine at Wake Forest College, and its adjacent, expanded hospital affiliate, the North Carolina Baptist Hospital. As for what explained the dramatic rise in PDC visits, much of it could be attributed to the prosperous wartime economy: more people had more money to spend on private health care.

If Davison acknowledged these realities and the evidence from Hanes, he was also determined that the PDC adhere to the commitment at the core of its creation: that teaching always take precedence over private practice. To Davison the PDC had been a necessary measure for retaining faculty during the Depression. He rarely (if ever) saw a private patient himself, and he initially staffed his Pediatrics Department with part-time professors who had private practices in Durham—faculty, that is, who did not have PDC privileges. Hanes, for his part, shared Davison's desire to keep private practice in its proper place, but the PDC also meant money for his department and power for him. Although Hanes practiced at the PDC, he was so wealthy that he usually gave his fees to the Department of Medicine and donated his entire salary to the Anna M. Hanes Research Fund. The man for whom the PDC meant the most was its founder, Dr. Deryl Hart, the chairman of the Department of Surgery. Like Hanes and the other clinical chiefs, Hart combined a fixed salary as department head with the power to control the PDC incomes of his faculty by "taxing" private practice fees for use in development, department, and research funds. Unlike Hanes, however, Hart saw private patients almost all day long—mainly in the operating room—and not, it seems, for personal gain (although that was possible). Rather, Hart worked tirelessly to maintain, in the absence of the surgeons who were away at war, the department's revenue from PDC receipts.

EXPANSION VERSUS CONSOLIDATION

By 1944 Davison found himself struggling to control not only the PDC and DUMC's expanding research but also the different plans that he, Hart, and Hanes had for Duke Medicine's future. All three men agreed that DUMC's

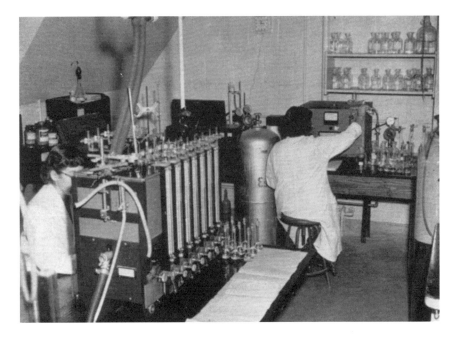

4.4 Technicians at work in the laboratory of Dr. Walter Kempner. *Duke University Medical Center Archives.*

monopoly days were over; in addition to competition from the new medical center at Wake Forest College, the University of North Carolina appeared poised for expansion of its medical program and facilities. A Hospital and Medical Care Commission appointed by the state's governor had recently made the creation of a public four-year medical school and a large associated teaching hospital top concerns, and UNC's supporters were determined to have both established in Chapel Hill.

Yet DUMC's leadership triumvirate did not agree on what these developments meant or whether and how to respond to them. Hart envisioned a competitive future that was best anticipated, he believed, by expanding the hospital with more private beds. With more private beds, Duke could train more surgeons and internists. It could also increase thereby the salaries of existing faculty and staff and have additional funds to recruit exceptional talent for teaching and practicing the "specialization" that would give Duke Medicine a competitive edge in the future. Expanding the hospital, however, was not what Davison and Hanes wanted. Nor did they consider specialization important to Duke Medicine's future. They believed that the size of the hospital should be determined by the needs of the medical school and that the medical school did not need a larger hospital.

The principal purpose of the medical school for Davison (his obsession, in fact) was to train general practitioners, not specialists, and to train them well—something that could not be done if the medical school grew too large or the PDC interfered with teaching. So deep and sustained was the demand for general practitioners, moreover, that competition seemed not to be an issue. North Carolina, the South, the nation—all needed as many well-trained general practitioners as medical schools could produce. Thus, by focusing on general practitioners, DUMC was serving the basic health care needs of the vast majority of Americans while also facilitating the specific regional goal of The Duke Endowment's hospital section: to create small nonprofit, community-owned hospitals equipped with several pieces of essential technology and staffed by well-trained general practitioners.

Hanes sympathized with Davison on the matter of general practitioners, but he also believed that competition was coming and that the best way for Duke to meet it was to establish a reputation for research and scientific training among its medical students, graduates, and staff. He not only opposed Hart's idea for more hospital beds, he also wanted all of the clinics moved out of the existing building and into a new building funded by The Duke Endowment. With the crowded confusion of the clinics thus out of the house, the space they abandoned could be occupied by the medical school for additional teaching and research.

SALARY POLICY AS A MEANS OF CONTROL

In the spring of 1944 Davison decided to do something about what he perceived as the clinical faculty's excessive moneymaking in private practice. After discussing his plan with Hart and Hanes, Davison fixed at $2,500 the basic annual salary the university would pay to all faculty who engaged in private practice. Whatever additional income they received (from either the PDC and salary supplements or both) was between them and their respective department heads. Hanes knew Kempner was one of Davison's main targets, and he also knew how Davison planned to use the money saved on the salary cutbacks. "It has been the constant policy of Dean Davison to have as large a house-staff as could be employed profitably," Hanes wrote to Alan Gregg, "and he tells me that he plans to increase this staff, after the war, by 50 per cent, God and the tax laws permitting." At the same time, Davison knew that Hanes had pledged matching funds from the Department of Medicine for Gregg's new Rockefeller project to aid the "training of young doctors coming home from the war."[48] [Figure 4.4]

The new salary policy affected more faculty in Hanes's department than in any other department at DUMC. Hanes assured Davison he was "not opposed" to the change, only that it be applied "*without any exception* to all men doing private practice" in every clinical department. Hanes likewise considered it

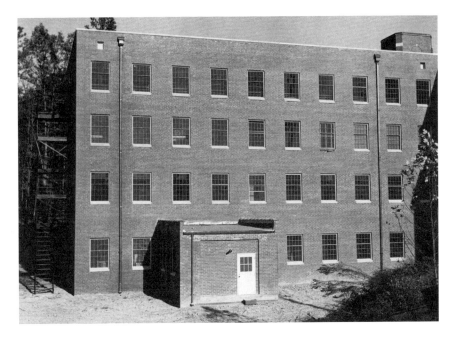

4.5 The Bell Research Building under construction (1945–47). *Duke University Medical Center Archives.*

imperative that each department head have a "competent associate." Whether the departments accomplished this voluntarily or at Davison's insistence didn't matter, Hanes stressed. But it was "doubly important under the present accelerated program, for unless men get relief now and then the quality of teaching will suffer greatly." Finally, Hanes responded to the salary change with an explanation of the PDC that became part of the standard argument for its value to Duke Medicine and Duke University. Hanes wrote to Davison on May 31, 1944: "The Private Diagnostic Clinics have been well run and the Hospital and University have profited greatly from their excellent work. Without private practice our teaching would collapse at once, or else salaries would have to be greatly increased; so I don't think it just to hold it against our teachers that they do private practice. I regret the volume of this practice, but it may well be evidence of work well done. As a matter of fact, medical teaching of high order is obtained by this school at very cheap rates, due solely to the existence of private practice."[49]

BUILDING FOR RESEARCH

The same day that Hanes wrote to Davison about the advantages of private practice at DUMC, The Duke Endowment approved funding for a building Davison had been referring to dismissively as the "dog house." Eventually named for William Brown Bell, Cyanamid's president and an Endowment trustee, the building was not the new clinic facility Hanes was promoting. Nor did it have the hospital beds that Hart considered crucial. And it certainly was not what Davison wanted. It was a building designed specifically for research, and when completed the following year, at a distance of several hundred yards from the main building, the two-story brick construction would make it the first West Campus building without Duke's distinctive Gothic stone architecture. There was, in fact, no hint of "nostalgic modernism" about it. It was a plain, red-brick building. [Figure 4.5]

In calling the building the "dog house," Davison was alluding not only to its small size and distance from the master's mansion, as it were, but also to the fact that Beard would continue teaching there the course in operative surgery using dogs. Yet the building also showed the muscle of the converging forces Davison could not control. On the most basic level, the "dog house" reflected a compromise between the competing research and teaching needs of Beard, Kempner, and other DUMC faculty. Beard received much of the space in the new building, and Kempner and others got laboratory space vacated by Beard on the fourth floor of the Medical School. In addition to Beard's new virus research laboratory, the building provided space for his course in operative surgery, a laboratory for the Department of Surgery, laboratory space for the preclinical departments, and additional new space for research animals.

On a deeper, long-term level, the building portended the powerful intertwining of Duke Medicine's inherited and developed networks with the emerging opportunities for federally funded biomedical and scientific research. Hart later described the building as "the first example of interdepartmental and widespread Medical Center cooperation in obtaining a much needed facility when adequate funds otherwise were not available." The Duke Endowment provided $100,000 for the building, the Dorothy Beard Research Fund put in more than $50,000, the Departments of Medicine and Surgery each contributed $10,000 (from funds generated by the PDC), and the Rockefeller Foundation's International Health Division gave another $10,000. Simultaneously, moreover, with passage of the Public Health Service Act of 1944, the foundation was established for the strong and mutually beneficial relationship between Duke Medicine and the National Institutes of Health.

As a result of the 1944 act, the National Cancer Institute became a division of the (then singular) National Institute of Health, which itself had become part of the Public Health Service in 1943. Among other things, the 1944 law defined the shape of medical research in the postwar era, giving the head of the Public Health Service, the U.S. surgeon general, the power to "make grants in aid to universities, hospitals, laboratories and other public or private institutions, and to individuals." One year later, in September 1945, two-thirds of the wartime grants made by the Committee on Medical Research were transferred to the Public Health Service, and the following year the grants program of the National Cancer Institute was expanded to the entire NIH (which became the plural "Institutes" in 1948). Not only were Beard and Kempner among the earliest recipients of NIH research grants; DUMC also received, between 1948 and 1956, several large NIH construction grants that were combined with PDC funds from the Departments of Medicine and Surgery and with funds from the Dorothy Beard Research Fund to add three additional wings to the Bell Building. The relationship has proved to be a fruitful one for both NIH and Duke Medicine, which continues today as one of the nation's leading recipients of NIH grants.

Davison eventually recognized the importance of the "dog house," and he even supported some of the later NIH construction grants. But the whole thing took some getting used to. As Hanes's successor, Dr. Eugene Stead, later wrote. "Dean Davison was so unsympathetic that for years the approach to Joe's building (named the Bell Building) was by a dirt trail that turned to mud with each rain."[50] With massive federal aid for biomedical research, however, that primitive trail soon grew into a road paved with gold.

THE "SLOW DIFFUSION OF PSYCHIATRY" AT DUKE

The collapse of Duke's Department of Neuropsychiatry in the early 1950s coincided with the resignation of its first chairman, Dr. Richard S. Lyman, with the retirement of Alan Gregg as director of medical sciences at the Rockefeller Foundation, and with the end of Rockefeller funding for the foundation's program in psychiatry. During the preceding years, however, the department had established an admirable record of community outreach. It had treated and trained war veterans, it promoted interdisciplinary studies on campus, and it was one of the major reasons why the Rockefeller Foundation suggested Dr. Eugene A. Stead Jr. as Fred Hanes's successor in the Department of Medicine at Duke. Stead was not only an outstanding teacher, he was also doing groundbreaking work in cardiology, he held the liberal racial views the foundation promoted, and he was a devoted practitioner of "whole-person" medicine.

Richard Lyman had exactly what Alan Gregg favored in the psychiatrists and physicians Rockefeller promoted, especially in the South. He was a racial liberal and community activist who was also a skilled researcher, teacher, and therapist. Although Lyman had expected to postpone his start at Duke because of research related to the war, the army delayed establishing its medical laboratory at Wright Field, and Lyman instead pushed ahead with his plans to ripple psychiatry slowly outward through DUMC, the university, Durham, the state of North Carolina, and the South. He started with a small budget, a small staff, a new hospital ward, an outpatient clinic, and the Highland Hospital in Asheville.

He also started with an unusual arrangement. He was assured by the university's president that he could have consultants on his staff from the Department of Psychology and the Department of Sociology. Lyman later explained his request: "I felt that, particularly in North Carolina where rural problems are frequently met, psychiatry would have to be prepared to understand this life. . . . I expected to work with and to exchange information with those in other fields which have active interest in helping people to live adequately. I wanted an opportunity to teach some one or two psychologists and sociologists what I could find out about our patients, and, in turn, to be taught about these patients and their ways of life by my colleagues."[51]

Within the medical center itself, Lyman relied heavily for teaching on Drs. R. Burke Suitt, Maurice H. Greenhill, and R. Charman Carroll. Both Suitt, 34, and Carroll, 39, were closely connected with Highland Hospital. Suitt had practiced at Highland for five years before moving to Johns Hopkins in 1938, where he served as an assistant in psychiatry until his appointment at Duke in September 1940. Carroll, a native of St. Louis, had been adopted by Highland's founder, Dr. Robert Carroll, while studying nursing at the hospital between 1929 and 1932. After becoming a registered nurse, Carroll had taken her A.B. degree at Duke University and had pursued her medical studies at the University of North Carolina and then at the University of Colorado, where she had received the M.D. in 1939. She spent the following year with Davison, interning in his Department of Pediatrics, before becoming the first resident in Duke's Department of Neuropsychiatry in the fall of 1940. Just how deeply she shared her adoptive father's hopes for Highland are not known, but by 1941 Dr. Robert Carroll was doing everything possible to enlarge the hospital's "work by associating it with a Children's Psychiatric Hospital and the Pediatric and Psychiatric Departments at Duke."[52]

Dr. Maurice H. Greenhill was the one psychiatrist Alan Gregg wanted on Lyman's staff. Greenhill, 32, had just completed several years as a resident and Rockefeller fellow in Boston, where he had worked in the neuropsychiatric clinic of Harvard's Dr. Stanley Cobb, one of the nation's leading practitioners of psychosomatic medicine. Not coincidentally, Gregg had selected Cobb and his group at Massachusetts General in 1933 as the foundation's "showpiece treatment center for mental disorders."[53] The core of that project, a 20-bed inpatient neuropsychiatric service, was still being funded by the foundation in 1940, when Gregg suggested that Lyman consider Greenhill to run the new 15-bed Meyer Ward at Duke Hospital. Greenhill arrived at Duke in January 1941, and by February Lyman was assuring the Rockefeller Foundation that Dr. Greenhill had "filled the bill admirably."[54] [Figure 4.6] Con-

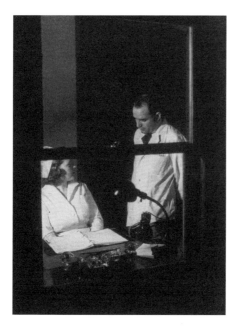

4.6 Dr. Maurice H. Greenhill confers with Miss Schmitt, head nurse in Psychiatry. *Courtesy of the Rockefeller Archive Center.*

veniently, too, Greenhill's wife was a trained medical social worker, as was Lyman's, and the two women worked together in DUMC's division of social services—Mrs. Greenhill "temporarily" and Mrs. Lyman in "volunteer work, assuming responsibility for the social work in the Children's Syphilis Clinic."[55]

Lyman and his staff pursued at Duke the larger Rockefeller goal of overcoming the professional isolation of psychiatry by linking it to medicine through the general hospital and the teaching clinic. This meant educating faculty and staff in addition to teaching medical students. As Lyman wrote to the foundation early in 1941, "Our emphasis is that of a slow diffusion of psychiatry into the other services, working through the out-patient clinic. . . . It is my hope that as time goes on, more and more psychiatry will actually be done by the younger internists themselves."[56]

Adding research and therapy to the department's activities was also important to Lyman but the situation demanded patience and a focus on teaching. The only staff member then engaged in the "experimental aspects" of the field was Dr. Hans Lowenbach, a German-born neurophysiologist who had trained in Europe and at Johns Hopkins. Since coming with Lyman to Duke, Lowenbach had developed work within DUMC and at Dorothea Dix, the state mental hospital in Raleigh, "running a rather busy laboratory . . . in his work with electric shock, the brain waves, vestibular studies, etc."[57] [Figure 4.7] As for therapy, there wasn't much; not only did Greenhill lack nurses, orderlies, and attendants on the 15-bed inpatient ward but Hanes also discouraged psychiatric therapy with outpatients. "In my first interview with Dr. Hanes," Lyman later wrote, "he advised me to hold patients here only for diagnosis and discharge the patients to their local doctors who could then do the treatment. I never undertook to follow his advice."[58] But he really had little choice at first. Lyman and his colleagues had to spend their time "predominantly" on teaching: "1) for undergraduates and junior members of other services in dealing with the more easily-handled psychiatry which comes their way . . . ;

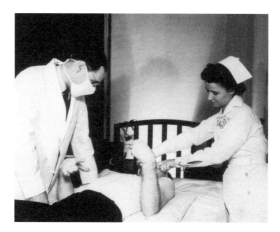

4.7 Dr. Hans Lowenbach observes a patient's reaction to electroshock therapy. *Courtesy of the Rockefeller Archive Center.*

2) for a very few graduates in neuro-psychiatry, working on our unsolved problems in applied physiology and in formulating our approach to the individual in this community."[59]

DEMANDS OF RESEARCH AND STAFFING

The demands of teaching notwith-standing, Lyman's main interest was in research, particularly "the opportunity for studies on the social aspects" of the department's psychiatric work. In March 1941, Lyman visited New York to discuss with both the Rockefeller Foundation and the General Education Board his first proposed research project at Duke. He described the course he was preparing as "an experiment in social distance-closeness in which intelligent negroes take part in dealing with white psychiatric patients."[60]

Under Lyman's plan, "24 carefully selected college students, 12 white and 12 colored, divided equally between the sexes, will be given a six months' intensive course, including lectures in psychology, sociology, etc., and practical work on the wards. Detailed observations will be made of the reactions between patient and student, with particular attention to racial factors. The white students will come from Duke, the Negroes probably from Fisk. (Fisk is chosen over the North Carolina colleges on the ground that the students are more nearly comparable to those at Duke.)" Tuition, housing, meals, transportation, uniforms, and a "substantial stipend for incidentals"—everything would be given to the students free. Lyman needed $5,000 of the estimated $13,000 for the project while Duke would cover the rest.[61]

Lambert considered the whole thing "a costly and futile scheme, which has not been thought through." No college graduate, white or black, was going to aspire to a career as an orderly, he objected, though some needy students would eagerly participate "because of the attractive financial side. Duke students are now being used as attendants at $25 (?) a week. Particularly good recruits are found, Lyman says, among football players in the off season." Lambert spoke for the foundation in turning Lyman down. "There is no chance of the project's being given favorable consideration, and I don't think he will expect any further word from us about it."[62]

Lyman's plan reflected a genuinely creative attempt to deal with a fundamental problem: the lack of trained psychiatric personnel. There was only one psychiatric nurse available to Greenhill on the inpatient ward and only one psychiatric social worker in DUMC's division of social services. Highland had been expected to contribute staff, at least in part: it had a hospital training school for nurses and "a training school especially licensed for affiliate and postgraduate psychiatric nursing."[63] Yet by 1941 Highland had, apparently, lost the trained personnel who could teach the specialty. What was more, with the general mobilization of nurses in connection with the war, Highland's program in general undergraduate nursing was generating almost as much revenue as was patient care.

At the same time, problems were emerging between Duke and Highland. Carroll had used all of Highland's earnings to remodel its central building, and The Duke Endowment refused his requests to reimburse the hospital for its charity care.[64] As Lyman noted, "It soon became evident that some radical change would have to take place to bring the Durham and the Asheville units together, or else they would drift apart."[65]

Lyman had his hands full just keeping things together in Durham during the war. He lost the one faculty member he had inherited in psychiatry, Dr. Raymond Crispell, who entered the navy in the spring of 1942. (Lyman filled his spot with Dr. Leo Alexander, an Austrian émigré who would later investigate German psychiatric atrocities during the war.) Lyman also brought in the Chilean-born psychoanalyst, Dr. Ignacio Matte-Blanco. Lyman considered Matte-Blanco "a great addition to the staff" and wanted to keep him after his appointment ended in July 1942. Lyman offered $1,000 of his own personal funds to keep Matte-Blanco if Davison could find another $1,000 from "some source, possibly in New York, for help along these lines." Davison found the money, and Matte-Blanco remained until the following spring, when he went back to Chile, to became that nation's leading psychoanalyst.[66]

By the spring of 1942, Lyman was desperately seeking a solution "to the organization of teaching psychiatric nursing." He wanted to institute "adequate teaching" for undergraduate students at Duke and establish a graduate school for "advanced psychiatric training at Asheville." He had added nursing students to his own "experiment in which trial of negroes is being compared to use of Duke students, on the one hand, and girls presumably of high school education, on the other." But that was clearly not enough, especially as Highland's "integration" with the department's program appeared headed for another blow, this time from Duke's dean of nursing, Margaret Pinkerton. "Without the present undergraduate nursing school of the Highland Hospital," Lyman wrote to Davison, "the finances of that institution would be so strained as perhaps to even close it, and yet the school must be closed as an undergraduate school in order to comply with the standards Miss Pinkerton wants, and incidentally with the standards advised by a report from the national nurses association."[67]

Psychiatric Care in North Carolina

Psychiatric care was in poor condition throughout the state. A series of articles had appeared in the North Carolina press containing complaints by two former patients against the state mental hospital at Morganton, eliciting an immediate response from Raleigh. Governor Melville Broughton appointed a five-member board to investigate the complaints and recommend changes.[68] Almost all of the complaints the board investigated, as well as the recommendations it made, echoed those compiled in the Rockefeller report submitted to Governor Ehringhaus six years earlier. Indeed, the principal recommendation of both was to establish "a unified Board of Control to have oversight of all the hospitals for mental disease in the state, with a psychiatrist at its head."[69]

Early in 1943, the state legislature approved Broughton's recommendation, and in July the newly appointed board met with Broughton for the first time. One of the board's first tasks was to study the Rockefeller report. According to a reporter at the *Durham Sun*, the board's assignment raised "the pertinent question of why this report had not been more profitably studied and used years ago." Davison sent Alan Gregg a copy of the article, which argued that the state's mental patients appeared to "have been victims of neglect because of political exigency." Gregg thought the "commentator expressed some rather shrewd guesses, and I believe that out of his comments there is a possible lesson. In any event," he responded to Davison, "I am glad that the situation in North Carolina on the point of the care of mental diseases has finally been reorganized and thus the main objective of our grant has been at least reached."[70]

CHALLENGES AND INNOVATIONS IN NEUROPSYCHIATRY

Gregg's associate director, Robert Lambert, was visiting Duke as the legislature approved Broughton's mental health proposals. He found Lyman "as intense as ever and a little more cadaverous." Rather than leave Duke as previously intimated, Lyman had been taking on every aspect of the psychiatric work and "shows the strain," Lambert reported.[71] Indeed, as Lyman himself described his schedule, he gave lectures "eight hours in the quarter for first year students, fourteen hours for second year, Tuesday and Saturday rounds for third year, seminars once a week for internes, eighteen hours this present quarter for nursing students, and six hours a week for the school of attendants. In addition I must see patients and do research."[72]

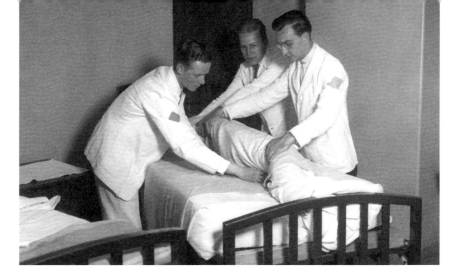

4.8 Conscientious objectors working on Meyer Ward. *Duke University Medical Center Archives.*

Lyman's schedule reflected both his sense of responsibility and his status as one of the most popular and creative teachers in the medical school. As Hanes told Lambert, "in spite of his oddities, Lyman is a very effective teacher. Students are enthusiastic about him. Through movies, talkies, etc. L[yman] has made psychiatry attractive. Students applaud him. He is a terribly earnest person." Lyman had been filming his patients since his days in Peking with the Rockefeller Foundation, and he was now combining a variety of audiovisual techniques to create a collection of "canned cases" for concentrated teaching. He was using phonograph records to store "the patient's history," Lambert wrote. "The history as told by the patient himself and motion picture film is made whenever indicated. There are always photographs, of course." By coordinating these elements into prepared lectures on general and specific psychiatric conditions, Lyman was able to ease his heavy teaching load.[73]

Lyman was also continuing to recruit faculty and staff who represented diverse cultural backgrounds and therapeutic interests, from social adjustment and individual psychotherapy to shock and group therapy. There was Lowenbach, the German-born electroencephalographer, and two psychiatrists from Vienna, Dr. Otto Billig and Dr. Charlotte (Frisch) Walker, who joined the department shortly before Lyman brought in Leo Alexander, the Austrian neurologist. After Alexander joined the army, Lyman replaced him with Dr. Herman H. de Jong, a specialist in electroshock and catatonia. And in 1943, following Matte-Blanco's return to Chile, Lyman brought in a Chinese psychoanalyst from Fisk, Dr. Bingham Dai, who had worked with him in Peking. Lyman then used his own personal funds to bring in from Harvard Dr. Alexandra Adler, the Vienna-born daughter of Dr. Alfred Adler, the founder of individual psychology. Adler, in addition to interpreting and systematizing her father's work, was a specialist in child guidance.[74]

Lyman's personal interests and departmental needs were also carrying his search for diversity into uncharted territory. In yet another experiment to staff the Meyer Ward effectively, Lyman convinced a Methodist bishop to send him 20 conscientious objectors for training. After being "carefully selected" from among their fellow objectors at the Methodist Camp, the men were trained to take patient histories and do psychological tests in addition to their duties as orderlies and attendants. Lyman "has taken a special interest in the young men," Lambert wrote in April 1943, "inviting them to his home for social gatherings and taking the risk of public disapproval for so doing." In fact, Lyman "succeeded in getting two other professors to open their homes to the group."[75] [Figure 4.8]

More dangerously diverse still were Lyman's actions across the color line. He "has become more and more interested in Negroes," Lambert reported. "Encourages the young radicals to talk over race question with him. Says every Negro is race conscious, though it may take several interviews before you can reach a point of frank conversation on the subject." The Rockefeller officer also found Lyman deeply interested "in mental disease among the colored" and attempting to do something about it. Though he could not admit blacks to Meyer Ward, which had "no beds for Negroes," Lyman had arranged "for a few to be admitted to the Lincoln Hospital." So far, Lambert wrote, Lyman had seen "35 colored patients. They show no distinctive pattern of mental disturbance, though there are apparently certain differences in reaction."[76]

Lyman received crucial assistance in this work from two African American women. One was Nola Mae Cox. Cox worked briefly with Lyman during the orderly-attendant experiments and then saw him regularly in her role as the social worker at Lincoln Hospital. He formed a closer, professional relationship with Ethel J. Wiggins, whose husband served on the staff of the North Carolina College for Negroes. Wiggins assisted Lyman "in making contacts with Negro psychiatric patients and also in getting the histories and making the medical examinations, and in some instances even carrying out some of the details of psychotherapy." Just who paid Wiggins's salary is not clear, but she worked with Lyman from 1942 until the summer of 1943, when she applied to work in the psychiatric wards in Haiti. In the years that followed, Wiggins continued to turn to Lyman for recommendations and advice as she pursued her career at the University of Chicago's School of Social Service Administration and at the United Charities of Chicago.[77]

Revealingly, Lyman gave Wiggins lead-author status on the article they published together in the *American Journal of Psychiatry*. The article dealt with their use of psychodrama as a therapeutic tool in the case of Charlie W. Lawson, a 57-year-old black man whose manic behavior prompted his family to bring him to Duke. Lyman recorded Lawson's entire life history on tape, and Lawson, after a short stay on a regular ward in Duke Hospital, returned to his farm, where Wiggins photographed him and his family reenacting the incidents prior to the onset of his manic episode. "This reenactment was said by the patient and his children to have had a beneficial effect on his feelings about his psychotic experience." Wiggins and Lyman also pointed out in closing that Lawson's case was "only one of many which have been 'canned.' Either lantern slides or moving pictures preserve more or less of the appearance and activity of the patient. Sound records add the patient's account of himself. The combination can then be used simultaneously or seriatim to present the clinical data considerably more vividly, we believe, than can be done from the written records."[78]

The pressure to do something about Highland Hospital was an additional strain on Lyman during the spring of 1943. In March, The Duke Endowment rejected a second request from Carroll to have Highland reimbursed for its charity cases. Carroll had made this one under Highland's new charter as a nonprofit corporation, and under changed circumstances. "Numbers of patients are being referred from the psychiatric unit at Duke to be treated here at reduced rates," Carroll had explained, "and this has definitely reduced the relation of our income to expense for the year, a loss which can only be met by assistance from your Endowment Fund or by the closing of our doors to free patients." Rankin, in his response for the Endowment, assured Carroll that while he wanted to do everything he could for Highland, the focus of the foundation was "the general hospital" and it could not set a precedent by contributing to a psychiatric hospital. "The Trustees cannot consider an appropriation for the Highland Hospital without being willing also to receive and consider favorably applications from other psychopathic institutions, a number of which, as you know, we have in North Carolina."[79]

Lyman then proposed moving to Asheville with Bingham Dai and Herman de Jong to make Highland "headquarters for psychiatry instead of Duke Hospital."[80] But Carroll himself opposed the change, and Lyman had finally had enough. He joined the Office of Strategic Services in January 1944. Neuropsychiatry was put in Greenhill's hands.[81] Shortly afterward, Carroll met in Durham with Greenhill and Davison. Also at the meeting were G. R. Henricksen, Duke's assistant treasurer, and Edwin C. Bryson, a member of the Law School faculty who was also on faculty of the School of Medicine. The meeting produced several recommendations for dealing with the Duke-Highland relationship after Carroll's lease expired on September 1, 1944.[82]

Yet Greenhill ignored Highland as he mobilized the department to collaborate with the federal government on a project to treat psychiatric disor-

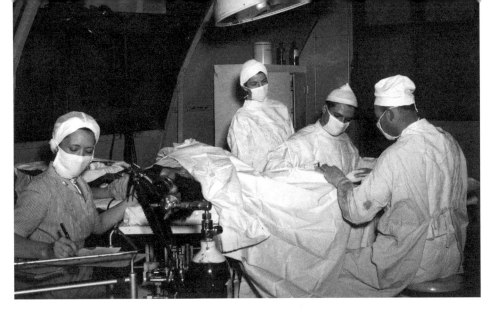

4.9 Operating room of the 65th General Hospital, in Botesdale, Suffolk, England, 1944–45. *Duke University Medical Center Archives.*

ders among returning veterans. The Duke Rehabilitation Clinic opened in July 1944 in downtown Durham, at the same time that the G.I. Bill of Rights was passed. The clinic was the only one of its kind in the South, and one of only three in the nation, and between the summer of 1944 and the spring of 1946, Duke psychiatrists treated some 1,200 North Carolinians referred to the clinic under contract from the Veterans Administration. Significantly, the clinic's success became a major reason for Durham's selection in 1946 as the site of a large VA hospital adjacent to Duke, and for the VA's simultaneous designation of DUMC as the site of a regional veterans residency program in neuropsychiatry.

The 65th General Hospital and Blood Transfusions

D uke's 65th General Hospital cared for the men of the Eighth Air Force returning from their bombing raids over Germany. In February 1944, after four months in Malvern, Worcestershire, the 65th was suddenly ordered to Botesdale, in Suffolk, 70 miles north of London. It was sent there, it seems, not only to prepare for the intense bombing campaign ahead but also to pacify several Air Force generals increasingly dissatisfied with the existing medical service of the station hospitals. The 35-hut compound soon became a designated specialty center in eastern England for neurosurgery, thoracic and plastic surgery, burns, and hand injuries.[83] In addition to daily casualties from the heavy bombers, the 65th received shipments of wounded from the ground troops in Europe. With a 0.4 percent mortality rate for treatment of fresh battle casualties, the unit was known for keeping soldiers alive, and in the course of treating more than 17,250 patients in England, the 65th earned an enviable reputation as one of the most successful general hospital units in the European theater of operations. [Figure 4.9]

The unit's chief of surgery, Lt. Col. Clarence E. Gardner Jr., later became chairman of the Department of Surgery at Duke, while the unit's chief of neuropsychiatry, Dr. Leo Alexander, became a consultant to the War Crimes Commission at Nuremberg. Gardner later recalled the procedure he developed during the war for treating certain chest injuries affecting the lungs. "What you had to do was to open up the thorax and peel that clot off of the chest wall, and also off of the lung. The lung would expand and the clot would not be in the chest wall any more, and that was called a decortication. And, I did a lot of those."[84] For the unit's youngest officer, Dr. Ivan W. Brown Jr., the war experience was transformative. In addition to his duties as the unit's neurosurgeon, Brown was sent by Gardner to study the British system of blood banking, and after adapting the system to the needs of the 65th, Brown helped shaped the system of blood banking used by general hospitals in the United States Army. Returning to Duke at the end of the war, Brown became one of the world's leading authorities on blood transfusions. He also became one of the world's first open-heart surgeons, and in 1957, his heat and blood exchanger, an invention for lowering and raising a patient's body temperature, became part of the pathbreaking heart-lung machine used to sustain patients during open-heart surgery.[85]

Brown's wartime interest in blood, blood banking, and transfusions was shared by Lederle Laboratories. The company's medical director, Dr. Arthur F. Coca, had stepped aside from the Blood Transfusion Betterment Association in 1940, after 12 years as its medical director, to be succeeded by Dr. Charles R. Drew, a black Rockefeller fellow who had just completed his dissertation at Columbia University. Drew's mission as the association's new medical director was to help plan and administer the Plasma for Britain Project, a dramatic pilot program supported by the American Red Cross and designed to investigate the shipment of blood plasma to the British Isles. As a result of the program's success, the American Red Cross decided to set up donor stations to collect blood for the American armed forces. Drew became the first director of the new program in 1941 and organized the first collection unit in New York.[86]

In the meantime, Coca worked closely with Ralph Wyckoff, Beard's horse virus colleague, to mobilize Lederle Laboratories for the production of plasma from the blood collected by the American Red Cross. By 1942, Lederle was the largest producer of blood plasma in the United States, and in the spring

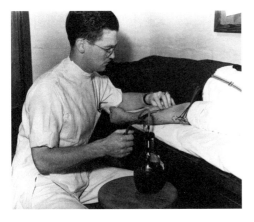

4.10 Physician with a patient at the Duke Hospital Blood Bank. *Duke University Medical Center Archives.*

of 1943, the company received the army-navy "E" award for its meritorious service in providing plasma and other blood products to the nation's armed forces.[87] Dean Wilburt Davison also did some valuable blood work of his own. As the physician responsible for tropical diseases at the National Research Council, Davison located the individual whose serum contaminated a yellow fever vaccine given to American troops. Over 50,000 troops became jaundiced, and some 60 died, after receiving the hepatitis-infected vaccine. Davison was "greatly chagrined" to discover that the source of the infection "was a Hopkins student."[88] [Figure 4.10]

New Players and New Connections

The chairman of the American Red Cross, Basil O'Connor, appointed Davison in October of 1944 to "a special medical and health committee composed of eleven men, prominent in their respective fields, to survey current Red Cross medical and health operations and to recommend plans for the post-war period." Davison's Red Cross connections included a number of familiar links, including the committee's chairman, Dr. Lewis Weed, and committee members Alan Gregg and Thomas Parran Jr., the U.S. surgeon general.[89] The following January, moreover, O'Connor, as president of the National Foundation for Infantile Paralysis, notified DUMC's School of Physical Therapy that it had been awarded a grant from the foundation to study the "mechanics of muscle action in health and disease." The grant was the first of many Duke Medicine received from the foundation over the next decade and a half, including a five-year $200,000 grant in 1946 for fellowships in orthopedic surgery.[90]

In addition to signaling the pattern of Davison's postwar professional activities, these developments reflected the expanding private and public networks of which Duke University and Duke Medicine were a part. Haiti, Cuba, and Puerto Rico; Germany, Japan, and China; Washington, New York, and Oak Ridge, Tennessee—from his official government business and private meetings to his medical conferences and Doris Duke's foundations, Davison began spending as much time away from Duke and Durham as he did at DUMC. "I soon earned the rather doubtful distinction of traveling from the Raleigh-Durham airport more than any one else," he later wrote, "with an annual average of thirty out-of-state trips, usually including one or more out of the country, and some years exceeding 50,000 miles annually. These journeys, usually at taxpayers' expense, were caused by the splendid cooperation of our government and universities on national and international committees and councils required by the expanded influence of the USA in world affairs."[91]

STRATEGIC SERVICES AND THE DEFENSE INDUSTRY

On a deeper, more clandestine level, several Duke and DUMC faculty also worked with the Office of Strategic Services during the war and then remained connected with the nation's security and intelligence networks after the war, especially the Central Intelligence Agency. The key figure in these networks was Calvin Bryce Hoover, chairman of Duke's Department of Economics, and the nation's leading authority on the Soviet and Nazi economies. He served as economic adviser to the secretary of agriculture and was a key figure in the intelligence section of both the Office of Strategic Services and one of its successor agencies, the CIA. Between 1946 and 1960, Hoover was one of the most powerful faculty members at Duke University.[92]

Several faculty members of Duke's Departments of Neuropsychiatry and Psychology also worked closely in the Office of Strategic Services during the war and then on campus following the war. The cross-campus connection was closest between Lyman and Dr. Donald K. Adams, a member of the Psychology Department. Adams was one of Lyman's interdisciplinary consultants before the war, and the two served together in the Strategic Services during the war. After the war, Adams recruited Dr. Louis D. Cohen, a child psychologist who had worked with Adams and Lyman in Strategic Services. Lyman's closest collaborator in the Office of Strategic Services, however, was his old friend and new departmental colleague, Bingham Dai, the psychoanalyst from China. In 1945, for example, the two men traveled through China and Indonesia to help the U.S. Army select "Chinese recruits" for the intelligence services of the Nationalist Chinese forces fighting against the communist troops of Mao Tse Tung.[93]

Beyond campus, Duke also had strong connections with the nation's security and intelligence networks. In Durham, for example, there was George Watts Hill, grandson of the Watts Hospital founder and an early Blue Cross partner with Davison. Hill was a wealthy banker and insurance executive who became an early recruit, like Calvin Hoover, to Roosevelt's Coordinating Office on Information. Hill then served as the special equipment officer for the Office of Strategic Services intelligence during the war. Another old Duke connection was Huntingdon Gilchrist, an "executive" with American Cyana-

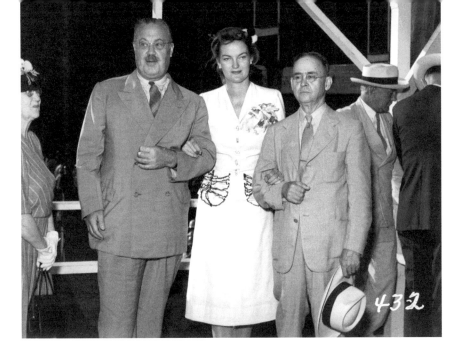

4.11 Left to right: Dr. Wilburt C. Davison, Doris Duke, and Dean William H. Wannamaker at the Jones Construction Company shipyard, Brunswick, Georgia, June 19, 1944. Doris Duke had just christened the company's new Liberty ship, the *James B. Duke*. *Duke University Archives.*

mid between 1928 and 1955. Gilchrist helped the United Nations select the site of its New York headquarters and worked closely with Allen W. Dulles, first at the League of Nations, then in the Office of Strategic Services, and later at the CIA; he also worked directly with Duke's Calvin Hoover on the Marshall Plan for postwar reconstruction in Europe.[94]

Proving equally influential were Duke's connections in the atomic research and defense industries. The principal owner-operator of one of the nation's largest construction companies, the J. A. Jones Construction Company of Charlotte, was Edwin L. Jones Sr., a graduate of Trinity and a trustee of Duke University. During the war, the company built everything from military bases and shipyards to the ships themselves. In 1943, the company built, in Oak Ridge, Tennessee, the largest single power plant ever conceived, and then received the largest construction contract ever awarded. The plant was one of three to effect atomic fission and produce the atomic bomb as part of the Manhattan Project. For the next 50 years, the company was at the center of the military-industrial complex, constructing huge civic, military, and industrial projects throughout the world. During that time, its owners gave generously to Duke University, including the lead gift for the Edwin L. Jones Basic Cancer Research Building, a basic cancer research facility that was completed in

1976 with a combination of private gifts and $4.4 million from the National Cancer Institute. [Figure 4.11]

Duke's Oak Ridge connections became numerous and important following the war. The head of Duke's Department of Chemistry, Dr. Paul M. Gross, took the lead not only in incorporating the Oak Ridge Institute of Nuclear Studies but also in negotiating its contract with the Atomic Energy Commission. The production of radioisotopes for scientific research and medical treatment became a major activity of the Oak Ridge facility, and in 1948 the Veterans Administration began a research program that employed radioisotopes at VA hospitals affiliated with medical schools. Though the Durham VA hospital was not completed until 1953, DUMC established, through an Institute of Nuclear Studies contract with the Atomic Energy Commission, a radio-isotope research program in 1948. At the same time, Duke University also became one of four regional training centers established and subsidized by the Atomic Energy Commission for training postdoctoral fellows in the use of radioisotopes in biology and medicine. Finally—in an irony that was especially poignant for Duke—Davison and other members of DUMC's staff, both past and present, became involved with the Atomic Bomb Casualty Commission, a long-term study of the survivors of the atomic bombs dropped on Hiroshima and Nagasaki in 1945.[95]

Pressures to Build

Early in 1945, Fred Hanes sent a letter to the chairman of The Duke Endowment, George Allen. Enclosed with the letter was a note Hanes had prepared for his colleagues on the "Building Committee, which is studying the need of the medical school and hospital for new construction." With the Bell Building still under construction, the committee's original expansion plans had become "muddled," and Hanes considered it "wise" to restate his reasons for offering to build a new nurses' home. "Please let me make clear that I have no interest in the building of a nurses home as such, but only as part of the larger plan which I have submitted. The imperative needs are these: (1) Nurses Home (2) Clinic building, which in turn will release space on first floor of present building for scientific work (3) Staff House (present Nurses Home) (4) Cafeteria (present nurses' dining room) (5) Addition to present building of the Medical School to facilitate better teaching and research." Hanes was especially concerned with "the need for more space for the development of scientific work. Among certain members of the faculty of Duke Medical School the idea seems firmly embedded that the clinical staff is little interested in this phase of the School's work, despite the fact that the clinical side has been as productive of scientific work as the so-called preclinical men, with only half as much laboratory space at their disposal. Any such division of scientific work into 'clinical' and 'pre-clinical' is artificial; all workers need much more room if our reputation as a scientific institution, and not as a repair shop, is to be maintained and to progress in the years to come."[96]

Hanes made it clear to Allen that Duke would benefit financially if these expansion plans were adopted. Put simply, in return for adopting his plans Hanes would give Duke additional shares of R. J. Reynolds Tobacco Company stock for construction of the nurses' home. "Under the conditions which have been discussed Mrs. Hanes and I will furnish 22,000 shares of Reynolds 'B' stock. Under the same conditions I am willing to increase to 25,000 shares of Reynolds 'B' stock, *provided that the whole plan be adopted for present and future development*."[97] Allen made it equally clear in his reply to Hanes, however, that DUMC's plans had to be considered within the context of the larger university. Allen appreciated Hanes's "continued interest in Duke University. I use the word 'university' advisedly," he wrote, "because I like to think that all of us are as interested and will continue to be interested in the development of the University as a whole rather than in any one particular department thereof." Noting that Hanes's proposed plans were "comprehensive as well as quite extensive," Allen wanted time to study and discuss them with Davison and the university's president, Robert Flowers. "To me it seems highly desirable to have a well-rounded, top-notch medical school which would involve necessary hospital facilities needed to that end, but personally feel that we should guard against hospital facilities there beyond that point."[98]

Hanes responded firmly but politely: "Nothing in the note I submitted calls for more hospital beds." His plans called for a nurses' home, a staff house, and "above all, more room for scientific developments. In the near future we are going to have strong competition," Hanes stressed, "which is good for us." The University of North Carolina had already constructed a large, new laboratory building and it appeared likely that the university would also soon get a four-year medical school and a large teaching hospital. "It pains me to think that the present school at Chapel Hill has far better facilities for scientific work than we have here at Duke," Hanes wrote. "We are going to stand or fall as an institution upon the scientific work done here. . . . I do not want us to have more patients but better facilities for scientific work."[99]

Financial Uncertainties and Plans for the Future

In the meantime, Duke was ignoring both the patients and the facilities at Highland Hospital. By the spring of 1945, Lyman was out of the country and Dr. Robert Carroll was reporting a "serious help shortage" at the hospital. The government had taken 25 percent of Highland's "best workers," Carroll reported, "and 50 per cent of our Negro help, including some who have been with us for many years, have moved on upward from the salary point of view to Moore Hospital and other government agencies." Worse still, Carroll saw "not the least chance that Duke [would] undertake further responsibilities which would require any type of personnel. Duke has decided to maintain Highland Hospital under a revised charter." "Our old board of directors has been practically superseded by a complete Duke membership," he noted; "I am retained as a hired man until some type of replacement can be found." As for Highland's future, Carroll was not sanguine: "[I am] afraid our gift to the university did little to inspire them to further investment. I think they are interested chiefly in being the object of donations rather than in initiating any campaign for funds. I do hope that my ideal of a children's psychiatric hospital will some time be attained, and that Asheville will be its location."[100]

Underlying much of this uncertainty, both in Durham and in Asheville, were the economic challenges faced by Duke and DUMC's largest funder, The Duke Endowment. Two of the foundation's largest investments—in tobacco and Alcoa securities—had been hampered by antitrust litigation during the war, while its largest investment, in Duke Power securities, had not taken up the slack. More than 1,000 Duke Power employees entered military service during the war, forcing the company to relocate and retrain its personnel, and not until 1946 did the federal government lift its wartime restrictions on utility construction. A verdict in the epic Alcoa case was finally reached in March 1945, and over the next five years, the government-financed aluminum plants built, staffed, and managed by Alcoa during the war were sold off to Alcoa's fledgling competitors. The tobacco cases, tried by a jury in 1941, had resulted in the conviction of 13 executives from the industry's three largest concerns—R. J. Reynolds, Liggett & Myers, and American Tobacco—on charges of monopoly and price fixing. The companies were still filing appeals at end of the war; these were finally dismissed by the United States Supreme Court in 1946.[101]

It was a disgruntled Fred Hanes that Lambert vacationed with in the fall of 1945. Davison was cutting positions and reducing salaries at the medical center, and Hanes, while he had agreed to reduce Kempner's university salary, had refused to cut it as drastically as Davison had proposed. Davison disliked the fact that Kempner was making a lot of money treating patients with the rice diet and that information about the diet was constantly being requested by such popular national magazines as *Good Housekeeping*. Davison wanted no such information released, however, and Hanes and Kempner had agreed not "to have anything put in the lay press before January 1946."

Yet it was Hart, not Davison, who was bothering Hanes the most. As Lambert described it, Hanes was "troubled over the insistence of some of the clinicians at Duke, led by the professor of surgery (Hart), to enlarge the hospital, adding a private pavilion." Hanes considered the hospital addition a bad idea; with 600 beds already, Duke's hospital was large enough to meet the needs of undergraduate teaching, which was the only reason for its existence. A private pavilion would "leave professors with less time for teaching and research," Hanes believed, and also augment the hospital's deficit, "thus taking from endowment money that should be devoted entirely to academic purposes." As for the arguments advanced by Hart and his colleagues: "The proponents of the project say that with more private beds, more young surgeons and internists can be trained,—incidentally incomes of professors and part-time staff will be upped, which Hanes thinks is the real objective of the proponents of the scheme. Even under present conditions, H[anes] says some of the assistant professors at Duke are earning from $15,000–$20,000 a year."[102]

That was the last vacation Lambert spent with Fred Hanes. Hanes began having chest pains early in December, and on December 14, 1945, he signed his will. In addition to bequests for his wife and close relatives, Hanes designated DUMC as the beneficiary of his residual estate: some $700,000 in securities. In the meantime, Lyman decided he wanted to return to China to organize a psychiatric unit there. Duke now needed a different kind of person, he believed, "someone who can go out and raise money." And in anticipation of leaving, he released Leo Alexander, Herman de Jong, and Alexandra Adler, "whose positions would be uncertain under another head."[103]

Hanes was still alive in early March when Lambert made his annual Rockefeller visit to Duke, and he was still "critical of Davison's economic policy," claiming that the dean was "always ready to let go any faculty member who is drawing a substantial salary." And yet in meetings with Hanes and Davison, Lambert found them both in agreement on one thing: there was no need for the proposed four-year medical school at Chapel Hill. Though North Carolina needed "a thousand more physicians," Davison doubted that a four-year school at Chapel Hill would "contribute materially toward such an increase." He believed, in fact, that "a statistical inquiry would show that most of the two-year students at U. of N. C. who go elsewhere to complete the course eventually return to the State." Hanes said simply "that in the minds of the University of N. C. constituency, the quest is not that of the need of such a school; it is simply that whatever Duke has, N. C. must have."[104] Fred Hanes died two weeks later at his home on West Campus.

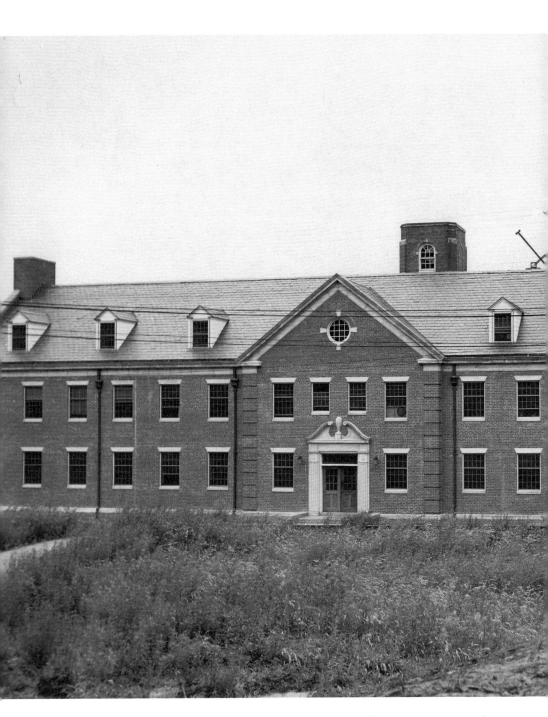

5.1 The Hanes Annex, originally the nurses' home, then the offices of the Department of Psychiatry, and now the John Hope Franklin Center for Interdisciplinary and International Studies. *Duke University Medical Center Archives.*

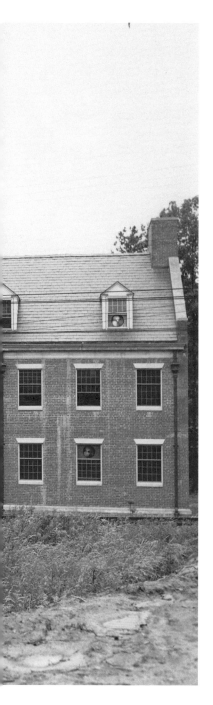

CHAPTER 5:

After the War: The Politics of Duke Medicine, 1946–1950

Politics and federal funding deeply affected the course of Duke Medicine after World War II. Several of the most important developments occurred in 1946: Willis Smith became chairman of Duke University's board of trustees, and Dr. Eugene Stead accepted the chairmanship of Duke's Department of Medicine. Both Smith and Stead then proceeded to do battle with Dean Wilburt Davison: Smith to prevent Davison from becoming Duke's next president, and Stead to prevent the dean from controlling him and the Department of Medicine.

It was also in 1946 that Congress passed the Hospital Survey and Construction Act, commonly known as the Hill-Burton Act. Hill-Burton dispersed federal funds to states for the planning and construction of health care facilities, and North Carolina became particularly aggressive in attempting to provide health and medical services for its citizens. Hill-Burton also elicited ambitious expansion plans from both the private medical center of Wake Forest

College in Winston-Salem and the promoters of the state-supported medical school at the University of North Carolina in Chapel Hill. Wake Forest College announced in 1946 that the college itself was moving to Winston-Salem, while UNC's supporters prepared legislation to fund the expansion of the university's two-year medical school to a four-year school and to build a large teaching hospital to accompany it. The Duke Endowment supported Wake's expansion plans but bitterly fought the UNC proposal in the 1947 session of the state legislature. The fight challenged almost a decade of cooperation between the two universities, particularly in the fields of health and education for blacks, and it also helped fuel a split within the liberal wing of the state's Democratic Party. As a result of that split, Duke trustee Willis Smith became a leader of the party's conservative faction and Dr. Frank Porter Graham, UNC's former president, led the party's liberal wing.

DUMC itself was one of the most progressive institutions in the American South. Its Department of Neuropsychiatry was especially dedicated to helping individuals and groups on the local, state, and national levels, among blacks and whites, children and adults, and veterans returning from the war. Many of Duke's faculty and alumni, however, particularly the aging alumni of Methodist Trinity College, resented the medical center's growing power and political activism, and by the time Willis Smith challenged Frank Porter Graham in the 1950 Democratic primary for the United States Senate, some of these initiatives faced an uncertain future.

Willis Smith in the Aftermath of War

Willis Smith was in Germany in the spring of 1946 when he got word of the deaths of Fred Hanes and John F. Bruton, the long-time chairman of the university's trustees. As president of the American Bar Association, Smith was in Nuremberg to observe for the association the conduct of the trials of the principal Nazi leaders before the International Military Tribunal. He had been invited to the trial by the War Department and by the American chief of counsel at Nuremberg, Justice Robert A. Jackson, whose staff made certain that Smith and his fellow bar association traveler, Tappan Gregory, were properly provided for when not in the courtroom.

A number of other people associated with Duke were also at Nuremberg. Jackson's assistant was Sidney Alderman, a trustee of Duke University. Also on Jackson's staff was Dr. Raphael Lemkin, a Duke professor who coined the term "genocide" while drafting the United Nations' charges against the Nazis at Nuremberg. (Lemkin, in preparing Smith's introductions to European leaders, always referred to him as being from "my university.") The assistant of the alternate American judge, Judge John J. Parker (an old friend of Smith's), was Bob Stewart, a recent graduate of Duke University. Among the new acquaintances Smith made was the assistant chief of U.S. counsel at Nuremberg, Robert Kempner, the brother of Duke's rice diet inventor, Dr. Walter Kempner; Robert Kempner was in charge of research and examination of captured documents.[1]

Smith was elected chairman of the Duke University board of trustees after returning from Europe in the spring of 1946. A tall, neatly dressed man who smoked Lucky Strike cigarettes, Smith had played basketball at Trinity College and studied law there before establishing himself as a powerful Democratic politician and corporation attorney in the state capital at Raleigh. In 1945 he was elected by the American Bar Association as its president. Of particular importance for Duke and Duke Medicine, especially in the years ahead, was Smith's willingness to oppose The Duke Endowment Republicans who tried to rule Duke from 30 Rockefeller Plaza in New York. It was the search for a new president of Duke University that eventually divided Smith and the New York group. The New York trustees wanted Dean Wilburt Davison to become Duke's next president, but Smith was equally determined not to let that happen. The search began slowly, and very discreetly, after Smith's election as chairman of the university's trustees. The first move was made at 30 Rockefeller Plaza, when the secretary of The Duke Endowment, Alexander H. Sands Jr., visited the vice president and director of the General Education Board, Jackson Davis. Sands, a long-time officer of both the Endowment and Duke Power, had recently been appointed to the board of trustees of Duke University; specifically, he had assumed one of the three seats reserved for Endowment trustees on the seven-member executive committee of university trustees.

"Duke University is quietly looking for a president," Davis wrote in his diary. "A[lexander] S[ands] is thinking of Julian Boyd, librarian at Princeton, who is a graduate of Duke. I told him I thought Boyd would be an excellent person." Sands then displayed what many at the General Education Board had long regarded as the Endowment's imperious control over Duke University. "He said the Executive Committee of the Board consists of 7 persons and a small group of these 7 is really in control. He thinks it advisable for them to agree on someone and clear matters with President Flowers in order to prevent any division or rival efforts for favorites." Davis was not impressed. "I told him the usual practice was to appoint a committee." Willis Smith soon appointed—and headed—the search committee for a new president of Duke University.[2]

Responses to the Hill-Burton Act

S mith's election as chairman of the university's trustees coincided with
congressional passage of the federal Hospital Survey and Construction Act. The act, commonly known as the Hill-Burton Act, provided
the largest federal grant program ever made for health care and was modeled
in part upon The Duke Endowment's plan for funding community hospitals. The act required each state that applied for Hill-Burton funds to do so
through a state body formed specifically to identify that state's needs for hospital and health facility construction and to disperse the Hill-Burton funds to
meet those needs. In anticipation of Hill-Burton's requirements, the North
Carolina legislature had created the North Carolina Medical Care Commission in 1945. The purpose of the commission was "to provide for the licensing,
inspection, and regulation of hospitals; to authorize subdivisions of government to construct, equip, and operate, and maintain hospital facilities; and to
provide adequate medical care to the people of the State of North Carolina."
At the same time, the commission was also authorized to provide nonprofit hospitals with funds for charity care and to construct a four-year medical
school and teaching hospital on the University of North Carolina's campus in
Chapel Hill.[3]

Just how Duke Medicine might qualify for Hill-Burton funds was not
exactly clear at the time of the bill's passage. Davison had already discussed
one possibility with the head of The Duke Endowment's Hospital Section,
Watson Rankin, who was also a member of the North Carolina Medical Care
Commission. The project they discussed was Deryl Hart's plan to add a five-
story wing to Duke Hospital. The addition featured expanded and modern-
ized facilities for the Private Diagnostic Clinic, additional hospital beds for
private patients, and a large public clinic for indigent outpatients. On the eve
of Hill-Burton's passage, however, Rankin considered all such plans premature. "If it passes," he wrote to Davison on June 1, 1946, "the North Carolina Medical Care Commission under the provisions of the Act will have to
declare a set of priorities as a basis for approval of applications for Federal
assistance in the building of hospitals and related services." The commission
had not yet set priorities and thus had no applications for funding, both of
which would be "needed for the intelligent action of the Commission and also
for the information of the Public Health Service through which organization
or to which organization the application for Federal funds will be sent. Therefore," Rankin wrote, "my advice to you is to wait until the situation is further
clarified." Which was fine with Davison. "I shall not do anything about an
application for assistance with the clinic building until I hear from you."[4]

Davison had more pressing matters to attend to anyway. He needed to find a successor to Fred Hanes and to figure out what to do with Highland Hospital and the Department of Neuropsychiatry. The most promising candidate for the chair in Medicine was Dr. Eugene A. Stead Jr. of Emory. Not only was Stead an effective teacher and innovative researcher; he was also medically, and politically, correct. He had been born and raised in Atlanta, Georgia, in a family of evangelical Methodists, and he had obtained his undergraduate and M.D. degrees from Emory, a Methodist college in Atlanta. After internships at Harvard, moreover, both in medicine and in surgery, and a residency in medicine at Cincinnati General Hospital, Stead had returned to Boston as a research fellow and associate in medicine. There he had worked closely with Dr. Soma Weiss, the first Jewish professor of clinical medicine at Harvard Medical School and one of the nation's leading proponents of psychosomatic medicine.

One of Stead's most important assets, however, was the fact that he had been recommended by Robert Lambert. The Rockefeller officer had been visiting Stead since Stead's arrival at Emory in 1941 as chairman of its Department of Medicine, and he liked what he saw. Stead "looks upon buildings as secondary," Lambert wrote in 1944. "Men come first. He will, therefore, work for strengthening staff as the first need." Lambert also found Stead "applying the venous catheter technique to an average of a patient a day" and planning "to continue in the cardio-vascular field, attacking the problem of why cardiacs 'swell up'; that is, why salts and water do not get through the kidney as they should." Stead also showed in Atlanta the progressive community activism that the Rockefeller Foundation encouraged. He seemed "sure of his influential position in the hospital and community, as well as in the medical school. He has gotten into city politics to the extent of working on the mayor and others influential in municipal government—including labor leaders—to convince them of the value of medical training in promoting better care of the sick. S[tead] is writing an article for a local labor magazine on this theme." Additionally, Stead was so interested in what Lambert described as the "training of colored nurses" and "continued education of the Negro Physician," that he held several conversations on the matter with Florence Read, the president of Spelman College in Atlanta.[5]

Shortly before Stead visited Duke in June of 1946, Lambert discussed the situation "at some length" with Davison. What concerned both men was how Stead might view the PDC and the salaries at Duke. Most of Emory's medical faculty opposed organized faculty clinical practices like the PDC, and Stead, now also dean of the School of Medicine at Emory, was closely connected with that tradition.[6] His family physician since childhood, Dr. James E. Paullin, had also been his mentor at Emory, and Paullin, while recently serving as president of both the AMA and the American College of Physicians, had strongly opposed group practices like the PDC. In truth, Lambert and Davison hoped and expected Stead to feel the same way. Yet while Davison thought Duke could meet "any condition Stead may make about the private diagnostic clinic and staff salaries," Lambert wondered if that were true. The Rockefeller officer saw many "vested interests at Duke, where during the war, much to Fred Hanes' concern, the diagnostic clinic brought large salary supplements to practically all members of the clinical group. I understand some associate professors are earning over $25,000."[7]

Stead's interview at Duke coincided with a letter from the Life Insurance Medical Research Fund notifying him that he had been awarded a two-year grant of $32,000 for support of his work on "cardiac output and blood flow in various tissues." Duke then offered, and Stead accepted, the chairmanship of the Department of Medicine—an appointment that was to begin in January 1947. Close on the heels of his commitment, Stead was also asked to serve on the initial advisory panel for the Cardiovascular Section of the National Institute of Health. The panel was one of many associated with the 21 study sections recently established by the NIH's newly created Research Grants Office, the purpose of which was to provide technical advice and review grant applications from nonfederal institutions and scientists doing research in diseases and systems. Finally, Stead learned in September that both Davison and the insurance fund would approve the transfer of his grant from Emory to Duke.[8]

By then the dean had also laid the groundwork for Stead to fire Walter Kempner. Davison had started the process in August, asking Lambert if the Rockefeller Foundation had any objection to the university's "getting rid" of Kempner. According to Davison, Kempner was ignoring his research and teaching duties while making over $50,000 a year mainly treating wealthy patients, whose records he insisted upon keeping secret. And on top of that, Davison groused, nobody at Duke liked Kempner. Lambert responded simply for the foundation, "we have no claim on or for K."[9]

The matter came up again early in September while Lambert was vacationing in Roaring Gap, North Carolina, but this time Davison was focused on Highland Hospital, Dr. Richard Lyman, and the Department of Neuropsychiatry. Highland's founder, Dr. Robert Carroll, had resigned as the hospital's director, and Davison's hope that Highland "would provide enough income to replace the R[ockefeller] F[oundation] grant (as the Hospital did make money in private hands)," was not being realized. In fact, Lambert reported, "there is no net income as yet and probably never will be." Davison hoped the foundation might renew its psychiatry grant when it expired on June 30, 1947, but he was also well aware, Lambert wrote, that the foundation planned no "further support—that it was clearly understood Duke would take over at the end of the period."[10]

Although morale had remained low in the Department of Neuropsychiatry following the war, the department reached a turning point in the spring of 1946 with the creation at Duke of a Veterans Resident Training Program in Neuropsychiatry.[11] The purpose of the program was to prepare veteran physicians for board certification in neuropsychiatry and for service in the medical facilities of the Veterans Administration. Almost 60 percent of hospitalized veterans were receiving treatment for neuropsychiatric problems, and the VA expected heavy caseloads for the next 20 years, with 30 percent of its hospital beds projected for occupancy by psychiatric patients and thousands of other veterans needing outpatient care. At the core of the new training program were medical school residencies for veterans who were already board-certified physicians. The veteran residents were expected to spend part of their time in class and at least half of their time taking care of veterans in collaboration with a psychiatric team that consisted of a psychiatrist, a psychologist, a social worker, and a psychiatric nurse.[12]

The neuropsychiatry training program also reflected the federal government's new, wider role in improving medical care in the United States; specifically, it was part of the larger postwar effort to provide medical care and professional development for the nation's veterans through the cooperation of the VA with universities, colleges, medical schools, and medical centers. When President Harry Truman signed Public Law 293 on January 3, 1946, establishing the Department of Medicine and Surgery within the VA, the new department was charged with coordinating medical care for veterans, and, as the first step in that process, the department established professional divisions or services within the VA. One was the Neuropsychiatry Division, which contained separate sections for psychiatry, neurology, and clinical psychology. On January 30, moreover, just a week after plans were announced to construct a $4.5 million VA hospital on or near Duke's campus, the VA created a system of affiliations of veterans' hospitals with university medical schools. And critical legislation continued to emerge throughout the spring and summer of 1946: first, the National Mental Health Act (which called for the establishment of the National Institute of Mental Health), followed by the Hill-Burton act.

Duke established its veterans neuropsychiatry training program in March of 1946, after almost two years of treating veterans at the Duke Rehabilitation Clinic—a VA contract clinic—in downtown Durham. The clinic, like the training program, was initiated by Dr. Maurice Greenhill, and both were among the first such VA affiliates in the United States. The clinic had been one of

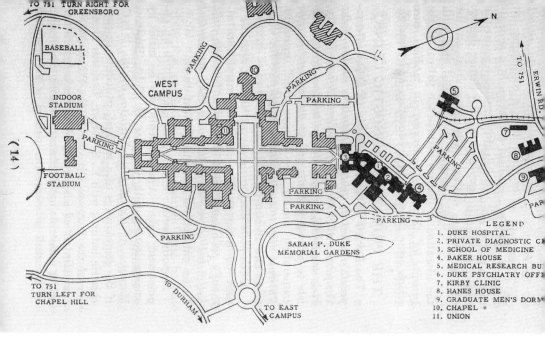

Within the map image, the following labels appear:

TO 751 TURN RIGHT FOR GREENSBORO

BASEBALL

INDOOR STADIUM

WEST CAMPUS

PARKING

PARKING

N

TO 751

ERWIN RD.

(14)

FOOTBALL STADIUM

PARKING

PARKING

PARKING

PARKING

PARKING

PARKING

TO 751 TURN LEFT FOR CHAPEL HILL

TO DURHAM

SARAH P. DUKE MEMORIAL GARDENS

TO EAST CAMPUS

LEGEND
1. DUKE HOSPITAL
2. PRIVATE DIAGNOSTIC C?
3. SCHOOL OF MEDICINE
4. BAKER HOUSE
5. MEDICAL RESEARCH BU?
6. DUKE PSYCHIATRY OFF?
7. KIRBY CLINIC
8. HANES HOUSE
9. GRADUATE MEN'S DORM?
10. CHAPEL
11. UNION

5.2 Map of Duke University and Duke Medical Center, 1956. *Duke University Medical Center Archives.*

only three in the nation when it opened in 1944, and now the training program was the seventh such affiliate established in the United States. Lyman selected his former colleague at Hopkins, Dr. Leslie B. Hohman, a specialist in child psychiatry, to run the program. The program "gave us our first chance to teach properly since the founding of the department," Lyman wrote. "All of us entered into the project, under the direction of Dr. Hohman. This teaching took first place in our efforts. The veterans did good work. It had the side effects of improving the care of many patients as well as of yanking up the quality of some of our civilian teaching."[13]

Unfortunately, the program was also poorly organized, at least initially, and created unwanted ripples across the campus, the state, and the VA bureaucracy. The major challenges involved record keeping, personnel, and space. As Greenhill explained to Lyman in April: "Some chaos is resulting in the clinical aspects of the veterans program because the Veterans Administration is dumping large numbers of cases on PDC and because we have no organized overall plan for the clinical aspects of the Residents Training Program."[14] Errors and abuses also flourished as a huge new bureaucracy emerged; double-billing became a major problem, as did the wide dispersal of the department's offices, personnel, and records. Patients were often seen by both Duke physicians and veteran trainees. Some were seen in downtown Durham (at the Duke Rehabilitation Clinic); others were seen in the PDC; and still others visited the department's small outpatient clinic, the Kirby Clinic, which, together with a surplus army building purchased by Lyman and Hohman, was located near the railroad tracks on Erwin Road. While most department faculty had offices in the Kirby Clinic, others shared the lone office on Meyer Ward or an office in the PDC, and there were no offices for the veteran residents in the neuropsychiatry program. Coordinating patient visits with record keeping and clinic staffing quickly became a logistical nightmare.[15] [Figure 5.2]

Many of these problems created additional tension among Davison, the Department of Neuropsychiatry, and the president of Duke University, Dr. Robert Flowers. As Davison later explained: "Leslie Hohman claimed that I had promised that Duke would repay him for a surplus army barrack purchased after the war and used as a temporary psychiatry office. Actually, I had told Leslie that Dr. Flowers, the president, said that Duke would repay him. Dr. Flowers did not keep his promise because he was furious because the Veterans Administration had accused the psychiatry department of charging double fees. It was a false charge but the newspaper headlines did not improve the situation."[16]

THE VA-DUKE COLLABORATION IN CLINICAL PSYCHOLOGY

Over on East Campus, the Department of Psychology more than doubled in size in 1946 when six new faculty members, and their first six graduate students (five male veterans and one woman), arrived under grants from the Clinical Psychology Section of the VA's Neuropsychiatric Division. The purpose of the program was to train Ph.D. students in clinical psychology. Both men and women were eligible for the program, veterans and nonveterans alike (with special consideration given to veterans). Trainees spent part of the four-year course in classroom work and part as government employees working in VA hospitals or mental hygiene clinics in collaboration with other professionals on the "psychiatric team." At Duke this collaboration took place both in the VA Mental Hygiene Clinic and in the Kirby Clinic. As one new clinical psychologist later recalled, the Kirby Clinic "was a place where the students in clinical psychology were able to obtain some experience in dealing with behavior problem cases."[17]

Duke's professor of clinical psychology, Dr. Donald K. Adams, led the new department section while also serving as chief clinical psychologist for the VA region that included North Carolina, Virginia, West Virginia, Maryland, and Washington, D.C.[18] The new program's most experienced clinical psychologist, Dr. Katharine M. Banham, was a specialist in child psychology (or child guidance, as it was then called). Banham, who remained at Duke until her retirement in the 1980s, later recalled that upon her arrival "the clinical section of the Psychology Department found a certain amount of opposition in the administration of the university at that time."[19] The dean of women, for example, had "a cautious attitude toward work in the clinical area of psychology work," while "the clinical psychologists were very much under observation as to whether their behavior was appropriate to the department and there were criticisms of faculty members."[20] Part of the problem, Banham believed, was Duke's denominational background: "Trinity College started as a Methodist College, with emphasis on theology." There were also the activities of Dr. Gelolo McHugh, one of the six new faculty brought in for the VA training program in clinical psychology. "He developed a self-report questionnaire which he called the 'Sex Knowledge Inventory,'" Banham noted, "and again this aroused a certain amount of questioning and apprehension in the Duke administration."[21]

Among the other psychologists recruited to Duke for the VA program in clinical psychology was Louis D. Cohen. Cohen had met Adams and Lyman in the Office of Strategic Services, working for the army as a clinical psychologist, and had initially registered as a Ph.D. student at Duke. Cohen quickly earned his degree and became a key link between the Departments of Psychology and Neuropsychiatry. He worked closely with Adams and Lyman to secure practicum facilities for training clinical psychology students in the medical school. He also took the lead in having a psychologist assigned for duty in the Department of Neuropsychiatry, in setting up the psychological services at Duke Hospital, and in initiating a pattern of joint appointments between the two departments. In 1957, after almost a decade of supporting collaborative and interdepartmental research activities within the medical school, Cohen became director of the new division of medical psychology at DUMC.[22]

This was just the kind of collaboration envisioned by the Rockefeller Foundation's Alan Gregg in supporting the VA training programs in psychiatry and psychology. His contribution to the process was applauded in 1946 by Dr. Florence Powdermaker, chief of the Psychiatric Education Section of the VA's Neuropsychiatric Division. "Your ears must be burning frequently," Powdermaker wrote to Gregg, "as we scarcely ever come together in two's or three's without quoting something that you have said that is pertinent to whatever the discussion may be. There is a deep appreciation by all of us, as you must know, for the help that you are giving us."[23]

Initially, however, there were simply too many people and too much paperwork to permit constant collaboration between the VA's training programs at Duke. What the participating faculty did share was a sense of community activism and a genuine desire to improve the mental health of all people, regardless of race, sex, age, and class. Likewise, both groups were also determined to demonstrate to the wider world that they, and those they trained, could provide valuable help to individuals and institutions. And in both departments, moreover, there was a deep interest in child psychology and in the potential of using Highland Hospital as a training facility for residents at Duke.[24]

Federal Funds and Institutional Pride

Both The Duke Endowment's Watson Rankin and Don S. Elias, owner of the *Asheville-Times Citizen* and a long-time trustee of Duke University, were at a special meeting of the North Carolina Medical Care Commission on August 8, 1946. The purpose of the meeting was to give commission members a chance to respond to a report from the National Committee for the Medical School Survey. Both the commission and the committee had been established by the General Assembly of 1945: the commission by legislation that anticipated Hill-Burton, and the committee through an amendment to legislation authorizing UNC's trustees to expand the university's medical school training to four years. As a result of the amendment, the National Committee had been charged with investigating not only the best location for the expanded school (and an affiliated teaching hospital) but also, at the insistence of Rankin, Elias, and other commission members opposed to the expansion at UNC, a study of whether North Carolina needed another four-year medical school. Although the National Committee agreed in its report that North Carolina needed to provide its people with modern medical care and hospital services, two of the committee's seven members included a "statement" in the report disagreeing with the majority's recommendation to expand the Chapel Hill school to a four-year program.[25]

The August meeting further fueled what one participant described as "a battle which raged throughout the state with considerable fervor—and sometimes with ferocity. Its effects were evident for some years following the action of the 1945 and 1947 General Assemblies, which finally passed legislation which implemented essentially all of the recommendations of the Medical Care Commission." Locally, this battle stalled the collaboration that had emerged between Duke and UNC, particularly in the health and education programs funded by the Rockefeller Foundation and the General Education Board. At the same time, the fight also fed issues and enmities that foreshadowed one of the most important events in North Carolina's modern political history: the 1950 Democratic primary for the United States Senate. Finally, in altering the relationship between Duke Medicine's inherited and emerging networks, the battle provoked an anti-Duke response among many North Carolinians that lasted for decades.

Just what was at stake in the August 8 debate was clear to the commission long before Hill-Burton passed on August 13. Under the terms of the act, which was designed to increase the nation's supply of hospital beds, especially in rural areas, North Carolina was eligible for hospital construction grants totaling some $3.5 million a year for five years beginning in 1947. Nationwide, the act authorized hospital construction grants to state agencies in the amount of $75 million a year for five years, plus $3 million a year for state surveys of hospital facilities. The guiding principle of the act, federal dollars without control, strongly appealed to most states, but especially to southern states seeking to maintain local and racial control. Hill-Burton contained a separate-but-equal provision that permitted hospitals receiving federal funds to continue existing patterns of racial segregation. It also allowed states to develop hospital plans that included segregated institutions—if, in the opinion of the state hospital-planning agency, those institutions provided adequate facilities for the population served. As the state's designated health-planning agency, the North Carolina Medical Care Commission was the conduit for federal Hill-Burton funds.[26]

OPPOSITION TO EXPANSION OF THE UNC MEDICAL SCHOOL

Rankin did not object to Hill-Burton. It reflected, in part, his own work at The Duke Endowment for the past 20 years. What bothered Rankin was the expansion plan pushed for Chapel Hill. He considered it a political move that threatened the twin pillars on which Hill-Burton—and his Hospital Section—rested: local control and small, nonprofit community hospitals. The Chapel Hill plan proposed coordinating and integrating the state's medical services through a network of local and district hospital units that would be linked together in a state-supported medical center at the top, including the proposed four-year medical school and teaching hospital at Chapel Hill. "I have some reservations with respect to the idea of centralizing influence and control over hospital activities from states through districts to local units," Rankin wrote to a hospital official in Chicago. "You, of course, can appreciate that this is a problem with many angles, because only a small per cent of our hospitals are tax built and tax supported. Most of our hospitals, as you know, represent community interest and church interest. Moreover, I confess that I have always had great respect for that principle of government that localizes in counties as compared with states and states with the nation primary responsibility and initiative."[27]

Rankin submitted a 24-page statement at the August 8 meeting "Opposing the Adoption of the Majority Report of the National Committee for the Medical School Survey." In it he challenged, with his usual eloquence and exquisite statistics, the committee's two major recommendations: that the state needed a third four-year medical school in addition to Duke and Bowman Gray, and that the school needed to be a unit of UNC and located on the campus at Chapel Hill. He then went on, in similar fashion, to attack the four major arguments "advanced from time to time" for another four-year medical school in North Carolina: that it would "more adequately provide for the indigent sick of the State," "bring about a more even distribution of physicians as between urban and rural people," "provide North Carolina boys with a place where they can obtain a medical education"; and finally, "the first, the very first, proposal of its kind ever seriously submitted as a reason or a basis for the development of a four-year medical school is [that it would] . . . *integrate* [link] the medical services of the State." Rankin's comment on the last argument was withering: "Sixty-nine medical schools in the United States and Canada, but not one ever yet organized and financed for the purpose of *integrating* the hospitals of a state or of a Canadian Province. So we are to be the guinea pig for the first experiment."[28]

What worried Rankin's fellow commissioner Don Elias was a quote attributed to Dean Davison and read at the August 8 meeting by a supporter of the Chapel Hill plan. "I gained the impression that you felt another four-year medical school was very much needed to assist in the expansion of our medical care program," Elias wrote to Davison. "I would be glad to have from you your views in the matter." Davison's quote—that "local medical schools have an important influence on the number of graduates who practice in the community and state"—had been offered in rebuttal to the central claim made by the Rankin-Elias group that "there is no evidence to support the conclusion that another medical school as such would add a single physician to the number practicing in the state." In responding to Elias, Davison said he realized his "personal opinion would be attributed to Duke rivalry, even though I am the proud possessor of an honorary degree from the University of North Carolina." As for the statement quoted in the report, it was correct; a local medical school did have an impact on the number of graduates who practice locally, Davison explained, but only if "the school can get local students. . . . Our situation is too few North Carolina students. . . . The presence of a four-year medical school in the State does not make the graduates practice there, but the number of local students, the economic situation and the availability of local hospitals are the important factors in attracting young graduates."[29]

OTHER INSTITUTIONAL CHALLENGES

A four-year medical school and teaching hospital in Chapel Hill, a new chairman of Duke's board of trustees, a new chairman of Duke's Department of Medicine, the VA residents training program at Duke, the proposed VA hospital, Hill-Burton—these were not the only turning points for Duke Medicine in 1946. There was also the decision to move Wake Forest College to Winston-Salem. The college had opened its four-year medical school there in 1941, as

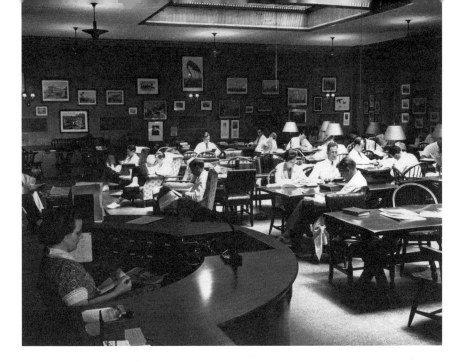

5.3 Circulation desk and patrons in the reading room of the Duke University Medical School Library, 1946. *Duke University Medical Center Archives.*

the Bowman Gray School of Medicine, and now, as one school official privately explained, "The Trustees of the Z. Smith Reynolds Foundation have this year made it advisable to move Wake Forest to Winston-Salem. . . . At present ninety percent of the institutions and the facilities of Higher Education are located in the Eastern half of North Carolina, which half includes only ten percent of the industry of our state. Our plans are to build a great Educational Center in the Western half of our state where ninety percent of its industry is located." As part of that build-up, moreover, Bowman Gray's widow now gave the medical school the manor house at her Graylyn Estate. (The house was soon turned into a psychiatric hospital at the urging of her son Gordon Gray, a graduate of UNC's Psychology Department.)[30]

It was also in 1946 that The Duke Endowment accepted a proposal from the Private Diagnostic Clinic that created financial and political problems for the next decade and a half. The deal was designed to fund construction of the private clinic and hospital addition that Hart had been promoting for the past two years and for which Davison hoped to seek partial funding from the Hill-Burton funds available to the North Carolina Medical Care Commission. As Dr. Deryl Hart explained the PDC's offer, "If The Duke Endowment would increase its proposed grants for expansion of hospital space for ambulatory patients from $600,000 to $1,000,000, the two divisions of the P.D.C. would assume responsibility for a $500,000 hospital addition for beds." The resulting agreement provided "that whenever $2 of Duke Endowment money was spent, we would be expected to put up $1 from the Development Fund. Since only $200,000 had been accumulated in the P.D.C. Development Fund, the Departments of Medicine and Surgery each agreed to loan to the Development Fund, without interest, $150,000 from their departmental funds. All departments, with the exception of one . . . doubled their percentage payments in the Development Fund . . . to continue in effect until the commitment toward this building was fulfilled." By the time construction began in 1955, however, "building costs of 1946 had at least tripled, the presidency of Duke had changed again, and the new president's policy meant less support to the Medical Center." Indeed, the PDC would need a $1 million loan from the university to meet its obligations.[31]

That Duke itself was nearing a turning point in 1946 was also suggested by a report from Jackson Davis at the General Education Board. The report brilliantly captured the growing tension between the university's traditional regional commitments to North Carolina and the South and its wider goal of achieving "a place of real leadership in the educational world," as stated in James B. Duke's indenture. "Duke is more like a Northern University than any other [I] visited," Davis wrote in his "Report on a Visit to Southern Institutions." "The interest in scholarly work and research is conspicuous. The faculty that I saw seemed to be primarily interested in fundamental questions and in broad national or international as opposed to regional or local problems." Davis considered this focus "a natural state of affairs among men of high standing in their fields. It is a state not to be overlooked in efforts to build up southern Universities to positions of leadership. The more outstanding they and their faculties become the less likely they will preoccupy themselves with purely regional and local problems unless work on these problems is the means to national reputations." Jackson considered Duke "one of the few outstanding universities in the South" and in possession of "a better foundation to build upon than most other universities of the South."[32] [Figure 5.3]

There were shortcomings, to be sure. Duke appeared to have "entirely too meager resources for research. Small grants predominate and no large projects came to my attention. It seemed to me that to organize research here in an institute to deal with Southern problems, as one might well do at the University of North Carolina, would be a mistake. A more fruitful method at Duke would be to underwrite specific projects for designated men or groups of men. Such arrangements would be less likely to divert the school from its chosen course and would be more compatable [*sic*] with its own conception of a university as an aggregation of great scholars pursuing fundamental research and teaching."[33]

Wilburt Davison was neither a great scholar nor pursuing fundamental research. He was, however, a great teacher and a strong supporter of Duke's collaboration with UNC in health programs funded by the General Education Board and the Rockefeller Foundation. That's why he was now among "a selected group" of some 20 individuals who gathered at the North Carolina College (for Negroes) in Durham, on November 7, 1946, for a discussion of Hill-Burton's potential impact on the college. The only woman at the meeting was the director of UNC's Department of Public Health Education, Dr. Lucy Shields Morgan, who for the past year had been directing a small group of public health students at the North Carolina College. Most of the state's leading black educators were also at the meeting, as were the president of the state's black medical society and the superintendent of Durham's Lincoln Hospital, the black hospital located near the college. In addition to Davison the white men at the meeting included Dr. Nathan C. Newbold, head of the state's Division of Negro Education, and Dr. George M. Cooper of the North Carolina State Board of Health.[34]

In his opening remarks to the meeting, the president of the college, Dr. James E. Shepard, noted that the meeting had been called "to discuss the present facilities and services of the health education program and to discuss the future needs of the health program of the North Carolina College." The statistics Shepard offered were sadly familiar to most of his listeners. "In 1940 there was one public health nurse for every 7,947 white persons of North Carolina, and in 1940 there was one nurse for every 32,303 Negroes. There are 54 counties in the state which have no hospitalization facilities for Negroes." Shepard wanted "the college to serve the State and the colored people of the State in a health program," and he asked the meeting's participants to "discuss all phases of the situation frankly and tell him what can be done and what ought to be done for the people of North Carolina and the other Southern states."

At the top of Shepard's own wish list was a new student infirmary for the college. "The General Education Board has given $20,000 for the equipment of an infirmary," he explained; "it is not known what the Legislature will do, but it has been requested to appropriate $100,000 for the erection of the infirmary." Shepard also noted that he had been instructed by the school's board of trustees—whose chairman, Dr. Robert Flowers, was also president of Duke University—"to continue plans for the establishment of a Department of Public Health Nursing" at the college. In fact, Shepard noted proudly, the National Nursing Association had just approved his nominee to head the program and "plans for the school will be released to the public as soon as they have been perfected."

Dr. Lucy Morgan then summarized the first year of Public Health Education at the black college. Ten students—seven from North Carolina and three from Mississippi—had taken the public health courses, and while only one scholarship had initially been offered by the State Board of Health, by the end of 1945 the school had secured General Education Board Scholarships for three other students from North Carolina. "This fall," said Dr. Morgan, "we are continuing with instructors from the University, guest speakers from all over the country. New Orleans, Louisiana sent a young man. We have G.I.'s enrolled—6 men and 5 women. We have only two young women who have not been placed, and we hope to place them soon."

The most important presentation of the evening was made by William Rich, the superintendent of Lincoln Hospital. Rich was chairman of the Medical Training for Negroes committee of the North Carolina Medical Care Commission, and he had plenty of ideas and plans for public health education at the college. To Shepard's earlier point on the availability of public health nurses, Rich now added the fact that only 149 black doctors were practicing in the state, "when according to population, there should be between 800 and 1,000." More telling still, the nation's two major black medical schools, Howard University Medical School and the Meharry Medical School, "have a waiting list of 1,200 and can admit only 150 students. What will happen to the 1,050 who desire to enter medical schools?" Rich asked. "Those problems are very serious and demand attention. In addition, we have 5 Negro hospitals with training schools for nursing. It is difficult to secure well trained superintendents, instructors, and directors of nursing education, because most well prepared persons in this field remain in the north and east, because of salaries."

Rich then reached the crux of his presentation. He was drafting a report in response to the recommendations made by the National Committee for the Medical School Survey and the North Carolina Medical Care Commission. The report would emphasize "the real need we have for training of medical post graduate and graduate students. Where can Negroes go for internship, residencies?" Rich asked. Then answered: "New York, Philadelphia, Detroit; they are lost to North Carolina. Facilities must be provided in North Carolina for the training of medical students and for post-graduate education. I have recommended that the State provide one school on the college level for Negro students and one good three-year nursing school, consolidating all facilities of the different schools into one excellent school." The National Committee had recognized "the great need" for such a school, Rich stressed, but its members "did not have a great deal" more to say about it in their report. "They are very much interested in Public Health Centers. I am interested in knowing what support a program of affiliation with the medical school of the University of

North Carolina would receive from the Government. Dr. Parran is very much interested in public health. Recently the Government gave Mr. Dent of Flint-Goodrich Hospital of New Orleans money for experimental work."

Davison sat quietly as Shepard asked Rich why North Carolina College "could not get some of that money." The week had not been an easy one for the dean. Robert Lambert had visited him, at Mrs. Hanes's request, to see what might be done to maintain her husband's interest in neurology at Duke. At the same time, Davison and Rankin had been publicly criticized for their opposition to the health plan of the North Carolina Medical Care Commission. In comments quoted in the local press, the president of the State Medical Society, Dr. William M. Coppridge of Durham, had asked the organizational meeting of the North Carolina Good Health Association: "Why should representatives of the Duke Endowment and Duke University find fault with a plan designed to spread better medical care over this State and impose upon the State university the duty of training more North Carolina citizens in the arts and sciences of medical care? Is their opposition to this program motivated by a sincere desire to promote better medical care among the people of North Carolina?"[35]

And now Rich and Shepard were promoting what? A big black medical center at North Carolina College? One that would be affiliated with the proposed four-year medical school at Chapel Hill? Although Davison had worked with Shepard for almost 20 years, he had also been given much of Shepard's financial power in the reorganization of Lincoln Hospital a decade earlier; indeed, the wounds from that battle had still not healed. As for Rich, the young black businessman brought in to superintend Lincoln's reorganization, he was held in "very high esteem" by blacks and whites, including Davison, Rankin, and Lambert.[36]

"As I listened to the discussion," Davison told the meeting, "several problems occurred to me: Health Education, in which I am tremendously interested, was the first." Davison considered it useless to build more facilities when those that existed were not fully utilized. "North Carolina," he told the group, "with its many clinics, and the like has the 38th highest infant mortality rate in the nation. We have facilities but do not use them. We need *public* health education." In other words, he believed that Shepard's college needed to educate the public on the health care already available. It needed to mobilize existing funds "for education in the field of public health, such as maternity clinics, and the like. Jobs can be created in the Department of Health to employ people trained in college here." And while training personnel was "very important," he said, he also warned that a "School of Nursing is a pretty expensive and complicated thing. The training at the University of Virginia, which can accommodate the largest number of students, is not utilized fully." Rather than build a nursing school, Davison advised sending students to existing schools, to "provide money for fellowships for students from this State." He also argued that "a college infirmary is a waste of money. We have from 20 to 100 beds empty, certainly 50% of the time, in the infirmary provided for women students at Duke University." And with that Davison turned to Shepard and said: "The problem here seems to me to persuade Mr. Rich to operate [the college infirmary] with you on a contract basis."[37]

Dr. George Cooper had been waiting to hear what the voice of Duke had to say. "The Children's Bureau is ready to aid, with funds," he announced, "any program which meets its approval, for the improvement of the health program, as it relates to North Carolina College. . . . What is the program you recommend for the training school for Nurses?" he asked Rich. "A Nurse Training School," Rich responded, "on the college level, located in North Carolina, affiliated with the Lincoln Hospital, or some good hospital." "I think the Children's Bureau could endorse that," Cooper said and then departed. Davison had essentially been overridden. The meeting went on for a good while longer, until Shepard finally appointed Davison and several others to a committee, chaired by Morgan, "to work out an all-inclusive program" for public health education at the North Carolina College.

THE POWER OF COMMITTEE AND FOUNDATION CONNECTIONS

Davison now began to stumble through a series of humbling developments, most of which were not of his own making. On the most basic level, he faced an end to the hospital and health care monopoly that Duke Medicine had inherited through its private business and philanthropic networks. Aggressive state elites now yearned to compete, using private, local, state, and federal funding. So determined were they to prevail, in fact, that they formed a public relations organization, the North Carolina Good Health Association, to mobilize voters behind the recommendations of the North Carolina Medical Care Commission. The campaign included band leaders and movie stars, with radio spots and newspaper ads, as the association blitzed the state in preparation for the 1947 session of the General Assembly.[38]

Equally portentous of the dean's changing status was Dr. Eugene Stead's handling of Dr. Walter Kempner. As Lambert learned in mid-December, the new head of Medicine at Duke "had decided to observe K[empner] for a year before deciding whether to ask him to leave Duke, as Davison and others wanted to do now. Mrs. Hanes, who cordially dislikes Kempner as a person— his Germanic manner *is* most irritating—felt that Stead was right in not taking immediate action, being convinced that K. has something. The basis of an ouster would be, 1) K's secrecy with case histories—a traditional Germanic characteristic; 2) excessive money-making—incompatible with a wholesome academic atmosphere. Mrs. Hanes adds a third, in the jealousy of less prosperous colleagues."[39]

As Stead soon discovered, however, Davison's networks ran deep and wide. The dean controlled DUMC's most important committees and chaired its most powerful body, the Executive Committee of the Schools of Medicine, Nursing, and Health Services, and the Duke Hospital. The executive committee consisted of the deans of the Schools of Medicine and Nursing, the superintendent of the hospital, the department heads, and, in rotation, four other faculty members (from the schools of nursing and medicine). The executive committee was "subject to the President, Vice-President, Comptroller and Trustees" of Duke University and it met "once each month or oftener if necessary," Davison explained. "All school policies and inter-departmental questions are decided there and anything which requires the action of the Trustees is transmitted to the Vice-President of the University." Finally, in addition to the executive committee, Davison also chaired the administrative committee for the hospital and the administrative committee for the School of Nursing, where, on October 1, 1946, Miss Florence K. Wilson became the new dean.[40] [Figure 5.4]

Further empowering the dean was his relationship with Doris Duke and her foundation, Independent Aid, Inc. Davison became a director of the foundation in January 1947, at a time when he was the university's strongest link to Doris Duke. Davison had been her friend and surrogate father for almost two decades, seeing Duke through the loss of her day-old daughter, Arden, in 1940, and then through the Reno divorce from her husband, James Cromwell, in 1943. The following year Davison had arranged a job for her at UNC, where she briefly did research on tropical diseases in the School of Public Health, and he had also escorted her to Georgia, to the docks of the J. A. Jones Construction Company, for the christening of the *James B. Duke*, the Liberty ship named in honor of her father.

Davison and Doris Duke corresponded directly with each other about grants, haggling over details. "I am back in New York until after Christmas," Doris Duke wrote to Davison in November 1946, "and hope to get the Independent Aid budget—among other things—straightened out for the coming year. You will recall, that in 1945, Duke took over half of the budget of the Medical Social Service Unit, thus lowering Independent Aid's contribution to the work there to $7,500. In the spring of 1946, you again applied for $15,000 since the program had completely outgrown the facilities. That amount was allowed for the current year with the understanding that for the year 1947 Duke might properly assume responsibility for $7,500.00, so that the contribution of Independent Aid could again be reduced to $7,500.00. I hope that it will be possible for Duke Hospital to work this out." Well, yes, Davi-

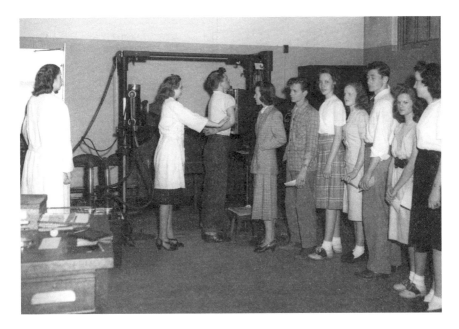

5.4 Members of Duke Hospital's nursing staff using portable x-ray equipment during a community clinic. *Duke University Medical Center Archives.*

son replied, "the reason I asked for $15,000 for the Medical Social Service Unit was because the work had trebled and we needed a total of $23,402.50. This amount was financed by the $15,000 from Independent Aid, $7,500 from Duke University, and from an unexpended balance from the previous year. Would it be possible to obtain $15,000 from Independent Aid for next year so that we could continue the program on the same basis?"[41]

It was through Doris Duke and her foundation that DUMC linked Durham and the state of North Carolina with some of the strongest, most progressive social welfare networks in the nation. One of the key connections was Miss Duke's earliest and dearest friend, Aleta Morris MacDonald, or "Leta," as she was called, the daughter of Lewis Gouverneur Morris. In December of 1946, she was elected to the board of Independent Aid along with Clarence Pickett, executive secretary of the American Friends Service Committee, and Sophie Van Theis, executive secretary for the past 30 years of the Child Adoption Committee of the State Charities Aid Committee of New York. At the same time, Independent Aid's networks also ran through MacDonald's husband, Byrnes MacDonald, a Catholic activist who served in the administration of New York City mayor Fiorello H. LaGuardia before the war and later worked for the Sinclair Oil Company.[42]

The Independent Aid director most intimately involved with Duke Medicine, Marian Paschal, had recently died, ending almost a decade of work

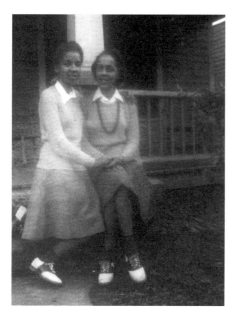

5.5 Clementine Amey, left, and Harriett Amey. *Doris Duke Charitable Foundation Archives.*

with Doris Duke, Davison, and the Department of Social Services at DUMC. Paschal had helped create the department in 1937, with funding from Independent Aid, and since that time, she had supported the department's aggressive outreach to public health and welfare agencies, to private family and childcare groups, and to religious, civic, and professional organizations on the local, state, and national level. Department personnel, many of whom Paschal recommended for their positions, were also assisting in medical studies on premature infants, helping unmarried mothers, and facilitating follow-up visits for syphilis patients. By demonstrating, moreover, what its personnel could do, the department was receiving numerous requests from state and local agencies for trained medical social workers. By 1946, the department's staff was playing "an active part in the progress of the Durham Social Planning Council" and sitting "on various committees and boards within the community and State, including the Durham County Association for the Blind, the Durham Children's Museum, the advisory cabinet of the Y.W.C.A. of the Woman's College of Duke University, the North Carolina League of Crippled Children, and the State Conference for Social Service."[43]

Paschal's most personal contribution to Duke Medicine was her interest in the education of Harriett and Clementine Amey, the daughters of North Carolina College business manager, Charles C. Amey. Paschal first heard about the girls during their father's fundraising visits to Independent Aid in New York; eventually, she exchanged Christmas cards and letters with them and developed a special interest in Harriett's training in medical social work at Boston University. Although Paschal died before Amey completed her training, she would have enjoyed seeing the young black woman cross the color line at Duke. In the spring of 1947, with a salary arranged by the Federal Security Agency in Washington, D.C., and Dr. George M. Cooper of the North Carolina State Board of Health, Amey was appointed to the staff of the Department of Social Services—the "first Negro worker" to hold a staff position at Duke University. [Figure 5.5]

Trustee Activism

In January 1947, as Davison prepared for his first meeting as a director of Independent Aid, Paschal's successor, Georgea T. Furst, received a 33-page report titled "A Suggested Plan for a Total Health Program at North Carolina College for Negroes." Furst wrote Davison for more information. "Dr. Shepard has sent me a report prepared by Dr. Lucy Morgan, head of the Department of Public Health Education at the University of North Carolina. This report outlines a plan for establishing a public health center and infirmary and a school of public health education," Furst explained. "It also includes the program for public health nursing and a school of social work. Dr. Shepard states that he has not fully gone into the costs of such a program or other details. However, he is sure that a great deal of money would be necessary to put through such a program. He states that he is certain that he could secure support for this program from the State Legislature if he could be assured that this organization [Independent Aid] and the General Education Board had given it their approval." The scope of Shepard's plan surprised Furst. It was "one of far greater magnitude than that about which he wrote us late in December," she wrote to Davison. "At that time he was asking only for assistance in setting up a school of social work." Furst hoped that Davison would "discuss the whole matter with the other members of the Board at the meeting on Friday."[44]

Shepard's plan was also part of the larger health care debate confronting the North Carolina Medical Care Commission as the state legislature prepared for the final hearing on the proposed expansion of UNC's medical school. To Duke trustee Don Elias the debate was critical, making him muster everything he had to get out of bed and over to the airport to catch his flight out of Asheville. Despite a painful infection in his trachea and lymph glands, the 58-year-old newspaper publisher was determined to join The Duke Endowment's Watson Rankin in Raleigh for testimony before the General Assembly's Joint Appropriations Committee.

The legislative chamber was packed for the February 13 hearing. The session was the last for public debate on the program recommended by the Medical Care Commission, and Rankin and Elias repeated their earlier arguments against expanding the two-year medical school of the University at Chapel Hill: the state did not need another four-year medical school, and if it insisted on having one, the school and its hospital should be located in an urban center like Charlotte or Greensboro and not in the village of Chapel Hill. But their arguments were rebuffed by the program's leading proponent, Major L. P. McLendon of Greensboro; he "expressed the gratitude of North Carolina to the Duke Endowment for its generous support of hospital construction and care of the indigent, but he also pointed out that no individual and no organization had—or should have—the power to tell the state of North Carolina what it should or should not do for the education or medical care of its citizens." According to the dean of UNC's medical school, many observers believed that "the statement and forthright manner of Mr. McLendon was the highlight of the afternoon's hearings."[45]

Don Elias returned to Asheville and crawled back into bed, where he was still confined a week later when he wrote to his fellow Duke trustee, Willis Smith, on another project dear to his heart: "I hope very much to be out next week and be at the Trustees' meeting as I want to talk with you and assist with things that you and I know need attention, but at the moment I can't make any predictions."[46] Elias and Smith had been talking for months with another trustee, Edwin L. Jones Sr. of Charlotte, about the "things" that needed attention at Duke. First and foremost were the retirements of the university's beloved president, Dr. Robert L. Flowers, and its popular vice president, William H. Wannamaker. Their curtain call had to be slow and graceful, however, with plenty of heartfelt applause and genuine respect for their years of leadership and devotion to both Trinity College and Duke University.

Needing more immediate attention was Jones's plan to "develop a notable research institute on the Duke campus." The plan was one of many being hatched by North Carolina's colleges and universities for taking advantage of the transformation of government-sponsored research that had emerged from World War II. In this case, the Davey Compressor Company of Kent, Ohio, had approached Jones about its interest in funding such an institute, and Jones, fresh from his Oak Ridge success on the Manhattan Project, was eager to promote the study and development of nuclear physics in the South. Jones envisioned two parts to the institute at Duke, a "greatly enlarged Physics Department" and a major "Research Laboratory" that would be "properly staffed, equipped, and managed" and that would serve "the industries of this section, such as Textiles, Tobacco, Chemicals, Woodworking, etc." Smith immediately arranged for the chairman of the Department of Physics, Dr. Walter Nielsen, to be put on the agenda for the trustees' semiannual meeting on February 27, 1947.[47]

WILLIS SMITH'S VISION FOR DUKE

The February meeting marked the emergence of a new vision of who should rule at Duke, in what ways, and for what purposes. Put simply, Willis Smith intended to reshape the way the university operated and was governed. He wanted less control by the Endowment trustees at 30 Rockefeller Plaza and more input from the trustees and alumni in North Carolina. He wanted to centralize the university's fiscal and administrative operations and to make them more efficient and consistent throughout the institution. And most important of all, he wanted to improve Duke's image within the state by recruiting and accepting more North Carolina students to the university, especially to its medical school. Smith was targeting, in fact, many of the things that had enabled Davison and Duke Medicine to flourish at the expense of the rest of the university. Davison and Duke Medicine derived their power from Duke's national corporate and political networks and, together with The Duke Endowment, were leading the opposition to the largest, most significant state health care plan in history. Duke Medicine also consumed half of the university's annual income from endowment, yet Duke Hospital was still running a deficit.

Smith's vision for Duke was deeply affected by his political ambitions and loyalties. He put politics and the Democratic Party above any sentimental sense of being "True Blue." He had encouraged the state's governor, R. Gregg Cherry, a fellow graduate of Trinity College and Trinity law school, to enter politics, and then had used that network in his own race for the speakership of the state house of representatives. Smith had twice considered running for governor but chose instead to work closely with the Cherry campaign and its manager, William B. Umstead. Umstead was also a graduate of Trinity law school, like Smith and Cherry, but unlike them, he was a graduate and trustee of UNC and had deep personal and professional connections with the Duke family and their business networks.

Smith and Umstead were associated with different wings of the state's Democratic Party: Smith was part of the liberal wing of the party, which was centered in Raleigh, while Umstead (like Cherry and Elias) belonged to the conservative faction. After three consecutive terms representing North Carolina's Sixth District in the U.S. House, Umstead had retired voluntarily in 1939 to resume his law practice in Durham. Yet ever since Cherry's victory, one newspaper reported, Umstead "had been regarded as a certain candidate for the Democratic gubernatorial nomination in 1948." Certain, that is, until December 17, 1946, when Cherry appointed him to the seat left vacant by the death of United States senator Josiah W. Bailey, one of Duke University's most loyal supporters. For Smith, the governor's office seemed his for the taking.[48]

North Carolina politics had reached a turning point, in fact, by the time the Duke trustees met in late February 1947. On February 7, the state's most powerful politician, former governor O. Max Gardner, died as he was about to embark for London as the new United States ambassador to Great Britain. For most of the trustees at the meeting, his death deepened the already intense political discussions occasioned by the current session of the biennial legislature and the upcoming vote on the program proposed by the North Carolina Medical Care Commission. Whether the Duke trustees officially discussed the program is not clear, but what happened next certainly bore the stamp of the Duke networks in action.

On March 10, a bill was introduced into the legislature calling for the establishment of a two-year medical school at the North Carolina College for Negroes in Durham. The bill's timing coincided with what one newspaper reported as the scheduled deliberations of the Joint Appropriations Committee "to consider the establishing of a four-year medical school at the University of North Carolina at Chapel Hill." Though the bill's author asked that it be placed before the appropriations committee, the speaker of the house passed it on to the education committee, where it died.[49] One week later, however, the legislature approved, without debate, the recommendations of the North Carolina Medical Care Commission. The denouement was described by the Raleigh *News & Observer*: "During the past ten days Governor Cherry, who had been regarded as lukewarm to the proposal, is reported to have swung his support squarely behind it. Cherry's move was believed largely responsible for the ease with which it passed the Committee."[50]

Local Politics and Its Repercussions

Among the repercussions of the approval of the UNC program was another crisis for psychiatry at Duke. Dr. Richard Lyman had grown impatient waiting for Duke to commit future funding for the Department of Neuropsychiatry, and frankly, too, so had Robert Lambert and Alan Gregg at the Rockefeller Foundation.[51] In March, Lyman presented the university with an ultimatum: provide at least $50,000 a year to the department or he was gone. Lyman saw two possible paths for the department to follow. One led back to Hanes's vision, "which consisted of *diagnosis* and *consultations without facilities for treatment*, with inadequate beds and very poor arrangements for any therapy other than electric shock and few other related procedures with some psychotic patients." The other route was to "pool our efforts chiefly with the extramural interests of mental health, the Veterans, possibly also the U.S. Public Health and other related agencies. . . . I do not see how the limitations of space, staff and money can permit both to be developed well." And on top of that, Lyman continued, with "Bowman Gray developing . . . and with the UNC medical school in the offing, it may be pertinent to wonder how Duke will be oriented as time goes on." While "hostile competition" from Bowman Gray appeared unlikely, that was not the case with Duke's Chapel Hill neighbor. "The UNC is by heritage and current interests the place where community and state interests in psychiatry should logically be fostered. They have an inside track which even a Governor with a Duke degree could not displace."[52]

That Duke quickly agreed to fund the Department of Neuropsychiatry after the Rockefeller grant ended appears closely related to the announcement on April 14 that staffing was now complete for the new Durham Child Guidance Clinic. The announcement was made by the clinic's president, W. M. Jenkins, who was also superintendent of the Durham County Schools. Jenkins told reporters "that through the cooperation of the Duke Medical School, the Duke Psychology Department and the Duke Hospital the services of three psychiatrists, one clinical psychologist and one pediatrician have been secured for the clinic." The clinic's psychiatry section was headed by Dr. Maurice Greenhill and included two of his junior colleagues in the Department of Neuropsychiatry; the clinic's psychologist was Dr. Katharine Banham of the Department of Psychology; and the clinic's pediatrician was one of Davison's favorite students, Dr. H. Grant Taylor, associate professor of pediatrics at Duke Medical School. Located on the third floor of the City-County Health Building in downtown Durham, the clinic soon opened under the guidance of a full-time psychiatric social worker, who also served as the center's executive secretary.[53]

Few of DUMC's local networks were more progressive and persistent than those connected with the development of the Durham Child Guidance Clinic. The clinic owed its origins to Durham's Junior League. One of its members, Estelle Markin Greenhill, and her husband, Dr. Maurice Greenhill, helped mobilize DUMC's Department of Social Services to work not only with the Junior League but also with Durham's Social Planning Council. The Junior League provided almost all of the funding for the clinic during its first two years of operation; eventually the clinic became a member of the Community Chest, receiving funding from that agency (and its successor, the United Fund), as well as from the city and county schools and the Public Mental Health Act, which provided grants for the training of students in clinical psychology. In addition to treating emotionally disturbed children and their families, the Durham Child Guidance Clinic also assisted other community agencies in the social, medical, and educational fields and helped train psychiatric residents at Duke as well as students in social work and psychology at Duke and UNC.[54]

Along with the new clinic and the new university funding, a grant from the United States Public Heath Service helped reinvigorate the Department of Neuropsychiatry's already considerable commitment to the Rockefeller Foundation's goals of interdisciplinary studies, psychosomatic medicine, and community activism. In addition to his colleagues in the Psychology Department, Lyman collaborated with several members of the Departments of Anthropology and Sociology. One such partnership was with the anthropologist Dr. Weston La Barre, whose wife, Maurine Boie La Barre, was a psychiatric social worker; she became executive secretary of the Durham Child Guidance Clinic in 1948 and later joined DUMC's psychiatry faculty in the division of child and adolescents.[55]

Like the La Barres, the Lymans and the Greenhills had marriages that brought together physician and medical social worker. Katherine Ham Lyman had volunteered in the Department of Social Services upon her arrival at Duke in 1941, taking responsibility for the social work in the children's syphilis clinic; in 1942, she was hired as the psychiatric social worker assigned to the Department of Neuropsychiatry. Estelle Greenhill arrived in Durham having completed her studies in medical social work at the University of Chicago; after briefly working with the Department of Social Services and the Junior League, she secured League funding for a campus nursery school and child study laboratory.[56]

The busiest nexus of Duke's new mental health networks was Dr. Maurice Greenhill. In 1944, while linking Duke to the VA through the Duke Rehabilitation Clinic in Durham, Greenhill had become the first psychiatric consultant appointed to the North Carolina State Board of Charities and Public Welfare in Raleigh. In 1946, he established the veterans neuropsychiatry training program at Duke, and, with the arrival of Dr. Eugene Stead at DUMC and the cooperation of the division of physical therapy, he organized a psychosomatic service to teach the psychosomatic aspects of medicine throughout the medical school and hospital.

SEGREGATION AT DUKE

It was Lyman, chairman of Neuropsychiatry, who pushed most aggressively to reform racial segregation both at DUMC and in Durham. He worked within the context of local racial cooperation, of course, which encompassed decades of close collaboration between the Duke family and Durham's black leadership. He also worked in one of the most integrated of the nation's segregated medical centers, and with one of the best black hospitals in the South. Unlike Durham's other two hospitals—the whites-only Watts Hospital and the blacks-only Lincoln Hospital—Duke Hospital admitted both white and black patients, but it then segregated them onto wards by service, sex, and race. Black physicians lacked admitting privileges at Duke Hospital, where all of the nurses, all of the medical students, and all of the faculty were white and generally segregated themselves by sex, service, and profession. Yet the color lines at Duke Hospital were of a peculiar kind. White physicians always cared for black patients, as did white nurses, while black housekeepers, orderlies, and assistants moved through and about every area of the hospital—except that they changed clothes in their segregated dressing rooms in the basement. [Figure 5.6]

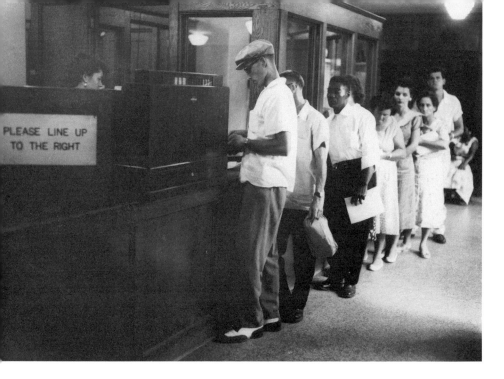

PLEASE LINE UP
TO THE RIGHT

5.6 The color lines were constantly shifting within Duke Hospital. Here, customers wait in line at the cashier's window. *Duke University Medical Center Archives.*

Lyman also had the luxury of pushing for racial reform within the most liberal local area in the American South—a place where, at least until then, public and private institutions had collaborated with state, local, and federal agencies to create health and education networks among Duke, UNC, the North Carolina College for Negroes, and Lincoln Hospital. While Chapel Hill had the largest collection of liberals around, and certainly the most celebrated ones in the South, those at Duke, especially in DUMC, lived their liberalism quietly: as in the first racially integrated college-level basketball game in the South, a secret 1944 contest between the regulars of the North Carolina College Eagles and a team of white medical students from Duke; as in the numerous Duke physicians who had worked regularly at the Lincoln Hospital since the mid-1930s; as in the hiring of Harriett Amey by the Department of Social Services; as in the training program Duke was about to start for black practical nurses; and as in "the fear that publicizing the hospital policy of upgrading Negroes would cause some wealthy donors to withdraw their support" for Duke University.[57]

Lyman had shown no such fear in an address to the Junior League on the "psychiatric problems among negroes of Durham." He began his presentation by saying that he knew of "very few places in Durham where psychiatric interests have been developed for negroes. . . . All the major clinical services at Duke have space allocated to negroes on wards except psychiatry. Medicine, surgery, obstetrics and gynecology, and pediatrics all have beds for negroes. There are no neuropsychiatric beds for negroes." Lyman considered this unacceptable: "I could not be satisfied to work anywhere in this country with such a gap in service to the community," he declared. "Accordingly, I have set out to fill the gap another way:—namely, by trying to build up some little negro psychiatry which does not require hospitalization on a psychiatric ward."[58]

Lyman then reviewed the "start" that had been made in "training a few persons interested in negro psychiatric problems" and in locating "enough patients to provide the training and to give some background of experience necessary to go on in this field." Lyman had worked so far with four black "collaborators," three women and one man, and was now planning "part-time contacts" to train another black woman who worked at the Lincoln Hospital. As for the future of black mental health professionals, Lyman ventured that it would "be carried out at least in part by the negroes, but not necessarily by negro doctors of medicine." He acknowledged that black physicians already had too much "pressure" from other work while "the lack of good financial return from most mental patients will discourage turning to psychiatry as a specialty." But he believed that his "lucky start here at Duke was just a sign of the way the wind [was] blowing on this whole subject. . . . Collaboration of white interests with negro workers . . . may very well give a significant incentive to the development of an organized Negro Psychiatry, to be taken over more and more by negroes as time goes on."

Davison as Candidate for the Presidency of Duke

At the same time that Duke's mental health community was mobilizing around desegregation, Dean Davison made a decision that he described in his *Reminiscences*. "In the spring of 1947," he wrote, "the medical school and hospital were running smoothly, and I finally became bored with dictating hundreds of useless letters (the average was one hundred and fifty per week), and attending three or more intra- and extra-state medical and committee meetings, so I planned to retire on my sixtieth birthday in 1952. I actually wrote my resignation on the 17th of April, 1947."[59]

Things were not running smoothly, of course, and Davison did not write his resignation because he was bored. He wrote it in anticipation of becoming the next president of Duke University—a matter not mentioned in his *Reminiscences*. During this critical period in the history of Duke University, Davison in fact received vigorous support for his candidacy from The Duke Endowment officers who wanted to control the university from 30 Rockefeller

Plaza. These men—George Allen and Alexander Sands—in addition to running the Endowment, also sat with their fellow Endowment trustee, William Neal Reynolds of Winston-Salem, on the seven-member executive committee of the university's board of trustees.

By 1947, the New York trustees considered the 55-year-old Davison the best man to replace president Robert L. Flowers at the center of the Duke's progressive health and education networks. Flowers, the son of a Trinity trustee, had graduated from the United States Naval Academy before joining the faculty of Trinity College in 1891 as a professor of mathematics. He had become secretary-treasurer and vice president for finance of the new Duke University in 1924; a trustee of The Duke Endowment in 1926; the Durham representative of Benjamin N. Duke and his family; and in 1941, the second president of Duke University. Through these connections, moreover, Flowers had maintained valuable networks as chairman of the board of trustees of North Carolina College, as a member of the board of trustees of Lincoln Hospital, and as a local leader with close ties to both the Liggett & Myers Tobacco Company and the city and county boards of education. By 1947, the 77-year-old Flowers controlled access to The Duke Endowment for all of Duke University, for the North Carolina College, for Lincoln Hospital, and for most of North Carolina. Indeed, through his state political connections Flowers, together with his son-in-law, Dr. Lenox D. Baker, an orthopedic surgeon at Duke, secured state funding for the North Carolina Hospital for Cerebral Palsy, construction of which began in 1948 on land donated by Duke.

If Davison lacked many of Flowers's connections, that feature appeared an asset to the group in New York. The dean's attachment to North Carolina was still more professional than personal, and his perspective on Duke mirrored that of 30 Rockefeller Plaza. It went on beyond Durham and North Carolina to embrace Washington, New York, and the wider world. Nor did the dean have any of Flowers's deep (and frequently inconvenient) attachments to the traditions and alumni of Trinity College. In particular, Davison ignored Duke's long association with rich Methodists and the poor Methodist Church; though a product of the Methodist parsonage himself, he saw little or no role for religion in his life and even less of a place for it on campus.

Davison ran DUMC as both a businessman and a missionary. He used the wealth and power of the corporate hand to extend the healing touch as far as possible. And to himself and his many supporters, both in New York and at Duke, the dean was still pioneering the Endowment's mission of providing well-trained general practitioners on the southern frontier. He had directed the selection of DUMC's original faculty, he had established its library, supervised the construction of its buildings, and kept it running through the Great Depression and the Second World War, all the while building its reputation as one of the leading medical facilities in the southeastern United States. To those who liked Davison, the university presidency seemed a fitting reward for his 20 years of dedicated service. As two of Davison's former students later wrote, "While he was dean of the School of Medicine, Duke was Davison and Davison was Duke."[60]

Davison continued to cultivate this loyalty during the second reunion of medical school alumni, April 24–26, 1947. The reunion was an important catalyst in creating the network of medical alumni that soon emerged as one of Duke Medicine's most important assets. Seven years had passed since the first such reunion, and now, some 300 medical alumni and 150 spouses attended professional presentations and mock clinics, a dinner-dance, and parties for the 65th General Hospital and other medical units that had served the country during the war. There was also the traditional beer and barbecue at Josh Turnage's restaurant, Davison's favorite local haunt, and an announcement that surprised many of the alumni: that they had commissioned a portrait of "the Dean" to be painted in early August.[61] [Figure 5.7]

Unfortunately, the entire celebration was marred by a series of mysterious fires and assaults at the hospital. Firemen and hospital workers "raced frantically from one end of the building to the other" extinguishing seven different fires on the day before the reunion began, and in nearby Duke Gardens, an unidentified assailant shot and injured a hospital nurse before robbing her male companion, a medical student from Texas. Early Saturday morning, moreover, on April 26, a nurse on the maternity ward followed the smell of smoke to the vast hospital attic where an unidentified man punched her in the face and then fled as she called for help. The workers who answered her call managed to extinguish the blaze and, according to a hospital spokesman, "the fires caused 'no real damage,' except to destroy some 10,000 x-ray films in the hospital's invaluable collection." Although observers "generally agreed the fires were an 'inside job' by someone familiar with the big, rambling hospital," the case was still under investigation a month later when yet another fire destroyed even more records. Yet no one, it seems, was ever caught and charged with arson.[62]

Willis Smith's Challenges to the Status Quo

In the meantime, Willis Smith moved firmly and strategically to implement the changes he envisioned for Duke, and this did not include installing Davison as the university's president. Smith's first move was a simple one; he sent the trustees a memo asking them to suggest individuals to fill vacancies on the university's board of trustees. Smith also asked Professor Calvin Hoover to evaluate his proposal for recruiting more North Caro-

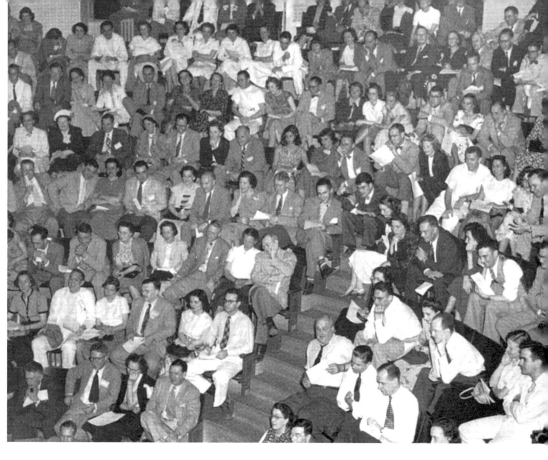

5.7 Duke University Medical School alumni reunion, April 27, 1950. The amphitheater is crowded for a mock clinic given by the medical students. *Duke University Medical Center Archives*.

lina students to Duke. Hoover wrote Smith that the "proposal that students from North Carolina continue to be charged the present rate of tuition while tuition be increased for out-of-state students appears to be both feasible and desirable. . . . While it is undoubtedly a matter for congratulation that Duke University draws its student body from the entire nation rather than from the local area alone, it is of first importance that we not lose our roots in the South and particularly our roots in North Carolina."[63]

Smith also used the local-student issue to launch his wider campaign to integrate the medical center more closely with the rest of the university. In suggesting in particular that the School of Medicine accept more North Carolina students, Smith elicited a positive response that reinforced his point. One trustee, a Methodist minister from Rocky Mount, wrote: "I am delighted to be associated with you in attempting to make Duke realize some of our dreams. Your statement before the Board of Trustees concerning admissions to the Medical School found an enthusiastic response in my own heart." (The minister's twin daughters had applied to the medical school a decade earlier, and though their applications were not denied, they were not well treated and went to another medical school, where they graduated in the upper third of their class. "I am proud of their records," the trustee wrote, "but it will always be an unpleasant memory to know that their applications were not received very graciously at Duke.")[64]

Smith also submitted his own test case to Davison, asking the dean for "favorable consideration" on an application from the nephew of a prominent judge. The judge, Smith wrote, had been a "friend for a good many years, serving in the Legislature with me and otherwise being friendly with me." The nephew, who was then a junior at UNC, wished "to enter Duke Medical School in the fall of 1948." Smith had made the judge's family aware that Duke's medical school was "anxious of course to take in only top-ranking students," so that the young man's chances of admission improved with good grades. And yet, Smith intimated, the case had the potential to improve Duke's political image within the state. Davison replied to Smith that, "in view of [his] recommendation," the admissions committee would give the student "every consideration." The student was admitted to the entering class of 1948.[65]

It was the medical center's finances, however, that Smith and his allies targeted most aggressively. University payments to the medical school had increased dramatically over the past decade, even as budget deficits had become a way of life at the hospital. At the same time, there had been a steady decline in the rates of return on the Endowment's investments, making it difficult not only to meet the increased costs of the university's maintenance and operations but also to fund such pressing needs as increased faculty salaries. Alarmingly, by the late 1940s medical center demands consumed more than half of the university's income from The Duke Endowment, and what made this appear inefficient and, perhaps, improper, at least to the few who were aware of the situation, were rumors of the great wealth being simultaneously generated by the PDC.

Smith began investigating DUMC's finances indirectly, in March of 1947, by having Duke's administrative assistant, Alfred S. Brower, prepare the university's application to the Endowment for charity assistance to Duke Hospital during the previous year. The application was so much better prepared than the usual Duke submission that one Endowment official wrote Smith to thank him for its thoroughness: "May I say that the detailed preparation of the 1946 application for assistance from Duke Hospital more nearly complies with the requirements of this office than any application heretofore submitted by Duke Hospital. We are very much gratified in that the information contained in the application is on a much more comparable basis with other hospitals applying to The Duke Endowment for assistance."[66]

Of more importance, Smith now appointed Don Elias as chairman of two new trustee committees: one to address student admissions and the other to deal with the medical school and hospital. Calls to "dig deep" into the medical center came almost immediately from a member of the Medical School and Hospital Committee, Eugene Newsom of Durham. Newsom was one of the seven members of the executive committee of Duke's Board of Trustees, and he prefaced his prescription with praise for the "wonderful work" being done by the hospital and medical school. "What we need to dig into is what becomes of the money in the Private Diagnostic Clinic. . . . The funds going into this 'pool' are tremendous," Newsom explained, "and those being paid out to those participating in the 'pool' are tremendous. It is my opinion that Duke University should be receiving a much larger percentage of the 'pool' than it is. It is also my opinion that many of those have drawing percentages from the pool far in excess of what they should have."[67]

Newsom considered the matter a "delicate" one embracing "the whole question of basic procedure," and he suggested that he, Smith, and the committee's chairman, Don Elias, investigate the PDC before the next board meeting.[68]

The Dean and the Rice Diet Doctor

In the portrait commissioned by medical school alumni, Dean Davison sits on a high stool with his tie askew and his collar unbuttoned, while around him, on shorter stools, with their backs to the viewer, are several attentive students. The dean's long white lab coat is buttoned at the waist. His pipe is held firmly in his left hand—Davison was smoking 15 bowls of tobacco a day; he was also drinking heavily and taking caffeine tablets.[69]

Within weeks of that August portrait sitting, U.S. president Harry Truman initiated a series of events that had the indirect effect of seriously diminishing Davison's power at Duke and of helping transform the university's medical center from a provincial facility of state and regional influence to an institution of national impact and international renown. On August 19, while Congress was in recess, Truman appointed Oscar Ross Ewing as administrator of the Federal Security Agency. As head of the huge agency, Ewing, 58, was responsible for supervising and directing 11 different governmental units, including the Office of Education, the Social Security Administration, the Food and Drug Administration, and the United States Public Health Service (home of the National Institute of Health). Ewing's appointment had a profound and lasting impact on Duke University and Duke Medicine, both during his five years as head of the Federal Security Agency (the precursor of the Department of Health and Human Services), and later, during his work with North Carolina governor Terry Sanford on the Research Triangle Park in Durham.

Oscar Ewing knew more than Dave Davison about Duke's wide legal and financial networks, and he and his wife also cared much more than Davison about the benefits of the rice diet developed by Dr. Walter Kempner at Duke. Ewing had studied law in Iowa under H. Claude Horack, a professor who was now retiring after 14 years as dean of Duke's School of Law. Ewing had also been intimately involved in defending Alcoa against the government's anti-trust suit as a partner of the law firm of Hughes, Hubbard, & Ewing in New York. When he resigned to head Truman's Federal Security Administration, Ewing's firm included George A. Burwell (a nephew of The Duke Endowment's president, George Garland Allen) and Wright Tisdale, whose future included the vice presidency of the Ford Motor Company and the chairman-ship of Duke's Board of Trustees.[70] [Figure 5.8]

Ewing's Kempner connection became critical from the day he was sworn in at the Federal Security Agency. Among the agency heads who visited him that day was the head of the Public Health Service, U.S. surgeon general Dr. Thomas Parran Jr., a close personal friend of Davison and The Duke Endowment's Watson Rankin. "We had a very nice chat," Ewing recalled, "and to make conversation, I told him of an experience that Mrs. Ewing had had. She had high blood pressure, hypertension, but had got wonderful relief from a Dr. Kempner who was at Duke University Hospital. When Mrs. Ewing first went down to Duke she couldn't walk three hundred yards, and by the time she left three months later, she could walk three miles a day. It was a miracu-lous improvement. . . . I told all of this to Dr. Parran who said, 'I think the National Institutes [*sic*] of Health are making Dr. Kempner a grant for some research he is doing.' And I answered, 'Well, that's very nice.'"[71]

Neither man was aware, it seems, that Kempner's grant application had recently been rejected by an NIH advisory panel—a panel on which the chair-man of Kempner's department, Dr. Eugene Stead, was serving. Stead him-self had voted in favor of funding Kempner's application. "From the begin-ning," Stead later wrote, "the students and house staff pointed out to me that Kempner with his rice diet did better than the patients treated by me with dig-italis, diuretics and moderate sodium restriction. My own observations sup-ported theirs." Stead also looked into the charges that Davison had long been whispering against Kempner, namely, that the rice diet records were not accu-rate. "I reviewed the charges against Kempner," Stead explained. "They were primarily directed against his method of record keeping. His records consisted of a minimum of verbiage and maximum of measurements to which a numeri-

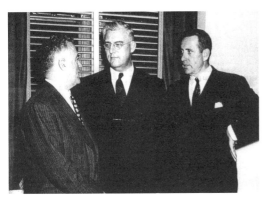

5.8 Left to right, Oscar Ross Ewing, Harold J. Gallagher, and Willis Smith at a banquet honoring the retirement of Judge T. D. Bryson and H. Claude Horack from the Duke Law School. May 28, 1948. *Duke University Archives*.

cal value could be assigned. These records, though they seemed strange at the time, are very similar to those that we now find profitable to store in the hospital." Stead came away convinced that "Kempner had the best records and the best followup of anyone in the institution. I checked the output of his laboratories and found the data of high quality."[72]

Yet it was not Kempner's records that Stead's fellow NIH panel members objected to. They rejected Kempner's proposal because it lacked control studies of various kinds—something that Kempner refused to set up, arguing that most of his "patients were too ill to tolerate extended waiting periods, that terminally ill patients in control groups would be unethically denied the benefits of the best available treatment, the rice diet, and that variations in the basic diet invalidated the information gained from monitoring that permitted the immediate conversion of scientific data into treatment regimens."[73]

Not coincidentally, perhaps, the chairman of Duke's board of trustees, Willis Smith, now began hearing from grateful patients of Dr. Kempner, who was the major economic engine of the medical PDC. While most physicians doubted the value of the rice diet and its German designer, hundreds of patients, like William K. Jackson, thought otherwise. "Dr. Kempner has done such a fine job on me that I think he is sending me home next Thursday," Jackson wrote to Smith from Duke Hospital. "I am convinced that if my doctors in the north had not been so uninformed and biased and had been willing to send me down here two years ago, when I first suggested it, my history would have been far different." Another Kempner patient, Herman Horneman, wrote Smith a few days later enclosing "a check of $5,000 for Duke University to be used by Dr. Walter Kempner for his research. Dr. Kempner through his research has helped myself and a great number of seriously ill patients."[74]

Both correspondents also let Smith know that Kempner and his patients needed improved facilities and better attention. "Having lived here at the hospital for twelve weeks," Jackson wrote, "it is inevitable that we should see the limitations and obstacles to the adequate care and treatment of Dr. Kempner's patients. He is a pioneer in medical science, and we hope can be given the proper facilities for developing his work." One obvious but unmentioned obstacle was the anti-Semitism of some of the hospital's nurses. According to one nursing supervisor, who arrived from Boston in 1947, Kempner's patients were "enormously wealthy, mostly Jewish people from New York," who "were neglected, strangely as it may seem, because the nurses mostly were white southern Baptists and they did not like Jewish people, or they did not like their stereotype of Jewish people, and they never tried to find out if it was true or not. They [the Jewish patients] were wealthy, which was another dreadful sin. Their rooms were a mess. They questioned everything. So, here were these wealthy people who were getting terrible care."[75]

Kempner himself wrote and congratulated Ewing on the agency appointment but made no mention of the failed NIH grant. Ewing, still unaware that the grant had been rejected, wrote Kempner back: "I understand the Public Health Service is giving you a grant and I'm very glad to hear that." To which Kempner immediately replied, according to Ewing, "No, the Public Health Service was not giving him a grant, that he had applied to the Public Health Service for a grant and also to the insurance companies for a grant. The insurance companies had made him a grant but not the Public Health Service." Ewing, confused, asked Parran to investigate the matter, and Parran reported back that the Public Health Service was indeed not giving Kempner a grant. "'Don't you think you ought to?'" Ewing asked the surgeon general. "'This is marvelous work he is doing.'"[76] The suggestion infuriated Parran. Not only had a panel of medical scientists rejected the grant but also, he snapped, the dean of Duke's medical school, Dr. Wilburt Davison, had disputed Kempner's research. Parran then accused Ewing of abusing his power. "This is the first time in the Health Service's long existence that a nonprofessional has brought pressure," the surgeon general fumed. And from that point on Parran was determined not to make the grant.[77]

Ewing was equally determined that the grant be made, however, and in the fall of 1947 he saw an opportunity to force the issue. Vacancies on several of the surgeon general's advisory boards—at the National Health Council, the Cancer Institute, and other NIH sections—needed to be filled; some of the boards had ceased functioning, in fact, because they could not muster a quorum. Additionally, this prevailing uncertainty had the potential to affect the proposed proliferation of new categorical institutes that would soon turn the singular NIH into the plural National Institutes of Health. When Parran tried to fill the vacancies, though, Ewing refused to approve the appointments. "As a result," Ewing recalled, "Dr. Parran came into my office one day mad as a hornet. He announced, 'You've got to approve these appointments.'" But Ewing refused: "I'm not going to until you can do something about this grant for Dr. Kempner." To which Parran allegedly responded, "I can't do anything.

That advisory group doesn't meet until the first of the year." "Well, all right," Ewing shrugged. "That's all right." He could wait till then if Parran could.[78]

A Role for Lyman

I n the meantime, as the two most powerful men in American medicine brought the nation's burgeoning health care bureaucracy to a virtual standstill because of their differences over a situation at Duke's medical center, Davison heard from Lyman, who was set to begin a year's leave that October. Lyman recommended that Duke sell Highland Hospital. There were just too "many obstacles" to integrate the hospital with the neuropsychiatric department in Durham, Lyman wrote, "of which the distance of Asheville from Durham is only one." And if selling Highland proved "positively impossible from a purely legal standpoint (not merely from the matter of expediency in view of Dr. Carroll's antagonism to sale), there is no alternative to the necessity to invest $150,000 into the Highland Hospital."[79]

Lyman had been trying to leave Duke for almost a year. He had visited the VA in Washington several times, asking for full- or part-time work, and the United Nations had asked him to join the Medical Training Center in Nanking, China. In both instances, however, Alan Gregg had made it clear that Duke could not be forgotten. As he reminded Lyman regarding Nanking: "Obviously my role in your decision would be balanced by the conflicting interests that I naturally have in the success of the enterprise at Duke and the needs of China in psychiatry." Gregg was more specific in a letter to the VA's Florence Powdermaker, noting that "Dr. Lyman's suggestion that he might work with you full time derives, I think, from one of his major interests, racial differences in psychiatry. . . . In the light especially of Lyman's attraction for younger men who might be thus drawn into Psychiatry," Gregg wrote, "I should regret his leaving Duke. I would doubt whether a full time post in the V.A. would result in quite as many or as valuable an effect as his present status of teacher and trainer would produce." As for part-time work, Gregg thought Lyman "could be very valuable to white psychiatrists who have no idea of how deep are the racial differences. And I am equally sure that Lyman could give and receive much from negro physicians needing advanced instruction in psychiatry. I would think that traveling to V.A. hospitals with considerable negro N.[euro-] P.[sychiatric] populations Lyman could be of great value and metabolize some of his restlessness as well. Of course if Lyman has a ward of negroes at Duke you could assign personnel for short periods there and the effect would be even greater."[80]

But since Lyman wasn't about to get a ward for black veteran psychiatric patients in Duke Hospital, and the Nanking matter was still unsettled, he accepted a temporary job offered by the VA. He took a year's leave of absence from Duke to do a six-month consultantship at the black Veterans Hospital in Tuskegee, Alabama. There he worked with Dr. Charles Drew and others to plan and supervise a training program for black psychiatrists.[81]

Davison, the Duke Endowment, and a New President for Duke

Between 1948 and 1950, Duke Medicine found its progressive community outreach both aided and arrested by university, state, and national politics. The process began early in 1948 as the chairman of Duke's board of trustees, Willis Smith, prepared to meet in New York with George G. Allen, the chairman of The Duke Endowment and a member of the executive committee of university trustees, about such issues as funding and the choice of the next Duke president. Early in January Smith received a letter from Allen's nephew, George A. Burwell, on stationery that still contained Oscar Ewing's name as part of the firm's letterhead, "Hughes, Hubbard & Ewing." "I don't know whether Mr. Allen has written you directly or whether he is counting on my doing it for him," Burwell wrote to Willis Smith. "However, in any event, I know that he is planning on your spending the night of February 6th at his apartment. The address is 820 Fifth Avenue in case you do not have it in your records."[82]

By the time Willis Smith visited New York, he knew he would not be the next governor of North Carolina. Smith's decision not to run had been a good one, for on February 6, 1948, North Carolina's commissioner of agriculture, W. Kerr Scott, announced he would run against Charlie Johnson for the Democratic nomination for governor. Backed by a coalition of white farmers and organized labor, by blacks, women, and the Chapel Hill community, Scott had the political pundits agog for the first time in decades. As Raleigh's liberal *News & Observer* put it: "By one brief statement the gubernatorial campaign has been changed from one which attracted little interest to a campaign that promises to be one of the most lively in the state's history. That is a wholesome and welcome development."[83]

Smith was in New York to press for what he considered wholesome and badly needed changes at Duke University. In addition to planning a long-range fundraising campaign, he had come there to discuss with the New York trustees the results of a faculty poll on the question of Duke's next president. Smith knew the Endowment trustees wanted Davison for president, but he was equally determined for that not to happen. Rather than keep the selection process closed and quiet, confined only to the executive committee of university trustees, Smith had convinced Sands and Allen to let him appoint a search committee of nine university trustees, including Sands and Smith himself, to nominate the new president. Also, instead of ignoring faculty opinion completely, as Sands and Allen had wanted to do, Smith had arranged for the faculty to select five of their number, including at least one woman, to consult with the trustee search committee. Davison was one of the five, as was Calvin Hoover of the Economics Department, and in the days before Smith left for New York, the advisory committee passed him the faculty responses to the poll.

The poll was bad news for Davison. The faculty preferred either a recognized scholar for president or someone with an established academic reputation. At the same time, the faculty also "considered the matter of Wannamaker's successor as vice president for education and dean of the university to be inseparably connected with the matter of the presidency." Almost three-quarters of the faculty favored an external appointment for president—that is, someone from outside the university—while also favoring an internal appointment to fill Wannamaker's position. "Just why the majority of the faculty preferred an external appointment is not certain," one close observer has written, "but it may have been that faculty members in arts and sciences feared precisely what [the Endowment's] George Allen and Alex. Sands wanted: to see Wilburt Davison, the highly successful and popular dean of the medical school, made president." It was not that the nonmedical faculty disliked Davison; they were simply wary of him out of "fear that the medical school, already one of the most outstanding components of the university, would be developed further and faster than the other parts of the institution."[84]

Smith was hardly back from New York when Davison suffered another setback to his power and presidential prospects at Duke University. On February 12, President Harry Truman announced that he would not reappoint Dr. Thomas Parran Jr. as surgeon general of the United States. The news was both a personal and professional blow for Davison; in addition to sharing a long friendship with Parran, the two men served together on a variety of national boards and committees associated with private and public health care networks, including various Rockefeller philanthropies. "Thomas Parran organized the NIH to pioneer in *clinical* medical research," Davison later noted to himself, "fostered Hill-Burton aid to build Hosp.—spent a week in 1940(1) [with] Rankin, Reynolds & me studying the D[uke] E[ndowment] Hosp. program—1946 started World Health Organization & invited me to its charter mtg."[85] Indeed, the *New York Times* described Parran as "the originator of New Deal policies in the field of health."[86]

At a press conference the following day, Parran's former boss at the Federal Security Agency, Oscar Ewing, explained the surgeon general's departure as a matter of job rotation. "If you don't rotate it, you, to a certain extent kill ambition," Ewing said of the position. Others believed Parran was ousted for opposing the Truman administration's national health care agenda. Congress was already considering the administration's proposed Health Law, which called for compulsory health insurance, and on February 14, at Truman's request, Ewing announced a national health assembly in early May "to set up national health goals for ten years."[87] Yet Ewing himself later recalled that he passed over Parran because of the Kempner matter. "That whole experience annoyed me so much that when Dr. Parran's term as Surgeon General expired the following May, I did not recommend him for reappointment. I recommended Dr. Leonard Scheele. The President knew Dr. Scheele and was very happy to appoint him."[88]

Duke and Davison got more bad news early in March when nine women died in a fire at Highland Hospital. The fire was the third at the hospital in less than a year, and among those who perished in the blaze was Zelda Fitzgerald, the widow of novelist F. Scott Fitzgerald. The *New York Times* reported the tragedy, as did newspapers across North Carolina, and in the months that followed the press continued to follow the investigation of the fire. In responding to the disaster, the directors of Highland Hospital, Inc., most of whom were Duke University administrators, made DUMC's Dr. Charman Carroll (the daughter of Highland's founder, Dr. Robert Carroll) the hospital's new director. Yet not until the following spring, near the time of Robert Carroll's death, did Highland's nonprofit corporation settle all of the lawsuits arising from the deadly fire.[89]

The fire at Highland fueled an already intense lobbying campaign that had emerged in anticipation of the March 20 meeting of the university trustees' presidential selection committee. The nine-member committee was evenly divided between those who shared Smith's opposition to Davison and those who wanted the dean to emerge from the meeting as the candidate recommended for the university presidency. On March 15, Willis Smith registered his disgust with both the PDC and the hospital in a letter to Clarence H. Cobb, business manager of the medical division of the PDC. Smith had reviewed the complaints of a friend who considered her sister's hospital bill excessive, including the PDC fees charged by her sister's psychiatrist, Dr. Charman Carroll. This matter, Smith explained, had been brought to his attention "some time ago" by the woman—a secretary who had worked for him and for his father-in-law. And though Smith admitted he was "not in a position to evaluate a doctor's services in a matter about which I know so very little," he did hope the bill might be adjusted to relieve the pressure on the already financially strapped family. "I hear so many complaints against our hospital," Smith griped, "and particularly the Private Diagnostic Clinic, with respect to what a great many call extortionate charges, that I have been very much concerned. The hospital, and for that matter the Private Diagnostic Clinic, ought to be assets of good will for the University, but I fear that they are anything but that."[90]

That same day Smith heard from a professor in the Divinity School who was "frantic" at the prospect of Davison becoming president. Included in the communication was a copy of the professor's recent letter to Benjamin F. Few, a nephew of Duke's first president and one of Davison's supporters on the trustee nominating committee. In writing to Few, the professor noted he had "heard that the New York members of our group are backing the Dean of the School of Medicine for president of the University" and he wanted to raise "several objections" to Davison's candidacy.

On the most general level, the professor considered Davison "not sufficiently well known in the academic world to meet the approval of the regular faculty." Nor, in the professor's opinion, did Davison have "sufficient reputation and influence in the social and civic life of the country. He is not known for advocacy of any line of social or civic reform nor is he largely influential in public life." And most damning of all, the professor considered Davison "not at all acceptable to the group who are interested in religion." This group believed James B. Duke "meant what he said when he placed religion first and foremost among the great interests which he wished developed here at Duke," and the group was simply "not at all pleased with the prospects of having the institution headed by a man who could not by the wildest stretch of the imagination be called a churchman."[91]

When Smith arrived at the March 20 meeting, Davison was also there, in his role as a member of the faculty advisory committee, and Smith handed the dean a long, stern letter. The letter explained in great detail why the medical school should not have rejected the recent application of a graduating senior at Duke University. Not only had the student made the dean's list; he had also roomed with Smith's son at prep school and was part of several important families with strong connections to Trinity, Duke, and Smith himself. Of particular importance to Smith was the fact that the "boy's great uncle was Senator Josiah W. Bailey, who until his recent death was an ardent friend of Duke University, as well as one of the protagonists for Trinity College when it needed friends." Smith continued: "When Senator Bailey prepared his will, he donated to Duke University and its Library all of his official papers and documents in his offices in Washington. Recently his son, Mr. James Hinton Pou Bailey of Raleigh, at my suggestion turned over to Mr. Powell of the Duke Library all the remaining papers of his father here in Raleigh, which Mr. Powell was interested in." Smith believed that ignoring "these things would be tantamount to saying that we were not interested in our friends, but would much prefer taking strangers from a far distance who themselves were likely not interested in the history or tradition of Trinity College and Duke Univer-

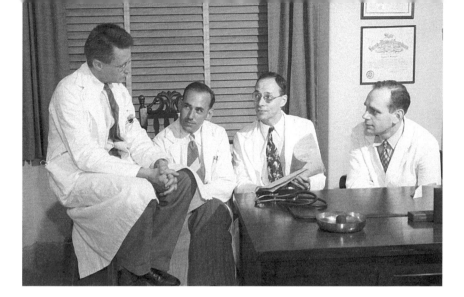

5.9 Left to right, Drs. Jack D. Myers, Walter H. Cargill, John B. Hickam, and Eugene A. Stead Jr. *Duke University Archives*.

sity. If that policy should be continued or pursued," Smith warned, "then we cannot expect to receive at the hands of North Carolinians much support."[92]

Smith exhibited similar tactical ability when it came to the president search. With the proxy of his friend Sidney Alderman in ready, Smith knew he had five votes against Davison on the nine-member trustee selection committee. But he didn't call for a vote. As he explained to George Allen at 30 Rockefeller Plaza, "I realized from the first that there would be very serious opposition to Dr. Davison, although I am personally exceedingly fond of him and appreciate the good work that he has done. I do not believe, though, that he has every [*sic*] fully realized the value of good will in North Carolina. Many Trustees have, without any solicitation on my part, expressed the same opinion and in opposition to Dr. Davison." Actually, Smith intimated, he had done the New York trustees a favor by avoiding a vote. "Mr. Sands suggested early on in our consideration that he thought whatever recommendation went from our committee should be unanimous, and I quite agree to that. Last Saturday when I saw the vote was going to be five to four, I did not put the matter to a formal vote, as I felt further consideration might enable us to agree upon someone without any adverse action by the committee."[93]

EUGENE STEAD'S RESIGNATION

If all of this was not enough to diminish Davison in stature and spirit, he also had to deal with Eugene Stead's resignation as chairman of the Department of Medicine. So urgent was the matter that Robert Lambert flew into the Raleigh-Durham airport from New York at 4 A.M., Saturday, May 1. The visit was one of Lambert's last to Duke before retiring from the Rockefeller Foundation, and by 7 A.M. he was at the medical center looking for Davison. Finding the dean away, however, Lambert called on Stead. "With sadness in voice and appearance S[tead] tells me at once that he has submitted his resignation to be effective June 30, 1949." The news didn't surprise Lambert, who summarized Stead's remarks in his Rockefeller diary. "Knowing I've had the story already from Mrs. Fred Hanes, he doesn't go into detail. Says simply that he and the dean couldn't agree on certain broad questions of policy. Calls himself a failure in what should have been a splendid success. Has no plans for the future, but thinks of returning to practice in Georgia—not Atlanta."[94]

Stead had refused to fire Kempner, as Davison had wanted him to do. Parran meanwhile had lost his reappointment as surgeon general, and Kempner had received two NIH grants, one for 1948 and the other the disputed grant of 1947. Both were approved by the NIH advisory panel on which Stead served. At the same time, Stead was perplexed at having Davison oppose him on the issue that provoked his resignation: creating a Department of Medicine staff that was strictly full-time (as opposed to the existing "geographic" full-time plan, which allowed faculty to supplement their income through private practice). Full-time, after all, was the old missionary approach of Flexner, Rockefeller, and Alan Gregg to keep moneymaking—private practice—out of medical education. As Lambert explained it, "The conflict, which was really between S[tead] and the senior clinical group with Davison supporting the latter, derived from S[tead]'s determination to make his full-time staff, mostly young newcomers, responsible for both teaching and research."[95]

Stead's "young newcomers"—Frank L. Engel, James V. Warren, Jack D. Myers, and John B. Hickam—had come with him from Emory. "I had brought with me to Duke four young men," Stead later wrote, "all destined for bright careers in academic medicine. I knew that they would all in due time leave Duke, and I wanted to give them as rich an experience as possible. I knew the senior clinicians at Duke performed well without me and that, because of their level of income, they would never go to another academic institution. I therefore, as part of my educational program assigned the new faculty members to run the Department and chair key committees when I was out of town. It never crossed my mind that this would create anxiety or resentment."[96] Unfortunately, it did. What set things off was when Stead tried to supplement the salaries of the newcomers by taking away the small annual salaries (of $2,500 to $3,000) that the university paid the senior clinicians for their part-time positions. According to Lambert, several part-time faculty "were to be relieved of teaching duties and consequently of their $2,500 part-time salaries. This was the issue which led to the break following several round table discussions in which a lot of accumulated bitterness found expression."[97] [Figure 5.9]

Stead's "difficulty" made it appear to some observers that he was "trying to accomplish at once by decree what he could have obtained in a year or so by patience and tact." He "is admired and appreciated here as a great teacher and productive investigator," Lambert explained, "but he has aroused widespread antagonism based in large part on fear of more drastic changes. It is to be expected that his resignation will be accepted, though there is a possibility that a mutually acceptable compromise will be worked out."[98] Two days after submitting his resignation, in fact, Stead was visited by Dr. Wiley Forbus, chairman of the Department of Pathology. Forbus "came by to teach me a few of the facts of life," Stead later recalled. "He reviewed the opportunities that lay in front of me at Duke. He recounted the times he had made errors in judgment and had had to back down. He showed me that in the end these episodes had been beneficial to him and had facilitated his growth as a person. He urged me to withdraw my resignation. I did so in a letter to Dave. He replied that he had no power to allow me to withdraw the resignation. The Executive Committee would have to vote to accept the resignation or decline to accept it."[99]

The Rockefeller Foundation certainly hoped Stead stayed. It was Lambert who had recommended that Duke take a look at Stead, and Stead was closely linked to the foundation's teaching programs in psychosomatic medicine at DUMC and at the University of Rochester's School of Medicine. The essence of both emerging programs were teaching liaisons between the Departments of Medicine and Psychiatry. The psychiatric teaching liaison at DUMC, Dr. Maurice Greenhill, had worked closely with Stead and the Department of Social Services in setting up and running a psychosomatic service. "While the purpose of this teaching is for the medical staff," the head of social services wrote, "it is recognized that the social worker can be of help to many patients in their adjustment of social problems which in some way have some bearing on the patient's personality and disease."[100]

Indeed, in the month before Stead's resignation, the Department of Social Services added a staff member specifically for the Psychosomatic Service. The department reported that "Mrs. Beatrice Cooper, major in Psychiatric Social Casework, New York School of Social Work, became a member of the staff with the approval and financial cooperation of the Mental Hygiene Program in North Carolina and the Department of Psychiatry, Duke Hospital." In addition to Cooper, moreover, who was working full-time with the Psychosomatic Service, "two medical social workers regularly assigned to the Medical Service have also carried selected cases for the Psychosomatic Service under Mrs. Cooper's supervision. In addition to being of direct assistance to her patients, Mrs. Cooper has made a valuable contribution in emphasizing the psychic and social aspects of illness, adjustment, and rehabilitation in the teaching of house staff physicians who are assigned to the Psychosomatic Service."[101]

It was not until much later in the year that Dean Davison decided to take up the matter of Dr. Eugene Stead's resignation again. Stead later recalled that the matter had been put "on the agenda of the next Executive Committee meeting. Dave was not yet ready for the vote and he managed to have an Executive Committee meeting where one or another key person was missing, so that a vote would not be called for. After a few months he decided to face the issue. In characteristic fashion he spent most of the afternoon on trivia but finally asked for a vote on my resignation. The swing vote was cast by Lyman, the professor of neuropsychiatry." In other words, Richard Lyman's vote enabled Duke Medicine to keep Dr. Eugene Stead—the single most important clinical physician at Duke for the next two decades.[102]

MORE DIFFICULTIES FOR DAVISON

Stead's resignation coincided with Lyman's return from Tuskegee and the first of two major disappointments in Duke's search for a new president. Lyman quickly became embroiled with the VA on two back-to-back fronts: settling up past accounts with the veterans neuropsychiatry training program and negotiating new ones. The most pressing matter was Duke's alleged double-billing of the VA, something that Lyman denied and that the VA tried to use as leverage, it seems, in negotiating a continuation of the training program at Duke. Late in May, moreover, Duke came within a hair of naming Dr. Ernest C. Colwell as its next president, before Colwell, the president of the University of Chicago, decided to stay on there.

If Colwell's decision brought talk of an inside appointment, specifically of Davison, those who opposed the dean remained mobilized behind Willis Smith. One Durham attorney, a Trinity alumnus, wrote to Smith: "For my part I wish that the Duke Medical School and the Duke Hospital was located somewhere else other than Durham, and most certainly I wish that it had not been located on the University campus." What worried him most—and it was a feeling, he claimed, that was shared by "scores of others"—was that they were "fast getting at Duke Hospital a John[s] Hopkins set-up. The tail will soon wag the dog, if it is not already doing it. Everything at John[s] Hopkins has been submerged to the advantage of the Medical School and Hospital." This seemed to him to be exactly what the New York group wanted at Duke, especially Alex Sands, Davison's chief supporter. Sands was "thinking about the matter from a business angle only," the attorney complained. "He never went to Trinity college nor Duke University and he can't possibly have the same feeling, not by a hell of a lot, that I have. Trinity College is fortunate to have a man like Mr. Sands connected. His money and his monetary connections will help, but only that. Colleges and universities will never be made and fine traditions built up by that detached group."[103]

Willis Smith now knotted the dean's purse strings through the university's new comptroller and business manager, Alfred S. Brower. Brower warned the dean in early June against reaching any deeper into Duke's endowed pockets: "I cannot stress too strongly that it will be impossible for the University to continue to increase its allocation from its endowment revenue for the purpose of the Medical School and Hospital as it has in the past, and you may expect this action to be typical of that which will necessarily follow in future years." Brower also reminded Davison that there had "been little increase in the income from the endowed funds in the past few years and the rate of return on these funds has been steadily downward. While this has been true, the Medical School has increased its draft upon the income of the university in an almost steady progression from $296,000 in 1939–40 to $456,000 in 1947–48. This increased provision now results in the School of Medicine and Hospital absorbing more than half of the entire income from the Duke Endowment."[104]

Davison was away in New York when Brower's warnings arrived. He was there meeting with the board of Doris Duke's Independent Aid foundation, assisting several Duke faculty with their funding requests. Calvin Hoover had asked the foundation if it might consider a funding request from Frank McCallister, a socialist labor organizer with the Georgia Workers Education Service. Davison considered aid doubtful, however, as he did not "know anything about the organization." Another query had come from Dr. Harold A. Bosley, the dean of Duke's Divinity School: would Independent Aid fund a fellowship for a divinity student who wanted to take a master's degree at the New York School of Social Work? Although Davison presented the request to the foundation, he suggested that funding was unlikely and that the student check with "Dr. Martha Eliot of the Children's Bureau," who might "know of funds available for this type of training."[105]

While Davison was in New York, the American Pediatric Society published a study Davison had been shepherding for the past four years. The title of the 20-page booklet, published on June 10 in Washington, D.C., with funding from Independent Aid, was "How Well Does North Carolina Provide for the Health of Its Children?" The *New York Times* answered briefly in the headline for its story: "Health Study Cites Physician Shortage, High Infant Mortality, Facilities Lack." The reporter described the booklet as "a sampling of what this country can expect in a state-by-state revelation of child health needs" and as a "pilot study in a country-wide survey conducted cooperatively by the nation's pediatricians, the Children's Bureau, and the Public Health Service,

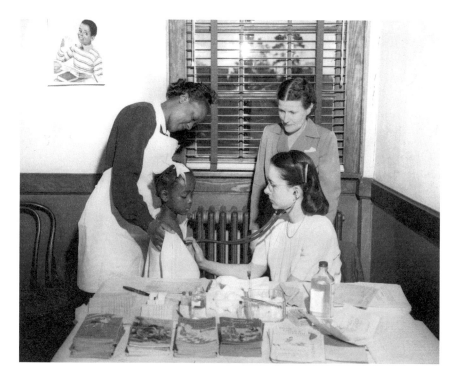

5.10 A member of the nursing staff of Duke Hospital examines a child during a visit to a community clinic. *Duke University Medical Center Archives.*

using both public and privately contributed funds." Although the shortcomings listed by the study were depressingly long, an aggressive response was promised. "The North Carolina Pediatric Society, which conducted the study, has announced that it will 'take responsibility for implementing the findings' and that it has 'adopted a vigorous program which it intends shall result eventually in better medical care for children regardless of race, creed, color, financial status or geographic location.'"[106] [Figure 5.10]

Davison completely ignored Brower's warnings in preparing DUMC's budget, and at the end of June, he was summoned to a meeting of the university's budget committee. There he "was told in very positive terms by me," Willis Smith wrote to one trustee, "seconded in person by Mr. Sands and Mr. Allen, that he and everyone else at the Medical School and Hospital were expected to observe the budget requirements." Yet when Brower called DUMC the following day, to work on the budget with Davison, he found the dean "had left the campus for about a month." So provoked was Smith that he investigated the situation further, discovering "that the whole Medical School group have given the Treasurer's office trouble heretofore in failing to observe many of the business requirements of the University. . . . Personally," Smith confided, "I feel fairly confident that this situation developed because Dr. Davison felt that he could go over the heard [*sic*] of Dr. Flowers and everybody else on campus. I think Mr. Sands and Mr. Allen now realize this without having to make it a point. Mr. Allen was quite positive in saying to Dr. Davison that he expected him to cooperate."[107]

Davison was still out of town when Duke and DUMC took a hit on Sunday, July 11, in the *Greensboro Daily News*. Headlined on the front page of the newspaper—"Duke Loses 'Overpayments'; Contract Revision Threatens VA Medical Program"—was a story on disagreements between Duke and the VA over double-billing in the veterans neuropsychiatry training program. For the most part, the long, detailed story provided an accurate account of the matter. There was some hyperbole, to be sure, as in the story's claim that "out of the VA-Duke controversy may well come a government-sponsored reexamination of the Veterans Administration's entire medical program." And there were also signs of political shenanigans, as when the newspaper pointed out that "the VA's regional office in Winston-Salem is expected to announce in the next few days the establishment of a mental hygiene clinic at Bowman Gray Hospital in Winston-Salem. Bowman Gray will then conduct most of the VA-ordered neuropsychiatric examinations for which Duke has been collecting $20 and, under a reduction volunteered by Duke some months ago, $16."[108]

Though the story reverberated from Washington to Durham, and from VA officials to the president of Duke, a new agreement was soon reached. The neuropsychiatry training program was continued at Duke, still under the leadership of Dr. Leslie Hohman, with Drs. Lyman and Greenhill as consultants. The VA did make one important change, however. It terminated its lease on the building next to the Kirby Clinic at Duke and rented space for its clinic in downtown Durham. The change left Lyman and Hohman with a building that Dr. Robert Flowers, angered by the recent revelations, refused to pay for.

SOME SUCCESSES

Davison was in New York when the VA story broke, working with Basil O'Connor and the National Foundation for Infantile Paralysis. The number of polio cases had been climbing nationally since May, presaging the epidemic that had arrived in June; by July, North Carolina led the nation in polio cases reported. On July 6, the foundation accepted Duke's offer to establish at Duke Hospital an isolation ward for acute polio cases. "The Red Cross volunteered and the battle began," one newspaper reported. "Special 'polio nurses' were flown in, local nurses volunteered, staff physicians were assigned to full-time duty in the polio ward, and the children's surgical ward was converted into a special 26-bed unit for severe cases." Over the next three months, the spe-

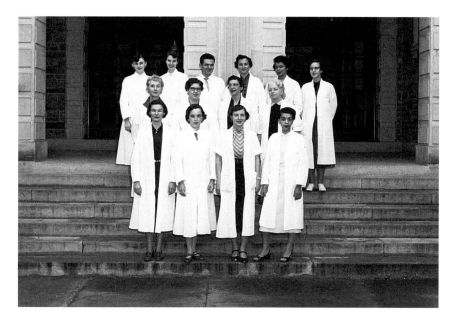

5.11 The Department of Social Services at Duke Hospital, ca. 1950. Harriett Amey is on the front row, extreme right. *Duke University Medical Center Archives.*

cial ward treated 126 patients, most of whom were between the ages of 2 and 10 years, and only four whom died, all within 48 hours of being admitted. This was excellent service Duke was rightly proud of, and in October, when the special unit closed, the university announced in the press the number of patients and their days of care for each of the 28 counties DUMC had served during the epidemic.[109]

While DUMC made certain that the polio story was widely covered, two other major developments at Duke received little or no publicity. One was the expanded commitment of some at DUMC to move from opposing racial segregation to actually promoting integration. Their activism was partly spurred by the success of Harriett Amey's "demonstration" project as the first black staff member of the Department of Social Services. Amey had been given "the responsibility for services to Negro patients on Obstetric, Gynecologic, and Pediatric Services. She has been well accepted in the hospital by all members of the staff," one supervisor reported, "and is performing an excellent quality of service to patients."[110] Moreover, in September of 1948, a black woman who trained as a technician at North Carolina College, Nell Cooke Jones, joined the laboratory staff of Dr. Walter Kempner. The most significant development at DUMC that fall was the program launched by Duke Hospital and the Durham city schools for training black practical nurses. Funded with a grant of $10,000 from the Durham City School system, the State Vocational Educational Department, and Duke Hospital, the program included three months of study in the basic sciences and nursing arts at Hillside High School (a local black school), followed by nine months of practical experience at the Duke University Hospital.[111] [Figure 5.11]

ANOTHER ATTEMPT TO FIND A PRESIDENT

Also unheralded at Duke that fall was the university's second failed attempt to secure a new president. Since July, the search committee had focused on the vice president of the Massachusetts Institute of Technology, James R. Killian Jr., a native of South Carolina who had attended Trinity College in the 1920s. Deeply interested in the position at Duke, Killian had gone so far as to visit the campus with his wife before notifying the university in September that he would remain at MIT, where, a month later, he became its president. In the meantime, Smith revisited a recommendation made earlier by Ernest Colwell, the president of the University of Chicago, who had suggested that the search committee give A. Hollis Edens a look. Although Edens was then working for the General Education Board in New York, Colwell had lauded him "as my number one candidate for the Presidency of Duke."[112]

It was fitting perhaps that Duke's first interview with Hollis Edens was arranged by men whose offices were only a few floors apart in the RCA building at 30 Rockefeller Plaza. Early in October, Alex Sands of The Duke Endowment met with Robert Calkins and Fred McCuistion of the General Education Board. Their meeting focused on the new physics building going up at Duke. Although The Duke Endowment had given $1 million to build and equip the new building, increased construction costs had driven up the cost of the building alone to $1 million. The building was on course for completion in March of 1949 but Duke now needed $200,000 to equip the building for "molecular structural problems bordering on biological science," for "low temperature apparatus—liquid air and liquid helium," and for "nuclear physics and cosmic ray research."[113] Sands wanted the General Education Board to help fund the equipment. The Duke Endowment's annual income was now about $5 million, he explained to Calkins and McCuistion, "of which about $1,280,000 goes to Duke University. Not all of the funds appropriated [to the Hospital Section of the Endowment] for hospital service have been utilized during the past few years. These unspent balances have been placed in a reserve fund which has been drawn upon for the physics building."[114]

Sands also learned from Calkins and McCuistion that Edens planned to visit Duke with them early in October. Both General Education Board officers considered Edens "qualified for the job [at Duke] although they had hoped that he would spend at least five years with them before undertaking such an assignment."[115]

Willis Smith, Truman, and a Proposal for National Health Insurance

W illis Smith wanted to meet Edens as soon as possible, but he had a more important mission to complete first. President Truman was coming to Raleigh, and Smith had been drafted by Governor Cherry to plan the ceremonies surrounding the president's unveiling of a monument to North Carolina's "Three Presidents": Andrew Jackson, James K. Polk, and Andrew Johnson. Truman also planned two campaign speeches during his October 19 visit, one at the unveiling and another at the state fair, after which Smith would entertain "the President's little family" at his home in Raleigh. Truman's supporters hoped the visit would counter the view of conservative Raleigh Democrats such as Pou Bailey, son of the late U.S. senator Josiah Bailey, who believed that the state would "go Republican on the national ticket and . . . elect a Republican Senator."[116]

What seemed to Bailey a disaster in the making, however, appeared to Smith and other Democrats as a promising political future. In the Democratic primary for United States senator, former governor Melville Broughton had defeated the conservative Democratic appointee, Senator William B. Umstead, and now appeared certain of besting his Republican opponent in the race to fill the remaining four years of the unexpired term of senator Josiah Bailey. Even more exhilarating was Kerr Scott's defeat of Charlie Johnson, the dynasty's man, in the Democratic gubernatorial primary.

The president gave a rousing address to the crowds he mixed with at the fair. "Today big-money Republicanism is on the march," Truman warned, "and to beat it we've all got to stand together. That's where we Democrats belong—together—shoulder to shoulder. We are the great middle-of-the-road party of the farmers and the workers and the small business men and the party of the younger people. We all belong together."[117]

Truman defeated his Republican opponent, Thomas Dewey, on November 2, 1948, and carried the state of North Carolina by a vote of 459,070 to 258,572. "Your friends in North Carolina are rejoicing at your great triumph," Smith telegrammed Truman. "My congratulations and best wishes." For the present at least, a new political era seemed to be emerging in the state.[118]

Over the next week or so, several prominent Truman supporters entered and left Duke Hospital as happy patients. The president of the United Auto Workers, Walter Reuther, departed from the hospital on November 10, one day before federal security administrator Oscar Ewing and his wife arrived. Reuther was leaving the hospital after exploratory arm surgery by Duke neurosurgeon Dr. Barnes Woodhall. "I received excellent care at Duke Hospital and want to express my admiration and thanks to Dr. Woodhall and his associates and the nursing staff," Reuther told the press. In addition to feeling he had "really been among friends" during his stay, the union leader sensed a "fine spirit" that was making something special happen in the state. "North Carolina is making tremendous progress on the economic and social problems which the American people showed on Nov. 2 they intend to solve in the democratic way."[119]

Ewing, after describing his admission to Duke Hospital as a regular two-year "check-up," announced that he would speak the following day at the hospital amphitheater on "socialized medicine." The theater was packed the next day as Ewing made his case for the National Health Insurance Plan, which he said "was included in the health program which he proposed to President Truman recently." In advocating the program, Ewing noted, "Each year more than 325,000 persons die who could otherwise be saved by the medical skill and knowledge we have. This does not include the losses in income or pain and suffering." Under the administration's proposed program, insurance premiums would be "deducted in a manner similar to the social security deductions now in use" and the "only difference in payment of doctors is that they would receive fees out of the insurance fund instead of from the patient directly."[120]

As for the arguments being made against his program, Ewing responded, "The best answer is to balance the health of 70,000,000 persons against the interests of some 180,000 doctors; decide for yourself on which side the social responsibility lies." Indeed, Ewing argued, under his proposed program, more doctors, nurses, and technicians would be recruited; aid to medical research would triple; medical schools would be expanded; more scholarships would be given for medical training; rural public health services would be improved; the number of hospital beds would be increased, especially in rural areas; and "an integrated system of hospitals, especially on a state basis, would be established." Finally, Ewing said, "There is great progress being made today in the medical profession, but the tragedy is that the benefits are not evenly distributed."

The Appointment of a New President of Duke

Business did not stop while the university's trustees were preparing to ask one of the General Education Board's officers, Hollis Edens, to become Duke's next president. Dr. R. Taylor Cole of Duke's Political Science Department was pressing Edens for a decision on whether to submit a request to the Rockefeller board for funding 30 to 40 top-ranking European students at Duke. "I remember very pleasantly our conversation at Lexington, Kentucky," Edens wrote to Cole on November 5, "and I have not forgotten

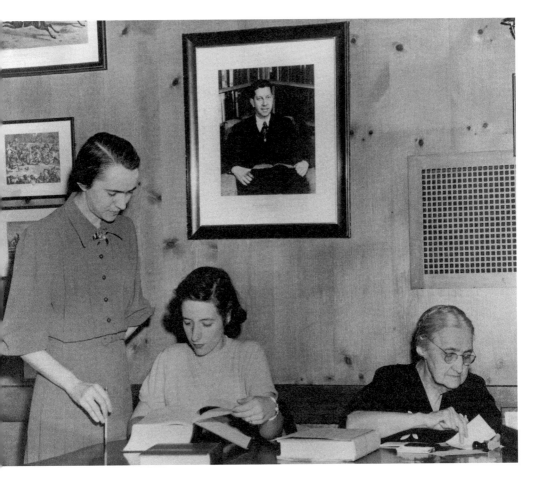

5.12 Left to right, Judith Farrar, librarian; Mary Duke Biddle Trent, chair of the library committee; and Mildred P. Farrar, assistant librarian, working in the Duke University School of Medicine Library. The photograph behind them is of Dr. Josiah C. Trent. *Duke University Medical Center Archives.*

that I promised to write you concerning the advisability of presenting to the General Education Board a request for a grant toward bringing foreign graduate students to Duke University. I have discussed the idea informally with the other officers, and it is agreed that we are not yet clear in our own minds that you should be encouraged to submit such a request."[121] Likewise, the Endowment's Alex Sands was pressing the General Education Board for a decision on equipment for the physics building. On November 10, he called Robert Calkins at the board "to report that Nielsen wished to submit the Duke request for funds for science equipment in the new physics building." Calkins suggested, though, "that in view of the possible changes in administration at Duke they might prefer to hold this request until Edens had determined whether or not he wished to submit it to the Board." Yet Sands appeared "anxious to have the board consider the request now."[122]

Duke's physics and political science requests were still pending at the General Education Board on November 19, when Hollis Edens was elected as the university's third president. Though Dave Davison later complained that "Edens was elected president by the trustees without referral to the faculty committee appointed by the trustees to help select a president," the dean had assured Willis Smith of his support for Edens before the appointment.[123] Most Duke supporters welcomed the selection, including Mary Duke Biddle Trent, the granddaughter of James B. Duke's brother, Benjamin N. Duke. "We just want to add a word of thanks to you and the board of trustees," she wrote to Smith in late November. "The announcement about the new president has thrilled us all, and Joe and I know how hard you have worked to secure this splendid man. He sounds like a person who will give distinction to Duke's future, and we know that it has a great future." Less than two weeks later, Trent's husband, Dr. Josiah Trent, died of an inoperable brain tumor, leaving behind his widow and their four young daughters.[124] [Figure 5.12]

Duke Medicine and the Promise of Progressive Southern Politics

T ruman's election represented a high point of the progressive promise in American health care reform. National health insurance was at the forefront of the new administration's agenda, and at DUMC the push for racial integration was already under way. North Carolina appeared poised, moreover, to create a new day in southern politics, with the election of a liberal governor by a New Deal coalition of organized labor, blacks, women, and rural white farmers.

Early in March of 1949, however, as Washington buzzed with the national health care debate, North Carolina's newly elected senator, Melville Broughton, died. Two weeks later, the state's new governor, Kerr Scott, made a decision that transformed the image of Duke, DUMC, and North Carolina for years to come. He appointed UNC president Dr. Frank Porter Graham, one of the South's leading liberals, to the seat left vacant by Broughton's death. To many observers, Graham's appointment seemed to furnish North Carolina with the leadership for a new day—a new day economically, politically, educationally, and medically for all of the South.

To other observers, however, like High Point radio commentator Bob Thompson, the appointment appeared fraught with danger. Thompson was particularly worried about Graham's past affiliations with allegedly subversive organizations. "We all know that Frank Graham is a friend of the little man, a friend of the Negro, a friend of labor—and we would not have him act otherwise," Thompson told his listeners. "We all know that he does believe in a paternalistic if not semi-socialistic federal government and though many of us do not agree with him, we respect his beliefs. But there is a great difference between being a liberal—a liberal who feels the weight of the responsibility of seat in the United States Senate—and being a fellow who goes chasing after will-of-the-wisps, lending his name to every organization with a high sounding title regardless of how subversive may be the control of said organization."[125]

Within days of Thompson's broadcast, Willis Smith received a letter from Don Elias. "Bob Thompson sent me a copy of the broadcast about which you talked to me," Elias wrote. "It does not give quite all that you heard he said on the air, however, here it is for whatever it is worth." Across town, Pou Bailey was outraged at the thought of his late father's Senate seat being occupied by Frank Graham. And he was determined to fight the senator if Graham decided to stand for election in 1950. "As you no doubt apprehend," Bailey wrote to Virginia senator Harry Byrd, "the appointment of Dr. Graham to the Senate caused severe political upheaval down this way. . . . The initial reaction among most of our old time political leaders was one of anger and a determination to insure Dr. Graham's defeat in 1950." Bailey then described in detail for Byrd the "very bad political situation in North Carolina," pointing to the importance of 1950. "To sum up," he wrote, "it is generally accepted among the conservative people in North Carolina that 1950 will see the battle lines very tightly drawn."[126]

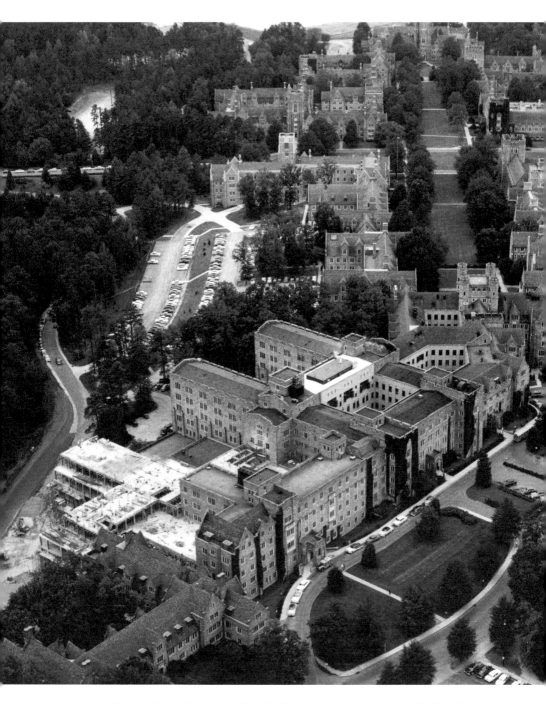

6.1 The new Private Diagnostic Clinic building under construction, 1955. *Duke University Medical Center Archives.*

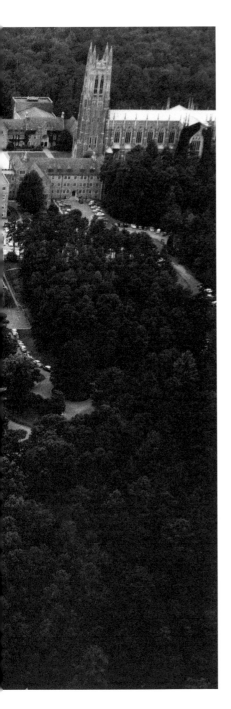

CHAPTER 6:

Duke Medicine at the Crossroads, 1950–1960

D uke Medicine passed through two fairly distinct phases in the 1950s. Between 1950 and 1955, DUMC was more acted upon than actor, as it fell subject to the political and institutional goals of Willis Smith, the chairman of Duke's board of trustees, and his ally, university president Hollis Edens. Smith and Edens tried to curtail DUMC's autonomy and power, especially the expansion plans of the Private Diagnostic Clinic, as they worked to foster Duke's cooperation with the statewide medical planning of the North Carolina Medical Care Commission and the North Carolina Hospital Study Committee. At the same time, Duke and DUMC were also influenced by the fear of communism and the Korean War, by the growing challenge to racial segregation and smoking, and by the activities of UNC president Gordon Gray. Not only was Gray secretary of the army when he agreed to become UNC's president in 1950; he was also a strong supporter of psychiatry and the emerging medical centers in Chapel Hill and Winston-Salem. It was also Gray who appointed the North Carolina Hospital Study Committee in 1951.

Gordon Gray resigned from UNC in 1955, however, and returned to Washington to serve as President Dwight Eisenhower's special assistant for national security affairs. By then, Willis Smith was dead, the Korean War was over, the Supreme Court had issued its *Brown* decision outlawing racial segregation in public schools, and a new federal bureaucracy—the Department of Health, Education and Welfare—was responsible for many of the governmental units previously administered by Oscar Ewing at the now defunct Federal Security Administration. For the next five years, 1955–60, DUMC became more actor than acted upon as it defined much of the path it would follow for the next several decades. Its liberation resulted in part from the developments noted above, but also from generational and programmatic changes within both the Rockefeller philanthropies and the Duke ensemble of interests. At the same time, the Private Diagnostic Clinic expanded at Duke Hospital and created numerous clinics in surrounding counties, while most of the DUMC's medical faculty mobilized behind Philip Handler, chairman of the Biochemistry Department, and Paul Gross, Duke's vice president, in support of the Research Training Program. This program featured a cross-campus alliance in the basic and physical sciences that was linked to a variety of public and private funding sources, particularly the U.S. Public Health Service (including the National Institutes of Health) and the United States military.

The Smith-Graham Race of 1950

The defining event of the decade for Duke was the 1950 Democratic primary for the United States Senate. In January of that year, the incumbent, Senator Frank Porter Graham, filed to run in the primary, leaving Willis Smith to ponder the question, Should he run against Graham in the Democratic primary?

Willis Smith had spent much of his life leading the liberal wing of North Carolina's Democratic Party, the wing now backing Graham, and it was also clear that Graham had the support of the Truman administration. "Dr. Frank" was widely identified as the foremost southern liberal of his time. He was an original member of Truman's civil rights committee and the first president of the interracial and integrationist Southern Conference for Human Welfare. He was also one of only three southern senators to oppose the filibuster against Truman's Fair Employment Practices Commission, and one of only a few southern politicians of the period who dared to endorse the eventual abo-

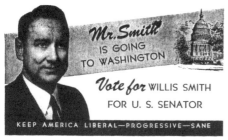

A Vote For Willis Smith
Is A Vote For
SOUTHERN DEMOCRACY

6.2 Campaign postcard for Willis Smith, 1950. *Rare Book, Manuscript, and Special Collections Library, Duke University.*

lition of racial segregation (though even he opposed federal compulsion to secure that end).[1] [Figure 6.2]

Late in February 1950, Willis Smith filed to run in the Democratic primary, and in May, with the support of the conservative wing of the party, he ran second to Graham in a four-way contest that saw Graham fall just short of the votes needed to avoid a runoff. Smith was on the verge of conceding to Graham, in fact, when on June 5 the United States Supreme Court handed down several decisions that challenged racial segregation. The court ruled that black Americans had the right to equality of treatment before the law and that railroads and graduate schools (at public universities) must integrate their facilities or implement strict equality within a segregated system. The following day, June 6, a young radio announcer at WRAL in Raleigh, Jesse Helms, asked station owner A. J. Fletcher to sell him some airtime that night. Helms wanted to broadcast a spot urging Smith to call for a runoff, and Fletcher, one of Smith's strongest supporters, agreed to split the cost of a 30-second commercial. The commercial ran 8 or 10 times between 6 P.M. and 9 P.M., with a staff announcer, not Helms, urging listeners to gather at Smith's house as a sign of support. Many observers believe that the size and enthusiasm of the crowd that night persuaded Smith to call for a runoff.

The Supreme Court rulings catalyzed white racial opinion and stirred many of Smith's supporters to reshape his campaign in the second primary. Whereas Smith had focused less in the first primary on Graham's relatively liberal racial record, and more on the senator's past affiliations with allegedly subversive organizations and Truman's "socialist" policies, race became the dominant issue in the second primary. Helms has long been accused of creating some of the Smith campaign's worst racist materials, but none of those claims has ever been proven. And if Smith himself was ultimately responsible for the actions associated with his campaign, nothing in his background suggests he was capable of the racist gutter dredging that now took place.[2]

Among Smith's most important allies in the second primary was Raleigh attorney James Hinton Pou Bailey. Bailey himself had just completed a successful primary race for a seat in the state senate, and his campaign platform captured many of the major concerns of Smith and his conservative supporters. Bailey was "particularly opposed to the idea of a welfare state which embodies socialization of industry, medicine, and of utilities. If elected," he promised, "I shall exert all of the influence which I have to halt the progress of these ideas. Nor will I support any legislation which would tend to extend the state government into those fields which typically belong to free enterprise."[3]

Buoyed by victory in his own campaign, Bailey worked tirelessly for Smith behind the scenes in the runoff. Operating mainly through his personal contacts, Bailey solicited and received substantial cash and in-kind contributions for Smith's campaign from wealthy individuals throughout the United States. Among the largest contributors were two physicians closely connected with the American Medical Association and strongly opposed to Truman's recently defeated national health care plan—a plan that Graham supported. One of the physicians, Dr. R. B. Robins of Camden, Arkansas, was feuding publicly with the federal security administrator, Oscar Ewing, over the issue of national health care.[4]

Willis Smith won the June 24 runoff by 21,086 votes and went on to defeat the Republican candidate for senator that November. His victory had a lasting impact on North Carolina's modern political culture, even as it cast Duke as a bulwark of southern conservatism. "From 1950 right into . . . the 1990s," historian William E. Leuchtenburg has said, "people are Frank Porter Graham Democrats or they are those who lined up with Willis Smith against him. It not only divided the Democratic Party, but it led to a movement of a number of Dr. Graham's opponents into the Republican Party—most conspicuously, Jesse Helms."[5] One Graham supporter, Terry Sanford, was particularly distressed by the election results. During a visit with Graham in the wake of his defeat, Sanford, who became governor of North Carolina in 1961 and president of Duke University in 1969, told Dr. Frank that the campaign was not over. "I told Frank Graham that he gave me and a great many others in our generation a real dedication to do something, to get even, to rectify that injustice. I felt all his boys had benefited," Sanford recalled, "and had certainly been renewed in their desires to do good things by his defeat. His defeat spurred us on to somehow rectify the error of the people."[6]

The Aftermath of Smith's Election

But what impact did Smith's victory have on DUMC? How did it affect the development of Duke Medicine? The simple answer is, it gave Smith additional power to advance his agenda at Duke. Smith had been working since 1946 to make Duke University a regional center for applied research in physics, chemistry, medicine, and engineering—a laboratory, as it were, for southern industry. Smith expected DUMC to help make this happen by cooperating with the rest of the university and with the state, especially given the competing political demands from the growing medical centers at UNC and Wake Forest College. Indeed, in addition to the expansion plans proposed for the medical centers in Durham, Chapel Hill, and Winston-Salem, plans for a collaborative regional research center emerged simultaneously at UNC, where the master of regional studies, sociologist Howard Odum, "proposed several research center formats that incorporated the idea of cooperation among research organizations." It was from this local crucible, in fact, that the idea for the collaborative Research Triangle Park emerged after 1955—after Smith and Odum had died and after Gray had resigned from UNC to return to Washington.[7]

Equally important to DUMC's development was Smith's expanded influence over the dispersal of federal Hill-Burton funds through the North Carolina Medical Care Commission. Even before his election as senator, Smith, as chairman of the university's board of trustees, held considerable sway in determining which of DUMC's proposed construction projects would be submitted to the state commission (and also to The Duke Endowment for matching funds). Now, as a United States senator, Smith wielded strong influence over which of the state commission's recommended projects were actually approved for Hill-Burton funds by the Federal Security Administration. Significantly, Oscar Ewing still headed the sprawling bureaucracy, which included among its many huge operating units the largest single source of funding for research and training at Duke University: the United States Public Health Service and its National Institutes of Health.

Smith was always more concerned with Duke's relationship to North Carolina and the Democratic Party than he was with facilitating the growth of Duke Medicine and the PDC. He was already the principal powerbroker at Duke by the time of his election to the senate. He had foiled the efforts of the New York trustees to make Davison president of Duke, and in doing so he had earned even greater respect at the university among the faculty and the North Carolina trustees, many of whom were affiliated with the Methodist Church and the state's textile industry. Smith had also forced Davison to adhere to the university's budgeting process, a change welcomed by many faculty and administrators alike, and Smith was deeply concerned with what he perceived as the PDC's negative impact on Duke's reputation in the state. Smith loved Duke and was dedicated to it as an institution, but he also viewed it within the context of his own political ambitions and goals. He was certain to face fierce opposition for reelection in 1954 (at the end of the term he had been elected to complete), and he needed to cooperate with the state's Democratic leaders to have a chance of winning.

Smith used DUMC and the PDC to pursue his own political and institutional goals, and he received crucial support in the process from Hollis Edens, the university's new president. According to Dean Davison, DUMC suffered "eleven lean years" under Edens's leadership. "Only by the strenuous efforts of the medical faculty and Paul Gross was the medical school able to maintain some of the standards which had been established before Edens' arrival and to prevent *Lux extincta est* (the light has failed)."[8] Indeed, by threatening Duke Medicine's autonomy and economic power, Smith and Edens soured the relationship between DUMC and Duke University for decades to come.

Hollis Edens arrived at Duke steeped in the tradition established by Abraham Flexner at the General Education Board, that is, that medical school faculty should not engage in private practice. According to the PDC's founder, Dr. Deryl Hart, Edens came to Duke "having been convinced that an absolute full-time system such as that at Hopkins or the University of Chicago was highly desirable." Edens and Smith then proceeded to make things difficult for the PDC, especially for its expansion plans at Duke Hospital. Not only did rising building costs delay the hospital addition for a decade, "but the presidency of Duke had changed," Hart later explained, "and the new president's policy meant less support to the Medical Center. The hospital section of The Duke Endowment would make a grant only when requested by the administrative head of an institution."[9] Only after Smith's death, in fact, in June 1953, did the PDC's expansion plans resurface, prompting Edens to threaten the "disclaiming by Duke University of all financial responsibility for Duke Hospital after 1956," and also, it seems, to advocate that the university take over the PDC.[10]

Willis Smith was particularly concerned with the public image of Duke created by its opposition to the expansion of the medical facilities at Chapel Hill. In the months that followed the incident, Smith heard from those who wanted the university to play a more aggressive role in improving Duke's image in the state. One Greensboro editor, Henry Kendall, complained that the university was "woefully behind in the realm of public relations. As you know," he wrote to Smith, "there is no one high in the administration who gets about much either in contact or leadership. I think that is one of Duke's big weaknesses now and it is costing heavily." To emphasize his point Kendall enclosed a clipping for Smith from the *Wilson Times*. The story quoted remarks made by a guest speaker at the annual meeting of the Wilson chapter of Duke alumni: "Outside of North Carolina we have always been received with a great deal of friendship but here at home in the state we are not very well liked."[11] Smith was naturally concerned with this image, and he took several steps to try to improve it. He put pressure on Davison, as previously noted, to accept more North Carolinians to Duke's School of Medicine, and

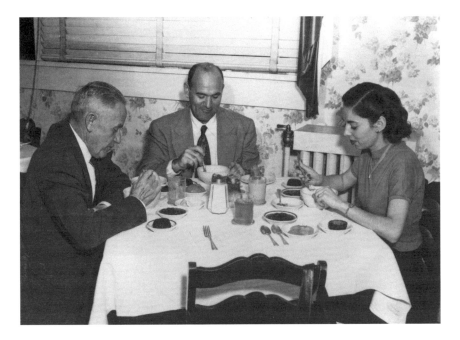

6.3 Rice dieters enjoy a meal together in Durham, North Carolina. *Duke University Medical Center Archives.*

he also spurred a reorganization of the university's public information bureau. The bureau hired an aggressive young director, a graduate of Duke, "to begin the 'contact and cultivation' of different newspapers throughout the state and beyond."[12]

Three months before filing for the Democratic primary, moreover, Smith had urged Duke's vice president for public relations, Charles E. Jordan, to facilitate a meeting between Edens and Kendall, the Greensboro editor, "for a conference on the general subject of public relations." Of more importance to DUMC was the letter Smith enclosed from Dr. Paul Whitaker of Kinston, North Carolina. Whitaker was a member of the North Carolina Medical Care Commission, a past president of the North Carolina Medical Society, and a prime mover of the North Carolina Good Health Association. "As you know," Smith wrote to Jordan, "Paul is one of the most popular men in Eastern North Carolina and one who can be of great service to the University. He has likewise been very much impressed with Dr. Edens, to whom I introduced him at one of the football games recently." Smith wanted Edens to follow up on the reference in Whitaker's letter to a "scholarship fund" for North Carolina students to attend medical school at Duke. "It is true that Dr. Whitaker was critical of the Medical School for not accepting more North Carolina boys," Smith explained, "but that same criticism was voiced by many members of the Board of Trustees and other loyal alumni not excluding the Chairman himself. I think that our friend Dave has finally seen the light and realizes that after all public relations do mean something even to the Medical School."[13]

Smith and the Funding of the Rice Diet Research

Smith wanted Davison to continue to see the light, however, and by the time he filed for the Senate Democratic primary, Smith had helped the dean's major nemesis, Dr. Walter Kempner, incorporate a private foundation and request tax-exempt status for it. The purpose of the Walter Kempner Foundation, Inc., was to raise funds to aid Kempner's rice diet research. Not coincidentally, perhaps, Smith filed the foundation's tax request on the day before *Collier's* magazine ran a cover story on federal security administrator Oscar R. Ewing. The article, titled "Mr. Welfare State Himself," mentions the role that Davison had played in the 1947 clash between Ewing and U.S. surgeon general Dr. Thomas Parran over the NIH cardiovascular grant to Kempner: "Parran explained that Dean Wilburt Davison of the Duke University Medical School, where Kempner was working, had himself advised against the grant."[14] [Figure 6.3]

The Walter Kempner Foundation published its first fundraising bulletin in the weeks that followed Smith's victory in the second Senate primary. The bulletin included a message from the foundation's president, John H. MacMillan Jr., a brief review of Kempner's use of the rice diet to control hypertension, and a section on the foundation's eight incorporators with a photograph and a biographical sketch of each. Duke's president, Hollis Edens, was among the incorporators, as were several prominent business, entertainment, and insurance executives. The purpose of the foundation, MacMillan explained, was "to secure funds for the continuation and extension of research now under way, as well as for facilities for the care of patients." Though Kempner had received public and private funding for the past several years, it was simply not enough to cover the expenses of laboratory personnel, equipment, test animals, and "the utilization of the masses of data" gathered from experiments. Kempner and his staff faced the difficult problem of "the lack of space for the two major activities that go on hand in hand—research, and the care of patients. Laboratory and office space, as well as examining rooms are at a premium in Duke Hospital," MacMillan wrote, "and the resulting congestion hinders the treatment of ambulatory patients as well as the utilization of voluminous files of records that must be kept at hand if they are to be of maximum value. Only seven hospital beds are available at Duke for Dr. Kempner's patients. They are always occupied, and on many occasions it has been necessary to house critically ill patients elsewhere in town."[15]

Smith's support for the Kempner Foundation had more to do with his own personal and institutional goals than with any specific interest in Kempner or the rice diet. Smith wanted Duke to benefit from the generosity and attention of the wealthy and powerful people Kempner was helping, including Oscar Ewing's wife, Helen D. Ewing. Smith was also deeply interested in Kempner's connections to the insurance industry. Between 1940 and 1944, the armed forces had rejected from military service some 165,000 men with high blood pressure, and it was hypertension that led to the massive cerebral hemorrhage that killed President Franklin Roosevelt in 1945. The insurance industry also knew from actuarial studies that high blood pressure was a major risk for cardiovascular disease, prompting many insurance companies to refuse to write policies for individuals with blood pressure above 140/90.[16] The president of the Kempner Foundation, John MacMillan, explained. "Dr. Kempner's research has been supported for the past several years by grants from the United States Public Health Service, the Life Insurance Medical Research Fund, and by Duke University, as well as by gifts from patients." Insurance companies were also among the largest clients of Smith's Raleigh law firm, while Smith himself had served as president of the International Association of Insurance Counsel (1941–43). Although Smith's personal connections to the insurance fund are not clear, the fund's impact on Duke Medicine is.

Between 1948 and 1956, the Life Insurance Medical Research Fund was second only to the American Cancer Society in the amount of research funding contributed by individual foundations to Duke University. The fund had been created in 1945, partly at the urging of Dr. Fred Hanes, and specifically for research on hypertension, heart disease, and cardiovascular drugs. The fund represented annual contributions from more than 140 insurance companies in the United States and Canada and it made grants to colleges and universities in both countries. One of the fund's first grants to Duke, if not the first, was made in 1946, shortly after Hanes's death, to DUMC's Phil Handler (in the Biochemistry Department) and Frederick Bernheim (in the Department of Physiology and Pharmacology) for research "on the role of protein intake in hypertension." Hanes's successor in Medicine, Dr. Eugene Stead, brought with him to Duke a grant from the insurance fund, and in 1947, the year that Ewing and Parran tangled over the NIH grant to Kempner, the latter received a $10,000 grant from the insurance fund for research: "on the effects of altering mineral metabolism by diet on the course of renal and hypertensive disease." In 1948, moreover, a substantial grant to Stead from the fund—for the "study of cardiac output and blood flow in various tissues"—drew the attention of the *New York Times*. "The Life Insurance Medical Research Fund," the *Times* noted, "the Scientific Director of which, Dr. Francis R. Dieuaide has headquarters in New York, has given several grants to the various departments at Duke University School of Medicine."[17]

By 1950, the Life Insurance Medical Research Fund had given out a total of $3.2 million in awards and had received the Lasker Award from the American Public Health Association for its contributions to the advancement of medical science and public health. Kempner, Handler, and Bernheim had all received additional grants from the fund by then, but Duke itself had still refused to issue any public statement on Kempner and the rice diet.[18] Davison's public embarrassment accounted for part of the silence, as did the time consumed by other groups of researchers testing Kempner's results—at least one of which appears to have been funded by the Life Insurance Medical Research Fund. Indeed, while Kempner's published research was setting the medical world ablaze, both with indignation and investigation, Duke remained silent on the subject until March 3, 1951. "The secrecy was lifted today from the rice diet for high blood pressure at Duke University," the *New York Times* reported that March. "For six years, the author of the diet, Dr. Walter Kempner, has maintained strict silence on the subject. Finally, the Duke bureau of public relations issued an authoritative report." Kempner had collected data on 1,800 patients suffering from high blood pressure between 1944 and 1950, and of those, 1,200 had experienced what he described as "marked benefit" from the rice diet. "A long medical controversy over whether [the] rice diet is worthwhile [is] swinging in favor of the Duke doctor," the *Times* explained. "The Rockefeller Institute, New York, and Columbia University studied patients on the diet for two years. They reported two-thirds received substantial benefit. A team of doctors who made a study for the British Medical Research Council reported that they confirmed the claims made by Dr. Kempner."[19]

Duke's Development as a Regional Research Center

Willis Smith's support for Kempner also reflected his unfolding plans to create a regional research center at Duke and the related efforts of Edens and the university's vice president, Paul Gross, to develop a 10-year, $10 million program for graduate work in 10 fields of study at Duke. By the spring of 1950, the General Education Board had pledged financial support for the graduate studies program but The Duke Endowment had not. As the board's director, Robert Calkins reported, Edens was considering eliminating the university's programs in the Education Department and was "quite hopeful that the Duke Endowment will be willing to come in with the GEB on the financing of the graduate education program. In all probability," Calkins wrote, "the Board will be asked for $500,000 instead of $600,000 for operating expenses over the first five years, and a million dollars toward \$3,000,000 endowment. We discussed at some length whether the endowment was strictly needed in view of the fact that institution may someday acquire the Doris Duke trust." Edens had reminded Calkins, however, that the university was merely a residual beneficiary of the trust and would not receive it if Doris Duke had children; in other words, Calkins reported, "the institution cannot, therefore, plan on receiving these funds, and certainly not within our lifetime. This leads [Edens] to conclude that Duke ought to build up its own endowment and especially endowment earmarked for graduate studies."[20]

While Edens worked with his old employer to support the graduate studies program at Duke, the university's vice president, Paul Gross, sought faculty support for the program and for Smith's larger, related plan to make Duke a regional research center. Smith's plan had first emerged in 1947 as a result of his collaboration with Duke trustee Edwin L. Jones Sr., the Charlotte contractor whose company had built the Oak Ridge gaseous diffusion plant for the Manhattan Project during World War II. Smith and Jones had mobilized Duke's trustees to fund "a greatly enlarged Physics Department" at Duke—to capture some of the "Millions of Government money" being spent on research in nuclear physics—and to lay the foundation for a "Research Laboratory" that "would draw support of Southern Industry to Duke University."[21] This plan directly affected the development of Duke Medicine and became the basis, in the years that followed Smith's death, for the plans promoted by Gross as chairman of the university's Long Range Planning Committee. Indeed, in the absence of Smith's mediating influence, these long-range plans caused a major split not only in the university's board of trustees, but also in the relationship between Edens and Gross (both of whom resigned in 1960), and in the relationship between the majority of the trustees and The Duke Endowment. It was from this conflict, in fact, that Dr. Deryl Hart, chairman of the Department of Surgery, would emerge as president of Duke University in 1960.

On Christmas Day, 1951, the university announced that its "research and development program which integrates the university's facilities with regional advances in science and health has been expanded to include engineering research needed to meet the rapid industrial growth of the new South."[22]

Duke's development program appeared to the *New York Times* to be a success. "Duke has developed as a regional research center in the fields of physics, chemistry, and medicine," the newspaper explained. The article gave details about projects under way in the Physics and Chemistry Departments and noted that "Duke Hospital conducts an extensive research program along with its treatment of patients and the training of physicians and nurses. Many of the hospital's research projects are national in scope and have attracted the services of leading medical scientists."[23]

The story in the *Times* also hints at the dispute that later erupted over Duke's development plans, especially the struggle between Edens and Gross. Edens, in the single quote attributed to him, focused on the expanded program's regional thrust. "Any region looks to its educational institutions for leadership," Edens said, "and Duke University is endeavoring to fulfill its obligations to the South by making its facilities available to industry." Gross mentions the regional context, too, but links it to Duke's national aspirations and to the fact that the university's "research and development program was also a long-term project that would require additions to the staff over a period of years." Gross told the *Times*, "It will help our university to serve more adequately the region in which it is located, and will keep our rank high with other schools that render service to the country."[24]

RESEARCH PROJECTS RELATED TO THE MILITARY

Smith's plan had its widest and most immediate impact on Duke Medicine through programs funded by the Atomic Energy Commission, the American military, and the nation's largest tobacco companies. These programs linked Duke to some of the key health and national security concerns of the day, including nuclear warfare, smoking, cancer, hypertension, and cardiovascular disease. Two studies linking smoking to lung cancer appeared in 1950, in the *Journal of the American Medical Association*, and from that point on, the public debate intensified as the tobacco industry launched a huge research and media campaign to challenge the link between smoking and cancer. The debate also provoked considerable worry among many different groups and individuals, including the American military and the Veterans Administration. The military had collaborated with the nation's tobacco companies to make free or cheap cigarettes available to American troops since World War I—a policy that continued during the Korean War (1950–53). But the increasingly heated smoking debate now raised several important questions: What was smoking doing to the long-term health of veterans? How was it affecting current and future medical costs at the VA? Who would pay those costs? How?

The growing concerns over the link between smoking and cancer also occurred at time when many policymakers assumed that the next war would be fought with atomic weapons—an assumption that posed critical questions for military physicians, defense planners, and the Atomic Energy Commission. What were the long-term effects of radiation? How would it affect soldiers, civilians, and atomic energy workers? What impact would it have on soils and crops? On the air that we breathe? On cancer? On the creation of a domestic nuclear power industry? At the same time, nuclear medicine was also offering such new and potentially useful tools as radioisotopes, which posed both exciting possibilities and fundamental questions regarding their use

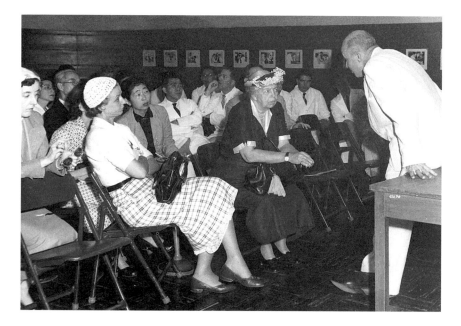

6.4 Dr. H. Grant Taylor, director of the Atomic Bomb Casualty Commission, responds to a question from Eleanor Roosevelt. Hiroshima, Japan. June 9, 1953. *McGovern Historical Collections and Research Center, Houston Academy of Medicine-Texas Medical Center Library.*

in basic medical research and clinical applications: how radioisotopes could enhance our understanding of human metabolism and metabolic functions, how they could be used to measure the distribution and excretion of atomic weapons fallout in humans, and how they could localize and possibly destroy certain types of tumors in the brain and lungs.

Duke's research on these questions situated the university at the nexus of global and local health concerns in the early 1950s. Although research on radiation's effects had started before the atomic bombs were dropped on Hiroshima and Nagasaki in August 1945, President Harry Truman issued a directive in 1946 authorizing the National Research Council (of the National Academy of Sciences) to undertake a long-term study of those who survived the atomic bombings. The Atomic Energy Commission funded the study, while the National Research Council's Division of Medical Sciences created the Atomic Bomb Casualty Commission to carry out the study in Japan.

The Atomic Bomb Casualty Commission was important to Duke Medicine for several reasons. Grants from the commission gave Duke staff and medical graduates the opportunity to study firsthand the impact of radiation on humans and also to conduct research on the topic. Davison himself was part of a group that went to Japan in 1951, at the request of the National Research Council, to help determine the future of the Atomic Bomb Casualty Commission. Davison was met in Japan by his favorite colleague and former student, pediatrician Grant Taylor. Taylor had taken a leave of absence as associate dean of Duke's medical school in 1949 in order to serve as the commission's deputy medical director for research in Japan and as a consultant for the Armed Forces Epidemiological Board in Korea. Taylor went on to serve as director of the commission between 1952 and 1954, before becoming a pioneer in pediatric oncology at the M. D. Anderson Hospital and Tumor Institute in Houston. The Atomic Bomb Casualty Commission continued to provide valuable research and data until 1974, when it was succeeded by the Radiation Effects Research Foundation, a private, nonprofit corporation created at the urging of the then president of the National Academy of Sciences, Philip Handler.[25] [Figure 6.4]

Duke's position at the crossroads of cold war research became particularly strategic after the Korean War erupted in June of 1950. Between 1950 and 1951, the Atomic Energy Commission increased its research contracts with Duke from $20,000 to $317,000, while research grants from the Public Health Service—usually the largest source of funding for research at the university—tumbled from $229,000 to $153,000. Just a month before the war began, in May of 1950, the *Journal of the American Medical Association* published the two articles linking smoking to lung cancer. The *New York Times* covered the story under the headline "Smoking Found Tied to Cancer of Lungs," pointing out that the *Journal* articles "warned that there appears to be a significant relationship between prolonged tobacco smoking and the development of cancer of the lungs."[26]

In the meantime, Smith, Gross, and Edens continued to expand the university's services as a research center. In January of 1951, the Department of Defense stepped up development and production of the Nike Ajax missile system in North Carolina and California, and in June the United States Army located its Office of Ordnance Research on the Duke Campus. The Army Research Office, as it came to be known, served as an administrative clearinghouse for proposals submitted to the service for covert funding of basic research. During its first eight years on campus, the office was located across the street from the president's mansion, in the large English Gothic residence formerly owned by Dr. Fred Hanes. The chairman of Duke's Chemistry Department, Dr. Marcus E. Hobbs, served as acting of director of the office until the permanent chief scientist took over. It was also in the spring of 1951 that Hobbs and Paul Gross began negotiating a five-year research grant with the American Tobacco Company and the Damon Runyon Memorial Fund, a philanthropy that specialized in cancer research. The plan called for American Tobacco to make the grant to the Runyon fund, which would then distribute the money to Duke's Chemistry Department—at $50,000 a year for five years—for research on the physical and chemical properties of tobacco smoke.[27]

Paul Gross was the principal scientific conduit for government- and industry-funded research at Duke in chemistry, physics, and several other fields. Gross had chaired the Chemistry Department at Trinity-Duke from 1919 until his appointment as vice president of the university in 1948. He had received the Herty Medal (for his research on tobacco) and the President's Medal for Merit (for developing a frangible bullet used by the Army Ordnance Department to train aerial gunners during World War II). He was also an internationally respected scientist and one of the incorporators of the Oak Ridge Institute for Nuclear Studies. The institute, which was created in 1946, was a cooperative program of higher education involving 19 southern institutions in a program "to further the development in the South of research in fields related to atomic energy."[28] The institute took its name from the Atomic Energy Commission's Oak Ridge National Laboratory, at Oak Ridge, Tennessee, which focused on radiochemical separations and the production of radioisotopes—radioactive versions of elements—for medical centers and research laboratories throughout the nation. By the late 1940s, the Oak Ridge laboratory was "the world's foremost source of radioisotopes for medicine, agriculture, industry, and other uses." Gross was elected president of the Oak Ridge Institute in June of 1949, after his predecessor, Dr. Frank Porter Graham, resigned to accept the Senate seat later occupied by Willis Smith.[29]

By 1951, Gross's handiwork with the Atomic Energy Commission was evident in several of Duke's departments, as well as in the university's medical center. The commission's influence was particularly strong in the university's Physics Department, where the chairman, Dr. Walter Nielsen, was also a founding member of the Oak Ridge Institute. "The department cooperates with Oak Ridge," one observer noted in 1948. "Its work does not duplicate but supplements work carried on at Oak Ridge. Nielsen hopes to maintain close cooperation with Oak Ridge, and in developing the work in physics at Duke to enliven the engineering department and maintain a closer and more active relationship between the two departments."[30] The Atomic Energy Commission also named Duke as one of four regional centers in 1948 for training postdoctoral fellows in the use of radioisotopes in biology and medicine. DUMC's Philip Handler, a biochemist, was put in charge of the program along with Nielsen and Dr. Jerome S. Harris, Davison's future successor as chairman of the Department of Pediatrics. At the same time, through a contract with the Oak Ridge Institute for Nuclear Studies, a radioisotope laboratory was established under Handler's control in the Biochemistry Department.[31]

The federal radioisotope program also connected Duke Medicine to the state's other medical centers and to the Veterans Hospital constructed next to

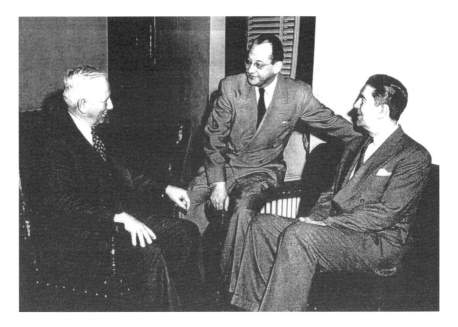

6.5 Dr. Paul M. Gross, left, and Duke president Dr. A. Hollis Edens, right, confer with Gordon Dean, chairman of the Atomic Energy Commission. *Duke University Archives*.

Duke's campus beginning in 1950. The Duke program was designed in part to foster collaboration among the state's medical centers and the state-supported engineering college at Raleigh. "While conceived as a joint enterprise with the University of North Carolina, North Carolina State College, and Bowman Gray School of Medicine," Wilburt Davison explained, "the actual program has been located at Duke, although a number of teachers from the collaborating institutions have participated in the teaching." Davison also pointed out that the radioisotope laboratory under Handler had "facilitated a series of metabolic studies using radioisotopes of phosphorous, calcium, carbon, sodium and potassium. Recently there was initiated a highly promising study wherein the positron-emitting radioisotope of copper is being used to localize brain tumors. This laboratory and its activities are to be moved to the Cancer Wing of the W. B. Bell Research Building when the latter is completed in order to expand its activities and to permit easy access to the isotope facilities of the Veterans Hospital currently under construction."[32]

DUMC's link to the Veterans Hospital and the radioisotope program suggests the extent to which Duke Medicine was influenced during the early cold war by overlapping concerns with radioactive fallout, cancer, and the health of veterans. Davison himself was appointed to the Oak Ridge Institute's Board of Medical Consultants in 1948, and at some point during his six years of service on the board, he became alarmed with his own tobacco habit. "On returning from one of my Oak Ridge trips, after seeing some advanced cancer patients, I noticed that my tongue was very red and sore. I suspected that my pipe might be causing a mouth cancer because I had smoked fifteen daily. . . . I stopped smoking for a week, and the redness and soreness disappeared. By that time, I had realized that the cause of the condition was not my pipe but some penicillin lozenges which I had been sucking because of a sore throat. I was so chagrined by my wrong diagnosis that I haven't smoked since."[33]

National concerns over the link between cancer, radioactive fallout, and the health of veterans became particularly acute in North Carolina in 1951 with development and production of the army's Nike Ajax missile system and with atmospheric testing of nuclear weapons in Nevada. Some of the Nike system's early rocket tests took place in North Carolina, on the Outer Banks; grants to Duke's Department of Physics (for microwave studies of materials and electronic communications) partly justified construction of the university's new $1 million physics building between 1948 and 1949.[34] By the outbreak of war in Korea, North Carolina was home to some of the nation's largest military bases, to numerous electronics plants making the ground systems and guidance units for the Nike Ajax, and to the Army Ordnance Missile Plant in Charlotte, where many of the Nike missiles were assembled.[35] [Figure 6.5]

That Duke Medicine deepened its commitment to the nation's veterans during the Korean War is thus not surprising. What is surprising is the impact of this experience on DUMC. Although the VA broke ground for its Durham hospital in January of 1950, on a site adjacent to DUMC, construction quickly became hampered by disputes between the building's contractors and local labor unions, and that was only the beginning. Politics, bureaucracy, and red tape delayed the building's opening until the spring of 1953—several months after the new teaching hospital was dedicated at UNC. While the VA hospital was under construction, moreover, DUMC eliminated its Department of Neuropsychiatry and helped facilitate the preservation and use of several of the largest and most important repositories of medical records and information in the world.

Veterans and the VA had emerged as central concerns for DUMC during World War II, but their importance to Duke Medicine increased dramatically in the decades that followed. Dave Davison was deeply involved in the national health system created for veterans, as was Dr. Barnes Woodhall, chief of Neurosurgery at Duke. Both men became associated with the National Research Council's Committee on Veterans Medical Problems after the war and with the committee's Medical Follow-Up Agency. Created as a permanent committee of the council in 1946, the Committee on Veterans Medical Problems was funded by the Veterans Administration and charged with two general purposes. It was to subsidize clinical research at veterans hospitals and

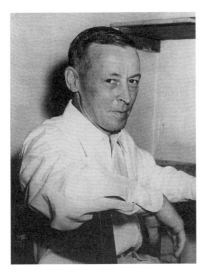

facilitate the use of the VA's vast collection of medical records. Systematic use of the records had first been proposed in the spring of 1946 at a conference on postwar research at the National Academy of Sciences. Barnes Woodhall had been among the 43 medical administrators and researchers who had attended the conference, as had John Whitehorn, chief of the Psychiatry Department at Johns Hopkins; Louis Dublin, a statistician with the Metropolitan Life Insurance Company; and Colonel Michael E. DeBakey, then a member of the army's Office of the Surgeon General. DeBakey's description of the VA records had served as the basis for discussion at the meeting. "It can fairly be said," he wrote, "that no similar amount of material has ever been accumulated, and it is doubtful whether a similar amount will ever again be available." DeBakey had suggested the material be put to "practical use by the establishment of a clinical research program, including a follow-up system to determine the natural and post-treatment history" of conditions and diseases treated during the war.[36]

Woodhall had then proposed one of the first studies undertaken by the Medical Follow-up Agency, a study of peripheral nerve injuries.[37] The Duke surgeon had handled many such injuries as chief of neurosurgery at the Walter Reed General Hospital in Washington, D.C., from 1942 to 1946. During that time, Woodhall had helped instruct "the American general surgeons who treated the majority of acute wartime neurosurgical trauma cases," and in 1945, together with Webb Haymaker, a neuropathologist, Woodhall had published *Peripheral Nerve Injuries: Principles of Diagnosis.* Woodhall's medical follow-up study was still under way, however, when the second edition of *Peripheral Nerve Injuries* appeared (1953), and by then the huge veterans study had consumed about a quarter of the funds received by the Medical Follow-up Agency. Finally published in 1957, the study involved 3,656 World War II injuries and the examination of three-quarters of the injured men at clinical centers in Chicago, Boston, New York, Philadelphia, and San Francisco. According to one source, "the study determined the optimal time for nerve suture and established the value of physical therapy during the time of nerve regeneration." Between 1958 and 1959, moreover, Woodhall served as a consultant to both the surgeon general and to the Veterans Administration and coedited and contributed to the two-volume history of neurosurgery in the army during World War II. Woodhall would succeed Davison as dean of Duke University's School of Medicine in 1960.[38] [Figure 6.6]

Dave Davison became head of the Committee of Veterans Medical Problems in 1950, and later that year, at the request of the VA, and after the outbreak of hostilities in Korea, he appointed himself and three others to a committee to investigate the cost effectiveness of the Medical Follow-up Agency. Their report, submitted by Davison in January of 1951, was very enthusiastic. "All of us have expected concrete, tangible, and useful results from the VA follow-up projects but none of us realized, until the meeting today, how excellent the progress has been and how important the reports are even in their preliminary stage," Davison wrote. The Duke dean believed that everyone concerned, from the VA and the military to the American taxpayer, would "all profit enormously" if the program were continued.[39]

Medical Libraries

D avison's work with the VA also reinforced his deep faith in the importance of medical libraries and in preserving medical information. One of his first requests to The Duke Endowment in 1927 had been for the authority to collect a hospital library, "for although buildings could be built and a staff assembled," he wrote in 1950, "a library had to be hunted in the four corners of the earth." The Endowment had funded Davison's search, and in 1950 he wrote that "The Duke Hospital Library probably is the most complete one south of Washington, and is increasing at the rate of 2,000 volumes per year."[40] The dean knew what he was talking about. He had been an honorary consultant to the Army Medical Library since 1943, and from 1950 to 1953 he was president of the Association of Honorary Consultants to the Army Medical Library. Davison was also familiar with the fabulous collection gathered by another honorary consultant of the Army Medical Library, Duke thoracic surgeon Dr. Josiah Charles Trent. Between 1939 and his death in 1948, Trent had gathered one of the finest and most extensive collections of rare medical books and manuscripts in the nation. He had also started the first blood bank at Duke and served as a member of the editorial board of the *Journal of the History of Medicine and Allied Sciences* and of the *North Carolina Medical Journal*. In 1956, Trent's private collection was donated to Duke University, forming the foundation of today's extensive Josiah Charles Trent Collection in the History of Medicine in the Duke University Medical Center Library.[41]

One of Davison's former students, Dr. Martin M. Cummings, later recalled that Duke had taught him "not only pediatrics but the value of libraries in medicine."[42] Indeed, Davison's support for the Army Medical Library helped shape Cummings's later career as director of the National Library of Medicine (1964–84). As Cummings wrote in 1972, at the time of Davison's death, a major concern of "Dr. Davison was to convert the Army Medical Library to the National Library of Medicine in name as well as in fact. New legislation was passed in 1956, creating the National Library of Medicine as the first specialized library with its own Congressional mandate."[43]

Davison also secured badly needed funding for the Army Medical Library from Doris Duke's first foundation, Independent Aid, Inc. Davison himself was a trustee of the foundation, and in 1951, as he prepared to visit the Atomic Bomb Casualty Commission in Japan, he asked Independent Aid to help the library with a grant. Davison noted in explaining his request that the library's honorary consultants assisted "the Regular Army in the operation of what probably is the finest medical library in the world. There are 100 of us in different parts of the country who help interpret the Army Library and also obtain help for it over and above the appropriations from Congress. For the first few years the Board of Honorary Consultants, who have served without salary or expense accounts, were financed by the Rockefeller Foundation for the secretarial and other expenses which occur. . . . However, when I became President this year the treasury was bare, and a thousand dollars would keep the wolf away for another year."[44]

The Dissolution of Neuropsychiatry at Duke

Back in Durham, Davison prepared DUMC to collaborate with the coming VA hospital by easing out Dr. Richard Lyman as chairman of the Department of Neuropsychiatry. Lyman took a leave of absence in 1950, ostensibly to accept a full-time appointment with the Veterans Administration. But he only took it, he claimed, so that Duke could free up his salary for visiting professor Dr. Willibald Scholz, director of the Neuropathology Division of the Deutsche Forschunganstadt für Psychiatrie (now the Max Planck Institute of Psychiatry) in Munich. Lyman also tangled with Davison by initially refusing the dean's instructions to appoint Dr. George A. Silver III to the VA planning committee; only later, after a "talk" with Silver, did Lyman "approve" the dean's appointment. Whatever the case, there was more than handwriting on the wall when Lyman submitted his resignation on February 21, 1951. Though he stayed on with the VA until the summer, he spent the rest of his career as visiting professor of neuropsychiatry at one of the nation's two black medical schools, Meharry Medical College in Nashville, Tennessee.[45]

Much to Lyman's chagrin, DUMC made no effort to find a new chairman before he left. Rather, Dr. Hans Lowenbach was made acting chairman of the department and the search committee suggested that Dr. Leslie Hohman run

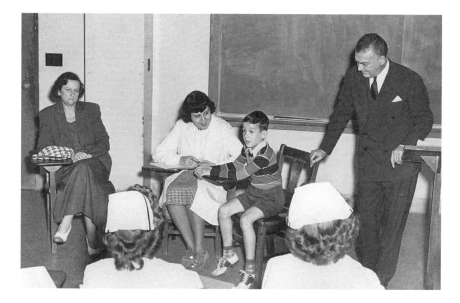

6.7 Dr. Leslie B. Hohman, standing, and Irene Cherhavy, a speech therapist, work with a young patient at the Child Guidance Center. *Duke University Medical Center Archives.*

the department for a period of some three years. Lyman was irate. He had recruited Hohman to run the veterans neuropsychiatry training program at Duke, but he now considered Hohman "virtually committed to tear down most of the things I have been trying to build up and his constructive work omits any attempt to round out the department and extend it into the community, so far as I have been let into it by His Highness, Hohman himself." Lyman warned Davison that either Dr. Maurice Greenhill or Dr. George F. Sutherland "must" be made acting chairman or there would "be serious disruption of the department, due to departure of men on the staff."[46] Though Hohman stayed on in the department, which was renamed the Department of Psychiatry in October 1951, both of DUMC's specialists in psychosomatic medicine, Greenhill and Sutherland, left before Dr. Ewald Busse arrived as head of the new department in the fall of 1953.[47] [Figure 6.7]

What happened? What explains this failure of the Rockefeller Foundation's great southern experiment in psychiatry and psychosomatic medicine? Why did psychiatry fail to flourish on its excellent foundations at Duke? Lyman may have suffered, as some have hinted, from mental illness himself. He certainly was an unusual person, and he liked to work all night, but the same could be said of many other physicians. Another explanation suggests race and the VA as factors. Lyman extended psychiatry into the community, and he did so without regard to race or, perhaps, with special regard for race—a risky pursuit, to say the least, given the fires of racial antipathy lit by the Willis Smith campaign. To be sure, Duke's mental health activists had by now retreated from the community. There was no more teaching of "Negro psychiatry" at Lincoln Hospital, at least not by physicians at Duke, and in 1952, the Durham Community Child Guidance Clinic moved from downtown Durham to a site on Duke campus, where it was completely reorganized and restaffed in 1953. Lyman had also angered the VA, as well as Duke's former president, Robert Flowers, in the double-billing incident with the VA, and Davison needed no such reminders while studying the cost-effectiveness of the Medical Follow-up Agency for the VA and preparing DUMC for collaboration with the new VA hospital.[48]

Nor could the Rockefeller Foundation exert personal and financial pressure to keep its experiment in psychiatry alive. Robert Lambert had retired from the foundation in 1948, shortly after Chester Barnard succeeded Raymond Fosdick as the foundation's president. Barnard had immediately initiated a reappraisal and restructuring of the foundation's programs, especially in its International Health Division. The division was merged with the Medical Sciences Division in 1951 to create a new Division of Medical Sciences and Public Health. But Alan Gregg was not its director; he was elected vice president of the foundation. The cold war also witnessed a generation of Rockefeller trustees intimately involved with foreign policy—including John McCloy, Dean Rusk, and John Foster Dulles—and an attendant shift in program focus beginning in 1952. "After disengaging from such areas as malaria control and psychiatry," one foundation historian has written, "a program was formulated centering around mental illness, human genetics and virology on the scientific side, and health care studies, professional education and population control on the applied side." Finally, in 1955, and possibly as Gregg's parting shot before he retired in 1956, the Division of Medical Sciences and Public Health was reappraised and split once again, with the appointment of directors for medical education and public health and for biological and medical research.[49]

The changing priorities in Rockefeller funding were already in evidence by the time of Lyman's resignation. In 1950, for example, at a time when the foundation made no new grants to DUMC, Alan Gregg spent a week in Chapel Hill discussing the opportunities and objectives of the University of North Carolina's new medical school. He also spent time with Duke president Hollis Edens discussing a possible grant from the Rockefeller Foundation to Dr. J. B. Rhine, head of the Parapsychology Laboratory in Duke's Department of Psychology. Though there was some hesitancy on the part of Edens, Gross, and others at the university about submitting a request for funding (mainly out of "concern over the scientific reliability of Rhine's methods"), the Duke president eventually agreed to accept the $50,000 grant, hoping also for some way "to validate Rhine's methods so that out of the grant might come a further substantiation of his work." In 1951, moreover, the only Rockefeller grant to Duke was to Dr. Frank A. Hanna, a member of the Department of Economics, for "Studies in Differences in State per Capita Income." Not until 1957, it seems, did the Rockefeller Foundation resume making grants to DUMC, and then it was a large, multiyear grant for creating a master's degree program in nursing.[50]

All of these factors combined with another, more important one to bring down Duke's Department of Neuropsychiatry. Much as Lyman predicted, the department fell victim to state politics. His resignation coincided with a $1 million appropriation from the 1951 General Assembly for construction at UNC of a psychiatric center that was to be part of what the legislature simultaneously designated as the North Carolina Memorial Hospital in Chapel Hill—"the state's memorial to the dead of all wars." UNC's new psychiatric center was designed to provide much of what Lyman had hoped for at Duke: "an outpatient clinic and wards for seventy-five beds for psychiatric patients, with research laboratories and office space." The primary purpose of the new UNC center "was for training more personnel for the mental hospitals in North Carolina and for the improvement of mental health in the state."[51]

Developments in Health Care Planning Statewide

The dissolution of Duke's Department of Neuropsychiatry reflected the wider efforts of Willis Smith to cooperate with North Carolina's political leadership. Delaying DUMC's expansion gave the state's other academic medical centers a chance to expand and compete with Duke Medicine. Between 1947 and 1955, Duke received only one grant from the North Carolina Medical Care Commission: an award of $372,240 in 1951 for construction of the Elizabeth P. Hanes House for Nurses. The local matching funds required by Hill-Burton for that project were provided by Mrs. Hanes herself ($473,760) and by Duke University ($60,000). The only other construction projects completed at the medical center between 1950 and 1956 were located outside of the original medical school–hospital buildings. A third wing was added to the Bell Research Building in 1952 (with funds provided by the U.S. government and the PDC), and in 1953, when the nurses moved down the street to their new dormitory, the PDC funded the conversion of the existing nurses' residence, Baker House, to PDC staff offices and a dormitory for house staff. Even more revealing, the only DUMC building to which The Duke Endowment contributed funds for construction between 1947 and 1955 was a hospital laundry.[52]

Beyond Duke, however, the combination of local, state, and federal funding significantly increased the number of hospital and medical facilities in the state. In 1950, for example, the North Carolina Medical Care Commission allotted funding for the expansion of Watts and Lincoln Hospitals in Durham, where three months later voters approved a $2 million bond issue to add to the commission's allotment. The North Carolina Memorial Hospital opened at UNC in September 1952, and in 1954, the first four-year class at Chapel Hill was awarded the M.D. degree. "In 1953–54," one historian has written, "the number of hospital beds in Durham and Chapel Hill increased 100 per cent with the opening of the Veterans Administration Hospital in Durham and North Carolina Memorial Hospital in Chapel Hill and completion of the expansion programs at Watts and Lincoln Hospital."[53] Over in Winston-Salem, moreover, a new 150-bed patient wing and other improvements were added to the North Carolina Baptist Hospital. Completed in 1954, at a cost of $1.7 million, the addition to Baptist Hospital was funded by the North Carolina Medical Care Commission and "by friends of the hospital, the Baptist State Convention, and doctors associated with the hospital and the Bowman Gray School of Medicine."[54]

It wasn't that Smith and Edens left DUMC entirely on its own to face this competition. Duke's trustees set up a special fund for Duke Hospital in 1952. As the university's financial report noted that year, "anticipating the more difficult operating conditions that will accompany the opening of the Veterans Hospital and the Memorial Hospital at the University of North Carolina a reserve for the stabilization of Hospital Income was set up and the sum of $84,694.03 was transferred to it."[55] Over the next several years, however, the hospital's budget deficits soared. From $5,272 in fiscal year 1950–51, the hospital's deficits climbed to $140,837 in 1953–54 before declining slightly to $138,513 during 1955–56.[56]

While Smith got help from Edens in controlling Duke Medicine's access to The Duke Endowment and the North Carolina Medical Care Commission, Smith wielded significant influence on his own, as a United States senator, in determining which hospital projects recommended by the commission were eventually approved for Hill-Burton funds. Smith's influence was recognized in 1951, for example, when the Federal Security Administration approved the state commission's recommendation for a new hospital laundry and boiler at Rex Hospital in Raleigh. In a letter to Smith objecting to the action, the president of the North Carolina Association of Launderers and Cleaners argued that "I do not think it was the intention when the Hill-Burton National Hospital Construction Act was passed to build hospital laundries in competition with already existing laundry plants. We already have too much government in business and too little business in government, to which we feel you will agree. We would appreciate very much any help you could give us in helping to stop the construction of this laundry at Rex Hospital."[57]

Smith also heard that same day from Frank Daniels, a Rex trustee who had anticipated the association's protest. "We respectfully hope that you will not interfere with the grant that has already been given us," Daniels wrote to Smith. "Medical Care has granted our request and 44% of the cost of this project will be met for the North Carolina Medical Care Commission with Hill-Burton funds." Smith wisely refused to interfere in the matter, noting in a letter to the laundry association "I am opposed to the Government going into business to compete with its citizens, but I do not feel that that policy should interfere with a hospital operating its own laundry for its own uses."[58]

Gordon Gray's National and Local Agendas

Among the many individuals with whom Smith and Edens cooperated in the early 1950s, none had a greater impact on Duke Medicine than UNC president Gordon Gray. Gray was a major figure in the nation's military and intelligence networks and one of the most adept and accomplished members of the "progressive plutocracy" that ran, and continues to run, North Carolina's corporate, political, civic, and cultural life. Gray was directly involved in the development of UNC's new four-year medical school, and his close personal ties to Winston-Salem's leading tobacco, textile, and banking families included a number of Duke's most powerful trustees and alumni. Gray was also deeply committed to the success of the Bowman Gray School of Medicine at Wake Forest College. Not only was the medical school named for his father, but Gray himself had helped convert the family's huge manor house into a clinical facility for the school's psychiatry department. It was from this strategic position at the center of the state's health care interests that Gray initiated a statewide planning effort that looked back to the Committee on the Costs of Medical Care (1927–33) and forward to the regional health care planning agencies of the 1960s, including the Research Triangle Metropolitan Health Planning Group, the Community Health Organization Committee, and the Health Planning Council for Central North Carolina.[59]

Gray had received a law degree from Yale after graduating from UNC with a degree in psychology. After briefly practicing law in New York, he had returned to Winston-Salem to become president of the Piedmont Publishing Company, which owned both local newspapers and the city's only radio station. Elected twice to the state senate before enlisting in the army as a private, Gray was a captain in the army's advanced intelligence headquarters in Europe at the end of the war. Following his return to Winston-Salem he was again elected to the state senate and had served in the 1947 General Assembly that approved the four-year medical school at the University of North Carolina.

Between 1947 and 1952, Gray became a central figure in making North

Carolina a key link in the Truman administration's domestic civil rights and foreign policy agendas. Gray held several powerful positions in the Truman administration. In 1947 he was appointed assistant secretary of the army under North Carolina native Kenneth Royall. Together the two men helped ensure that North Carolina became a major fortress of the cold war, involved in everything from making Nike missiles and hosting some of the nation's largest military bases to serving as a Voice of America relay transmitter site. In 1949, moreover, at a time when he was being considered for both the directorship of the Central Intelligence Agency and the presidency of the University of North Carolina, Gray succeeded Royall as secretary of the army.[60]

Gray was still secretary of the army when he agreed to become Frank Graham's successor as president of UNC, and by the time he resigned as secretary in April 1950, he had ordered the army to conduct its recruiting without regard to race. UNC had still not opened its doors to blacks, however, and plans had yet to be completed for its new 400-bed teaching hospital on the Chapel Hill campus. Gray's inauguration at UNC had taken place in September 1950, almost a year after Edens's at Duke, and two months later, in November 1950, Willis Smith had been elected to the United States Senate. From that point on, Smith and Gray began to define the split in North Carolina's Democratic Party. Smith aligned himself in Washington with conservative Democratic senators and sat with Nevada senator Patrick McCarran on the Senate Internal Security Subcommittee, where in 1951, in hearings before the committee, Republican senator Joseph McCarthy claimed to have a list of 205 communists then involved with shaping the United States government. Indeed, Willis Smith was presiding over the subcommittee during the session in which McCarthy announced the names.[61]

It was during this time that Gray made a speech to UNC alumni at Chapel Hill that worried many Duke alumni and supporters: "The University is the only agency of the State that can possibly have the continuity of mission, the continuity of obligation, the continuity of opportunity, the continuity of will, and the continuity of capacity to do the job and to serve as the general headquarters, if you will, of our fight for a happier citizenship, a healthier citizenship, and a more prosperous State. This University must become, and continue to be, the brain, the nerve center, the heart, and the conscience and the will of the State." Four days later, on April 24, 1951, Edward O. Diggs, a medical student from Winston-Salem, became the first black American admitted to UNC, and in June, UNC admitted three black students to its law school. It would be another 12 years before Duke admitted its first black medical student.[62]

On July 18, 1951, President Truman appointed Gordon Gray director of the recently created Psychological Strategy Board. The board was a high-level group working on broad strategy and coordination of the nation's psychological warfare and propaganda. Gray retired from the board late in 1951, but in the months that followed the Psychological Warfare Center was established at Fort Bragg, where in June of 1952 the army's first unconventional warfare unit, the 10th Special Forces Group, was established. Gray worked closely at the Psychological Strategy Board and its successor agencies with several of his intelligence colleagues from World War II, including C. D. Jackson, publisher of *Fortune* magazine and a vice president of Time, Inc., who had also served since 1948 as a director with Dave Davison of Doris Duke's Independent Aid, Inc.[63]

Gray also now expanded his national security concerns to the area of medical care and hospital costs. In September 1951 he accepted the chairmanship of the national Commission on Financing of Hospital Care. The purpose of the commission was to conduct a two-year study "to find the best ways of offering high-quality hospital care at the lowest cost" and also to evaluate "the current financial position of the country's hospitals." Created by (but independent of) the American Hospital Association, the commission on financing was scheduled to begin its work in January 1952 with a six-month pilot study in North Carolina. According to one newspaper report, the North Carolina study was to be conducted in cooperation with The Duke Endowment. "The 26-year record of uniform accounting encouraged by The Duke Endowment was a significant factor in the selection of North Carolina as the pilot study state."[64] Gray, in announcing the study, "stressed the need for attention to the present financial conditions of the country's hospitals because of the impact on the nation's health in the defense emergency." The information gathered from the North Carolina study was to be used "to develop recommendations that will have country-wide application in solving the problems connected with paying for hospital care. The study will take in Veterans Administration hospitals, Army and Navy hospitals, municipal, proprietary and voluntary hospitals."[65]

The financing commission was directly connected in several respects to the health services research group that had been so influential in shaping DUMC's early history, the Committee on the Costs of Medical Care (1927–32). Contributors to both groups included the Rockefeller Foundation and the Milbank Memorial Fund, with funding for Gray's financing commission also coming from the W. K. Kellogg Foundation, the National Foundation for Infantile Paralysis, and several other foundations. The staff and program director of the financing commission, Graham L. Davis, had joined the Kellogg Foundation after 15 years in Charlotte working at The Duke Endowment with Watson Rankin, a member of the 1927 research group. As a former president of the American Hospital Association, moreover, Davis represented another strong connection between Gray's financing commission and the earlier committee on medical care costs. The association's C. Rufus Rorem, a member

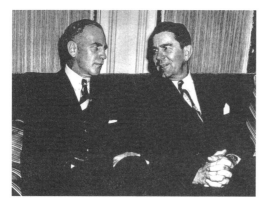

6.8 University of North Carolina president Gordon Gray and Duke president A. Hollis Edens. *Duke University Archives.*

of the 1927 group, had been the chief proponent of Blue Cross and Blue Shield plans, consideration of which, along with other group prepayment plans, was central to the Gray commission's agenda.[66] [Figure 6.8]

The numbers for Duke Hospital reflected many of the financing commission's concerns. Louis E. Swanson, the hospital's associate superintendent, noted that "the cost per patient per day in 1951 was $16.35, an increase of $2.20 a day from 1950 costs, and there is no indication that the upward trend of inflation will stop." Nor were the prospects good for meeting those increases. Forty-five percent of the hospital's patients were unable to pay the "full cost" of their stay, with the difference made up by Duke and other payers: "Duke University, 16.7 per cent; government and other contributors, 11 per cent; cities and counties, seven per cent." And the number of patients continued to rise. The hospital admitted a record number of patients in 1951 (17,170), while providing 170,878 days of medical care—1,003 more than its previous high. Patients came from 41 states, 85 percent from North Carolina (and within the state, from all the state's 100 counties, with Durham County topping the list at 4,036 patients). "This figure only applies to patients who occupied beds in the hospital," Swanson emphasized. "It does not include 156,820 visits (also a new high) to the out-patient and private clinics for examination and treatment. The Duke Out-Patient Clinic and Private Diagnostic Clinics," he explained, "have performed special services in helping patients in the earlier stages of diseases before hospital care was necessary."[67] [Figure 6.9]

The superintendent of Duke Hospital, F. Ross Porter, was one of 35 North Carolinians selected by Gordon Gray in December 1951 to serve on the financing commission's pilot study committee, the North Carolina Hospital Study Committee. The committee included blacks and whites, residents from the mountains, the piedmont and the coast, and representatives of state government, organized labor, hospitals, the media, industry, nursing, dentistry, and pharmaceuticals. Benjamin Duke's widowed granddaughter, Mary Duke Biddle Trent, was a committee member, as was William Rich, the black superintendent of Lincoln Hospital. There was a representative from each of North Carolina's Blue Cross and Blue Shield precursors, the Hospital Care Association (Durham and Duke), and the Hospital Savings Association (Chapel

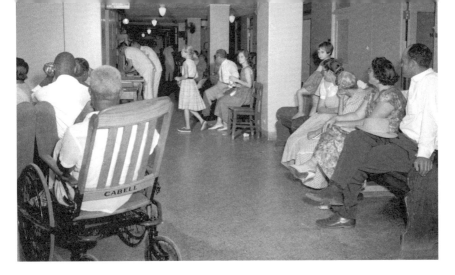

6.9 Crowded conditions in the Duke Out-Patient Clinic, 1957. *Duke University Archives.*

Hill). The president of the North Carolina Medical Care Commission, James H. Clark, was a member of the committee, as was the commission's executive secretary, former Rockefeller Foundation associate John A. Ferrell. And of course the Bowman Gray and UNC medical schools each had at least one representative on the committee. The committee's chairman, Major L. P. McLendon of Greensboro, was also president of the North Carolina Medical Foundation and chairman of the Medical Affairs Committee of the University of North Carolina's Board of Trustees. The state's governor, Kerr Scott, was the committee's honorary chairman.[68]

Integration at DUMC

The 1952 national elections also gave Duke's leadership new reasons to look beyond the university's regional economic and political allegiances. In November, the Republicans captured the White House for the first time since Duke Hospital opened in 1930. General Dwight D. Eisenhower and his running mate, Richard Nixon, were elected president and vice president of the United States. One month later, the *Pittsburgh Courier* ran a story in its Saturday magazine under the title "Duke University Hospital Takes the Lead in Integrated Training Programs." The story was written by Alex Rivera, a graduate of Durham's North Carolina College for Negroes, and it was accompanied by 10 of Rivera's photographs. "In the world-famous Duke University Hospital a revolution in Southern mores is occurring daily without fanfare or publicity," Rivera wrote. "More than 450 Negroes are employed in a variety of jobs and positions in the celebrated institution from menials to ranks of professional specialization." Rivera focused in particular on the successful training program for black practical nurses started by Duke Hospital and the Durham city schools in 1948. "Of the 125 Negro women who have been graduated from the course in practical nursing," he explained, "all have passed the board and seventy have been employed in the Duke Hospital. Others have been hired by Johns Hopkins, Cleveland's Nursing Hospital, Freedmen's, Bellevue and Lincoln Hospital, of Durham. It is privately admitted that so far the corps of practical nurses, both graduate and student, has been the only solution to a rapidly dwindling supply of white nurses which is constantly being siphoned off by industry and government."[69]

Rivera's story appears to have been prompted, at least in part, by the Republican victory in 1952. "Until very recently," he wrote, "there was the fear that publicizing the hospital policy of upgrading Negroes would cause some wealthy donors to withdraw their support, but the basic soundness and fairness of the Duke plan is now generally accepted by all progressive Southerners." The Duke plan had started in 1947, Rivera explained, when "Miss Harriett Amey, Boston University-trained medical social worker, was appointed to the Social Service Department." Since then, Duke had also trained, in addition to the practical nurses, a black x-ray technician, and numerous laboratory technicians. "The most completely integrated group is the corps of technicians working under Dr. Walter Kempner, world-famous for his rice treatment for high blood pressure. Four white technicians (two men and two women) and three Negroes (two women and a man) conduct the highly intricate experiments and tests to determine the effect of the rice diet on wealthy patients from all parts of the world." Rivera's powerful photographs include shots of individual black workers, integrated groups of children and working adults, and a class of black practical nurses. "In this region where the Negro question is virtually its prime frame of reference, economic, social and political, the philanthropy of James (Buck) Duke might be the instrument by which the South will find the cure of its greatest plague, the 'fits' of racial misunderstanding."[70]

The Political Arena

S ome aspects of the Republican victory were not promising for Duke. Early in 1953, and with the help of the Republican-controlled Congress, the new administration began a stringent review of budget requests from the Veterans Administration. Eisenhower also proposed, and the Congress approved, as the first reorganization of his administration, a Cabinet-level Department of Health, Education and Welfare. The new department was established that April with many of the agencies formerly administered by Oscar Ewing at the now disbanded Federal Security Administration. By May Davison was decidedly less upbeat about the prospects of the Medical Follow-up Agency; not only had the number of applications for research decreased but the VA had shown a decided preference for funding its own in-house research. Davison's report drew a warning from the National Research Council's Division of Medical Sciences. Unless the VA showed greater support for the agency, or unless some other funding agencies came forward, the Medical Follow-up Agency faced "a progressive scaling-down and ultimate termination of the operation."[71]

Senator Willis Smith, however, got along well with the new Republican administration. It helped, of course, that The Duke Endowment continued to sustain its powerful Republican connections, that North Carolina elected one Republican congressman, that Eisenhower garnered 44 percent of the state's presidential votes, and that Richard Nixon was, like Smith himself, a graduate of Duke Law School. Indeed, Smith's 1950 Senate victory had coincided with Nixon's own Senate win in California, and until Nixon assumed the office of vice president, he and Smith had occupied adjacent offices in the Senate building in Washington. Smith's administrative assistant, Jesse Helms, later recalled that Nixon's "office was next to Willis Smith's office when I was up there. . . . So that's when I got to know Nixon very well." By the spring of 1953, in fact, Smith's supporters were concerned over the senator's reelection chances and there was also speculation that Smith himself would join the Republican Party. He didn't. He died on June 26, 1953, of a heart attack.[72]

Smith's death signaled a battle for North Carolina's political soul and a major turning point in the history of DUMC and Duke University. Two of the most prominent politicians of the next quarter century, Richard Nixon and Lyndon Johnson, spoke at Smith's memorial service in Washington. Nixon presided at the service, and he also accompanied Smith's body to Raleigh afterward. In eulogizing the North Carolina senator, Nixon told their fellow lawmakers that he had counted on Smith "not only as a friend but as a counselor—a man to whom I could go for advice." Johnson, for his part, described Smith as one of the Senate's ablest members, whose record of achievement was "matched by few in public life." Johnson praised Smith's high standards of integrity and the fact that the North Carolina Democrat had been "one of the best known and most respected members of the American bar."[73]

Shifting Emphases Following the Death of Smith

Unfortunately for Duke, Smith had also been the key unifying force among the ensemble of Duke-related interests, and his death all but destroyed the sense of institutional oneness that he, Gross, and Edens had tried to foster at the university. Two-thirds of the university's 36 trustees were affiliated with (and to some extent selected by) the Methodist

Church, most of the remaining third were selected by the alumni of Trinity-Duke, and three Duke trustees were also trustees of The Duke Endowment. Of more importance, 7 of the 36 trustees, including the 3 from the Endowment, were also members of the university's executive trustee committee, the chief decision-making body for the university. Smith had controlled both the executive committee and the general board as chairman, and he had been aided in the process by Edens, who also belonged to both bodies.

In the wake of Smith's passing, however, the Endowment resumed its traditional efforts to control the university. Smith's successor as trustee chairman, Duke Power president Norman Cocke, was already a member of the trustees' executive committee, while Winston-Salem trustee, P. Frank Hanes, an attorney and former vice president of R. J. Reynolds Tobacco Company, was elected to fill the executive trustee seat left vacant by Smith's death. As one historian has noted, "Norman Cocke . . . was an original trustee of the Endowment, and at the same time that he was Duke Power's president in the 1950s, he served as chairman of Duke University's board of trustees. It was perhaps the high-water mark of the inter-locking relationships among the three major institutional legacies of J. B. Duke."[74] Unfortunately for Edens, this confluence of interests also significantly diminished his own power and influence at Duke. He had not been the Endowment's choice for the Duke presidency, after all; that honor had gone to Dean Wilburt Davison, whom Smith had aggressively opposed. Indeed, by the time Edens resigned in 1960, he derived most of his support from the religious faction of trustees and alumni who had opposed Davison.

Duke's post-Smith regime got its first real test early in 1954, when Davison asked the university administration to consider the 1946 proposal to expand Duke Hospital. In addition to new and expanded outpatient and PDC clinics, the proposed five-floor wing included rooms for private patients, new operating rooms, and other facilities. Though what happened next is not exactly clear, Edens apparently drafted a memorandum threatening to cut off university funding for Duke Hospital. Davison called up Edens to complain. "The disclaiming by Duke University of all financial responsibility for Duke Hospital after 1956 may not only change its tax and legal status," Davison warned, "but also may reduce the humanitarian good will which has been established among thousands of patients and their families and friends in this and other States. Many of the staff and I have put a quarter of a century of our lives into Duke Hospital, and my family and I have spent a quarter of a million dollars of our own funds, over and above my salary, for living expense during this period, so we hope that our efforts will not have been wasted. I hope that you will favorably consider these suggestions before the memorandum is adopted

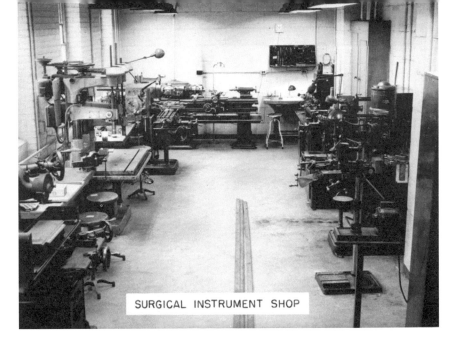

SURGICAL INSTRUMENT SHOP

6.10 The Surgical Instrument Shop was opened in 1949, in space paid for by the Department of Medicine and the Department of Surgery, for the fabrication of surgical and medical instruments. *Duke University Medical Center Archives.*

and published." Eight months later, Drs. Davison, Hart, Stead, and others signed a letter to Edens to "confirm previous commitments in regard to money for the building fund, whether or not additional funds are obtained from the [North Carolina] Hospital Care Commission or other sources."[75]

In the meantime, the PDC also began establishing referral clinics in a number of North Carolina communities. This effort was led by Dr. Lenox Baker, the chief of orthopedic surgery at Duke, and his eventual successor, Dr. J. Leonard Goldner, a specialist in hand surgery and clubfeet. "Doctor Baker had a map in his office with red circles with each circle demonstrating 50 miles," Goldner later recalled, "and he put these all over the state. And then he outlined where the clinics should be in order to take advantage of the doctors that he and we knew in community counties, as to how they could influence the town with an orthopedic clinic in order to have some hold on patient referrals. And it was through that, that he started the Clinton clinic and then on to Morehead, and then on to Ahoskie." Goldner himself started the clinic in Asheboro. "I felt it was a great opportunity because we were looking for patient referrals," he explained. "I never felt we should stay in the 'ivory tower.' . . . I thought we should get out into the community and that is the only way to get patients in. They just don't come to you when you sit here." Duke eventually established 18 community referral clinics, all of which became critically important to the success of the PDC and the formation of the Duke University Health System 40 years later.[76] [Figure 6.10]

Baker and Goldner also collaborated with the chairman of Duke's Anatomy Department, Dr. Joseph E. Markee, who was producing instructional movies for use in anatomy classes. Funded with grants from the National Foundation for Infantile Paralysis, Markee's movies earned him recognition from one knowledgeable observer as "the person who has probably done more to develop audiovisual methods in teaching anatomy in this country than anyone else."[77] One newspaper reported in 1951 that Markee's filmmaking program was spreading to other academic medical centers. "A Duke doctor is now at the Mayo Clinic setting up a similar program; another will launch one at the University of California's new medical school this Fall. A special Duke movie on the structure of the hand is now being distributed to all American medical schools."[78]

The hand film reflected Goldner's emerging specialization in hand surgery and the very real needs for such a specialty in North Carolina. Goldner remembered taking "advantage of Joe's opportunity to make the motion pictures to do the teachings. We had courses for physical therapists, occupational therapists, and we blended in the hand surgery that we had initiated. Well by 1952 or 1953," Goldner explained, "we had the only hand center in the Southeast and we were doing elective hands, we were doing hands for Liberty Mutual Insurance Company for the textile industry for various things. And I was on the governor's committee for prevention of injury and we were trying to work ourselves out of a job by putting safety switches on the [textile] rollers to keep their [the workers'] hands out of the fast moving machinery and so on, but that wasn't always successful. So we had a tremendous number of textile injuries and a lot of farm injuries."[79]

They also had a lot of Korean War–related injuries to deal with at the new Veterans Administration Hospital, which opened across the street from DUMC in 1953. Staffing of the hospital's medical and surgical services was controlled by Duke's Departments of Medicine and Surgery, and the VA, as it was called, quickly became important as both a teaching and recruitment tool for Duke Medicine. "In those days we had a very strong VA association," Goldner recalled. "After we had rounds at Duke on Wednesday—we would meet at 7 and have rounds from 7 to 9—and then we would all go to the VA from 9 to 10 and bring up x-rays. And bring up four or five patients for the whole staff from Durham Regional, which at that time was Watts Hospital. We would meet at the VA. So, the VA was a very close part of our relationship and the teaching was very strong and each staff member had a responsibility. So you know you are going to be at the VA one day a week for four hours or six hours, and you

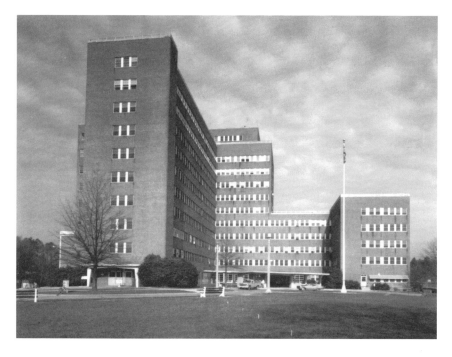

6.11 The Durham Veterans Administration Hospital opened in 1953 across Erwin Road from the Duke University Medical Center. *Duke University Medical Center Archives.*

know you are going to be operating certain days. And it was a teaching program. . . . It was important to our overall training and it was what we call a resident-run program but supervised by the faculty."[80]

The physician chosen to be the first chief of Surgery at the new VA hospital, Dr. William W. Shingleton, had all the right connections to improve Duke's image in the state. He was a native North Carolinian and a graduate of Atlantic Christian College in Wilson, North Carolina. He had earned his M.D. degree at the Bowman Gray School of Medicine, and he had done his internship and residency at Duke. Appointed to the Duke staff in 1950, after completing his residency in general and thoracic surgery, Shingleton was expected to fill the VA position when the hospital opened. However, after a three-month course at Oak Ridge on the "Techniques and Uses of Radioisotopes," Shingleton returned to Duke, where construction delays at the VA combined with his own newfound interest in surgical oncology to change his plans. He remained on the Duke staff in general and thoracic surgery and pursued the use of chemotherapy in the treatment of tumors. Shingleton's change of plans proved particularly fortuitous both for Duke and for his own career. As an early leader in the field of surgical oncology, he helped conceptualize the role of comprehensive cancer centers in President Richard Nixon's "war" on cancer in the early 1970s. Shingleton also served as a member of the National Advisory Cancer Board under presidents Nixon and Gerald Ford, and in 1971, in addition to attending the signing of the National Cancer Act, he became director of Duke's Cancer Center, one of 15 such centers to receive construction funds from the federal government. It was also Shingleton who helped the Duke center become a comprehensive cancer center in 1973 and to achieve the distinction of becoming the highest rated such center in the nation in 1977.[81]

Many of Duke Medicine's future leaders honed their clinical, laboratory, and administrative skills at the Durham VA, and professional appointments to the VA became an important part of the recruitment package offered to prospective Duke faculty and staff. In 1952, the first chief of Medicine at the Durham VA, Dr. James Warren, agreed to let Dr. E. Harvey Estes Jr. complete at Duke a fellowship and residency interrupted for Estes at Emory by his military service during the Korean War. "The VA Hospital was brand new," Estes recalled a half century later, "some of the floors had not even opened. And the department of medicine was just forming. So I stepped in at the end of my fellowship time as the first head of the cardiology division at the VA Hospital." Two years later, in 1955, both Estes and Warren moved back across the street to DUMC, where Warren became chief of cardiology at Duke and Estes a cardiologist in the PDC.[82] [Figure 6.11]

The shuffle at the VA that followed their move left vacant the director's position at the Radioisotope Unit there, a position controlled by Dr. Philip Handler. Handler offered the position to a promising young physician at the National Heart Institute, Dr. James B. Wyngaarden, who was then doing research in the underground radioisotope laboratory at the National Institutes of Health. Though Wyngaarden declined the VA position in radioisotopes, he subsequently accepted a joint appointment to the Departments of Biochemistry and Medicine at Duke in 1956. He also served at the VA in medicine. "I then received my first rounding assignment at the Durham VA Hospital where Joe Greenfield was my intern," Wyngaarden recalled. "In those days we rounded three days per week, eleven months per year."[83] Within a year of Wyngaarden's arrival, moreover, James Warren accepted the chairmanship of the Department of Medicine at the University of Texas in Galveston, and Estes returned to the VA as its chief of medicine. Estes then went back to the PDC in 1961, and in 1966, a year before Wyngaarden was appointed chairman of the Department of Medicine at Duke, Estes became chairman of the new Department of Community Health Services at DUMC.[84]

Within DUMC itself, the combination of VA duties and the planned expansion of Duke Hospital brought another important addition to Duke Medicine. In 1950, Dr. C. Ronald Stephen, an eminent Canadian anesthesiologist, was appointed professor and head of the division of anesthesiology in the Department of Surgery. To the existing certificate program for nurse anesthetists, Stephen added a faculty and a full academic program in anesthesiology. He also established a required clerkship in the division, a residency training program, and a reputation for the division as "a nationally recognized center for clinical investigation—especially for new anesthetic adjuvants and agents." As Stephen's successor, Dr. Merel H. Harmel, later wrote, "When the Durham Veterans Administration Hospital came into being, anesthesiology, with the other clinical specialties, mounted a teaching and research program that was to flourish until 1966 when Dr. Stephen resigned."[85]

A New Vision for Duke Medicine

W hy did teaching and research begin to flourish in Duke Medicine during the late 1950s? The simple answer is that Duke University linked its future to the military-industrial complex that invested heavily in research for national defense and health care between 1945 and the early 1990s. Yet that linkage only partially explains the expanding foundations of the medical center's excellence. The PDC also became a successful and generous business in the late 1950s, at a time when The Duke Endowment reasserted its traditional interest in supporting Duke Medicine. These developments did not go uncontested, however, especially in the years that followed Smith's death. Between 1954 and 1960, Duke Medicine was at the center of a struggle over the future of Duke University and its medical center.

Much of that struggle focused on the growing practice of the Private Diagnostic Clinic and the development of the Research Training Program at Duke. While most of the criticism of the PDC came from outside of DUMC—from Edens and the religious group of university trustees—there was also an undercurrent of debate within Duke Medicine regarding the PDC. The most important internal debate, however, concerned the future of its medical school: what should the school's objectives be and how should its curriculum and activities be designed to reach those goals? Both of the chief protagonists in this debate, Wilburt Davison and Philip Handler, offered programs that addressed the future of the medical school considering both the university's long-range development plans and the goal of more closely integrating Duke Medicine with the rest of the university. The Davison program offered little support, however, for the vision of research-oriented graduate studies pursued since World War II by Smith, Gross, and several of the university's leading trustees. Indeed, the Davison plan was rejected in 1954 by most of DUMC's faculty and by the rest of the university as well. But this was not the case with the Research Training Program, which was developed between 1955 and 1959 by Gross, Handler, and others at DUMC, including Drs. Eugene Stead and Barnes Woodhall. The Research Training Program received strong support from most of the medical school faculty. It was endorsed by the faculty of Duke's physical, biological, and mathematical sciences, and it was backed by The Duke Endowment and the university's most powerful trustees.

THE COMMONWEALTH FUND'S ASSESSMENT OF DUMC

Duke Medicine was clearly at a crossroads in the fall of 1955 when Drs. Charles Warren and John Eberhart visited DUMC for the Commonwealth Fund. The fund was making grants to American medical schools that exhibited "obvious needs for outside funds," and Duke was on the list for investigation. The case was a hard one to make for DUMC, however, for by the time Warren and Eberhart visited Duke, Edens had failed to terminate the university's support for Duke Hospital, and construction was under way on the long-planned, five-floor addition to the hospital. Funding for the new $4.6 million wing was provided by The Duke Endowment ($1 million), various PDC funds (over $3 million), and the North Carolina Medical Care Commission ($480,000). Significantly, too, the university struck a deal with the PDC to help finance the addition. As Hart later explained it, "since the costs exceeded the resources then available, the University advanced to the [PDC] Development Fund almost $1,000,000 at an interest rate of 4 percent." The loan signaled the deepening bond between the financial strength of the PDC and that of Duke University and its medical center.[86]

During their visit to Duke in September of 1955, Warren and Eberhart found a "medical school which is just now coming to the end of its first generation." Several members of the original staff were still teaching, but they would be "retiring sometime within the next ten years. In other words," Warren wrote, "the Duke Medical School was established a generation ago with sizeable private funds and a well qualified younger staff, and this period of its development will be drawing to a close within the next few years." After interviewing "numerous people" within DUMC and across campus, the Commonwealth observers believed they could be "fairly explicit in describing the conception which the school has of itself. On the whole it does not view itself as charged primarily with the responsibility of meeting community needs for health services. It views itself, on the other hand, as a national school and prides itself on enrolling, over the years, students from all the states in the country. Its graduates, too, disperse widely. On the other hand, it is not entirely neglectful of local community needs in that it puts a good deal of time and effort into training para-medical personnel, to use the term they employ, meaning laboratory technicians, x-ray technicians, nurses of course, nurse anesthetists, physical therapists, occupational therapists, dietitians, and other members of what they recognize as necessary constituents of the health team."[87]

What the Commonwealth observers found particularly striking were the power and autonomy that DUMC's clinical chairmen derived from the PDC. The "outstanding feature" of Duke's medical school, Warren noted, was "certainly the plan by which the School finances much of its work in the clinical departments by the income from the private practice of its 'geographical full time' staff. . . . On the other hand it has the clear disadvantage that the economic gulf between the preclinical and clinical faculty is widened with the ensuing resentment that is inevitable. These feelings are also probably accentuated by the fact that the clinical chiefs wield an extraordinarily large amount of power, which naturally is felt in the determination of overall school policies." So strong were the clinical chairs that they determined in large measure what Davison could do as dean. "It means in essence that the clinical department heads have a great deal of autonomy and indeed this seems to be a principle that applies pretty generally throughout the School. Dean Davison either does not seem able or is not interested, or both, in directing the major policies of the school through his own office." Although Davison had the power as dean to veto decisions of the Health Affairs Committee he headed, he "rarely" used it. "School decisions, in other words, are heavily weighted by a clinical group and the Dean himself has definitely limited power to direct policy."[88]

The Commonwealth observers also learned more about the PDC from its founder, Dr. Deryl Hart, whom they found "practically manic on the subject." Hart aggressively defended the PDC as an example both of "free enterprise" and of "a highly commendable plan" that other university medical schools, including Emory, were beginning to adopt. "It amounts to a procedure by which the medical school can greatly augment its income," Warren explained, "and it can operate at a level that it clearly could not do if it relied entirely on endowment, contributions and student fees for income." The new hospital wing, for example, had been funded mainly by the private practice of the PDC. "It also seems likely that this arrangement has attracted to Duke a number of highly capable clinicians who are probably also good teachers but who would be less willing to work in many medical schools where the financial arrangements are so much less attractive. A good deal of research in the clinical departments is financed this way," Warren continued, "and on the whole I cannot escape the feeling that the assets of the plan probably outweigh its deficits."[89]

The one faculty member who openly criticized the PDC was Davison's assistant dean, Dr. Kenneth E. Penrod. Penrod had arrived at Duke in 1950, as a member of the Department of Physiology and Pharmacology, and he had coauthored the curriculum development program recently rejected by the medical school and Arts College faculties. Penrod was described by one of the Commonwealth observers as "fairly young, serious, devoted to the medical school and students, humane and sophisticated in his approach to medicine. He was the one member of the staff who seriously criticized the 'free enterprise' system, as Dr. Hart called it, under which the geographical full time clinical staff earned the bulk of their incomes through the private diagnostic clinic. Dr. Penrod feels that the private practice tail may be wagging the educational dog."[90] Penrod pointed out to his visitors that "some of the men in medicine and surgery contribute very little to the educational program, even though the education of medical students is the only excuse for the existence of Duke Hospital. He sees little point in adding an 108-bed unit to the private diagnostic clinic when it is hard to keep the present 600 beds full. . . . Penrod granted that the clinical departments used the private practice income for such good uses as buildings, additional staff, etc., but added that such use of the funds generally tends to increase the money made by the private diagnostic clinic."[91]

Commonwealth's observers also summarized for the foundation the educational program titled "Preliminary Report of the Committee for the Study of Medical and Patient Care at Duke University." Written by Penrod and another Davison protégé, Dr. Samuel P. Martin III, the report made three general proposals. The first proposal combined an undergraduate curriculum in the arts and sciences with Davison's focus on producing as quickly as possible as many well-trained general practitioners as possible. Students would be accepted for medical school after one or two years of college and would then take two courses in their third year of college: one on "the basic concepts of chemistry and biology" and the other a course "in human behavior given by psychologists and sociologists." This proposal, Eberhart reported, "was rather widely discussed within the medical school and with representatives of the Arts College, but was not accepted. It would have required significant outside funds to support it and these were not in sight." At the same time, "the Arts College people were not entirely happy with the idea of a special undergraduate program for a limited number of premedical students, especially since other premedical students would have had to continue on the regular program."[92]

The second proposal reflected the tradition of psychosomatic medicine at Duke. It suggested the need within the medical school to "sharpen the interest of the staff and the students toward the patient as an individual." This meant giving medical students "responsibility for social, psychological and biological phases of patients early in their training and with equal emphasis, and that preclinical training should be spread out through the full four year curriculum and should be integrated." To help facilitate these developments, a change was also suggested in DUMC's outpatient departments, "so that students would have a longer and more continuous experience there and could be given increased responsibility for the continuous and complete care of the patients."[93]

The third and final proposal in Penrod and Martin's report concerned "the inclusion of more community aspects in patient care, including enlarging the contribution of the social service staff and the creation of housing facilities near the out-patient clinic so that ambulatory patients could be better provided for." Penrod saw little future for the proposals, however, as he confided to the observers for the Commonwealth Fund. "Dr. Penrod is not hopeful of immediate action on these proposals, although he says Dean Davison is quite in favor them. Other members of the faculty, whom he did not name, are apparently very firmly opposed and he does not expect significant movement until there have been some faculty changes."[94]

The Commonwealth observers left Duke believing they "had seen a good medical school," and "probably the strongest school south of Baltimore and east of St. Louis." They attributed much of the school's strength to its financial resources, both from endowment and "from the practice of medicine by its staff. But it has good men," Warren stressed, "and an educational philosophy that encourages an interest in patients as people and emphasizes the doctor's obligation to assume responsibility for more than just the acute physical breakdown of his patients." Yet Warren also noted that, in the particular case of Duke Medicine, "the price one pays for having it operate at the level it does and still remain essentially solvent is a situation characterized by a high degree of department autonomy exaggerated by the particularly powerful positions of the clinical departments. Obviously, overall University–Medical School relations cannot be optimal while this situation exists and there is little reason to think that any major changes will be made in these arrangements in the near future. This gets in the way of certain improvements, particularly curricularwise, that might be made in the educational program and perhaps raises the question of whether it is too big a price to pay for financial stability." Though neither Commonwealth investigator saw "any pressing need" to make a grant to Duke, Warren suggested that the school "be put on a deferred list for possible programmatic support later on."[95]

THE RESEARCH TRAINING PROGRAM AND SCIENCE RESEARCH AT DUKE

A year later the Commonwealth Fund received a grant request from Duke's Dr. Philip Handler, the chairman of Biochemistry, who asked for construction funds for a building to house a proposed research training program for medical students at Duke. Commonwealth declined the request, however, citing the fact that it wasn't funding "construction per se," so Handler sought funding in other directions for what he called an "Experimental Training Program in the Basic Medical Sciences." Plans for the new program were already under way, in fact, by the time Jim Wyngaarden interviewed at Duke in 1956. "So the idea was born—in fact, was in the conversation—when I first came to look at this position in 1956," Wyngaarden later recalled, "of starting a training program whereby a medical student could spend a full academic year in research training and thereby be exposed to a whole series of concepts, a whole series of techniques and perhaps conduct a limited research project with enough time to do it so that it had a fair chance of being successful."[96]

The Research Training Program was conceived by Handler and by Dr. Paul Gross, Duke's vice president, with the collaboration of Dr. Eugene Stead, the chairman of Duke's Department of Medicine, and several other faculty members of the university's medical school, including Dr. Barnes Woodhall. As Handler and Stead later described the program, it was designed as "an intensive training period of nine months in which students could enter at any time after completion of the first two years of medical school. The heart of the program was a central teaching facility, where students familiarized themselves with advanced research tools in a variety of fields by proceeding through a series of experiments under the guidance of specialists."[97]

By the time Handler reapplied to Commonwealth for funding late in 1957, he and Gross had mobilized a cross-campus alliance in the physical sciences behind the proposed program. According to Handler, the "entire staff" of the medical school had received the plan with a "unanimity and enthusiasm almost unique in the history of the institution." Equally important, Duke's Departments of Mathematics, Physics, Chemistry, Zoology, and Electrical Engineering had pledged their "complete cooperation" with the program, and the Graduate School had approved a Ph.D. plan for the program based upon "the merits of the interdisciplinary approach to the study of the biological sciences."[98] Gross made the case for the program simply and eloquently in his letter of support to the Commonwealth Fund. "The history of medicine," he wrote, "especially in recent years, clearly indicates that medical advances are frequently made through the application of advances made in the basic sciences underlying medicine only after a lapse of some years before these can be consolidated into the structure of current medical research, teaching and application. The program envisaged by Dr. Handler would put prospective clinical investigators in practical working contact, during the formative years of their career, with the advancing front of the basic sciences of chemistry, physics and biology."[99]

Handler and Gross made their appeal having already received major financial commitments from the Markle Foundation, the National Institutes of

Health, and Duke University for the estimated cost of the program's physical facilities. What the program needed from Commonwealth, Handler explained, was a grant for personnel, for until the program's operating expenses were covered, the commitments to construction funding would not be forthcoming. "Operation of the program will be a considerable 'teaching load' and may not, in all fairness," Handler wrote, "be added to the responsibilities of the present staff. Additional faculty personnel are required particularly in areas not adequately covered by our present staff, namely, biophysics, neurophysiology, electronmicroscopic cytology, microbial genetics, and pharmacology." Handler asked for $75,000 a year for five years from the Commonwealth Fund, "specifically to defray the stipends of the additional staff necessary under the program, the technicians, secretary, and special lecturers."[100]

Duke's Research Training Program reflected several mutually reinforcing developments both within the Duke ensemble of interests and within American society in general. The description of DNA's structure in 1953 ushered in a new era of biomedical research, while the 1957 flight of the Russian satellite Sputnik not only reshaped the curriculum of American schools to emphasize science and mathematics but also prompted passage of the National Defense Education Act (which provided millions of dollars for student loans, scholarships, and fellowships, and the purchase of scientific equipment for schools) and the creation of the National Aeronautics and Space Administration and the Advanced Research Projects Agency. In the meantime, the budget of the National Institutes of Health continued to skyrocket under the aggressive leadership of Dr. James A. Shannon, who became director of NIH in 1955. Between 1950 and 1955, for example, the NIH budget had increased from $52 million to $80 million; by 1960, it was $400 million. It appeared to one Commonwealth observer that Duke's proposed research training program complemented Shannon's efforts at NIH. "The plan then is to help along the development of clinical investigators particularly and we know that this is an area in which the National Institutes of Health is concerned with their broad thinking about the desirability of accelerating the development of graduate physicians as competent research workers." Likewise, Duke's Research Training Program was also closely tied to the evolution of North Carolina's Research Triangle Park, a planned research park created in 1959 and located between Duke University in Durham, the University of North Carolina at Chapel Hill, and North Carolina State University in Raleigh.[101]

Duke's Research Training Program was also designed to forge stronger links within Duke Medicine itself and between DUMC and the rest of the university. Both Handler and Gross made this point in their discussions with the Commonwealth Fund. "Clearly, it would afford an excellent opportunity to serve as a testing ground for experiments in medical education," Handler wrote regarding the program, "an opportunity to attempt a truly integrated, interdisciplinary approach to biological problems, and an opportunity to cement the relations between clinical and preclinical departments as well as those between medical school and university."[102] The foundation's principal investigator, Dr. Lester Evans, heard similar arguments during his visit to Duke in December 1957. Evans met with "some 35 or 40 persons representing all of the departments of the medical school, both junior and senior members of the departments, and representatives of a few of the central departments of the university. Further," Evans wrote, "I was able, both directly and indirectly, to secure what I believe is a fair estimate of the University's interest in the program and a very sane judgment by the University administration of the state of transition in which the medical school now finds itself. This program for training in research then is a direct expression of this beginning period of transition which is characterized by two factors: one, the deliberate effort to introduce interdisciplinary and inter-departmental teaching, and two, to strengthen the ties with the University through the basic science areas. Dr. Gross, the vice president of the University made this point quite clearly and said that before the University would approve the plan which we now have before us, it was discussed extensively in the major faculty groups and finally at the trustee level. There was full concurrence at every point in the proposal."[103]

BEHAVIORAL SCIENCE AT DUKE

There was no provision in the Research Training Program, however, for the recently renamed Department of Psychiatry—the one department that had done more than any other to promote interdisciplinary and interdepartmental teaching at DUMC and to strengthen ties with the university and the local community through the behavioral sciences. The new chairman of the renamed department, Dr. Ewald W. Busse, was recruited to Duke in 1953 by the Rockefeller Foundation, the Commonwealth Fund, and the Josiah Macy Jr. Foundation. Busse had arrived from the University of Colorado Medical Center in Denver, where he had been working as a specialist in electroencephalography and as chief of the division of psychosomatic medicine, and he brought with him a team of psychiatrists, none of whom, including Busse himself, initially practiced at the Private Diagnostic Clinic. Those who moved with him immediately were Drs. Robert H. Barnes and Albert J. Silverman, and they were soon joined by Dr. Sanford Cohen and Dr. Charles E. Llewellyn.[104] Another Colorado colleague, Dr. John A. Fowler, arrived in Durham in the summer of 1953, six weeks before Busse. "Fowler was the first trained Child Psychiatrist in North Carolina and was certified in child psychiatry by the American Board of Psychiatry," Busse later wrote. "Fowler was named the director of the Dur-

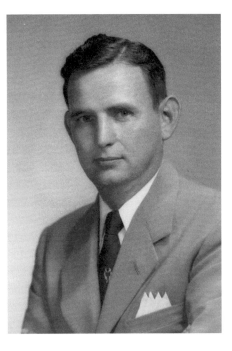

6.12 Dr. Ewald W. Busse. *Duke University Medical Center Archives.*

ham Community Child Guidance Clinic for children and youth as well as the Duke University Child Guidance Clinic."[105] One of Busse's first tasks had been to explore funding for their projects. "Commonwealth was so interested in psychosomatic medicine," he recalled. "Macy was interested in interdisciplinary. Rockefeller had—and I didn't know this until way after I got here—had put money into Duke to develop a Department of Psychiatry." (Like many people then and since, Busse seemed surprised at the Rockefeller connection.)[106] [Figure 6.12]

Evans, the Commonwealth investigator, recalled Busse well: "I recall very distinctly a long conversation he had with me before he accepted the Duke position and the questions he raised at that time. He was wondering whether it would be possible for good psychiatry to develop in the Duke environment but was able to point to such assets as the enlightened points of view in the departments of medicine and pediatrics with regard to psychiatry and the very evident good relationship which all of the school hoped for but had not had with the previous administration and teaching of psychiatry in the school." Evans reported approvingly on Busse's new programs: "On this visit, I found that the development of a good department of psychiatry had been a very potent influence in bridging some of the gaps which had been built up by departmental autonomy. One device has been the institution of a very extensive program of research in geriatrics which in all respects is interdisciplinary. I witnessed some of this work and found anatomists, physiologists, psychologists, psychiatrists, and internists worked together in the study of the process of ageing."[107]

While Busse accepted the department's traditional emphasis on psychosomatic medicine, he expanded its focus on child development and pioneered in the new field of gerontology. As Busse himself later wrote, "In 1960 the Division of Child Psychiatry was restructured to incorporate the Durham Child Guidance Clinic within its framework. This change was needed for several purposes including 1) acquisition of leased land on Duke University campus and the construction of a new building; 2) improved teaching and training program for child psychiatric fellows; 3) an increase in overall budget; and 4) improved services for the emotionally disturbed child and their parents in Durham County." The new child guidance center was constructed on the Duke campus in 1961, with 55 percent of the funding coming from the North Carolina Medical Care Commission (Hill-Burton funds), and the rest in equal amounts from The Duke Endowment, the Z. Smith Reynolds Foundation, and a bank note signed by Dillard Teer and Mary Semans. In addition, Busse noted, "an agency budget covering the Durham Child Guidance Clinic was established which permitted all funds to be received from any source including the United Way, state, federal, school, county tax, Duke University and private organizations."[108]

The achievement most often associated with Busse's tenure at Duke is the Regional Center for Research on Aging, later called the Center for the Study of Aging and Human Development. The foundation for the center was laid in 1955 with the formation of the Duke Council on Gerontology. The council, like the emerging plans for the Research Training Program, represented an effort in part to improve the relationship between the medical school faculty and other departments on campus. The council was chaired by Busse and designed, according to the Duke Hospital newspaper, as "a University-wide effort to contribute to the study of problems of aging by encouraging research, providing a central source of information on gerontology and disseminating information resulting from Duke research."[109] The next step came in 1956, Busse recalled, when the new U.S. surgeon general, Leroy Burney, decided to "develop five centers for the study of aging, and set up the money to do it. And we applied."[110]

Early in August 1957, at a press conference in Durham, Duke joined the U.S. Public Health Service in announcing the university's new gerontology center. Duke was to receive more than $1.5 million in grants from the National Heart and Mental Health Institutes over a five-year period, and during that time it was to establish "an experimental regional center for research on aging" as a pilot project. "If it is successful similar projects may be started in other parts of the country," the *New York Times* reported.[111] According to the monthly newspaper of Duke Hospital, the *Intercom*, the new center's research policies were to be determined by a panel on interdisciplinary research that included Drs. Busse, Stead, Handler, Woodhall, and Davison from the medical center; Dr. Eliot H. Rodnick, chairman of the Psychology Department; and Dr. Paul M. Gross, vice president and dean of the University. "Among the research projects being considered as part of the center's program is establishment of an interdisciplinary team involving psychiatry, internal medicine, surgery, nursing, psychology, social work and a consultant in sociology. This team will be concerned with alleviating the health problems of aging, study of preventive and therapeutic techniques in this field, and determination of the ideal composition of such an interdisciplinary health team."[112]

The surgeon general took pride in announcing the Duke center's "firsts." According to Burney it was "the first time that funds appropriated by Congress to the Public Health Service for aid to research have been awarded to help in the establishment of a large-scale regional research center." Burney also noted that it was "the first time, to my knowledge, that one of the leading institutions of higher learning in this country has set out, in a deliberate fashion, to mobilize its extensive resources in search of better understanding of the processes of aging—one of modern man's most challenging problems."[113] As an example of those problems, Burney pointed to the projected increase in the number of "senior citizens": from 14 million in 1957, their numbers were expected to increase to 21 million by 1975. And yet, Burney emphasized, "with all our successes in the control of infectious diseases and improvement of the environment, we have made little progress in extending the active life of older people."[114] As for the "extensive resources" Duke mobilized behind the new center, these were used to build a new Gerontology Building. Completed in 1960 at cost of $1 million, the Busse Building (as it was later called) was funded by The Duke Endowment ($562,000), NIH ($410,770), and the R. J. Reynolds Tobacco Company ($50,000).[115]

This public and private funding reinforced Duke Medicine's own internal commitments to rejuvenating the Department of Psychiatry. The department's PDC revenues, once on par with those of the clinical giants, Medicine and Surgery, had plummeted in the early 1950s as a result of the department's problems and the opening of the Durham Veterans Administration Hospital. The PDC now helped Psychiatry out, and according to Dr. Deryl Hart, it did so by using its funds in a novel way. "By 1956," he later wrote, "the resources in both the Development Fund and the departmental funds derived from private practice [at the PDC] increased in amounts sufficient to provide for construction of a major building [the Deryl Hart Pavilion]. . . . The first large interdepartmental aid from these sources was given in 1956–57 to provide facilities for Psychiatry, for which no provision had been made in the original plans and construction of the Medical School. This department was provided with offices and space for both public and private ambulatory patients in the new construction, and it acquired from Surgery in the original hospital the space occupied by 52 beds (18 children and 34 adult private patients) with their supporting services which had to be replaced for Surgery in the new construction."[116]

From that point on, however, Busse faced numerous challenges associated with the changing priorities of federal funding for mental health care.

In much the same way that Lyman had struggled earlier with the twists and turns of the VA's mental health programs (and that the Psychiatry Department would struggle later with diminished federal and private reimbursements for psychiatric care), Busse struggled with shifting bureaucracies and specialties: from the concerns with aging of the Eisenhower gerontocracy to the mental health and child development goals of the youthful Kennedys and the primary care programs of the Johnson and Nixon administrations. "I wanted and others wanted to really move child research," Busse later recalled. Duke's Department of Pediatrics was also "very interested, very cooperative," he explained, as was the division of neurology. "The difficulty was again funding."[117]

In investigating Duke Medicine for the Commonwelth Fund, Lester Evans discovered that the Research Training Program did not include the social and behavioral sciences at Duke. This decision was made, he reported, by Handler and the others planning the program, including Busse himself, who "stated very clearly that in their discussions of the past year he had expressed the view that the program should evolve around the broadest possible concept of the biological sciences at present and when the behavior and social sciences are more strongly established in the medical school, in part as a result of present efforts of psychiatry, that work in this area be included." It seemed clear to Evans that Busse and his Duke colleagues had given "very thoughtful consideration" to the whole matter before suggesting "that there be delay in the initiation of training in the social and behavioral sciences."[118]

Just how many university trustees even knew about the program, much less the absence from it of the social and behavioral sciences, is not clear. The program was undoubtedly approved, however, by the executive committee of university trustees, which was controlled in turn by the trustees appointed by The Duke Endowment. And these men definitely wanted Duke to follow the long-range plans that Willis Smith had developed and pursued since World War II.

DUMC AND OTHER UNIVERSITY RESEARCH PROJECTS

DUMC's cross-campus alliance with the physical sciences connected Duke Medicine with some of the best and most controversial scientific research at Duke. For years Paul Gross had associated the Chemistry Department with tobacco research funded by the General Education Board, the North Carolina Department of Agriculture, and the Liggett & Myers Tobacco Company in Durham. Also, the Damon Runyon Memorial Fund had made a large grant to Duke's Department of Chemistry in 1951 with funds contributed by the American Tobacco Company of New York. The grant was made for a general research program on tobacco smoke that was initially called "A Study of Air Pollution." Gross arranged it so that Duke dealt only with the Damon

Runyon Fund, "and thus, that there will be no direct support of research at Duke University by the American Tobacco Company." Gross was also assured by the tobacco company that "publicity with respect to this research activity, and the findings resulting from it, will be published from Duke University through the medium of standard scientific journals." And finally, Gross eliminated the possibility of "clinical studies" on tobacco smoke at Duke, confining the program to research on the "chemical and physical properties" of what he described as "aerosols." This approach, one company official wrote, was "more in line with Dr. Gross' experience and interest and would remove any fear of linking Duke University or the tobacco industry with cancer or any possible damaging effects of tobacco on health."[119]

In the months preceding the Runyon grant, moreover, Benjamin Few became president of the Liggett & Myers Tobacco Company. Few was the nephew of Dr. William P. Few, the university's first president, and he had served as a Duke trustee since 1941. He had also served on the trustee committee to select the new president and had joined the "New York group" in supporting the candidacy of Dr. Wilburt C. Davison. It was also Few, who, late in 1953, amid the growing public debate over the relationship between smoking and lung cancer, refused to attend a meeting with other tobacco executives to discuss hiring "a public relations counsel" for the industry. In explaining his actions, Few wrote to the other tobacco executives that he and his Liggett "colleagues felt the best policy for the industry to follow right now was to do nothing—that any kind of publicity released by the industry would add fuel to the fire, and that in the course of time the whole thing would blow over."[120] That didn't happen, of course; indeed, the "thing" blew all over Duke's president Hollis Edens just days later when he announced that Liggett & Myers had given the university a grant of $105,000 "to study anything in relation to the production of tobacco." The announcement drew several questions from the audience. "When he was questioned on whether the money would be used for research in lung cancer," the *New York Times* reported, "Dr. Edens replied: 'That's not what it was set up for.' Asked if Duke had any research under way aimed at the effect of cigarette smoke on human lungs, he declared: 'None that I know of. This Liggett & Myers grant is not for that purpose. I can assure you.'"[121]

The American Cyanamid Company was also keenly interested in the "aerosol" research being done by Duke's Chemistry Department. Cyanamid and its subsidiaries produced many of the chemicals used by tobacco farmers to grow and cure their tobacco. It also produced a number of chemicals that the tobacco companies used to flavor tobacco and to bind cigarette papers. Yet Cyanamid's concerns went beyond the composition of tobacco smoke to the potential impact of the industrial chemicals the giant firm was producing.

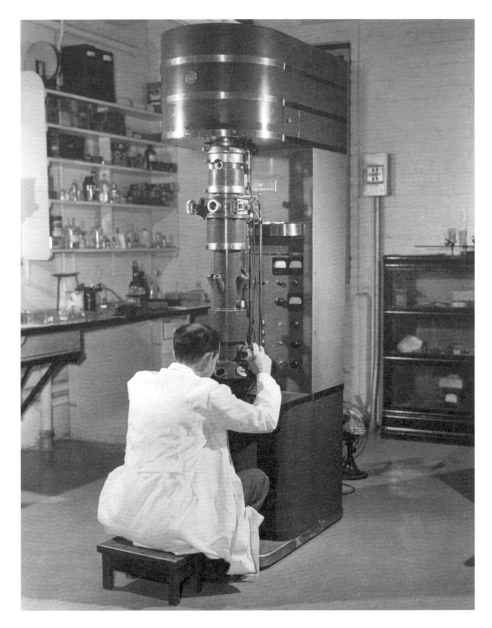

6.13 Dr. D. Gordon Sharp, a Duke biophysicist, using the new electron microscope installed in Dr. Joseph Beard's experimental surgery laboratory in 1950. *Duke University Medical Center Archives.*

How were these chemicals affecting the environment? How were they affecting human beings? And what about radiation? Could its impact be separated from that of tobacco smoke and other aerosols in the environment? These were the kind of questions that Paul Gross had Duke's Chemistry Department studying. Gross called his report to the Runyon fund "An Investigation of the Techniques and Methods for the Study and Evaluation of the Physical and Chemical Properties of Some Aerosols." Indeed, in 1961 the United States surgeon general would appoint Gross as head of the national Committee on Environmental Health Problems, the chief recommendation of which was that "a national center be established to undertake integrated research and other activities related to environmental health." In 1965, after an intensive lobbying campaign by North Carolina governor Terry Sanford, Oscar Ewing, and others, the surgeon general of the United States would announce that the National Environmental Health Sciences Center would be located in North Carolina's Research Triangle Park.[122]

By the time Handler proposed the Research Training Program, American Cyanamid had shifted its attention from Beard's work on animal viruses to funding scholarships, research, and graduate fellowships in Duke's Chemistry Department. The shift began in 1950, with the death of Cyanamid's president, William Brown Bell, and continued under North Carolina native Kenneth Towe, who served as president of Cyanamid (1952–57), as a trustee of Duke University (1954–63), and as a trustee of The Duke Endowment (1954–78). Beard, for his part, began receiving substantial funding from the American Cancer Society for his continuing research on the role of viruses in causing cancer.[123] [Figure 6.13]

The emergence of Duke's Research Training Program coincided with the growing influence of Benjamin Duke's granddaughter, Mary Duke Biddle Trent, in shaping the affairs of Duke University and The Duke Endowment. Mary Trent believed that Duke Medicine should embrace biomedical research and specialization as well as the practical medical education that Davison had always stressed in collaboration with the Endowment's original mission.[124] Trent herself was elected to Durham's city council in 1951, as part of a local coalition of black and white voters, and she was also a member of the North Carolina Hospital Study Committee appointed that year by Gordon Gray. Trent also served briefly as Durham's mayor before marrying her second husband, Dr. James H. Semans, in 1953. Semans, a urologist who specialized in treating the physical and psychological problems associated with erectile dysfunction, also taught and researched the topic and lectured on the subject to audiences throughout the world. In 1957, Mary Semans became a trustee of The Duke Endowment, and in 1963 a trustee of Duke University.

The Dean and the Doris Duke Foundation

The growing influence of Mary Semans at Duke coincided with Doris Duke's declining interest in and support for the university. Much of what Doris Duke did for the university she did for DUMC, and she did it through Wilburt Davison. Davison spent 25 years on the board of directors of Independent Aid and its successor, the Doris Duke Foundation, which was formed in 1951. Davison was one of four (and sometimes five) directors who dispensed grants several times a year from the foundation and from accounts Doris Duke described as her "additional 10% funds" and "20% Gross Income Fund." Miss Duke had her own favorite groups and issues, as did Davison and the other board members, and the foundation received unsolicited requests and inquiries from groups and individuals throughout the United States and around the world. Catholic charities were a foundation favorite, as were Planned Parenthood and several state and private organizations devoted to social welfare and the needs of children. The foundation also received a large number of medical and health-related requests that were passed on to Davison for his comments and criticisms.[125]

Most of the funding requests that Davison submitted to the foundation were for projects at DUMC, and in most instances they were accepted. In addition to annual grants to the Department of Social Services, which climbed to $30,000 a year, the foundation made grants at various times to the Departments of Pediatrics, Microbiology, and Radiology, and to the division of ophthalmology. All of the grants to DUMC, it seems, were made for equipment and personnel, as Davison took "a very dim view of private foundations contributing to research when there is so much research money available from federal sources."[126] The foundation also made grants to build a play room for children in Duke Hospital, and another for training nurses at Highland Hospital, which "not only does an excellent job for its own patients," Davison wrote, "but . . . is setting the pace for the state institutions, which all too often are custodial rather than restorative."[127] Duke's medical school even received through the foundation an appropriation by way of the California Paralyzed Veterans Association.[128]

Davison strongly supported the various grant proposals submitted to Doris Duke's foundations by Durham's YMCA and the city's black hospital. "Lincoln Hospital is near to my heart," Davison wrote to the foundation, "and a truly remarkable job is being done with inadequate support. Anything which can be given them will be wisely used." Davison was especially fond of William Rich, Lincoln's black superintendent, who on one occasion requested $1,000 "for books for the library in order that Lincoln Hospital can continue to be accredited by the American Hospital Association." Davison hoped the request would be "placed on the agenda because Mr. Rich is doing a splendid job in making the Lincoln Hospital one of the outstanding colored hospitals in this whole area."[129] Lincoln didn't always get what it asked for, however, and neither did Davison. When he spoke in favor of a large grant to Durham's new YMCA building, for example, the foundation's secretary replied that the request "left Doris completely cold. I gave her not only the formal request that had come but also your comments about the needs of the 'Y.'"[130]

Neither did Doris Duke and the Dean share the same sense of where medicine ended and quackery began. It was her money, and her body, and she could subject them to whatever treatment struck her fancy. The foundation gave a grant for "music therapy," for example, to the Hospitalized Veterans Service of the Musicians Emergency Fund. Duke herself occasionally received therapy from a physician who used VHF radiowaves to treat her joint pain. But it was the foundation's support for the Kirksville College of Osteopathic Medicine that most bothered Davison. Doris Duke was "friendly" with Drs. Isabelle and Josephine Morelock, osteopaths associated with the college, and between 1948 and 1954, the foundation gave the Missouri institution more than $20,000 in research grants. Davison usually avoided discussing the matter, either with Miss Duke or others at the foundation. But when queried about Kirksville on one occasion, he wrote to the foundation's secretary, "As an old legislator in Pennsylvania said, 'I see no reason for different licenses for osteopathy, naturopathy, allopathy and homeopathy. All of these paths just lead to the grave.'"[131]

Davison genuinely liked Doris Duke, and dealing with her idiosyncrasies was a small price to pay for the information and power the foundation provided him. Queries came to him from throughout the United States and the world, and he was able, through the wealth and reach of the foundation, to affect the lives of many people in many far-flung places. Grants went out to the Maryknoll Sisters' Clinic in Pusan, Korea, and there were grants for training technical assistants at the National Taiwan University. Grants also went to Operation Brotherhood in Vietnam, which was doing work among refugees there, and to the International Boy Scouts, the World University Service, and the Society of Brothers. Davison always kept in mind, moreover, the foundation's ability to shape public relations and the image not only of the United States but of Duke and DUMC specifically. In considering a grant to the Middle East, for instance, he wrote, "I believe it would be of great help in our relations in that area." In the case of the Durham YMCA, he "felt that a grant from the Doris Duke Foundation would greatly benefit the 'town-gown' relationships." In commenting on the Kirksville College of Osteopathic Medicine, Davison noted, "I have found because of public relations of Duke University, I must keep an 'unanswered file' in regard to osteopathic, chiropractic, minority students and other controversial subjects. I formerly answered most of them, but found that my replies sooner or later got into the newspapers and Duke University was embarrassed."[132]

Duke's new Research Training Program was not a beneficiary of the Doris Duke Foundation, however. Although Davison endorsed the program publicly, he lamented it in private and continued to push for the curriculum revisions rejected by the medical school and the university. "I really believe that we are making progress toward the goal of integrating and correlating the various disciplines of the medical school," he wrote to Commonwealth in endorsing Handler's proposed research program, "and are also training students to practice 'complete medicine' in which the patient and his environment, instead of his particular disease, are the center of the students' interest." Wilburt Davison did not like Phil Handler, however, and he did not like what Handler was doing to the Duke medical school. Davison believed that Duke Medicine should continue to focus on producing well-trained general practitioners through practical medical education. He described Handler as a "political" scientist who had "doomed practical medical education" and who, "except for training graduate students in bio-chemistry, had very little contact with medical education, and as far as I can ascertain that contact has not been beneficial to the students."[133]

The Commonwealth Fund approved a three-year grant to Duke for the Research Training Program in 1958, and the program began in the fall of 1959 under the direction of Dr. James B. Wyngaarden. (The program also received funding from Duke University, the John and Mary R. Markle Foundation, and the Atomic Energy Commission, but more than half of the $1.3 million in grants received by Duke for the program came from the National Institutes of Health.) [Figure 6.14]

Resignations and a New President for Duke

The Research Training Program moved into its home in a new wing of the Bell Building in January 1960, just as a battle erupted between the Gross and Edens trustee factions over Duke's long-term development plans. The clash led to the resignation of both men and to the selection of Dr. Deryl Hart to succeed Edens as president of Duke. What happened? What explains these developments? One answer points to the beliefs of the Methodist or religious faction of university trustees. Duke appeared to them to be growing not only too much too fast but also in the wrong direction. It was moving toward a Johns Hopkins type of set-up, in which graduate education was emphasized and, in this case, dominated and controlled by men connected with Duke Power, Big Tobacco, and the federal government. Gross

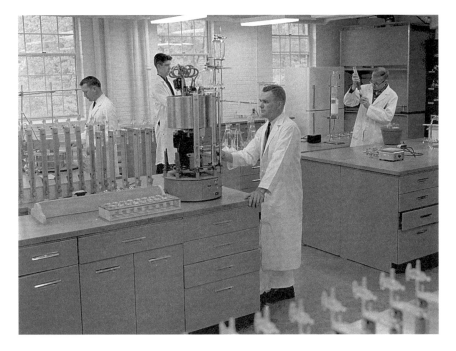

6.14 Faculty and students in the new laboratory of the Research Training Program, June 1960. *Duke University Archives*.

had followed up on the Commonwealth grant, for example, by submitting a funding request to the General Education Board. He requested $1 million "for an improved graduate program in the humanities, especially in language areas, at Duke University during the coming decade," and pledged Duke to a matching grant of $1 million.

Another possible spark for this trustee struggle was the raging debate over smoking and lung cancer. Many of the religious trustees had long opposed the use of tobacco, both on principle and for health reasons, and now, with increasing evidence that smoking and lung cancer were related, they were worried about the growing power of Big Tobacco in the affairs of Duke University. The fires of the smoking debate were raging close by, in fact, when the trustee confrontation erupted in February 1960. Specifically, Paul Gross was deposed for federal court proceedings that took place that spring and involved a suit filed against Liggett & Myers in 1954 by Otto E. Pritchard, a Chesterfield smoker who had lost his right lung in 1953. Gross testified for Liggett & Myers as part of the larger argument mounted by the company's attorney "that the medical profession does not know the cause of lung cancer. The profession has not accepted as proved any of the various theories of possible causes, including city life, industrialization, auto fumes, viruses, and radiation." According to the *New York Times*, legal observers expected the trial to "furnish a test case with nation-wide significance for the legal determination of the controversial questions of the cause of lung cancer and the liability of cigarette manufacturers."[134]

Gross's testimony was read to the federal jury and in it, the *Times* reported, he said that "Liggett & Myers Tobacco Company did no research on the physical effects of smoking between 1932 and 1953. . . . Dr. Gross said in his deposition that from 1932 to 1953 most of Liggett & Myers' research was done by Duke laboratories. He said it was confined to nicotine, the growing of tobacco and plant diseases. Dr. Gross said he had told Liggett & Myers that studies linking smoking and lung cancer were not conclusive." And Gross truly believed what he said, it seems. Not because his research was funded by the tobacco industry, but because he designed that research with the particulate composition of environmental pollution in mind, not the impact of that pollution on personal health.[135]

Edens submitted his resignation in February of 1960, and it was accepted in March, at the annual meeting of university trustees, where the religious faction also demanded and received Gross's resignation. "In brief," Gross wrote to the General Education Board that May, "the picture is as follows. A small, but influential, group of the Trustees who are anxious to have the University move ahead in connection with plans projected by a Long Range Planning Committee, of which I was the Chairman, decided that Edens was not the man to continue to lead the University during the development phase for the next ten years until his statutory retirement." Consequently, Edens, after negotiating a settlement with the executive committee of university trustees, had resigned.[136]

As far as Gross was concerned, his own resignation reflected the fact that Edens "had built up strong, but almost exclusively local support in alumni and church groups and among as much as two-thirds of our Board of Trustees who were in favor of keeping the institution more local and regional in character, as well as closer ties with the Methodist Church." Thus, when the full board accepted Edens's resignation at its March 23 meeting, Gross found that he too would have to resign: "As a counter move my resignation as Vice President was requested by the majority of the Board supporting Edens, as well as my resignation as Chairman of the Long Range Planning Committee. . . . An interim president, Dr. Deryl Hart, Professor of Surgery in our Medical School, has been appointed to take office July 1. He is a sound man and one whom I think can carry us through the next year or so and give time to look for the right leader for the long pull ahead, as well as to bring about badly needed changes in our administrative and organizational structure which are long over-due."[137]

The time seemed right to Dean Wilburt Davison for him to retire. "As the Medical School was now safe from presidential attack," he later wrote, "there was no need for me. Also, it was obvious to me and to most of the medical faculty that inasmuch as I must retire automatically at the age of 69 in 1961, and as I was becoming increasingly antagonistic to the eager research beavers (and vice versa), a new dean was needed. A committee considered several candidates and recommended the appointment of Barnes Woodhall, professor of neurosurgery. I asked for a sabbatical year from 1960 to 1961 so that I could resign as dean on July 1, 1960, and continue as James B. Duke professor of pediatrics, without any duties, but with full salary until September 1, 1961." Early in 1961, Davison was elected as a trustee of The Duke Endowment.[138]

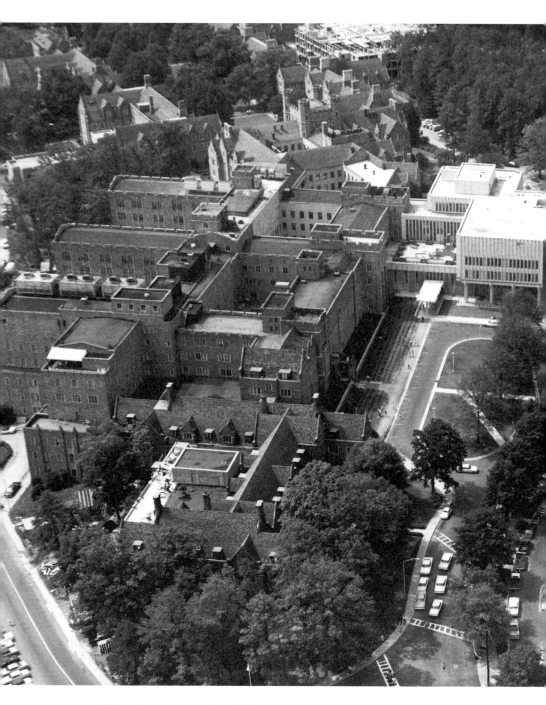

7.1 New main entrance to the medical center (white building, top), and adjacent Clinical Research II and Rehabilitation Buildings (top right), 1970.

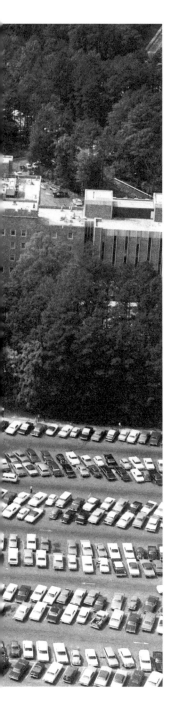

CHAPTER 7

Race, Place, and the Mission of Duke Medicine, 1960–1980

The years from 1960 to 1980 marked the ascendancy of surgeons, scientists, and liberals at Duke University. The founding chairman of Duke's Department of Surgery, Dr. Deryl Hart, served as president of Duke between 1960 and 1963 and was succeeded as president by Douglas M. Knight, a native of Cambridge, Massachusetts. Knight arrived at Duke with a decade of experience as a university president and with a proper Ivy League pedigree—three degrees and a faculty background in English literature at Yale.

Knight also arrived during the governorship of Terry Sanford, one of the most ambitious and innovative politicians in the South in the 20th century. Sanford won the Democratic nomination for governor in 1960, just a week before Hart's appointment as Duke president, and in the weeks that followed, Sanford defied the state's Democratic elders and backed a Massachusetts Catholic, Senator John F. Kennedy, for the party's nomination for president. Both Sanford and Kennedy won their elections in November 1960, and over the next four years Sanford established a number of progressive programs that not only improved life

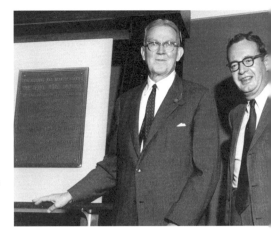

in North Carolina but also helped shape the "Great Society" of Kennedy's successor, President Lyndon Baines Johnson. Sanford then succeeded Knight as president of Duke University in 1969, and for the next 15 years his personal and political connections proved helpful in expanding DUMC's private and public networks. [Figure 7.2]

Within Duke University Medical Center, Hart's trusted colleague, Dr. Clarence Gardner, ran the Department of Surgery between 1960 and 1964 and was succeeded in turn by Dr. David C. Sabiston, a Hopkins-trained North Carolinian who ruled Duke's Department of Surgery for the next 30 years. Surgeons also took control of the administration of Duke's medical center. The chief of neurosurgery, Dr. Barnes Woodhall, succeeded Wilburt Davison as the school's dean in 1960, and in 1964 he was succeeded in turn by another surgeon, Dr. William G. Anlyan. Anlyan then became Duke's vice president for health affairs in 1969, following Sanford's arrival as president, and in 1987, under the university's new president, DUMC psychiatrist Dr. H. Keith H. Brodie, Anlyan was made Duke University's chancellor for health affairs. Indeed, between 1960 and Anlyan's retirement 1989, the administrative histories of both the medical center and the Department of Surgery ran very much in parallel.

Bill Anlyan proved to be one of DUMC's most adept fundraisers, administrators, builders, and recruiters. He came to Duke as a surgical resident in 1949, after earning undergraduate and M.D. degrees at Yale, and with the arrival of his fellow Yalie, Douglas Knight, as president of Duke in 1963, Anlyan became associate dean of the School of Medicine. There he worked closely with Woodhall in planning the future expansion of the medical center, and after succeeding Woodhall as dean, Anlyan converted their plans into buildings that cost millions of dollars and contained millions of square feet of space. Anlyan also found success as an excellent faculty recruiter for Duke Medicine. "I always looked for the best in the country or the best in the world," he later wrote in his autobiography, "and unless they made outrageous demands, in most cases we were able to meet their needs in terms of money, space, support, and administrative structure to recruit the people we wanted. I tried to look

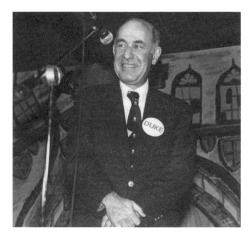

7.3 Dr. William G. Anlyan. *Duke University Medical Center Archives.*

for people who were thirty-five to thirty-eight and had their futures in front of them. They might be a little bit of a gamble, but they had to have chalked up an excellent track record. I did not want to recruit people who regarded Duke as a nice place to retire."[1] [Figure 7.3]

Drs. Eugene Stead and Philip Handler did some of the most creative and progressive work at DUMC between 1960 and 1980. According to Stead, Dean Wilburt Davison "always said he only made three mistakes in his life. He said 'I shouldn't have ever appointed Barnes Woodhall,' our distinguished neurosurgeon. He said 'Phil Handler was the worst thing that could have happened to everybody.' But he said 'the worst of all was Gene Stead.'" Where Woodhall went wrong, in Davison's mind, was in backing the research-centered curriculum changes pressed by Handler and Stead, first in the Research Training Program of the late 1950s and then in using that experience to reshape the medical school curriculum in the mid-1960s. Forty years later, in a passing reference to this internal friction, Anlyan noted that Davison, during his last years as dean, "became more interested in developing primary care services in North Carolina. He became disenchanted with Phil Handler, chairman of biochemistry, and with Gene Stead, chairman of medicine, because he had the feeling that the two of them were leading the Medical School and hospital in the direction of a tertiary-care, research-oriented institution, rather than paying attention to the general or family practitioner. Incidentally, I think he was right that we had not paid enough attention to family practice, and we paid the price for that in the 1960s."[2]

Handler and Stead did indeed speed the growth of science and research at DUMC, even as they reinforced the progressive political activism they shared with Duke's sixth president, Terry Sanford. Handler made his first political stand in the early 1950s, as the new chairman of the Department of Biochemistry, when he opposed giving vice president Richard Nixon an honorary degree from Duke—an award for which Davison had tried to mobilize support among the medical faculty. Handler also collaborated with Sanford in Democrat Hubert Humphrey's 1968 presidential campaign; while Sanford ran Humphrey's national campaign against Nixon, through the Citizens for

Humphrey-Muskie Committee, Handler led Scientists and Engineers for Humphrey in North Carolina. That was a year before Sanford arrived at Duke, and a year before Handler himself was elected president of the National Academy of Sciences, a position he held until six months before his death in December 1981. Yet Handler's political activism worried many of his fellow scientists and Duke colleagues, especially after Nixon's victory in 1968. "The 'morning after' many [of them] had misgivings," one observer wrote of Handler's pro-Humphrey involvement, "and possibly as a result of this involvement, President Nixon seemed especially reluctant to seek the advice of scientists and science in government. Eventually in 1972, he abolished the Federal Science Advisory Board."[3] [Figure 7.4]

Handler also pushed to expand interdepartmental and interdisciplinary research at Duke. Speaking at a campus lecture series in 1968, on the topic "Duke University and the Year 2000," Handler told the school's alumni that "it is literally in our hands to direct our evolution." From genetic manipulation to the "mind-body problem," Handler believed that the "unifying concept that all life is understandable in chemical and physical terms has made a mockery of many of the lines which separate the biological disciplines. In due time we will have to reorganize the life of the University to take cognizance of this. The barriers have fallen intellectually—we now have to remove them in terms of the administrative management." And yet, Handler continued, "these problems require solutions and decisions which should never be left to the scientists. Scientists are very competent in the laboratory, but they have no right to make the larger decisions which affect mankind. It is imperative in the University to create interdisciplinary operations, crossing the life sciences with philosophy, religion, government, and sociology, because these greater questions will have to be resolved. If they are not resolved deliberately, the events will run away with themselves; and whenever that happens, you can be certain mankind will suffer."[4]

Links to NAS and NIH

If Handler proved prescient regarding the evolution of interdisciplinary studies and administrative management at Duke, his economic assumptions as president of the National Academy of Science were wildly optimistic. Handler was elected to the position in 1969, at the peak of the "golden age" of academic medicine, and according to one scientist, it was Handler's "contention that federal funding of science would increase indefinitely at 15 percent a year. . . . [H]is argument was that scientific research had such a small base, and that the economic growth of the country would be such

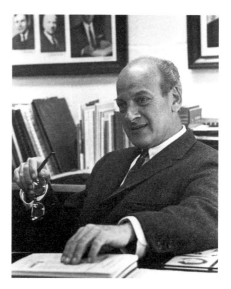

7.4 Dr. Philip Handler. *Duke University Archives.*

that the 15 percent increase would be fueled continually by growth from a small base."[5] Handler had years of evidence to support his assumptions, including his experience at Duke, and by the time he began his presidency at the National Academy of Sciences, Medicare and Medicaid had combined with increased spending for the war in Vietnam to drive the bottom line for medical and scientific research off the top of the charts.

Despite the economic decline of the 1970s, Handler supported a number of important and lasting developments at NAS. One was the Institute of Medicine. The institute was established in December 1970, during the first Nixon administration, as a tool to help the National Academy of Sciences influence national policy on the larger problems of medicine and health care.[6] In 1977, moreover, as Handler testified before a Senate subcommittee in support of the controversial new field of gene splicing, word came that scientists in California had used recombinant DNA to grow in bacteria a protein normally produced in animal and human brains. Handler described the achievement as a "scientific triumph of the first order," and offered it to the subcommittee as evidence "that gene splicing research does have great potential." Which turned out, of course, to be an understatement; within a decade the company that had backed the research, Genentech, ruled the new field of biotechnology.[7]

Handler also worked closely with Dr. Eugene Stead to expand and strengthen DUMC's existing networks with NIH. A key figure in their collaboration was one of the golden boys of the golden age of academic medicine, Dr. James Wyngaarden. Recognized early for his exceptional mind and laboratory skills, Wyngaarden was especially interested in the problems of purine metabolism as related to gout and other conditions. Between 1948 and 1951, he held an internship and residencies at the Massachusetts General Hospital in Boston, where he also assisted in some of the earliest clinical trials involving the use of steroids to reduce the inflammation associated with arthritis. Wyngaarden was also one of only 12 men selected nationally by Dr. James A. Shannon, then associate director for research in the National Heart Institute, to serve on the original staff of the new Clinical Center at NIH. (This service came to be called the Clinical Associates Program.) From 1952 to 1953, moreover, while waiting for the new clinical center to open, Wyngaarden worked as a visiting investigator under Dr. DeWitt Stetten at the Public Health Research Institute of the City of New York. Significantly, Stetten was then collaborating with Handler and two other scientists on the first edition of what became one of the most widely adopted biochemistry textbooks for both graduate and medical students, *Principles of Biochemistry*.[8]

By the time the textbook was published in 1955, Wyngaarden was a clinical investigator at NIH, Stetten was an associate director of the National Institute of Arthritis and Metabolic Diseases, and James Shannon was director of the NIH. "About that time," Wyngaarden later recalled, "Stetten mentioned to me that Phil Handler . . . was looking for someone [to become] . . . director of the Radioisotope Unit of the Durham VA Hospital. . . . I doubted that I would have any interest in that particular position, but I had heard exciting things about Duke University and both the Departments of Biochemistry and of Medicine . . . and I had never met Eugene Stead." Wyngaarden visited Duke and came away "tremendously impressed" with the medical service under Stead. He was also intrigued. "It was a small and, by comparison with the Boston experience, a rather primitive place," Wyngaarden remembered. "The hospital was perhaps half the size of Massachusetts General, if that; the staff was much smaller; far less an investment in biomedical science at that time; but clearly it was a place that was unfolding with a very bright future. It already had a splendid reputation."[9]

Wyngaarden turned down the VA position, but joined the Duke faculty in 1957 with a joint appointment in the Departments of Biochemistry and Medicine. He then served as executive director of DUMC's new Research Training Program between 1959 and 1965, when he accepted the chairmanship of the Department of Medicine at the University of Pennsylvania. Returning to Duke in 1967, he succeeded Stead as chairman of the Department of Medicine and remained there for the next until 1982, when he was appointed director of the National Institutes of Health by President Ronald Reagan.[10] [Figure 7.5]

Ralph Snyderman's Rise to Chancellor

Among Wyngaarden's many contributions to Duke was his recruitment of Dr. Ralph Snyderman. Snyderman had completed his internship and residency at Duke between 1965 and 1967, and in the years that followed he had made an important discovery at NIH—one with major implications for Wyngaarden's own specialized research interests. This was "the discovery of C5A as a chemotactic factor for leukocytes," Snyderman later

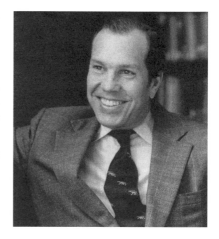

7.5 Dr. James B. Wyngaarden. *Duke University Medical Center Archives.*

explained. It was a discovery that was "much more important than I knew at the time," he continued, "of identifying one of the major mediators of inflammation as a specific, well-defined peptide." His discovery was also part of a much larger body of research, which identified a mechanism "by which inflammatory media is degenerated. . . . [P]utting . . . a small part of the field of inflammation into modern biochemistry and biology was something I was being credited for."[11]

Wyngaarden helped lure Snyderman back to Duke in 1975 after aggressively competing to recruit the young scientist. He made Snyderman an assistant professor of medicine at Duke and chief of rheumatology at the VA Hospital. He also made him a Howard Hughes investigator and gave him space in the Bell Building laboratory once directed by Dr. Frank Engel, the brilliant endocrinologist who had come with Stead from Emory in 1947. Wyngaarden "gave me that very laboratory with some additional space as well," Snyderman recalled. Wyngaarden also appointed Snyderman chief of the division of rheumatology at Duke in 1976—a position previously held by Wyngaarden himself. "I remember asking him 'What do you expect of me as division chief?' And Jim was very specific," Snyderman explained. "If I hadn't asked, I don't think he would have told me. I remember him telling me that he expected me to be financially responsible, to hold the division together, to make sure that the people within the division were happy and cohesive, to provide the leadership for that. And, the other thing that really influenced me is that he wanted me to be the best rheumatologist in the division. . . . I took that seriously, and I spent a lot of time to make sure that I was a good clinical rheumatologist." Snyderman would succeed Bill Anlyan as dean of Duke's medical school and chancellor of Duke University in 1989.[12]

Wyngaarden's resignation from NIH occurred at the same time as the selection of Dr. Ralph Snyderman as chancellor. Though Snyderman had left Duke two years earlier, to work at Genentech in California, his appointment reflected years of nurturing in Duke Medicine. "I had a long history with the institution," he later recalled; "they certainly knew me and I knew the institution, fifteen years on the Faculty and my house staff training." Duke had been on Snyderman's mind since his days as a medical student at Downstate Medical College in Brooklyn. During summer breaks at Saranac Lake, while working

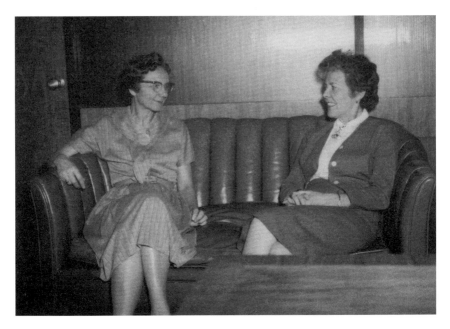

7.6 Thelma Ingles, left, with Virginia Arnold, nursing adviser for the Rockefeller Foundation. *Courtesy of the Rockefeller Archive Center.*

with a small group of handpicked medical students, Snyderman conducted research and "essentially read through all" of the 1960 textbook coauthored by Jim Wyngaarden, *The Metabolic Basis of Inherited Diseases.* The book taught Snyderman "a tremendous amount about basic science and its application to medicine" and also gave him, he recalled, "an exalted view of Jim Wyngaarden, and that influenced [him] to some degree to come to Duke [as an intern]." As did the Research Training Program that Wyngaarden had directed. It was "a very innovative program," Snyderman later recalled in an interview at Duke. "That had a lot to do with bringing me here. It distinguished this place from others."[13]

Eugene Stead's Initiatives

Another feature that distinguished Duke Medicine for Snyderman was the friendship between his mentor at Downstate Medical College, Dr. Ludwig Eichner, and Dr. Eugene Stead at Duke. To Snyderman the road to Duke seemed "an easily identifiable path because of the friendship of the chairmen of medicine at Downstate and at Duke."[14] Snyderman found Stead as exhilarating and transformative as he was exhausting. "Stead was a tough man. He still is," Snyderman noted in 1990. "He has a characteristic

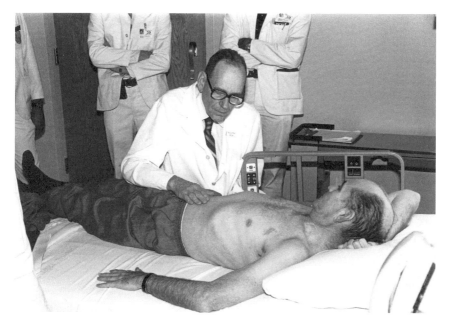

7.7 Dr. Eugene A. Stead Jr. examining a patient. *Duke University Medical Center Archives.*

about him which I don't understand. And that is, when people are around him, at least the kind of people that were around him at that time, he drove them to exceed any potential expectations they ever had for themselves. I never worked so effectively."[15]

Similar sentiments were expressed by Duke nursing professor Thelma Ingles, who spent a year studying with Stead as "a kind of guinea pig student in a pilot study of our projected program leading to the Master of Science in Nursing." The purpose of the program was to improve the clinical practice of nursing by having nurses work in close association with the medical staff. The program was funded jointly for seven years (1957–64) by Duke University and the Rockefeller Foundation, and though it was denied accreditation three times by the National League of Nursing— which asserted that "it was at least inappropriate and perhaps dangerous for nurses to assume medical tasks"— the program was applauded by the foundation and by Ingles alike. The director of medical education at the foundation, John Bugher, noted "that one cultivates a plant where it seems to grow. The only school which has had the initiative and foresight to do the groundwork involving both medicine and nursing which is necessary to formulate an adequate curriculum of this kind has been Duke University." As for Ingles, who had started the program "fully aware that [she] entertained some pretty unpleasant feelings towards doctors in general," she soon discovered that her "close work" with numerous doctors did "much to eradicate these feelings." And her relationship with Stead was especially enlightening. "He actively is a friend of nurses," Ingles wrote in 1961. "It's sad that some nurses don't want doctors for friends."[16] [Figure 7.6]

Between 1961 and 1963 Stead also actively pursued a faculty position at Duke for Dr. Louis Sullivan, the black hematologist who in 1989 became President George Bush's secretary of health and human services. Stead wanted Sullivan to direct a new residency program for African Americans at Lincoln Hospital; though Sullivan himself would be based at Lincoln, he was to have a full-time faculty position in Duke's Department of Medicine. The Duke Endowment funded the Lincoln program and Duke's Department of Medicine directed it. Unfortunately, and for reasons that are still not clear, a university administrator refused Stead's request for Sullivan's appointment. The decision infuriated Stead, who considered resigning (again), and it also stunned the other department heads, many of whom considered the action a threat to their traditional authority and power.[17] [Figure 7.7]

Stead conceived his most widely recognized contribution to Duke and American medicine in 1964: the physician assistant program.[18] Stead's idea for the program emerged in response to the conditions that had shaped his vision for improving the clinical skills of nurses: the disparity between increased demand for health services and a shortage of personnel to provide them. After first considering Durham firemen for his program, Stead turned to highly trained military veterans who had served in the medical corps during the war in Vietnam. The purpose of the physician assistant program was to train these former corpsmen to a level more advanced than medical technician but less than that of physician. A 1965 grant from NIH—which until then had only supported M.D. and Ph.D. candidates—got the program started, and major grants followed from the Josiah Macy Jr. Foundation, the Rockefeller and Carnegie Foundations, and the Commonwealth Fund. By 1980, the program was firmly established and standardized, and by 2004 there were more than 45,000 practicing physician assistants in the United States and more PA training programs than medical schools.[19]

Duke's physician assistant program reflected a change in Stead's assumptions regarding the training of specialists and general practitioners at Duke. One former house officer, Dr. Melvin Berlin, recalled discussing the matter with Stead in the 1950s. "I said 'Dr. Stead wouldn't it be really great if a great institution like Duke would institute some type of rotation to train general practitioners or whatever you want to call them?' And he said 'Mel, there is no place in modern medicine for the general practitioner.' That's what he said then. He later changed his mind but at that time—and he was not the only one. I remember being told that by Dr. Sam Martin who became dean at the University of Florida. He said the same thing . . . that American medicine needed specialists."[20]

Stead, apparently, changed his mind after the creation of Medicare and Medicaid in 1965. America now needed as many general practitioners and primary care providers as the nation's academic medical centers could train. There was no fully organized training program in North Carolina for general practice, and with a shortage of physicians in rural areas throughout the state, demands for family medicine programs had become persistent and loud. The outcry was especially strong in eastern North Carolina, where Leo W. Jenkins, president of the newly named East Carolina University, was making speeches every day for the creation of a medical school at his university. Only in 1974, however, after years of opposition from UNC supporters in Chapel Hill, did the General Assembly appropriate the funds for a four-year medical school at East Carolina University. The mission of the new school, which enrolled its first class in 1977, was "to increase the supply of primary care physicians to serve the state, to improve the health status of citizens in eastern North Carolina, and to enhance the access of minority and disadvantaged students to a medical education."[21]

Changes to the Curriculum

It was in this context of the Johnson administration's "Great Society" programs and the social revolution of the sixties that DUMC became embroiled in an internal debate not unlike the one that had occupied it in the mid-1950s: What were the objectives of Duke Medicine and how should the curriculum embrace those goals? Should Duke Medicine devote itself to training general practitioners or should it concentrate on creating specialists and physician-scientists? Much as had happened a decade earlier, external developments deeply influenced the debate within Duke's medical center in the mid-1960s. Yet equally important to the debate, and to the future of Duke Medicine, were the new "elective system" of undergraduate medical education, the creation of the M.D.-Ph.D. program at Duke, and the professional goals of Drs. David Sabiston and James Wyngaarden, both of whom emphasized specialization and the training of physician-scientists. Sabiston succeeded Dr. Clarence Gardner as chairman of the Department of Surgery in 1964, and Wyngaarden succeeded Stead as chairman of the Department of Medicine in 1967.

The major curriculum reforms of the 1960s, the introduction of an "elective system" of undergraduate medical education and a medical scientist training program (M.D.-Ph.D.), were in large measure a fulfillment of the long-term program in graduate studies launched at Duke by Willis Smith, Paul Gross, Edwin L. Jones, and Phil Handler after World War II. Handler offered his ideas for curriculum reform in the spring of 1961, in a 12-page memorandum to Duke's new medical school dean, Dr. Barnes Woodhall. The title of the memo is "Development of the basic sciences at Duke Medical School," and in it Handler argued vigorously for making Duke Medicine a national leader in research in the basic sciences. "Their development has not kept pace with the vigor of our clinical endeavors," he wrote. "This has been true largely for financial reasons, viz., the growth and expansion of our clinical departments have been largely self-financed. But as we enter upon this second phase of our development with the opportunities generated by the appointment of new departmental chairman in Pathology and Physiology, and the expectation of increased support from the Duke Endowment and the Federal Government, it would be well to consider where we are going."[22]

Handler challenged his colleagues to adopt a broader vision of medical education and training. "We must unshackle the fetters of the concept that the 'prime role of the Medical School is teaching undergraduate medical students.' Our prime concern must not be that restrictive. Our business is information about human biology in health and disease. In our library we accumulate it; in our laboratories we increase the sum of information; in our hospital we utilize it; and in our academic pursuits we disseminate it. No one of these functions can properly be stated to be any more important than the others," Handler argued. "Our role is not so much to teach as it is to provide an atmosphere which facilitates learning, while we attempt to arouse the interest and enthusiasm of our students." Handler had no intention of deemphasizing the importance of teaching undergraduate medical students or of relaxing "our efforts in their behalf." What he wanted was for the house staff to benefit from further training; for the basic scientists to train more basic scientists; and for Duke Medicine to place as much emphasis on basic research as it did on teaching and private practice.[23]

An initial plan for curriculum reform emerged late in 1961 with the help of the new chairman of Pathology, Dr. Thomas D. Kinney, who succeeded Wiley Forbus in 1960, and the new chairman of Physiology, Dr. Daniel C. Tosteson, who was recruited by Wyngaarden from Washington University Medical School in St. Louis. Kinney, a graduate of Duke medical school, was recruited from the Western Reserve School of Medicine; familiar with Western's recent curriculum experiments in interdisciplinary teaching methods, he joined Handler, Stead, Tosteson, and Dr. Jerome Harris, chairman of the Department of Pediatrics, in presenting the faculty with a proposal for curriculum reform late in 1961.[24]

The reformers' goals remained fairly constant even as American medicine was being reshaped by the War on Poverty (1964–68), the Civil Rights Act of 1964, and Medicare and Medicaid (1965). Duke's reformers wanted their medical students to become lifelong learners and to have not only a variety of professional pathways to choose from but also the freedom and experience to make an informed choice. It took more than three years of planning, however, as well as significant financial support from Duke University and The Duke Endowment, before the faculty put forth a curriculum one observer described as "so excellent that it is difficult to describe it other than in superlatives." In February of 1965, with a grant from the Commonwealth Fund for additional faculty, the new curriculum was announced for the fall of 1966.

In place of the traditional curriculum, which divided medical school into two years of preclinical (or basic science) laboratory courses followed by two years of clinical (or patient contact) work, Duke's "new model of medical education" exposed students to both patients and career choices sooner. "Its first academic year included presentation by each basic science department of the core of principles and information deemed essential for any physician. In the second year students entered the wards of medicine, surgery, obstetrics and gynecology, pediatrics, and psychiatry as clinical clerks. The third and fourth years were given over to elective courses, equally divided between basic science and clinical subjects, chosen in accordance with the individual student's career goals and with the guidance of an advisor from each of these general areas. A particular objective of the basic science program in the third year was to provide each student with an opportunity to investigate a limited subject area in depth." This third-year elective in basic science offered students many of the same opportunities originally provided by the successful Research Training Program.[25]

A New Chair of Surgery

The new curriculum was still not fully funded in 1964 when Dr. David Sabiston was appointed as the third chairman of Duke's Department of Surgery. Sabiston was an intense, ambitious surgeon with the kind of connections preferred by the old and new Duke Medicine alike. A native North Carolinian, he held an undergraduate degree from UNC, and both he and his wife came from prominent families in eastern North Carolina. He was a graduate of the Johns Hopkins School of Medicine and had done his internship and residency there. He was also a Howard Hughes medical investigator and an accomplished surgeon who was doing pathbreaking research in cardiovascular physiology and the use of radioactive isotopes in lung scans for pulmonary emboli. Sabiston had been first on the list of the surgeons suggested for the Duke position by Dr. Alfred Blalock, who was retiring as surgeon-in-chief of the Johns Hopkins University Hospital and as professor and director of the Department of Surgery of the medical school at Hopkins. Blalock recommended the 39-year-old Sabiston in a letter to Dr. William G. Anlyan

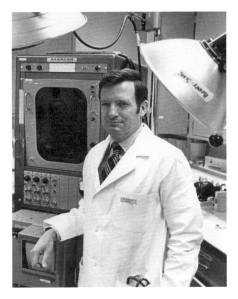

7.8 Dr. David C. Sabiston Jr. *Duke University Medical Center Archives.*

in January of 1964: "My first choice would be David Sabiston, who, as you know is my right-hand man in the Department of Surgery here. It was a great surprise to me that he was not named as my successor as Director of the Department here. It is my understanding that the final choice here was between Sabiston and [George D.] Zuidema. Hopkins practically never chooses a person who is on the staff at the time, and certainly the committee followed the policy in the present decision."[26] [Figure 7.8]

Blalock's description of Sabiston foreshadowed the latter's outstanding career as a teacher, researcher, and administrator at Duke. "I have a great admiration for Dave," Blalock wrote of Sabiston. "He is a fine gentleman, he is thoroughly honest, he has modesty and humility, and yet he is forceful. He is the best administrator I have ever had as an associate. He is an excellent teacher and clinical surgeon, and he has a real flair for investigative work. He has the loyalty of the students, the house staff, and of his associates. In fact, I do not know of any weaknesses in his makeup. I regard his bibliography as the best of those under the age of 40 who have been associated with the department here. I am quite confident that he would run an excellent department and that he would do it in a quiet and dignified, yet effective manner." The recommendation was important to Blalock, both for his allegiance to Sabiston and to Duke. Blalock counted Deryl Hart and Joseph Beard as among his oldest friends. "I have great admiration and affection for the Duke Medical School and Hospital," Blalock wrote to Anlyan. "A number of my best friends such as Deryl Hart were chosen on the original faculty, and I have followed the remarkable development of Duke with great interest."[27]

Sabiston's selection genuinely pleased Dr. Deryl Hart, who had recently retired as president of Duke. "As you know I was not on the committee that selected him but was pleased with their selection," Hart wrote to Blalock, "therefore I did not communicate with you in any regard to your opinion of Dave since this was out of my area. Mary [Hart] and I have known Dave and Aggie [Sabiston] for a good many years and as individuals we like them very much indeed." Hart also promised not to interfere with Sabiston's future course. "As you probably know I come up to my official retirement on September 1 and will not in any way intrude my ideas on Dave's running of the department. I have been asked to stay on as a consultant to the Private Clinic, have told Dave I do not want to be a thorn in his side or cause him any trouble and that I will not want to stay on any longer than I can be of some help."[28] Much to Hart's delight, Sabiston quickly demonstrated a loyalty to and enthusiasm for Duke Medicine's "basic organizational pattern and [its] relationship with the University," especially the "substantial private practice (which is recognized by the University as the prerogative of the staff) and is carried on within the Medical Center complex under the favorable conditions provided by the Private Diagnostic Clinic." Hart had nothing but praise for the Department of Surgery's "renewed drive" under Sabiston and he predicted that the department's "'golden years' lie in the future, during which it will play an important role in the further development of the Medical Center and University."[29]

A New Chair of Medicine

Jim Wyngaarden was on a sabbatical in Paris at the time of Sabiston's appointment. He was studying the "regulation of gene function" under the distinguished molecular biologist François Gros at the Institute de Biologie-Physiochemique. "All of that was largely under the aegis of the NIH," Wyngaarden later said of his year in Paris. "I had obtained research grants for the support of the laboratory [in rheumatology at Duke] and had become a career investigator of the NIH, which would have provided salary for as long as I was a faculty member." What Paris made possible for Wyngaarden was the practical experience in genetics that Duke's Research Training Program could not yet give him. "I chose to spend that year that way in order to become much more conversant with the whole emerging field of molecular biochemical genetics," he explained. "I had learned a great deal about this from the theoretical side as a member of the RTP faculty, but I never worked in that field, and the techniques were new and exciting."[30] Also contributing to the significance of Wyngaarden's experience in Paris was the fact that he was introduced there to recent Nobel laureate James Watson, one of the co-discoverers of the structure of DNA, whose "penetrating intellect made a lasting impression" on the young physician-scientist from Duke.[31]

Wyngaarden returned to Duke in the fall of 1964 where the unspoken but obvious expectation was that he would succeed Stead as chairman of the Department of Medicine. Yet by the time the new curriculum was announced in 1965, Wyngaarden had resigned from Duke to accept the position of chairman of the Department of Medicine at the University of Pennsylvania. "About that time the University of Pennsylvania position came along," Wyngaarden explained. "I found it uncomfortable to be in the position that I perceived myself to be in. It had never been really stated, although when Pennsylvania came along, there was some pressure to name the future chairman in the department even though Gene [Stead] was not going to retire for a couple of years. I found that very uncomfortable, even to have the question raised. And so, with a lot of wrench in the decision, I did take the job in Pennsylvania with the expectation that I would stay there. I had no expectation at that time of returning to Duke, and I went there then in the summer of 1965."[32]

Wyngaarden's departure also reflected the growing tension associated with finalizing plans for the new curriculum, establishing the Medical Scientist Training Program, and honoring the parting requests of Dr. Eugene Stead. As part of the inquiry into the new curriculum, Wyngaarden, as chairman of a committee on genetics, wrote "a report recommending that we set up a genetics department." Genetics, he believed, had achieved "its own identity"; others disagreed, however, and for a combination of financial and institutional reasons, his recommendation was ignored. Following Wyngaarden's departure for the University of Pennsylvania, Stead spearheaded two developments that Wyngaarden considered tangential at best to his own vision of the future of Duke's Department of Medicine. One was funding for the training program for physician assistants and the other was the formation of the Department of Community Health Sciences in 1966. Stead then "decided to follow through on his idea of retiring at sixty," Wyngaarden recalled. "No one could dissuade him from that, and I was invited to come back. I actually met with Bill Anlyan and Dave Sabiston at the La Guardia Airport, I believe, in New York, a supposed secret that fooled no one, either at Penn or at Duke. It was widely known that we were meeting." Wyngaarden accepted their invitation to return to Duke and agreed to succeed Stead as chairman of the Department of Medicine in 1967.[33]

Wyngaarden knew by then that the Research Training Program would be phased out as such and replaced by an M.D.-Ph.D. program funded by the NIH. Wyngaarden himself had been a member of the original NIH committee that set up the M.D.-Ph.D. program—the Medical Scientist Training Program, as it is called. "By that time, the NIH had started M.D.-Ph.D. programs," Wyngaarden explained years later. "Duke was one of the originals of that. More and more schools wished to have M.D.-Ph.D. programs. The NIH really couldn't justify two very expensive introductory training programs at Duke while not funding other quality programs at other institutions. So in a way, they gave us our choice, and we opted for the M.D.-Ph.D. program." The purpose of the program was to produce physician-scientists who, through their training both in medicine and the basic sciences, would serve as "faculty for the many new medical schools throughout the country."[34] The Duke program was one of the first three established by the NIH in 1966, and since that time it has produced more than 270 graduates—more than from any other such program in the country.[35]

It was at this point, in the months before Stead retired, that he visited Dr. Harvey Estes, head of the recently created Department of Community Health Sciences at DUMC. "Well," Estes recalled, "he came to me and said, 'Now, look, I've got this PA program in the Department of Medicine. . . . My successor, Dr. Wyngaarden is not interested in the PA program. It doesn't fit his mission. It doesn't fit his future. It does fit yours, because it's a solution to rural communities. And so I'd like to transfer, before I retire, to your department and give you the responsibility, the duty of taking care of it.' . . . Well, we quickly agreed that this is a logical fit with my new department, and it was not with Medicine. So at that moment I took over the new PA program, and our department has had it ever since."[36]

Medical Care for All

If Wyngaarden saw no place for the physician assistant program in the Department of Medicine, David Sabiston believed that there was no place at Duke for the training of general practitioners. For Stead, Estes, and their colleagues, however, the realities that had shaped the PA program—a shortage of nursing and allied health professionals—became coupled with the critical need for GPs in rural North Carolina and the goals of President Lyndon Johnson's Great Society, including the creation of Medicare and Medicaid. Stead called their vision "The Duke Plan." "The Duke plan accepts the fact that public assistance will always be a necessary component of our society," Stead wrote in 1969. "Indeed, we anticipate that more, and not fewer, persons will need public assistance in the future. . . . The health field is the best area in our society to create jobs which can give real satisfaction to the worker who is limited in education or work skills."[37]

Stead saw many formidable challenges, to be sure. "How to give public assistance with dignity; how to share the cost of public assistance between the private and public sectors of our society; how to create useful jobs for that portion of society who can work but who, if paid the minimum wage, cannot return a profit to their employer; how to give home services to the rich and poor of all races in times of need so they can live in security outside of nursing homes; how to create for the unskilled career ladders which have sufficiently small steps to be realistic; how to prevent the recycling of dependency by appropriate attention to the young; how to build a home support system which will allow professionally trained women to work and maintain their homes. These are some of the burning questions of our time. The Duke University Medical Center is developing a program which will give new answers to these difficult problems."[38]

It was in this emerging mission of the Department of Community Health Sciences that one finds not only a source of internal debate at DUMC but also a source of external competition with the medical center at UNC. Duke created its Department of Community Health Sciences in the summer of 1966, just two months before UNC announced the creation of its long-planned Division of Education and Research in Community Medical Care.[39] Yet Duke initially had no intention of training general practitioners; according to Estes, the department's original chairman, "the general idea was that we would form a department that would use disciplines such as sociology and economics and computers and management in order to solve the problems of rural North Carolina without actually creating a generalist."[40]

Creating generalists soon became important at Duke, however. As Estes wrote several years later, "it was obvious the public was interested in a more accessible type of medical practitioner, who was able to offer preventive maintenance, continuity of care, and a correlative function between the patient and his family and a complex medical system. In 1970 the Family Medicine Program began. This new program added a very useful clinical focus to the activities of the Department," Estes wrote in 1980, "and the program now offers a new and much needed role model for the medical students. In 1978, to more accurately reflect these activities, the Department name was changed to Community and Family Medicine." Indeed, by 1980 the department was actively engaged in the community. In addition to the physician assistant program, which it operated at the Durham VA Hospital, the department was also operating a Family Medicine Center on the campus of the new Durham County Hospital, where it was training GPs in family medicine and competing for patients with the PDC at Duke.[41]

Growing Reputation and Growing Reach

Along with the new departments, new faculty, and new missions at DUMC, other important developments between 1960 and 1980 included the expansion of Duke's reputation for producing excellent physician-scientists and the intertwining of medicine and race at every level of government. This last development delayed construction at DUMC of a badly needed hospital in order to facilitate the larger goals of the new curriculum and of racial integration and regional health care planning, which were being promoted by the individuals and institutions interested in these aspects of Duke Medicine's evolution. Wilburt Davison, Mary Semans, Doris

Duke, Watson Rankin, Barnes Woodhall, and Bill Anlyan were all part of this group, as were the federal government and the nation's largest private foundations, particularly The Duke Endowment, but also the Rockefeller, Carnegie, and Kellogg Foundations and the Commonwealth Fund. DUMC continued serving, in short, as a laboratory for progressive experiments in teaching, research, and patient care.

The numbers for new faculty and department additions were mentioned in 1978, in a book of essays contributed by DUMC staff and faculty titled *Undergraduate Medical Education and the Elective System: Experience with the Duke Curriculum, 1966–1975*. Between 1960 and 1966, the authors noted, "eight new department chairmen were named. By 1970 four additional chairmanships had changed hands and two new departments had been created." The number of medical school faculty also more than doubled between 1966 and 1975, from 204 to 472, while the number of students in each entering class grew from 80 to 115, and the total number of students increased from 330 to 460. Closely paralleling this big bang in bodies was the rapidly expanding universe of knowledge and needs. As DUMC's reformers pointed out in 1978, the new curriculum had served the changing needs of the larger society. Planning for the curriculum had taken place "during a period in which high national priority was placed upon biomedical research, implementation occurred during the era of emphasis upon medical manpower production, and currently the curriculum serves students and a society concerned about the adequacy of health care and health care delivery."[42]

NEW BUILDINGS FOR DUKE MEDICINE

To help Duke accommodate these expanding populations and pursuits, the NIH provided substantial funding for several new buildings north of, and separated from, the original, self-contained hospital/medical school. NIH funding was particularly important for two buildings that emerged from President Richard Nixon's "war on cancer." The Edwin L. Jones (1976) and Edwin A. Morris (1978) Buildings became the research and clinical components respectively of the Duke Comprehensive Cancer Center—which, with the important leadership of Dr. William W. Shingleton, was one of the first such centers established under the National Cancer Act of 1971. While the lead gifts for both buildings came from private sources, principally from the namesake families and their corporate interests, NIH provided more than half of the funding for both structures. NIH played little or no direct role, however, in funding Duke Medicine's two new basic science buildings, the Nanaline H. Duke (1968) and Alex H. Sands Jr. (1973) Buildings; in both cases the major contributors were Duke University, The Duke Endowment, and the Private Diagnostic Clinic. As for other major buildings constructed during this time—the Marshall I.

Pickens Building (1969), the Civitan Building (1970–71), the Duke Eye Center (1973), and the Seeley G. Mudd (medical library) Building (1975) and its companion structure for continuing education, the Searle Center (1978)—all were built with some combination of private and Duke-related funding.[43]

Finding the massive funding required to construct a new hospital at DUMC was a different matter entirely. The desperate need for such a facility was stressed as early as 1961, in the long-range plan prepared for the medical center by the consulting firm of Booz, Allen & Hamilton. "The pressure of demand for hospital beds in the Duke Hospital has reached a point of severity," the firm warned in its three-volume report. "The increased number of beds and the supporting departments required to service them adequately should be provided by constructing a new hospital. The hospital should be designed to accommodate initially 400 beds and their supporting services with an expansion potential for an ultimate capacity of 1,050 beds."[44]

Booz, Allen & Hamilton also suggested that "Deluxe and Negro Private Accommodations" be provided in the new hospital. The deluxe rooms would be "larger than the regular private rooms, approximately one and one-half times the size." The private rooms for African Americans would be something new; though blacks had always been admitted to public wards at Duke Hospital, they were barred from occupying private rooms. To attract blacks who could afford such accommodations, the report recommended space in either the existing or the new hospital for "about 50 beds in private and semiprivate rooms for private Negro patients. This is an urgent need as there are no private inpatient facilities in the area for Negro patients. It is believed that there are a number of well-to-do Negroes in the area who would take advantage of such a service at Duke. These facilities, in addition to providing a needed patient service, would assist in providing medical students with a reasonably full range of needed socioeconomic and sociocultural backgrounds in the patients they treat."[45]

By the time Dean Barnes Woodhall received the Booz-Allen report in August 1961, the color line was being redrawn at DUMC. All of the hospital's waiting rooms and employee locker rooms were already integrated, and all hospital personnel were hired on the basis of their qualifications. The university's trustees had voted that April to admit qualified students to the graduate and professional schools at Duke University without regard to race, creed, or national origin. Duke's undergraduate colleges were opened to African Americans the following spring, and in June of that year Duke Hospital began offering private rooms to African Americans. In 1963, W. Delano (Del) Meriwether, a track star from Washington, D.C., became the first African American admitted to Duke's school of medicine, and in 1967, its first black M.D.[46]

In the meantime, the push for a new hospital was delayed. That it took

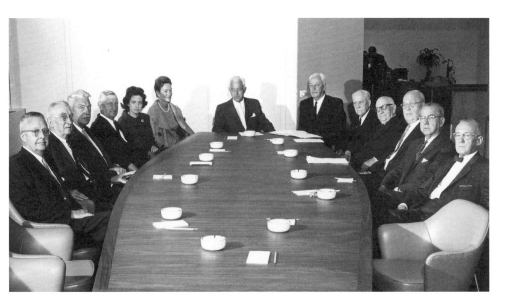

7.9 The board of trustees of The Duke Endowment. October 6, 1961. Left to right: Thomas F. Hill, Walter Smith O'Brien Robinson, Philip Heartt, Benjamin F. Few, Mary D. B. T. Semans, Doris Duke, Thomas L. Perkins, Marshall I. Pickens, Dr. Watson S. Rankin, Norman A. Cocke, Dr. Wilburt C. Davison, Kenneth C. Towe, R. Grady Rankin. *Photo Courtesy of The Duke Endowment.*

almost 15 years after the Booz, Allen & Hamilton report before Duke began constructing a new hospital raises the question, why did it take so long? The new curriculum and faculty changes were obvious factors. And yet The Duke Endowment had the wherewithal to help fund the hospital at any point its trustees so desired, and the trustees eventually took the lead in having the Endowment fund the 1980 building. Likewise, DUMC's clinical department heads eventually used the PDC's expanding building fund to match the Endowment's financial pledge to the new hospital. Bill Anlyan, the man in the middle of it all, does not address the question directly in his memoirs; after noting that planning for the hospital got started "around 1962," Anlyan writes that "Dr. Woodhall as well as the consultants—Booz, Allen & Hamilton—got a lot of faculty involved in the planning process. Unfortunately, the project did not move along, and many of the faculty were disappointed with what turned out to be a futile exercise. So when I became dean in 1964, one of the lessons I had learned from the previous deliberations was not to mobilize people in a program that was not going to come to fruition any time soon."[47]

But why didn't the project move along? What made it an exercise in futility? Put simply it was subordinated to the larger racial and health planning goals of Triangle leaders and the Endowment trustees most closely associated with Duke Medicine: Mary Duke Biddle Trent Semans, Dr. Wilburt C. Davison, Doris Duke, and Dr. Watson Smith Rankin. DUMC needed two things to build a new hospital, and both of them depended on the Endowment. It needed permission from the university's trustees, and it needed the financial support of the Endowment, which, through its three representatives on the seven-member executive committee of university trustees, wielded significant control over what Duke's trustees approved.[48]

Dave Davison served as an Endowment trustee between 1961 and his death in 1972, and to him the question of a new hospital was inseparable from his own efforts to maintain the original size and purposes of the medical center. "The Dean" seems never to have gotten beyond the original plans that he and Endowment trustee Watson Rankin had devised for the medical center in the late 1920s. Davison viewed the medical center as one big building with a hospital and a medical school; as a place that trained general practitioners from and for the South, especially North Carolina; and as a place where the clinical and preclinical departments were associated both geographically and by the number and kind of patients who visited DUMC. Davison never abandoned the idea that when a medical school got so big that it had to have a new hospital, it was time to start another medical school. [Figure 7.9]

EXPANDING CARE FOR AFRICAN AMERICANS

Ultimately, however, it was a combination of tradition and local needs that delayed the decision to build a new hospital at Duke. The tradition went back to the 1890s, to the racial cooperation established between Durham's white elites, particularly the Duke family, and the black businessmen then emerging as leaders within their local community. Nurturing this cooperation had been especially important to Washington Duke and to his sons, James and Benjamin Duke, both of whom provided critical political and financial support to the North Carolina College for Negroes, to the city's black hospital (Lincoln Hospital), and to the School of Nursing at Lincoln. By the time Duke University was created in 1924, its president, Dr. William P. Few, had adopted "the cause" of making Durham a hospital, medical, and public health center for both white and black people. And when Duke's new hospital and medical school were completed in 1930, they joined the all-black Lincoln Hospital and the whites-only Watts Hospital as the foundation for the future City of Medicine.

Doris Duke continued to nurture and strengthen this tradition in the decades that followed, as did Wilburt Davison and others affiliated with Duke University, especially Mary Duke Biddle Trent Semans. Semans, the granddaughter of Benjamin Duke, became a trustee of The Duke Endowment in 1957 and a trustee of Duke University in 1961. As a member of the Duke family, a graduate of Duke, the wife of a Duke surgeon, and, briefly, a Durham politician herself, no one was more committed than she to Duke, DUMC, Durham, and the Duke family legacy. From 1953 on, moreover, she and her second husband, Duke urologist Dr. James Semans, made community activism a large part of their life. "We always felt very strongly about fighting prejudice and this sort of thing," she recently recalled, "so we took various stands in the community. Race relations were very important to us, and wherever we saw a hole we'd try to fill it and sort of do what we could for the people in the community."[49]

Mary Semans saw an opening in the early 1960s, and together with George Watts Hill, the grandson of Watts Hospital founder George Washington Watts, she joined a regional health care planning initiative that included a racially integrated public hospital in Durham. The initiative was led by Hill, a wealthy Durham banker and insurance executive, who was also a powerful figure in Durham's Chamber of Commerce and chairman of the UNC board of trustees' subcommittee on health affairs. In June of 1963, Hill and the dean of Duke's medical school, Dr. Barnes Woodhall, asked the Long-Range Planning Committee of Durham's Chamber of Commerce to look at local health facilities and, according to one historian, Hill then "followed the lead provided by national health planners for evaluating area health facilities when he took the initiative in organizing the preliminary Research Triangle Metropolitan Health Planning Group." Those invited to discuss the health facilities initiative included representatives of Watts, Lincoln, and Duke hospitals in Durham, the North Carolina Memorial Hospitals in Chapel Hill, and the Research Triangle Institute, the Research Triangle Regional Planning Commission, and the Durham Chamber of Commerce. Among those who accepted the invitation were Dr. Barnes Woodhall and Dr. William Anlyan, the new dean of Duke's medical school, as well as Dr. James E. Davis, a surgeon at Watts Hospital and eventual president of the American Medical Association, and John Wheeler, Durham's most powerful African American leader.[50]

The health facilities plan was conducted by the Research Triangle Regional Planning Commission and was called "Medical Personnel and Facility Needs of Durham-Orange County." In addition to forecasting the future deterioration of clinical services at Lincoln Hospital, the plan recommended "calling for the creation of an independent Durham-Orange Medical Care Authority empowered to develop a coordinated plan for area health facilities." On January 1, 1964, the Health Planning Council of Central North Carolina was created, and in October, the trustees of Watts Hospital voted to open the hospital and its staff to both races. In the meantime, 15 people from Durham, Orange, and Wake Counties were appointed to the council, which was incorporated in June of 1964. John Alexander McMahon was elected as chairman of the regional council, which received funding from The Duke Endowment, the

United States Public Health Service, and other interested parties "to conduct surveys of area health facilities and gather data, and then to listen to hospital representatives describe expansion projects."[51]

The result was that Durham's voters, after rejecting a bond referendum for a new hospital in 1966, approved a second referendum in 1968. Watts Hospital was eventually closed, Lincoln Hospital was converted to a primary care facility, and a new, taxpayer-owned hospital, Durham County (later Regional) Hospital, was opened for all in 1976. The new Durham hospital had both an immediate and long-term impact on DUMC. Not only did it complicate plans for a new hospital at Duke, delaying construction there for almost 15 years; it was also subsequently acquired by Duke in 1998 (more than 20 years after it was completed) as an important component of the Duke University Health System.[52]

THE NEW DUKE HOSPITAL

Mary Semans was vice chairman of The Duke Endowment and a member of the executive committee of university trustees in 1972 when Anlyan, in the aftermath of Wilburt Davison's death, requested permission to begin detailed planning for Duke's new hospital. Anlyan's request was complicated, however, by a "protracted and acrimonious" debate among the state's economic and political elites over the question of creating a four-year medical school at East Carolina University. The new UNC board of governors had asked a panel of nationally recognized medical consultants to evaluate the need for another medical school as part of the UNC system, and the panel had recommended that the board of governors develop a plan for "a statewide system of medical and health education, based in hospitals in all regions of the state and organized in such a fashion to provide resources to enable the Duke University School of Medicine and the Bowman Gray School of Medicine to share with the University of North Carolina at Chapel Hill School of Medicine in the task of implementing the plan, using the expertise, experience, and educational resources of all three institutions in an organized fashion, integrated into a statewide effort." Funding for East Carolina's new school of medicine was provided as part of a larger $24 million appropriation by the 1974 General Assembly. The implications for Duke Medicine were profound.[53]

With these developments in mind, the executive committee of the Duke trustees granted Anlyan's request for a new hospital, and in 1975, in an area north of the original hospital, Anlyan and university president Terry Sanford turned over some soil for the groundbreaking ceremonies. The choice con-

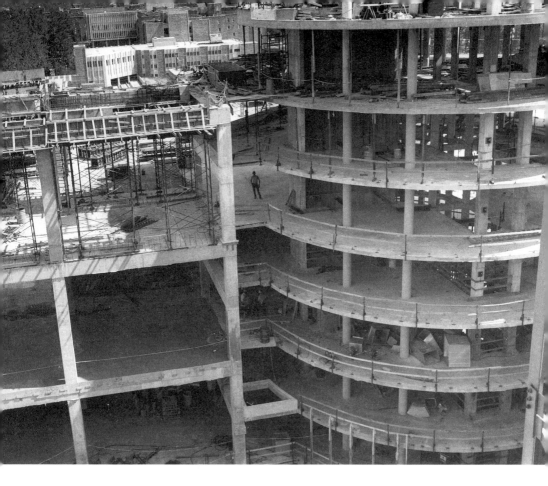

fronting DUMC—for either a partial or complete replacement of the existing hospital—came down to costs. "As I recall," Anlyan later wrote, "the total replacement would have cost $150 million, whereas the partial replacement—leaving ob-gyn and psychiatry in the existing hospital and somehow connecting the two buildings—was around $95 million."[54]

The university trustees accepted the partial plan with the condition that DUMC raise $40 million of the $95 million. A private bond offering would cover the difference. The Duke Endowment pledged $10 million to the project, and Anlyan received another $10 million in pledges from the clinical departments, including $5 million from the building fund of the PDC. "Obviously," Anlyan explained, "the clinical departments were going to be the beneficiaries of the new hospital, which would generate more income for them. They concurred. Some of the clinical faculty referred to the hospital project as 'Anlyan's folly,' and I am not sure that the project would have been approved had I put the matter to a vote of the clinical faculty. Nevertheless, I decided to go ahead with the project. It was one of the few times I had to proceed undemocratically."[55]

It was also one of the defining moments in the modern history of Duke Medicine's relationship with the rest of the university. Financing the new hospital "was the largest capital investment that Duke had ever made," recalled the hospital's former chief operating officer, William J. Donelan. "It was the first time the university had undertaken debt, particularly major debt, around a capital project." Part of the concern was the way the new hospital's debt was structured: the bonds sold to finance it were "backstopped by the full faith and credit of Duke University," Donelan explained. "Which meant that ultimately if the hospital performed so badly that it was defaulting on the bonds, the university endowment was pledged to backstop the debt. That was a point of high anxiety with the faculty of the general university and the academic council and the executive committee of the academic council." Indeed, from that point on, their concerns were such that "any time there were significant proposals for initiatives in the clinical program at Duke, it raised a whole set of questions in the academic community of the general university about whether that was really the right thing to do, which was really not a healthy design. So there was an anxiousness on the campus then, around particularly Duke Hospital and the clinical activities of the medical center, in financial terms."[56] [Figure 7.10]

A Community Health Center for Durham

Harvey Estes was the only Duke physician who had sat with Mary Semans and four other prominent Durham citizens on the 1966 Committee to Study the Watts Hospital Proposal. The committee's report, issued in March of that year, had recommended expanding Watts on the assumption that it would admit patients from Lincoln Hospital. Also, in connection with a suggestion that Watts might have its function "modified" in the future, the report had recommended that a single board of trustees should be created to govern both hospitals. The report had irritated Durham's chief black powerbroker, John Wheeler, who, despite years of collaboration with Semans and others on the matter, had dismissed the report as a fulfillment of long-held assumptions that Lincoln Hospital should be shut down and Watts Hospital expanded. Estes had responded by addressing many of Wheeler's concerns, giving particular stress to issues of equality in training opportunities, admissions, and employment at any new hospital. That November, however, Wheeler had successfully mobilized the Durham Committee on Negro Affairs to help defeat a bond referendum based in part upon the committee's report the previous spring.[57]

Duke's Department of Community Health Sciences had been created only months before the referendum was defeated, and over the next two years, the department's chairman, Harvey Estes, worked with the movement for a new public hospital in Durham. In the spring of 1968, for example, through the staff of the North Carolina Regional Medical Program, Estes helped facilitate the work of Lincoln Hospital's two strongest supporters, John Wheeler and Dr. Charles DeWitt Watts, in preparing a grant proposal to the federal Office of Economic Opportunity for the creation of a neighborhood health center at Lincoln. Though the office turned down the request, the goodwill and publicity generated by these efforts contributed to passage of the hospital bond referendum in November of that year. The following April, Estes was appointed to the projected hospital's Medical and Dental Advisory Committee, the purpose of which was to provide advice on the architecture and education programs of the new public facility. And in 1970, after Lincoln was successful in obtaining an Office of Economic Opportunity grant to establish the Lincoln Community Health Center, Estes recommended Dr. Eva Salber, a native of Cape Town, South Africa, for the position of administrator at the new Lincoln center. Salber, who was then at the Martha Eliot Community Health Center in Boston, became a part-time administrator at the center and a professor in the new Family Medicine Program of Duke's Department of Community Health Sciences.[58]

Major Figures in DUMC's Local Network

Estes also worked closely in Durham with the chairman of the regional Health Planning Council, John A. McMahon. McMahon embodied in a number of respects the continued impact on Duke Medicine of several of its earliest influences, particularly the American Hospital Association, the Blue Cross and Blue Shield program, and regional planning. After graduating from Duke in 1942, McMahon earned his law degree at Harvard. Returning to North Carolina in 1948, he had succeeded Terry Sanford on the staff of the Institute of Government in Chapel Hill. He had left the institute in 1959, however, and for the next five years, during a period that roughly bracketed Sanford's term as governor, McMahon served as legal counsel and lobbyist for the North Carolina Association of County Commissioners. It was during this time that McMahon joined the hospital movement in Durham; in 1964 he became chairman of the Health Planning Council, and, in 1965, he accepted a position as "vice president for special development" with the Hospital Savings Association, the Blue Cross and Blue Shield affiliate in Chapel Hill. It was this association, of course, founded with help from both The Duke Endowment and the state medical society, that had been competing since the mid-1930s with the Hospital Care Association, the slightly older Durham-based Blues affiliate started by Dr. Wilburt Davison and George Watts Hill in 1933. McMahon's "special development" was to merge the two local Blues and to become the merged company's first president in 1968.[59]

Though McMahon had left Durham and moved to Chicago, he had become a trustee of Duke University in 1970 and chairman of its board of trustees in 1971, a position he would hold until 1983. McMahon was also a member of numerous Blue Cross and Blue Shield and other health-related committees, both state and national, private and public. He was a director of the Research Triangle Foundation in North Carolina's Research Triangle Park and a member of both the Veterans Administration Special Medical Advisory Group and the Institute of Medicine of the National Academy of Sciences.[60]

McMahon also became president of the Duke Alumni Association in 1968, and as such, was a member of the search committee to find a successor to Douglas Knight as president of Duke University. Though McMahon had clashed with Mary Semans at a critical point in the Durham hospital negotiations, both were now of one mind as to who the university's next president should be. Mary Semans had met Terry Sanford in 1960, during his campaign for governor, and as governor he had appointed her husband, Dr. James Semans, as the first chairman of the board of trustees of the North Carolina School of the Arts. Duke's trustees elected Sanford as the university's sixth president in December of 1969, and, according to one source, Mary Semans had "high hopes" for him. Indeed, her hopes sounded much like those of Willis Smith 20 years earlier. While walking with Sanford "across the campus one evening she told him that her ambition for his administration was to reconnect Duke with its heritage and base in the Carolinas, where the Dukes had made their money. She told him that while she loved the school she could not abide its estrangement from the state: 'It simply is snobbish. It's not acceptable and it has not opened up its doors to the state and the people around it who are just terribly important.'"[61]

Duke Medicine benefited from Sanford's personal and political networks in a variety of ways. One important link—a link that had little precedent at Duke—was Sanford's connection to John W. Gardner and the Carnegie Corporation of New York. After leaving the governor's office in 1965, Sanford led a study, based at Duke and funded by Carnegie and the Ford Foundation, on the role of America's states in the nation's future. Later that same year, Gardner had resigned as Carnegie's president in order to become secretary of the Department of Health, Education and Welfare under President Lyndon Johnson. Gardner, as secretary (1965–68), had transferred to the Office of Civil Rights the power to enforce Title VI of the 1964 Civil Rights Act, which prohibited racial discrimination in all federally assisted programs, including NIH and other health programs. Though Gardner did not return to Carnegie after leaving his position at HEW, the foundation joined the Commonwealth Fund and the Rockefeller Foundation in making a large grant to Duke's Department of Community Health Sciences in 1970 for "support of an imaginative project for the better delivery of health care." According to the Rockefeller press release, the project would focus on the physician assistant program but would also use "the physician's assistant in a new way: as the liaison between a community worker and a doctor in deprived rural or urban neighborhoods. . . . It is hoped that this will bring the services of the whole medical system to people who have been out of touch with it for generations."[62]

Duke Medicine also benefited from its collaboration with Sanford's long-time legal adviser and fellow political activist, Joel Fleishman. Although Fleishman had returned to Yale after Sanford's term as governor, the new Duke president lured him back to North Carolina in 1971 to establish the Institute of Policy Studies and Public Affairs at Duke. Among the first projects for which the new institute received funding was one developed by Fleishman and Estes in 1972. The "multidisciplinary" Center for the Study of Health Policy, as it was called, was funded by a grant from the Commonwealth Fund and was designed to conduct political, economic, and legal analysis of health services delivery and financing. Among the strengths of the new center, according to its founders, were its ties to the law and medical schools at Duke, which gave it "a most advantageous position to apply its research, experimentation, and training activities to the design of a better health service delivery system for the Southern region." Yet the center's vision was to be as much national as it was regional. "The health care system in this country is inequitable, mismanaged, and inadequate. By conducting in-depth research in the areas of health services delivery and financing, and by offering substantive policy instruction at the undergraduate, graduate, and professional levels, the Duke Center for the Study of Health Policy can be expected to make major contributions to the reform of our national health care system."[63]

A Better Health Plan

The three-year grant for Duke's new center coincided with construction and completion of the Durham County General Hospital. When dedicated in October of 1976, the $20 million, seven-story facility included 326 private beds, 134 semiprivate beds, 12 operating rooms, and intensive care units for medicine, surgery, and cardiology. Among those singing the hospital's praises at the dedication was J. Alex McMahon.

Between 1972 and 1986 McMahon was president of the American Hospital Association, an organization with long, strong ties to Duke Medicine. In the

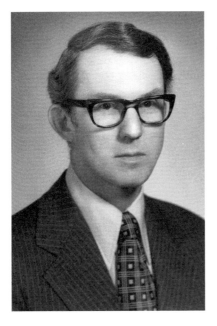

summer of 1977, just months after Durham's new public hospital was dedicated, he announced that the association had adopted "a universal health insurance plan" at its annual meeting in Atlanta. According to the *New York Times*, McMahon pointed out that due to "the financing aspect of the new plan, it was being called 'universal health insurance' instead of 'national health insurance' because the latter term was generally viewed as a government program totally financed by taxes." The goal of the association's plan was to provide "equal financing and accessibility to services for all segments of society" through "the establishment of multiple financing systems, independent regulatory agencies, copayment plans, and community delivery systems."[64]

By 1977 Harvey Estes was working on some of the same issues as chairman of a distinguished national committee appointed by the National Academy of Sciences' Institute of Medicine to study "manpower policies for primary health care." Originally appointed in September of 1975, the committee submitted its final report, "A Manpower Policy for Primary Healthcare," in May of 1978. And in November of that year, Estes, in a "Dean's Hour" lecture at the recently completed Searle Center, discussed the report with his colleagues at Duke. No one in the room, however, including Estes himself, could have foreseen the extent to which the committee's findings anticipated and shaped the central role of primary care providers in reforming America's health care system under health maintenance organizations, the formation of which were promoted in legislation signed by President Nixon in 1973.[65] [Figure 7.11]

What the committee from the Institute of Medicine approved, and recommended continuing, Estes said, was the "wide variety" of practitioners, practice arrangements, and payment systems then available. The committee also recommended several measures to facilitate "a shift in the numbers of physicians that are going into primary care as opposed to specialty and subspecialty medicine." These measures included establishing good training and residency programs at medical schools, as well as the creation of at least one clinic associated with each medical school that delivered exemplary primary care. "Now, I don't think these are outlandish or terribly far out recommendations," Estes commented, "and I don't think they've aroused very much controversy, but there has been some isolated controversy about them."

Creating much more controversy were the recommendations made by the Institute committee regarding "the reimbursement mechanism for primary care physicians." The committee recommended paying general practitioners and specialists the same thing for a given task. While there would always be "complicated problems" only a specialist could, and should, handle, Estes noted, in those cases the committee recommended a system governed by the "'gatekeeper' concept." In the gatekeeper system the specialist would be paid "a much higher fee for his special services, but in order to get that much higher fee, it would be necessary that those services be called for by the primary care physician." And when the gatekeeper made that call, Estes explained, the committee recommended "that the third party payer pay that entire fee, but it would require two things: I refer the patient to the specialist, and second, that that specialist have credentials that indeed qualify him to give those extra services."

Estes ended his presentation by briefly mentioning the one insurance plan in the country using a "very explicit" gatekeeper concept. The plan, based in Seattle, was proving "quite effective in being accepted by the patients in the area," he noted. "It's been quite successful in gaining physician acceptance in [that] about eighty percent of the primary care physicians in the area accept it and participate in it, and it's been quite effective in saving money for the subscribers because it saves quite a bit in hospitalization by making the primary care physician not only actually responsible, but he bears a little bit of the financial risk. If he is an over utilizer of specialty services, he bears some financial penalty for that."

The Debate over GPs versus Physician-Scientists

Estes' young department was already frowned upon by the old giants at DUMC, the Departments of Medicine and Surgery, and the Institute of Medicine recommendations only made things worse. There "were department chairs here who actively expressed their vehement opposition to the idea of training generalists," Estes later recalled. "Dr. Sabiston, head of Surgery, has said this in my presence, that he could not stomach the training of generalist physicians. That Duke was at the cutting edge, and that to go back and train generalists, was to go back to 1920s medicine. He felt this very strongly. But others shared that opinion."[66]

The chairman of the Department of Medicine, Jim Wyngaarden, was not entirely opposed to the training of general practitioners at Duke. What concerned him were the implications of the matter for teaching, research, and patient care. "The primary issue when the Department of Community Medicine was established was its role within Duke Hospital," Wyngaarden later explained. "The issue was giving or not giving beds in Duke Hospital (from the Department of Medicine quota) to the new department, and allowing its residents to rotate on the Medical service alongside or in competition with those of medicine. I was strongly opposed to establishing a second system of inpatient care and training in Medicine in Duke Hospital not under the control of the Department of Medicine. We successfully prevented that from occurring. . . . They eventually made arrangements for inpatient training at the Durham Regional, a much more appropriate setting than at Duke which is a predominantly secondary-tertiary care hospital."[67]

Wyngaarden was also deeply concerned with the declining interest in biomedical research and the decreasing number of M.D.'s applying for scientific training—trends completely at odds with the goals he had advocated for Duke Medicine since the late 1950s. Wyngaarden had noticed these trends while serving on a 10-member NIH committee appointed to evaluate the need for additional medical scientists in every field, especially in relation to the goals of President Richard Nixon's "war on cancer." It was while serving on this committee, in fact, that Wyngaarden, in a 1979 speech as president of the Association of American Physicians, described the disturbing trend of "The Clinical Investigator as an Endangered Species." His speech, subsequently published in the *New England Journal of Medicine*, proved prescient of the modern-day shortage of physician-scientists. "It is far and away the most quoted paper I ever wrote," Wyngaarden later noted with a laugh. "And I'm still referred to as the person who spotted that [trend] twenty years before it became a crisis. And people still ask me where that insight came from. Well, it wasn't such a remarkable insight. . . . It came out of that work on that committee."[68]

The debate at DUMC over general practitioners and physician-scientists reflected a combination of external social forces and the choices made by the medical center's leaders between 1955 and 1965 to couple Duke Medicine's original mission of primary care to a future that emphasized specialization and biomedical research, specifically, publicly funded research through the National Institutes of Health. By the time Dr. Wilburt Davison had retired from Duke in 1960, Wyngaarden had been directing the new Research Training Program there—in a new wing of the Bell Building. And from that point on, but especially after the introduction of the new curriculum and the M.D.-Ph.D. program in the mid-1960s, Duke Medicine focused on producing physician-scientists for its own faculty, for NIH, and for other academic medical centers while also maintaining the mission originally designed for it by The Duke Endowment and Davison, namely, to produce well-trained general practitioners for North Carolina and South Carolina.[69]

By 1980, however, Duke Medicine's reputation rested more on training specialists and physician-scientists for national and international service than it did on producing general practitioners for primary care and family medicine in the Carolinas and the American South. To many physicians and students alike, Duke was best known as the source of essential textbooks for the teaching and practice of medicine, including both new texts and the original and updated versions of "classics" in a variety of different fields. Also contributing to the lofty reputation of Duke Medicine were the awards, national appointments, and outstanding achievements of its faculty; its production of leaders for other institutions; and the contributions of its faculty as teachers and biomedical researchers.

Dr. Eugene Stead trained more than 30 physicians who became department chairmen at other institutions, and 2 who became chairmen at Duke, Harvey Estes and Stead's own successor, Jim Wyngaarden. Wyngaarden himself then continued this tradition with an impressive list of his own; some 25 of his trainees became department chairs, deans, chancellors, or vice presidents; one even became a university president. In the Department of Surgery, moreover, Dr. David Sabiston trained 134 chief residents during his 32-year chairmanship, and of those, 10 became departmental chairs and 31 held divisional chief positions in university departments.[70] Other faculty who were recognized for their professionalism and compassion as teachers included Drs. Donald B. Hackel and Edward S. Orgain. Hackel, a pathologist, joined the Duke faculty in 1960, and over the course of his long career in Duke Medicine, this much beloved laboratory instructor received three Golden Apple teaching awards, a lifetime Golden Apple for excellence in teaching medical students, and a distinguished teacher award from the Duke Alumni Association. Orgain, a cardiologist, came to Duke in 1934 and was made a professor of medicine in 1952; in addition to pioneering a drug therapy for hypertension, he was said "to treat all his young people as colleagues of equal status regardless of how green behind their ears they were. His gentlemanly but firm approach towards young people earned him the nickname of 'Easy Ed.'"[71]

Biomedical Research at Duke

By 1980, Duke Medicine enjoyed an excellent reputation for significant contributions to biomedical research. The foundations for this excellence lay in the combination of private and public support for the research of Dr. Joseph Beard in virology and immunology and of Dr. Walter Kempner in the treatment of hypertension. This interaction had begun in the late 1930s, expanded during World War II, and become institutionalized in the decades that followed, giving Duke Medicine its modern foundation in the government-sponsored research of the NIH. Although Kempner and his colleagues continued their research beyond his retirement in 1972, by the late 1950s, advances both in drug therapies (such as those on which Orgain worked) and in surgical procedures (like the sympathectomies performed by Dr. Keith S. Grimson at Duke) had made the treatment of hypertension much more immediate and convenient for patients than the rigorous regimen required of them—and Kempner—by the rice diet.[72]

Yet Kempner's practice continued to grow, expanding to include patients with diabetes and nephritis and, eventually, patients with marked obesity and the attendant medical and psychological problems that often accompany it. "More than any other single individual Dr. Kempner has made Duke Hospital an international Medical Center," Jim Wyngaarden wrote to Terry Sanford in 1972. "His achievements are based upon his professional competence, his charismatic and authoritative personality, and a team approach to patient care. Dr. Kempner included 'physician assistants' in his team well before the program at Duke was established." Wyngaarden also noted that Kempner's legacy included numerous "Rice Houses" in Durham, facilities at Duke, and all of his professional fees, "which have been handled through the Medical PDC office. His total income has been subject to the usual percentage deductions for clinic overhead, and the Medical Center Building Fund, and also to the usual 'research tax' which supports the Department of Medicine. In addition to these very substantial direct financial benefits to the University, his patients have contributed importantly to the growth of the Medical Center as a whole through the use of our facilities, and to the economy of Durham." Indeed, such contributions continue today through a variety of diet and wellness programs descended from Kempner's original work.[73]

Joseph Beard had a deeper, longer-lasting impact than Kempner on the nature and course of research at Duke. Much of this influence stemmed from Beard's continuing work on virology and immunology, especially the relationship between viruses, cancer, and the immune system. Between 1958 and 1959, Beard and his associates not only identified two cancer viruses that cause leukemia in chickens; they also provided tangible evidence of the link between viruses and human leukemia. One can trace the persistence of this immunological research through several departments at Duke, through the HIV/AIDS research pursued by Beard's student Dr. Dani P. Bolognesi and, later, by Dr. Barton F. Haynes, as well as in the research of several of Duke Medicine's top scientists, including D. Bernard Amos, Ralph Snyderman, and Robert J. Lefkowitz.[74] As Wyngaarden recently explained, "immunology relates to every disease category. I'm not saying every disease is immunological, but every one of these subspecialty groups has medical conditions—patients with medical conditions—in which the immune system is disturbed."[75]

Duke's research in immunology took on added significance in the years after Dr. Bernard Amos arrived as professor of immunology in 1962. Shortly thereafter, Beard broke both of his legs in an automobile accident and Amos became chief of DUMC's new division of immunology. Amos was also made professor of experimental surgery, the position originally created for Beard, who now became professor of virology at Duke. In 1964, moreover, Amos's division of immunology was combined with the Department of Microbiology to form the new Department of Microbiology and Immunology. Beard, after retiring from Duke in 1972, eventually moved to St. Petersburg, Florida, where, as the head of the commercial Life Sciences Research Laboratories, he supplied research laboratories with purified reverse transcriptase as part of a National Institutes of Health–National Cancer Institute program. As one admiring student later wrote, Beard "was a pioneer in molecular biology. He shipped virus all over the world that produced an enzyme, reverse transcriptase, which acted on bacteria. This virus in simple terms recombined DNA or caused gene splicing. His work in this field resulted in laboratories being established all over the world of a biogenetic nature."[76]

In the meantime, Bernard Amos continued to build on the fundamental contributions he had made to the conceptual understanding of the antigen system before joining the faculty at Duke. Amos was, according to one source, "the first to use serologic tests for histocompatibility to select sibling donors for optimal kidney transplantation, which dramatically enhanced graft survival. These serologic tests guided the first kidney transplant performed at Duke University in 1965. Through these discoveries and their application, Dr. Amos fathered and contributed enormously to the critically important area of organ transplantation, which he guided from fledgling to pivotal status." As a result of this research, Amos established one of the world's leading clinical and research transplantation centers at Duke University, and in 1980 he was elected president of the American Association of Immunologists—the organization which in 1939 had rejected the membership applications of Beard and his collaborator at the Rockefeller and Lederle Laboratories, Dr. Ralph W. G. Wyckoff.[77]

Some of Duke's earliest and most sustained immunological research also grew out of the interests of the faculty in allergies and asthma. One of Duke Medicine's 10 original professors, Dr. Oscar C. Hansen-Pruss, started the Allergy Clinic in 1930, but it was faculty in Davison's former department, the Department of Pediatrics, who focused on the subject. Dr. Susan C. Dees, professor of pediatrics from 1939 to 1978, led the way. As one of the first women appointed to the medical school faculty at Duke, Dees established the pediatric allergy training program in the early 1940s and served as chief of the division of allergy-immunology in the Department of Pediatrics between

7.12 Major figures in the history of Duke Medicine. *Duke University Medical Center Archives, unless otherwise indicated.*

D. Bernard Amos
Jay M. Arena
Dani P. Bolognesi

Ivan W. Brown Jr.
Rebecca H. Buckley
Duke University Medical Center
F. Bayard Carter

Norman F. Conant
Susan C. Dees
Sara Dent

Wiley D. Forbus
Irwin Fridovich
Clarence E. Gardner Jr.

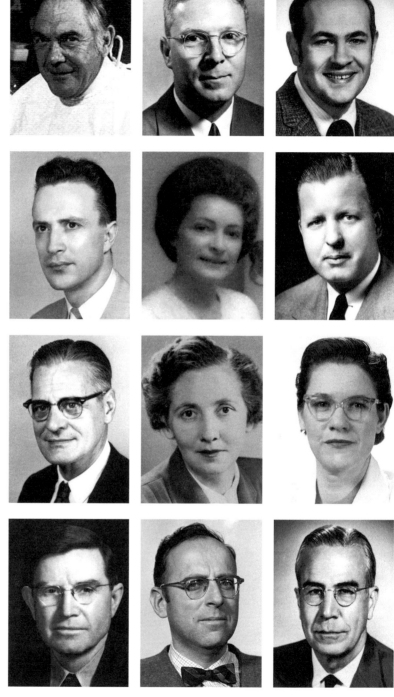

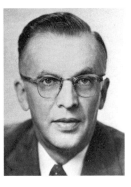
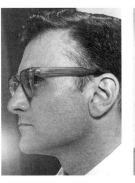
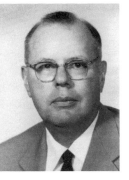

Keith S. Grimson
Donald B. Hackel
Edwin C. Hamblen

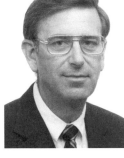
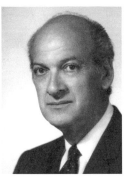
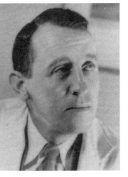

Charles B. Hammond
Philip Handler
Oscar C. Hansen-Pruss

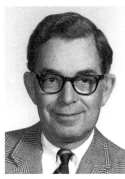
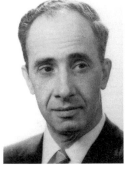
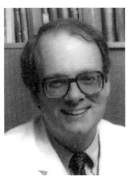

Merel H. Harmel
Jerome S. Harris
Barton F. Haynes

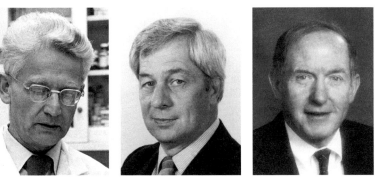

Albert Heyman
Robert L. Hill
Edward W. Holmes Jr.

Wolfgang K. Joklik
Samuel L. Katz
Walter Kempner

Robert J. Lefkowitz
Robert Machemer
Joseph E. Markee

Joe M. McCord
Blaine S. Nashold Jr.
Edward S. Orgain

Roy T. Parker
J. David Robertson
Allen D. Roses

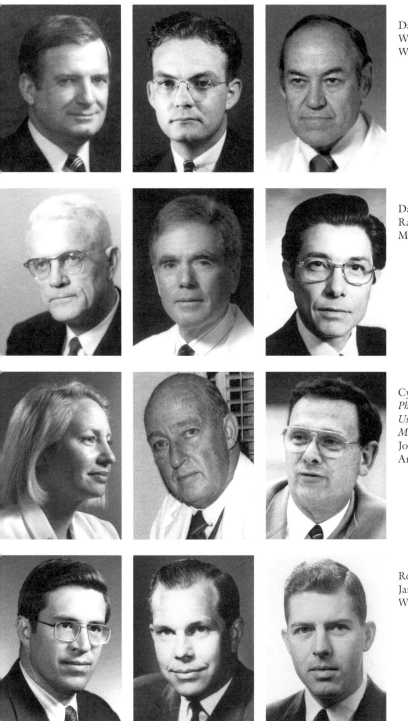

David C. Sabiston Jr.
Will Camp Sealy
William W. Shingleton

David T. Smith
Ralph Snyderman
Madison S. Spach

Cynthia A. (Cindy) Toth
*Photograph by Butch
Usery, Duke University
Medical Center*
Joseph A. C. Wadsworth II
Andrew G. Wallace

Robert H. Wilkins
James B. Wyngaarden
W. Glenn Young Jr.

1948 and 1974. She was also one of the first clinicians to recognize the immunological deficiencies associated with Wiskott-Aldrich syndrome and the fact that gastroesophageal reflux could trigger asthma.

Susan Dees also helped train more than 60 fellows in pediatric allergy-immunology during her tenure at Duke, including Dr. Rebecca H. Buckley, a Duke graduate who received her medical degree from the University of North Carolina. By 1980, Buckley was professor of pediatrics and immunology at Duke, chief of the pediatric division of allergy, immunology, and pulmonary diseases, and director of Duke's Asthma and Allergic Diseases Center. She was also embarking on the pioneering research that would enable her to develop a treatment for severe combined immune deficiency (or SCID). This once-fatal disease (known as the "bubble boy disease" during the 1970s and 1980s) was converted to a treatable condition by Buckley and her colleagues through the use of bone marrow and thymic transplantation.[78]

Duke's focus on immunological research was further reinforced in 1968 with the arrival of Dr. Samuel L. Katz as chairman of the Department of Pediatrics and Dr. Wolfgang K. Joklik as chairman of the Department of Microbiology and Immunology. Katz, a graduate of Harvard Medical School, arrived at Duke after more than a decade of research in virology and infectious diseases at the Boston Children's Hospital, where he had developed, with Nobel laureate Dr. John Enders, the attenuated measles virus vaccine. The use of this vaccine throughout the world is estimated to have decreased the number of childhood deaths from measles from around 7 million a year in 1974, when the vaccine was first widely implemented, to around 800,000 today. While Katz continued to engage in research at Duke, he became increasingly involved in developing national and international organizations active in vaccine policy development and pediatric HIV/AIDS research and care. Retiring from Duke in 1990, after 22 years as chairman of Pediatrics, Katz was succeeded by an internationally recognized physician-scientist, Dr. Michael M. Frank, who, as a specialist in allergy and infectious diseases, had served as clinical director of the National Institute of Allergy and Infectious Diseases at the National Institutes of Health.[79]

The Department of Microbiology and Immunology was only four years old when Wolfgang Joklik became its chairman in 1968. The department was the result of a merger, as noted above, between Amos's relatively new division of immunology and one of DUMC's original departments, the Department of Microbiology. The original chairman of Microbiology, Dr. David T. Smith, had served in that position from 1930 to 1958, and had been succeeded by one of the world's leading mycologists, Dr. Norman Conant, who had joined the department at Duke in 1935. By the time of Joklik's appointment, Smith and Conant had edited and updated several editions (including, along with Joseph

Beard, the 1952 edition) of Hans Zinsser's classic *Textbook of Bacteriology*, and Joklik would continue to lead this tradition for the next three decades, working with Smith, Amos, and others at Duke on the textbook *Zinsser Microbiology*. According to Dr. William Anlyan, dean of Duke's medical school, "Joklik was in the mold in which I recruited people: he was first and foremost a university and medical center citizen, and secondly charged with building the department he headed with the resources that were available. He was also the key chairman to develop the basic science component of our comprehensive cancer center."[80]

Joklik described in 1980, in "The Scope of Modern Microbiology and Immunology," the exciting crossroads his department had reached. Where microbiology had once been primarily an applied field, concerned with "controlling those microbes that affect man's health and wealth," it was now "at the forefront of the study of the control of the expression of genetic information, the molecular mechanisms of active transport, differentiation, and cancer—to name only a few." As for microbiology's connection with immunology, this stemmed, Joklik explained, "from a time when microorganisms were the only readily available and medically important antigens, and when immunology provided the only defense against diseases. This too has now changed," he argued, "and immunology has evolved into a distinct discipline which far transcends its traditional role; today it is an equal and essential partner with many other disciplines. Thus, at the molecular level, an understanding of the mechanisms of synthesis of antibody is providing clues in the quest to understand differentiation, while an understanding of antigen-antibody interactions is clarifying the nature of complementarity; at the biological level, an understanding of cellular immunity offers one of the brightest hopes in the fight against cancer; and at the clinical level, an understanding of the factors involved in transplantation immunity will surely usher in a new era in medicine."[81]

Immunology was not the sole focus of research at DUMC, of course. One of the most accomplished physicians at Duke, pediatrician Dr. Jay M. Arena, retired in 1979 after a career that included membership in the first graduating class of Duke Medical School, important studies in toxicology, the creation of a poison control center at Duke, and the development of the child-proof safety cap.[82] Dr. Jerome Harris, chairman of the Pediatrics Department from 1954 to 1968, was a biochemist who strongly supported the Research Training Program at Duke and also collaborated in the pediatric cardiology research of Dr. Madison S. Spach. Spach, a native of Winston-Salem, North Carolina, took his undergraduate and medical degrees at Duke. He then continued at DUMC as a resident in pediatrics and a pediatric cardiology fellow before becoming the first chief of the division of pediatric cardiology at Duke in 1960. Spach subsequently trained more than 30 pediatric cardiology fellows at Duke, many of whom assumed leadership roles there and at other leading medical centers, and he also made a number of important contributions to the field of pediatric cardiology, particularly in the area of electrophysiology (or electrical conduction) in the heart. "Overall," one source notes, "the body of work from Dr. Spach's laboratory has provided key insights into the nature of electrical conduction in the heart, the mechanisms of cardiac arrhythmias, action of clinically used antiarrhythmic drugs and the susceptibility of the diseased heart to potentially lethal cardiac rhythm disturbances."[83]

Research on the fundamental architecture of cell membranes, as well as on the transmission of electrical impulses within and between cells, was the specialty of Dr. J. David Robertson. Robertson, a Harvard M.D. with a Ph.D. in biochemistry from the Massachusetts Institute of Technology, arrived at Duke in 1966 to succeed Dr. Joseph Markee as chairman of the Department of Anatomy. Where Markee had pioneered in the production and use of films for teaching general anatomy, Robertson, 42, was an electron microscopist whose elegant electron micrographs were helping elucidate the patterns and structures of cell membranes. Building on his earlier success in applying electron microscopy to the study of nerve tissues, Robertson had recently discovered the structural basis of electrical transmissions across the synaptic "gap junction" of adjacent cell membrane channels. Robertson now added the teaching of electron microscopy at Duke to his already pivotal role in research, "skillfully bridging the gap between purely technical people who were interested in developing new instrumentation and new preparative protocols, while also supporting a variety of medical people who wanted simply to apply the electron microscope to problems in cell biology and pathophysiology."[84]

Contributing further to Duke's reputation for biomedical research and the training of physician-scientists were several developments within its Department of Biochemistry. The most important was the election of Philip Handler, Ph.D., as president of the National Academy of Science. Handler left Duke for Washington in 1969, and was succeeded by Robert L. Hill, Ph.D., a specialist in protein research whom Handler had recruited to Duke almost a decade earlier. It was also in 1969 that one of Handler's former Ph.D. students, Irwin Fridovich, and one of Fridovich's own Ph.D. students, Joe M. McCord, announced their discovery at Duke of an enzyme, superoxide dismutase, that catalyzed the elimination of superoxide, a free radical form of oxygen in the body. This important discovery gave rise to the "free radical" hypothesis of aging and chronic diseases and stimulated a wide and persistent stream of research (more than 22,000 articles since 1969) on the role of superoxide in a number of diseases, including heart attack, stroke, arthritis, and neurological diseases such as amyotrophic lateral sclerosis.[85]

The introduction of the new medical school curriculum also made research an integral part of the Department of Obstetrics and Gynecology and of two new departments, Ophthalmology and Anesthesiology. During the 34 years of Ob-Gyn's first chairman, Dr. Bayard F. Carter, the department's leading researcher was Dr. Edwin C. Hamblen, a world-renowned endocrinologist. A more specific research mission was defined by Dr. Roy T. Parker, a North Carolina native, who succeeded Carter in 1964 during the final planning stages of the new curriculum. As Parker wrote in 1980, "The pedagogy inspired by the new Duke Medical Curriculum, of which the new chairman had been a part, . . . caused the Department to reexamine its objectives. . . . Reproductive biology was established as the basic science orientation of the Department."[86]

The professional development of Dr. Charles B. Hammond, the most accomplished clinical investigator in the Department of Obstetrics and Gynecology, reflects one of the major career trajectories envisioned for physician-scientists trained in Duke Medicine. After completing his M.D. at Duke, Hammond did an internship in surgery there, as well as a residency in obstetrics and gynecology, before completing a year in Duke's Research Training Program. Hammond then did a two-year stint in endocrinology at the National Cancer Institute before joining the faculty at Duke where, from 1968 on, he played a leading role in directing clinical trials involving the use of chemotherapy to treat gestational trophoblastic disease, a devastating malignancy associated with pregnancy. By the time Hammond succeeded Parker as the department's chairman in 1980, the Southeastern Regional Trophoblastic Center at Duke was experiencing remarkable success in converting this malignancy to a highly curable disease. And Hammond and his colleagues would continue to improve the center's treatment during his 22 years as chairman, even as they continue to do so today.

When it came to the new Department of Ophthalmology, however, ramping up for research took longer than Dean William Anlyan envisioned. Research was not a strength of the department's founding chairman, Dr. Joseph A. C. Wadsworth II, whose 1965 appointment was as much political as it was professional. Wadsworth "had all the credentials to be a leader in clinical ophthalmology," Anlyan later explained, "although there was no research component in his career. It was my judgment that this new, small department needed as its highest priority to develop its clinical base and to look at a subsequent generation for leadership in research." Unfortunately, Wadsworth, having fulfilled his main mission—raising money for a new eye center—fought against his retirement and the appointment of Dr. Robert Machemer as his successor in 1978. Unlike Wadsworth, Machemer specialized in research; he is often referred to as the "father" of vitreoretinal surgery in honor of a revolutionary specialty he developed while at the Bascom Palmer Eye Institute in

Miami, Florida. As chairman of Duke's Department of Ophthalmology until 1991, Machemer would pioneer in macular translocation surgery at Duke—a specialty that his colleague, Dr. Cynthia A. (Cindy) Toth, has continued to develop. Machemer's successor, Dr. David L. Epstein, has broadened this new generation of leadership in eye research; a specialist in glaucoma and glaucoma laser surgery, Epstein has been chairman of Ophthalmology since 1992.[87]

The chief of the division of anesthesia, Dr. C. Ronald Stephen, resigned in 1965 after being refused his request to separate the division from the Department of Surgery and make it an independent department. The request was one that neither Anlyan, the surgeon-dean, nor Sabiston, the new chair of Surgery, was ready to grant. According to one departmental history, "the ensuing five years were difficult ones. The residency program atrophied, research declined, and the faculty gradually diminished in the face of increasing clinical responsibilities." During this time, Dr. Sara Dent, a specialist in cardiac anesthesia, "held the department together under the most trying of circumstances. It was not until 1970 when anesthesiology was made an independent department that the situation changed."[88]

In 1971, Dr. Merel H. Harmel, professor and chairman of anesthesia first at the SUNY New York Downstate Medical Center in Brooklyn and then at the Pritzker School of Medicine at the University of Chicago, joined the Duke faculty as the founding chairman of its Department of Anesthesiology. The department flourished under Harmel's leadership; between 1971 and 1980, the number of faculty increased from a total of only 6 members to 27 clinical anesthesiologists alone. There were also 13 scientists engaged in full-time research by then, both as M.D.'s and Ph.D.'s, and Harmel had reinvigorated the department's teaching and research programs at the VA Hospital. By 1980 the Department of Anesthesiology had expanded to eight divisions "principally oriented to the specialties: obstetrics, ophthalmology, cardiovascular-thoracic surgery, neurosurgery, pain, pediatrics, hyperbaric medicine and more recently critical care. In addition," Harmel noted, "there is a bio-engineering division devoted to instrumentation, measurement and the computer interface with anesthesiology."[89]

Expanded Research and Specialization in Surgery

Underlying much of Anesthesiology's rapid expansion was the explosion of research and specialization in Duke's Department of Surgery. Harmel shared with surgery's chairman, Dr. David Sabiston, the continuing impact on Duke of physicians trained at Johns Hopkins University. Sabiston had been a second-year medical student at Hopkins when his future mentor, Dr. Alfred Blalock, had performed the first "blue baby" operation; Harmel, as one of the first physicians to specialize in anesthesiology at Hopkins, had worked with Blalock during the procedure. Harmel later recalled this "extraordinary experience of being the first to anesthetize a blue baby, a child afflicted by a fatal heart malformation. The operation—making a bypass for the blood to get to the lung—had never been done. This was a very dramatic procedure, a world event. It was 1944 and people came from all over the world to see Dr. Blalock operate. That colored my career, you could say."[90]

Dr. David Sabiston blended the coloring of his own Hopkins career with the verdant opportunities at Duke for unprecedented public and private support in the training of physician-scientists and specialists. By the time Harmel arrived at Duke, Sabiston was requiring his surgical residents to spend at least two years in full-time basic research, either with a faculty member, a research group, or in another laboratory elsewhere. Sabiston was also establishing a record by then for teaching, fundraising, and patient care that would eventually rank him among the world's top surgical educators of the 20th century. According to one of his former students, Sabiston, by 1969, "had obtained over 2.4 million dollars in National Institutes of Health support for the Scholar in Academic Surgery Program. . . . His NIH funded Academic Surgical Research Training Program then supported 18 research fellows either in cardiovascular, oncologic, or transplant surgery as Duke Teaching Scholars in Academic Surgery. Between 1982 and 1987 alone, this program yielded 170 peer reviewed papers in cardiovascular surgery."[91]

Sabiston eventually received all of the major teaching awards at Duke and DUMC—several times—and was honored throughout the world for his achievements. "He was the Principal Investigator for the NIH Surgical Teaching grant . . . that extended from 1966 until 1998, as well as the large coronary revascularization grant from the NIH that was funded at Duke for over 30 years. Upon his retirement his extramural funding for clinical and basic research still exceeded over $6 million with a total life funding record of over $15.3 million. Yearly departmental extramural research funding increased from $400,000 in 1964 when he arrived to nearly 20 million dollars in 1994 at the time of his retirement. During his later tenure the Duke Department of Surgery led the list of academic surgery departments nationally in NIH support, and this trend continues today [2003]."[92]

Sabiston's own personal research interests, in cardiac and thoracic surgery, fit strategically with those of several of his new colleagues at Duke. Will Camp Sealy, Ivan Brown, and W. Glenn Young Jr. were all doing pioneering research in cardiothoracic surgery by the time Sabiston arrived. Brown's invention of a heat and blood exchanger had enabled him to become one of the world's first open-heart surgeons in 1957, and during the decade that followed he, Sealy, and Young published pioneering work in extracorporeal circulation and the use of hypothermia in cardiac surgery. Young himself performed the first coronary artery bypass grafting at Duke University, and in 1963 he accomplished the first aortic valve replacement for acute bacterial endocarditis.[93] Sealy made his most significant contribution to Duke Medicine more than 30 years after his arrival at Duke on July 1, 1937. "I was the first Surgical Resident assigned to the new surgical laboratory [under Dr. Joseph Beard]," Sealy later wrote. "Having expected to do experiments on dogs that require great surgical skill, I was taken aback when I found that the new laboratory's work was to be in virology."[94] In 1968, Sealy, after extensive collaboration with cardiologists Andrew G. Wallace, Madison S. Spach, and John P. Boineau in the Department of Medicine, performed the first successful surgical cure of the Wolff-Parkinson-White Syndrome (WPW) and its associated tachycardia.[95]

The operation earned worldwide recognition for Sealy as "the father of arrhythmia surgery" worldwide, and it also stimulated a number of important developments at Duke. These included a high volume of referrals for WPW surgery, the creation of a large clinical research project, and the addition of a clinical electrophysiology laboratory for Duke's relatively new Coronary Care Unit. In addition, Andrew Wallace explained, "Duke's work with WPW and other cardiac arrhythmias catapulted our electrophysiology program to international prominence. As a result we attracted large numbers of extraordinary trainees from the U.S. and abroad. If you look at the world's leaders in clinical electrophysiology after, say, the early to mid 1980s, I think it is fair to say that no one institution produced more than Duke in the decade of the 1970s."[96]

This combination of specialization and collaboration was becoming increasingly common by 1980 both within and between the departments of Duke Medicine. In the division of neurosurgery, for example, the specialty of Dr. Blaine S. Nashold Jr., stereotactic surgery, was about to experience a rebirth. Use of this surgical method, which combined Cartesian measurement principles with a special frame for the head, had become dormant after the introduction in 1968 of L-dopa, a drug used to alleviate some of the symptoms of the principal movement disorder treated by stereotactic surgery: Parkinson's disease. With the advent of computer-based imaging, however, such as computerized tomographic (CT) scans and magnetic resonance imaging (MRI), the stereotactic method was soon used for "the management of intracranial tumors, the rapid development of new surgical hardware, and the rediscovery of old methods and evolution of new ones for the treatment of movement disorders."[97]

Plans were also in place by 1980 for the division of neurosurgery to share a floor in the new Duke North hospital building with neurology, a division of the Department of Medicine. According to the chief of neurosurgery, Dr.

Robert H. Wilkins, the move was expected to "facilitate the continuing cooperative development of the clinical neurosciences at Duke."[98] To the chief of Duke's neurology division, Dr. Allen D. Roses, the prospects for teaching and research appeared especially promising. "With the current explosion of knowledge in the neurosciences," Roses wrote in 1980, "the Division of Neurology is in an excellent position to participate in and take early advantage of clinically relevant research opportunities and developments. Since much of the growth of Neurology has occurred after the development of the 'new curriculum' in the late 1960s, the Division's exposure to medical student teaching has been limited."[99]

Neurology was, in fact, the one division of Duke Medicine in which research had always held sway over teaching. This emphasis had emerged under the division's first chief, Dr. Frederic Hanes, and had continued with his successors, especially Dr. Albert Heyman. Heyman had started his Duke career in 1954, at the VA Hospital in Durham, where, as associate professor and chief of neurology until 1961, he had engaged in national epidemiological studies involving stroke-related incidents in women and African Americans. In 1965, moreover, while chief of the division of neurology at Duke, Heyman had been named director of the Duke–Veterans Administration Hospital Stroke Center—a position he held for the next 15 years. Finally, in 1979, after the arrival of Roses as division chief, and as a portent of the explosion in knowledge in the neurosciences, Heyman helped establish at Duke the first Alzheimer's support group in North Carolina. To be sure, Alzheimer's soon become the major research focus of Roses, who would resign from Duke in 1998 to become head of the worldwide genetics research program of the British pharmaceutical giant Glaxo Wellcome.[100]

Wyngaarden's Legacy

D uke Medicine was thus a national leader in training physician-scientists by the time Jim Wyngaarden left Duke to become head of NIH in 1982. Among his own personal accomplishments in the Department of Medicine, Wyngaarden took special pride in the research tradition that he and his colleagues, Dr. William H. Kelley (later professor of medicine at Michigan and then dean of the medical school at the University of Pennsylvania) and Dr. Edward W. Holmes Jr. (later chancellor of the University of California at San Diego), had developed. The tradition had started with Wyngaarden's own research interests "in purine metabolism in gout but also in the fundamental biochemical mechanisms that led to the reduction of nucleotides, purine nucleotides like adenylic and guanilic acid. And the regulatory mechanisms. The three of us worked on the regulatory mechanisms,"

Wyngaarden recently recalled at Duke. "I started it, and Kelley took them over, and Holmes took them over. And so for fifteen, maybe twenty years, we were sometimes referred to as the purine capital of the world because of our work on the regulatory mechanisms. And a number of foreign fellows would come and spend a year or two here: from Australia, Israel, some of them. And both Bill and Ed made enormous contributions to that over the years."[101]

To the wider evolution of Duke Medicine, moreover, Wyngaarden also continued to contribute his knowledge and power in shaping the direction of academic medicine in the United States. In addition to his many and influential roles at NIH, Wyngaarden had served since the 1960s on the five-member advisory board of the Howard Hughes Medical Institute. The board had two major functions: to designate categories for biomedical investigation and to select what were then called Howard Hughes medical investigators. Prior to 1985, there were only three major categories of investigation: immunology, genetics, and metabolic regulation. Duke was strong in immunology, of course, as it was in Wyngaarden's own field of metabolic regulation. "We were fortunate in being in on that from the beginning," Wyngaarden recently said of the Hughes scholars at Duke. "And at one time or another Allen Roses was a Hughes scholar, Ralph Snyderman was, Nick Kredich was, Bob Lefkowitz was. Those are a few of them that come to mind."[102]

What Duke didn't get in on from the beginning, however, was genetics. Although Wyngaarden had tried for years to establish a genetics department at Duke, his efforts had failed by the time he left for NIH. "We didn't have the resources to do a lot of it," Wyngaarden explained, "and I was aware that after I left, while I was at the NIH, there was a lot of inquiry about genetics. And we didn't go that route. I think there were entrenched physicians, chairs, at that time, who felt that genetics would take a lot away from what they viewed as their department's purview. And it didn't happen. As a consequence, Duke made no important contribution to the genetics revolution. None."[103]

The Fate of Family Medicine

It was in this context, after Wyngaarden left for NIH, that the issue of training general practitioners flared up again. And this time the confrontation got nasty. By then the Department of Community and Family Medicine had built and occupied its own Family Medicine Center at Durham County General Hospital. It was "a brand-new building," Harvey Estes recalled, "better than anything we've ever had since. It was designed for exactly what we were going to do. We quickly became one of the most popular programs in the country, and we always got our choice of residents. . . . Our department attracted young women. One year we had thirteen new residents, and eleven were women. . . . [M]any of them viewed their role as a more nurturing family doctor rather than a hard-nosed specialist who was treating patients and sending them back to the generalist physician."[104]

"Now," Estes continued, "that leads to the next phase, and that's how family medicine came to be a sort of thorn in the side of Duke, and this led to an attempt to remove it, and a very serious attempt. That's an interesting story which begins with one patient. Our clinic at Durham General was a clinic that signed on with some of the new HMOs in the area. And we quickly began to recruit a group of very loyal patients who came there and saw their family doctor. Our doctors, including the faculty, were not allowed to use Duke Hospital. But they were on the staff of Durham General."

The attempt to remove the thorn of family medicine from Duke was one of the many painful episodes that would convulse Duke Medicine in the 1980s. The Bayh-Dole Act, the genomic revolution, changes in the economic structure of research, the rise of "big pharma," the business ethos of the Reagan administration, a Duke psychiatrist as Terry Sanford's successor and a physician-scientist as Anlyan's—it was enough to crack even the most excellent of foundations.

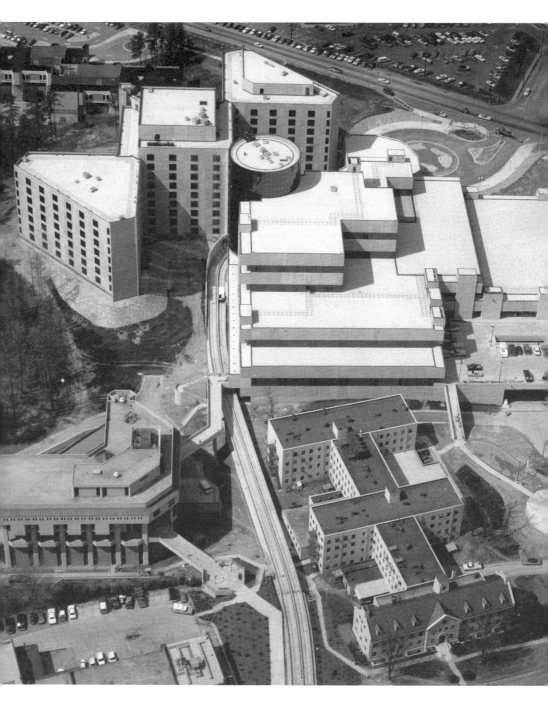

8.1 North Division of Duke Hospital with the Bell Building in the foreground, ca. 1980. *Duke University Medical Center Archives.*

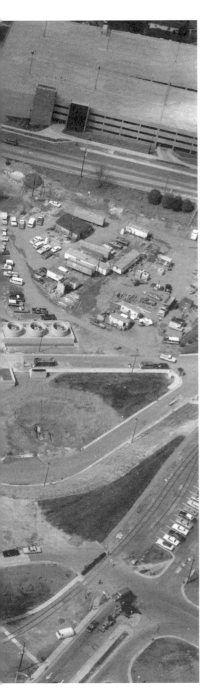

CHAPTER 8:

Duke Medicine and the Concept of Oneness, 1980–1989

By the fall of 1981 some of Duke's most faithful supporters were calling for Terry Sanford's head. The ambitious Duke president wanted the university's most famous alumnus, the disgraced Richard Nixon, to locate the Nixon presidential library on the Duke campus. Among the professoriate, many were outraged. Among the principal powerful trustees, however, opinions about Sanford (and the Nixon library) were more accommodating. Although they eventually conceded on the library issue, the Duke trustees announced that fall that Sanford, rather than retire in 1982 at the age of 65, had agreed to stay on for three more years. He also agreed to fill the post of university chancellor with his likely heir apparent, and in May of 1982 he asked the chairman of Duke's Department of Psychiatry, Dr. H. Keith H. Brodie, to become chancellor. Brodie accepted, and three years later, in 1985, he became the seventh president of Duke University.[1]

Challenges for the New President

For the next eight years Keith Brodie tried to maintain the progressive southern laboratory that Sanford, Mary Semans, and others had been experimenting with over the past quarter of a century. Yet Brodie found himself challenged at almost every turn by widespread political, moral, and economic changes that reshaped, resized, and rejected some of Duke's traditional webs and networks. These changes proved particularly disruptive at DUMC, where, in addition to a leadership crisis, Brodie faced increasing anxiety over the federal government's retreat from its generous funding of health care and medical research. At a time of increasing cost and inequity in the nation's medical system, the Reagan administration focused on cutting costs associated with Medicare and Medicaid programs. It introduced "diagnostic-related groups" that categorized and fixed prices for specific hospital treatments. It ended subsidies for the training of physicians. It cut funds for neighborhood health centers. And it pushed for deeper cuts in NIH funding. At the same time, many of Duke's brightest young scientists were demanding that the university make a deeper commitment not only to science in general but also, in particular, to the mutually reinforcing revolutions in genomics and business.

All of this was undoubtedly on Brodie's mind when he discussed the idea of institutional wholeness with Dr. Ralph Snyderman. The occasion was Snyderman's decision to become Duke's new chancellor for health affairs in 1989. "Keith Brodie, who is very articulate, had told me about the concept of oneness," Snyderman recalled in 1994, "one University, the Medical Center a part of one University. I had no objection to that, I never felt it should be other than that, and I still feel the same way. A lot of it, then, relates to what does that oneness mean? I always thought of the oneness as one family, and I'm not sure what Keith thought, but I think it was more like one individual. I think that there were some inherent differences in how Keith Brodie and I viewed the relationship between the Medical Center and the University."[2]

Keith Brodie's concept of oneness was based largely on the institutional and intellectual traditions he inherited at Duke. Both of his closest advisers, Terry Sanford and Mary Semans, promoted a closer integration of Duke Medicine with the rest of the university, and an expanded role for the university in the life of Durham, the Triangle area, and the state of North Carolina. The Department of Psychiatry that Brodie inherited in 1974 also had one of the most progressive, peculiar, and disappointing records in the history of Duke Medicine.

With passage of the Mental Retardation Facilities and Community Mental Health Centers Construction Act of 1963, Dr. Ewald Busse had bet Psychiatry's PDC funds on constructing a new facility with matching federal grants. The act authorized $329 million in grants over a five-year period for help in building mental retardation research centers and community mental health centers and also for training teachers to work with mentally retarded and other handicapped children. One month after the act was passed, however, President Kennedy was assassinated. "Without going into all of the details of it," Busse later remarked, "that whole effort just suddenly collapsed after his assassination. And so we'd already started building and then what happened, I [was] at a complete loss to understand, but it just didn't come out right for us. But we had built a building and fortunately we could use it for lots of things, but it remains something that—as far as I'm concerned—a place that didn't come out like I'd hoped."[3] Not until 1970 in fact was the first floor completed in the Civitan Building (the "Facility for Mental Retardation and Child Development"), and only in 1976, two years after Busse retired as chairman of the department, was the second floor completed. The Department of Psychiatry bore the entire cost of the second floor, at approximately $1 million, while the costs of the first floor were shared by the Department of Psychiatry ($337,000), the Department of Pediatrics ($47,800), the North Carolina Medical Care Commission ($150,000), and the Civitan Club ($100,000).[4]

Tangling Busse further in knots were the loose strings at Highland Hospital. The situation began to unravel in 1963 with the death of the hospital's director, Dr. Charman Carroll. In addition to the staff changes and administrative problems that followed, the situation was further complicated by disagreements at Duke as to what should be done with the facility.[5] "We did for a while send up residents," Busse later explained, "and that worked out reasonably well. But it was really a burden for us, with very little compensation."[6] By the time Keith Brodie succeeded Busse in 1974, the Highland load had grown even heavier. Highland Hospital had used all of its cash reserves to purchase the Asheville Christian Academy. "The purchase was in order to expand Homewood School, a program for adolescent therapy," Busse later wrote. "Teachers, not therapists were partially paid by the Department of Education of Asheville. When it opened in 1968 it had 24 students, but by 1972 it had 137 students. One of the serious problems was reimbursement because many of these patients were indigent behavioral problems (delinquents) referred by Asheville Public Schools. The financial loss was serious."[7]

Keith Brodie tried to improve the situation in Asheville but soon made the same recommendation Lyman had made 30 years earlier and for many of the same reasons: cut the cord to Highland. "We found it difficult to manage an entity that was four hours away by car," Brodie later explained. "The residency program there had come on hard times. We were able to send some of our own residents and some of our own med students up to Highland. But . . . at the end of the day [in 1979] the university sold Highland Hospital to the Psychiatric Institutes of America. They ran it for a few years. They were merged with another for-profit entity. And the long and the short of it is that ultimately it ceased to exist as a hospital and was shut down."[8]

Dr. Keith Brodie was everything that Busse wasn't as a networker. He was young, personable, and New England prep. He communicated well with his students, patients, and colleagues, and he spoke eloquently at all times—on his feet and on the spur of the moment. He also embodied in a powerful way the traditions at Duke of psychosomatic medicine, physician-scientists, and connections with NIH and the great foundations. He was Psychiatry's equivalent to Ralph Snyderman, the young NIH scientist Wyngaarden soon recruited to Duke. Brodie had entered the College of Physicians & Surgeons of Columbia University after graduating from Princeton with a degree in chemistry. "I decided I wanted to become a psychiatrist," he later explained. "It seemed to me that the future of that field was going to be quite exciting, that there would be a lot of chemical and biological breakthroughs. And so my interest lay in the biochemistry of mental illness, and I chose a residency that would equip me in that field by returning to Columbia-Presbyterian Medical Center after a year of medical internship in New Orleans."[9]

BRODIE'S EARLY EXPERIENCE

Brodie found success as a young physician-scientist in the late 1960s, much as Snyderman did, through a government alternative to combat service in the military. He was commissioned as an officer of the United States Public Health Service and assigned to NIH, where he worked, he explained, "for two years studying the biochemistry of affective disorders, principally bipolar disease; manic-depressive psychosis is what we called it in those days." Brodie's research focused on the psychopharmacology of treating the disease. "And my work there was with lithium and understanding the basic biology, the genetics, the pharmacology, the neurochemistry of that illness. And that attracted the attention of a couple of med schools, such that when I finished up my two years of service, I was recruited to join the faculty at Stanford and a few other places. But chose Stanford."[10]

Brodie organized and taught a multidisciplinary course in the Human Biology Program at Stanford and served both as chairman of the Medical School Faculty Senate and as director of the General Clinical Research Center. He also earned the support and admiration of his department chair, Dr. David A. Hamburg. Hamburg had recruited Brodie to Stanford, and it was also Hamburg who first suggested Brodie as a possible successor to Busse at Duke.[11] Within a year of Brodie's arrival at Duke, moreover, Hamburg was elected president of the Institute of Medicine of the National Academy of Science, and in 1983, a year after Brodie's appointment as chancellor of Duke University, Hamburg was appointed president of the Carnegie Corporation of New York. Hamburg then became intimately involved with the Education Commission of the States, an organization created 20 years earlier by Terry Sanford with grants from Carnegie and the Ford Foundation. Indeed, by the time Brodie succeeded Sanford as president of Duke in 1985, Hamburg was cochair with recently retired North Carolina governor Jim Hunt of the "Committee of 50," the organizational precursor of the Carnegie Forum on Education and the Economy and, eventually, the National Board for Professional Teaching Standards.[12]

If Hamburg suggested that Duke consider Brodie, it was Anlyan who decided to recruit the young psychiatrist. Disappointed with the search committee's recommended candidates, Anlyan "thanked the committee and took the book with the resumes home . . . for a weekend." Brodie was the kind of candidate Anlyan liked to see at Duke. "He was thirty-five years old, which meant that he had his career ahead of him. . . . He had also become the secretary of the American Psychiatric Association, which meant that he had some recognition, and his field of research was biological psychiatry and not the therapeutic type." And yet, Anlyan explained, there was a problem. "The criticism I had from some of the other chairs was that he [Brodie] was too young and that he would be in the palm of my hand and would not stand on his own in terms of taking positions that would be good for psychiatry. This proved to be wrong. He seemed to be a team player as well as a good chairman for his department. He was elected to the Academic Council [at Duke] and subsequently to the council's executive committee. Anytime I had a VIP patient I always went through the chairman of the appropriate department, and all the psychiatric problems of trustees, their families, and VIPs were sent to him."[13]

Brodie inherited a department at Duke that had grown under Busse from a combined total of 50 faculty and staff in 1954 to 59 faculty members and 26 house staff in 1966. By the time of Brodie's arrival in 1974, the department had 120 full-time faculty members participating in various ways in 35,208 outpatient visits and in 26,000 inpatient care days for 1,085 patients admitted for psychiatric care at Duke Hospital. "It was a department that was nationally recognized as one of the leaders in the psychosocial field," Brodie reflected. "Dr. Busse had not only built a strong clinical department with clinical teaching programs and psychoanalysis and group therapy and psychopharmacology, but he'd also built an aging center and used the Department of Psychiatry to bring faculty in to work in the field of aging. So Duke was really ahead of its time in identifying geriatric psychiatry. It was the case that many of the

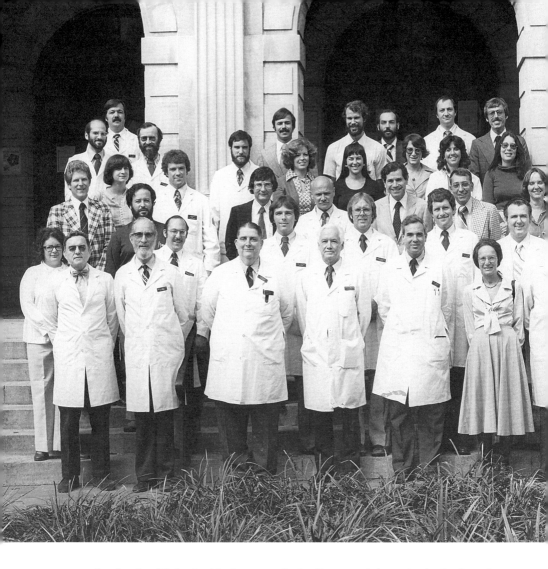

faculty that I inherited had come principally to work in geriatrics in the aging center. And as a result, the Department of Psychiatry was the third largest in the university, behind Medicine and Surgery."[14] [Figure 8.2]

Brodie's goals for the department were initially hampered by the bed space available to the psychiatry department. "My goal was to increase the number of psychiatrists in America and to recruit aggressively into the residency those who would become future teachers, future leaders." Brodie's plans included recruiting "some additional biologically-oriented psychiatrists; expanding the psychopharmacology research base; developing a departmental interest in family therapy, family studies; and expanding the child program to embrace psychopharmacology of children, which was not then represented in

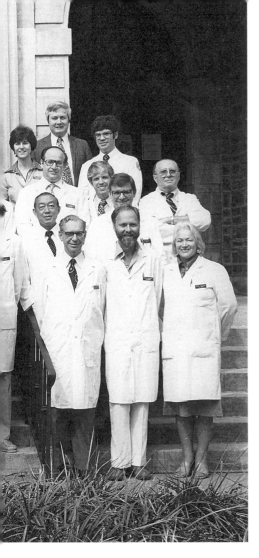

8.2 The Department of Psychiatry at Duke University Medical Center, ca. 1980. Department chairman Dr. H. Keith H. Brodie is on the front row, fifth from the left. *Duke University Medical Center Archives.*

the faculty skill set." Unfortunately, Brodie explained, "there were not enough beds to accommodate all of the patients that were clamoring to get into the psychiatry department. We had sixty beds. We had a waiting list usually at any point in time of about fifty patients. And doctors were financially dependent on their ability to treat patients in the hospital; that's where the money lay. And so there was tremendous pressure to expand. When I left the department eight years later, we had 120 beds. We added an adolescent unit, we added another adult inpatient unit, and we added a medical psychiatry unit which focused on providing mental health care to those who had distinct medical problems. . . . The income stream was substantial."[15]

Brodie also enjoyed a sense of wholeness or oneness at Duke that surpassed what he and his family had experienced in California. "And the South was a very welcoming part of this country for us," Brodie later said. "My wife comes from a fairly religious family, and her brother's a minister. So we found a welcoming spiritual dimension here which we had not totally experienced in California." Brodie was also able to offer a course at Duke that was similar to the one he had taught at Stanford. "But it wasn't until the W.D. Grant Foundation and the Commonwealth Fund began to show interest in catalyzing medical faculty teaching undergraduates," he later explained, "that we developed a bit of a program."[16]

Brodie learned his biggest lessons about the concept of oneness from Terry Sanford and Mary Semans. He was quickly exposed to Duke's big picture and given a role in planning the university's future. "And thus it was that I came, I guess, to the attention of Terry Sanford," Brodie recalled, "as I was a member of the Long Range Planning Committee for the university. And in that role, although I was at that time the chair of Psychiatry, I represented the medical center and provided some input to the overall formulation of the future of Duke." Sanford had always had Brodie's attention, of course. "Terry Sanford had run for president twice from the Allen Building and had been very active in politics, former governor of the State of North Carolina, a brilliant politician, a great leader of Duke, and a wonderful mentor for me," Brodie later emphasized. "Psychiatrists are taught to keep things private, and he knew the grand world of public relations and university relations and community relations. And worked hard to instill in me a broader vision of the place having to do with service, international, national, and local—the dimensions of which I had not really come to grips with in my past years."[17] [Figure 8.3]

Brodie also supported Mary Semans in her efforts to come to grips with a past that was very much alive in her city and family. He became a mentor, for instance, to Dr. Jean G. Spaulding, the first black woman to attend the Duke University School of Medicine. Spaulding's in-laws, Asa and Elna Spaulding, were two of Durham's most prominent black leaders; together with Semans, they had long symbolized the local tradition of interracial cooperation. Jean Spaulding received her M.D. from Duke in 1972, and in 1973, she began a three-year residency in the Department of Psychiatry. That assignment, she later recalled, helped her fulfill a decision she had made "in the 10th grade, to be a psychiatrist. That decision was supported and nurtured by innumerable individuals throughout my college years at Columbia University, throughout my medical school years at Duke, and most particularly by Dr. Keith Brodie during my years of residency and thereafter." Spaulding eventually started her own private practice in child, adolescent, and adult psychiatry and went on to become a member of the board of trustees of Duke University, vice chancellor for health affairs of Duke, and a member of The Duke Endowment.[18]

Brodie also supported Semans's larger interracial efforts at Durham County General Hospital. "When I got here in '74," Brodie recalled, "a new hospital was going to be built that would merge the two inpatient facilities, Lincoln and Watts, and I was asked to help plan a psychiatry inpatient unit for that hospital." The psychiatric unit became part of the new hospital, which opened two years later, in 1976. "And 6–2, which is what it was called, on the sixth floor of the new Durham County General Hospital, opened up," Brodie recalled. "We rotated three of our residents over there and put in a chief resident. They staffed the emergency room and did the treatment programs for them. Private docs on call on the service there. . . . It turned out to be the best teaching rotation."[19]

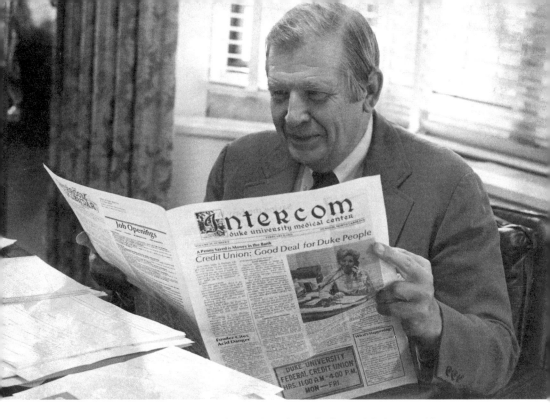

8.3 Duke University president Terry Sanford reading the medical center's in-house publication, *Intercom*. *Duke University Medical Center Archives*.

Brodie's appointment as chancellor of Duke in 1982 coincided with his presidency of the American Psychiatric Association and the appointment of Dr. Jeffrey Houpt as interim chair of Duke's Department of Psychiatry. Houpt had collaborated with Brodie in the early 1970s, in San Francisco, and in 1975 he had moved to Duke, where three years later he became head of the division of psychosomatic medicine. "In Jeff Houpt, who picked up as an acting chair when I left," Brodie said, "we had a consummate clinician who ran the consultation liaison service. And he was terrific. But for whatever reason, Dr. Anlyan didn't want to appoint him to the chair, and he left us and went to Emory. Became chairman there, then became dean there."[20] When Houpt left in 1983, Dr. Bernard J. Carroll, "the father of the Dexamethasone Suppression Test" (which was used to distinguish between biologic and stress-related depression) was appointed chairman of the Department of Psychiatry. But Duke had not seen the last of Dr. Jeffrey Houpt. Houpt would return to North Carolina in 1997, as medical school dean and vice chancellor for medical affairs at the University of North Carolina, and in 1998 he would be appointed CEO of the new UNC Health Care System.[21]

Anlyan's refusal to appoint Houpt marked the beginning, in fact, of an estrangement between Brodie and Anlyan that continued to grow during Brodie's years as president of Duke. One of Brodie's first tests as Duke's new president would be to try to stop Anlyan and the PDC from abolishing Duke's Department of Community and Family Medicine.

Recombinant DNA, the Research Triangle Park, and Ronald Reagan

The confluence of three major forces deeply affected Brodie's efforts to integrate Duke Medicine more fully into Duke University. In addition to continued reverberations from the cultural revolution of the sixties, these forces included the Reagan revolution of the 1980s and the growth of the biotechnology industry. While space permits only a cursory look at these forces and their impact on Duke, the important point is that the 1980s confronted Duke Medicine with a combination of far-reaching challenges and opportunities in politics, economics, research, and morality.

Perhaps the most crucial event in eventually transforming what many at DUMC thought about economic matters occurred shortly before Ronald Reagan was elected president in 1980. Congress passed the University and Small Business Patent Procedures Act, commonly known as the Bayh-Dole Act after its Senate sponsors, Birch Bayh, Democrat of Indiana, and Robert Dole, Republican of Kansas. Originally introduced in 1979, the act was one of a series of measures designed to improve the global competitiveness of American-owned high-tech companies by expediting the creation of new products based on tax-supported research. More specifically, by making it possible for universities and small businesses to patent discoveries arising from federally funded research, Bayh-Dole transformed the relationship between universities, the pharmaceutical industry, and the major dispenser of federal tax funds for medical research, the NIH. "Bayh-Dole gave a tremendous boost to the nascent biotechnology industry, as well as to big pharma," one observer recently noted. "Small biotech companies, many of them founded by university researchers to exploit their discoveries, proliferated rapidly. They now ring the major academic research institutions and often carry out the initial phases of drug development, hoping for lucrative deals with big drug companies that can market the new drugs. Usually both academic researchers and their institutions own equity in the biotechnology companies they are involved with. Thus, when a patent held by a university or a small biotech company is eventually licensed to a big drug company, all parties cash in on the public investment in research."[22]

The Duke connection with Bayh-Dole was less apparent than the link between Indiana senator Birch Bayh and his constituents. On one level, Bayh was linked with several Indiana natives whose networks had long bridged politics and health care on the state and national level, including Oscar Ross Ewing (federal security administrator, 1947–53), Leroy Burney (U.S. surgeon general, 1956–61), and Brodie's mentor, David Hamburg. Of more immediate importance were the potentially patentable discoveries made at Purdue University (from which Bayh had graduated) and the fact that the Indianapolis-based pharmaceutical giant, Eli Lilly and Company, was poised to reap the benefits of a licensing agreement with California-based Genentech, one of the nation's first and largest biotechnology companies. In Lilly's case the product was recombinant human insulin, which Genentech had produced in 1978. Lilly began marketing the Genentech-licensed insulin product in 1982—the first such recombinant product on the market.[23]

Duke trustee Elizabeth Dole, wife of Senator Robert Dole, was certainly one of Duke's most direct links to Bayh-Dole. Mrs. Dole had graduated from Duke in 1958, with a degree in political science, and had then earned a law degree and a master's in education at Harvard before pursuing government work in Washington. Serving first as a staff assistant in the Department of Health, Education and Welfare, where she handled indigent cases, she had moved on to become a consumer adviser to President Lyndon Johnson in 1968 and to President Richard Nixon in 1969. In 1970 Dole switched her party affiliation from Democrat to independent, and in 1973 she was appointed to the Federal Trade Commission. Married to Senator Dole in 1975, she continued at the commission until 1979, before joining the Reagan White House in 1981 as the president's assistant for public liaison. Mrs. Dole then served as secretary of transportation under Reagan, secretary of labor under President George Bush, and president of the American Red Cross. She is currently the senior United States senator from North Carolina.

North Carolina knew a good thing when it saw Bayh-Dole, and in 1981 it created the world's first government-sponsored biotechnology center. The North Carolina Biotechnology Center was not designed for laboratory research, however; it was designed to facilitate research, business, and education in biotechnology. It was also located in the Research Triangle Park, where it counted among its neighbors the recently completed Microelectronics Center of North Carolina, a research center focused on providing industry, academia, and government with the use of emerging electronic and computer-based technologies. By 1985, both of these state-supported centers had converted to nonprofit corporations and were the pillars of North Carolina's development strategy in information technology and biotechnology.[24]

By 1985, moreover, Duke and the Research Triangle Park were well-positioned to take advantage of Bayh-Dole and emerging scientific advances in drug therapy. Two of the most important links at the park, the Burroughs

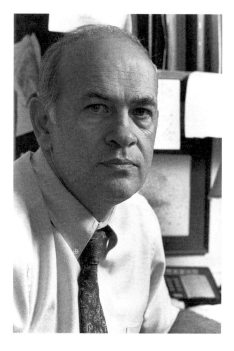

8.4 Dr. Dani P. Bolognesi. *Duke University Medical Center Archives.*

Wellcome Company and Glaxo, Inc., were subsidiaries, respectively, of the London-based pharmaceutical giants Wellcome, P.L.C., and Glaxo Holdings, P.L.C. Burroughs Wellcome had been in the park since 1971; Glaxo had arrived in 1983; and in 1995 Glaxo would acquire Burroughs Wellcome. Of particular significance to Duke Medicine was the fact that in 1984 Dr. Robert C. Gallo, the NIH scientist who codiscovered that the HIV virus was the cause of AIDS, contacted one of Dr. Joseph Beard's students at Duke, Dr. Dani Bolognesi. Gallo suggested that Bolognesi and his team of scientists switch their NIH-funded studies from animal viruses to AIDS, and according to one source, Bolognesi then put the matter to his Duke colleagues. "Bob [Gallo] said if we want to get into the field of AIDS research at all, this is the time to do it or we're going to be left behind. What do we want to do?"[25] [Figure 8.4]

They decided they wanted to focus on AIDS, and Burroughs Wellcome gave them an important opportunity. In November of 1984, scientists working at the company's facility in Research Triangle Park discovered that certain drugs could inhibit animal viruses in the test tube. The Duke group was asked to help in "screening about 300 compounds to see if any acted on the AIDS virus," one source reported. "Bolognesi's group had its own work to do, but it had the right equipment and know-how and agreed to help. One compound showed a lot of activity against the virus. Burroughs Wellcome developed it into AZT, the first AIDS drug, in 1987." In 1993, moreover, Bolognesi and his Duke colleague, Dr. Thomas Matthews, formed a biotechnology company called Trimeris to develop the "fusion inhibitor" process they developed at Duke to stop the AIDS virus from reproducing. Bolognesi stepped down as director of Duke University's Center for AIDS Research in 1999 to become CEO and chief scientific officer of Trimeris, which leased the technology from Duke. In 2004, after years of patient trials and collaborative work with the Swiss pharmaceutical giant, Hoffman-LaRoche, Trimeris received full approval from the U.S. Food and Drug Administration for the anti-HIV drug Fuseon.[26]

Duke's work with Burroughs Wellcome is just one example of how Bayh-

Dole combined with the revolution in computer technology to ignite the expansion of Research Triangle Park and transform Duke's relationship with the park and its companies. The park's first big boost had come in 1965 with the announcement that both IBM and the NIH's National Institute of Environmental Health Sciences Center would be located in the park. Among the initial benefits Duke derived from IBM's presence was a computer program designed to provide patient information to physicians in the new Department of Community Health Sciences at Duke. As for the Environmental Health Sciences Center, which Terry Sanford and Oscar Ewing had urged presidents Kennedy and Johnson to locate in North Carolina, the benefits came later. The center opened its permanent facility at the park in 1982, and since that time it has collaborated with Duke and the Triangle's other universities on issues affecting health and the environment. Between 1969 and 1979, the number of companies located in the Research Triangle Park increased from 21 to 39, and by 1989, 28 more companies had located there. The 1990s saw more than 40 new companies establish facilities in the park, and by 2004, it was home to more than 130 organizations employing some 40,000 people, almost all of whom worked in the park's 100 research and development–related organizations.[27]

Closely coupled with this growth were the tectonic shifts that Dr. Ralph Snyderman would initiate throughout Duke Medicine in the 1990s. Indeed, to many of his critics, Snyderman embodied the developments described by Big Pharma's biggest critic, Marcia Angell. Of medical schools and teaching hospitals, she writes, "These nonprofit institutions started to see themselves as 'partners' of industry, and they became just as enthusiastic as any entrepreneur about the opportunities to parlay their discoveries into financial gain. Faculty researchers were encouraged to obtain patents on their work (which were assigned to their universities), and they shared in the royalties. Many medical schools and teaching hospitals set up 'technology transfer' offices to help in this activity and capitalize on faculty discoveries. As the entrepreneurial spirit grew during the 1990s, medical school faculty entered into other lucrative financial arrangements with drug companies, as did their parent institutions."[28]

Family Medicine and the PDC

Bayh-Dole and biotech were growing blips on DUMC's radar screen when Keith Brodie became president of Duke in 1985. Brodie entered office focused on a nasty struggle that had spilled out from DUMC and across the state. Money was a major source of the trouble, as were the issues of leadership and power. With Sanford's departure, Duke found itself without

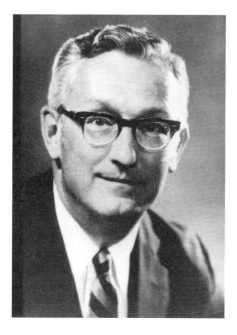

the hands-on approach of three of the most important figures in its recent history. Mary Semans had retired from the university's board of trustees in 1981 and become chairman of The Duke Endowment the following year. In 1983 Alex McMahon had stepped down as chairman and a member of the university's board of trustees, and also from his position as a director of the Research Triangle Institute. Within DUMC itself, Barnes Woodhall had retired from his various university duties and was suffering from the brain disease that would take his life in 1985.[29] [Figure 8.5]

The most powerful departments at the time of Brodie's election were Surgery, Medicine, Biochemistry, and Microbiology and Immunology. The chairman of Microbiology and Immunology, Wolfgang Joklik, was then in his 17th year as chair, while the chairman of Biochemistry, Robert Hill, was in his 16th year. The surgeon the VA patients called "The Man," Dr. David Sabiston, was in his 21st year as chairman of the Department of Surgery and had become one of the most powerful men at Duke University. The most important change among the big four departments had occurred in 1982; the chief of the division of cardiology, Dr. Joseph C. Greenfield Jr., had become chairman of the Department of Medicine when Jim Wyngaarden was appointed director of NIH. Greenfield and his predecessor in cardiology, Dr. Andrew Wallace, who had become CEO of Duke Hospital in 1981, had helped develop the concept of equipping and staffing coronary care units for patients needing specialized nursing care and prompt treatment of arrhythmias.

Among the first issues Brodie faced was that of Bill Anlyan's leadership during a confrontation between Harvey Estes's Department of Community and Family Medicine and the PDC giants, Drs. David Sabiston and Joseph Greenfield. The trouble began late in 1984, and while colored with disdain for the new brand of GPs that Estes was training—amid what Estes himself described as the "intellectual battles that were being waged between traditional academic medicine and this new upstart breed of people"—the core of the matter was money, power, and the PDC. Indeed, the incident set off a series of events that within a decade considerably diminished the traditional autonomy and power of the Departments of Medicine and Surgery at Duke. The deciding blows were delivered between 1993 and 1995, under Dr. Ralph Snyderman, when Greenfield stepped down and Sabiston retired. Simultaneously, in 1993, at a time when the PDC held some $160 million in its reserve fund, the practice abandoned its 1972 general partnership agreement and became a professional limited liability partnership. The PDC also adopted a revised operating agreement, and in 1995 consolidated into one office the business operations of the PDC's two divisions, surgical and medical.[30]

The forces Anlyan faced in the mid-1980s were almost impossible to reconcile. Estes and his upstart family practitioners were in the vanguard of change in the nation's health care system. They were the "gatekeepers" of the new HMOs—the primary care physicians who referred patients to specialists like those at DUMC. They were the generalists who worked closely with other primary care providers—the general internist, the general pediatrician, the nurse practitioner, and the physician assistant. They were the men and women who were learning how to run their practices as businesses; who were using computers and diagnostic technologies to improve cost effectiveness, precision, and efficiency; and who were emphasizing the least expensive forms of clinical care—health promotion and preventive medicine—that improved the bottom line of HMOs.

Yet Estes and his colleagues at the Durham County General Hospital were also competing for patients with the PDC and Duke Hospital. And that was one more uncertainty than some in Duke Medicine wanted. The Reagan administration had already cut more than $4 billion from Medicaid programs and had begun using diagnostic-related groups to reimburse treatment under Medicare. "That's a diagnostic-related group," one PDC administrator recently explained, "and what it means is if you come in for a heart procedure, they're only going to pay a certain amount. It doesn't matter if the hospital keeps you in longer or if they get you out quicker. . . . A DRG is a set payment, where in the past, the more widgets or labs or X-rays you did up in the ward, if they kept you in extra days, you could bill for a per-day charge and get paid for as much as possible." At the same time, many Blue Cross and Blue Shield plans, battered by the explosive growth in spending for medical care, were questioning physicians and hospitals on the issues of cost and quality, even as HMOs were negotiating discounted rates with hospitals and other providers in return for clients. "Increasingly," one observer has written, "liberal reformers (following the logic of prepaid, group health coverage) and conservative opponents (reasoning from a free-market model) agreed that the solution rested on managed care within HMOs and competition among them. HMO membership grew from under two million in 1970 to almost forty million (about 27 percent of the health care market) twenty years later. And commercial insurers adopted many HMO practices, including limits on the choice of provider and close utilization review."[31]

The trouble for Estes began when a faculty member at Duke, a man who could not find a primary care physician at DUMC, was seen by one in the Family Practice clinic operated by Estes's group at Durham County hospital. Admitted to the hospital with pneumonia, the patient, who had recently had surgery at DUMC, was examined by a staff urologist at Durham County General who had trained under the surgeon who performed the patient's surgery at Duke. As fate would have it, the urologist saw his former Duke teacher at a cocktail party and mentioned having checked the patient out at Durham County General. The Duke surgeon was irate. He "was incensed at this because his patient had been seen by a competitor across town," Estes recalled. "So he went back to his chief, Dr. Sabiston, and said, 'Do you know what's going on? Our Duke Family Medicine faculty are calling on Durham physicians that are our competitors to see our Duke patients. This is not right, and we ought to protest it.'"[32]

Sabiston disdained the training of GPs at Duke, and he moved quickly to mobilize complaints from the other departments. "This feeling was expressed in the meeting of department chairs," Estes explained, "and other departments were brought into the picture, because this same thing was happening in Medicine and other services. So behind the scenes and unknown to me, department chairs were getting together, talking about this, and they talked about it to the point that they came to see Dr. Anlyan and said this had to stop. 'We can't tolerate Duke being diluted this way or being competed with this way because this is becoming a significant financial loss.'"[33]

Medicine and Surgery were also concerned that the competition might spread to the PDC referral clinics in the surrounding counties. "The PDC was the engine to bring in the clinic business. It would bring in the patients," said PDC administrator Paul R. Newman. "And how did it do that? Our physicians would hold consultative clinics in pretty much eighteen key counties around us, where they would go on out—and if it was appropriate for that patient to leave the community, we'd bring the patient back here. Or the patient, because of the relationships doctors had set up—the referral relationships with other physicians in these communities—we would get those referrals. We would see the patient here, do the surgery or treat him on the inpatient [wards], and then send them back to the community." In other words, the primary care physicians trained by Estes and his department had the power, both as the new "gatekeepers" of American medicine and as staff of the PDC's referral clinics, to refer patients to specialists at many different hospitals, not just Duke.[34]

Anlyan could have responded to the situation "undemocratically," as he had in ignoring the clinical faculty's reservations about building Duke North. But he didn't. He hired Lewin & Company, a medical consulting firm, to study the matter both within DUMC and around the state. Lewin presented its report six months later, in the spring of 1985. The report, Estes explained, was evenhanded and either/or. "Lewin's conclusions were quite clear: You've either got to admit that this department [of family medicine] is part of you and begin to cooperate with it, or you've got to extrude it and wash your hands of it." The crux of the Lewin report was discussed at a special meeting of the department heads, including Estes, who recalled the choice the report described. While Duke Medicine was indeed training its own competition, the Department of Community and Family Medicine was also the "only countervailing force to this, because this department is training the generalists that are going out there who are seeing large volumes of patients and who are referring large volumes of patients. And if they are trained at Duke and they are favorable to Duke and they see Duke not as an enemy but as a friend, they will send their patients here. So there were both sides of this issue," Estes explained. "After this presentation, all of them except me went to a meeting to decide what they were going to do. And they came back and said, 'We've concluded that we need to get rid of family medicine.' And so Dr. Anlyan came in, and I think with some reluctance, told me that the other departments had voted that the Family Medicine Department would cease to exist."[35]

Estes resigned as chair of the department but decided "to stay as a member of the faculty and to fight it." Which didn't take him long, as most of the state's general practitioners were his allies. Not only was Estes a prominent figure in local, state, and national medical societies, but he was well connected with people whose opinion counted in the state. The state's most prominent general practitioner, Amos N. Johnson of Garland, North Carolina, and his black assistant, Henry Lee "Buddy" Treadwell, had served as Dr. Eugene Stead's models in launching the physician assistant program in the 1960s. Johnson, who died in 1975, had been president of the American Academy of General Practice and one of the most important supporters of the new four-year medical school at East Carolina University. In fact, Estes pointed out, the "Academy of Family Physicians in the state was actively cooperating with my new Division of Family Practice. They quickly contacted all the family doctors in the state and others, and it became widely known [that Duke had abolished its Department of Family Medicine]. So people began to write and say, 'If you do this, I'm never going to send another patient there.' So the weight of evidence was that not only was the department needed, but it was supported, and that there would be a price to pay if this were done."[36]

The result was that "Dr. Anlyan back-pedaled," and in June of 1985 his decision was reversed. "So the department stayed," Estes explained, "but I was no longer the chair. And George [R.] Parkerson [Jr.], who had been a faculty member for many years before that decision was made, took over as the chairperson. . . . But the program did shrink in size. It had been thirteen residents a year and went back to eight. So the election was to bring it back to Duke and to put it in the Pickens Building and to give up the building at Durham General, which was far better than Pickens as a place for our headquarters. So we paid a price, too," Estes conceded in 2004. "But the program is still there and still doing well, and I think the department has done well. But that's when I stepped down and became a geriatrician at that point."[37]

The Rise of Radiology

Keith Brodie became president of Duke in July of 1985 and immediately threw down the gauntlet to Bill Anlyan. He appointed the chairman of Radiology, Dr. Charles E. Putman, as vice chancellor for health affairs and vice provost of Duke University. To the existing order and its heirs apparent Putman represented a triple threat. He and Dr. Carl E. Ravin, the new chairman of Radiology, had turned the department into one of the most aggressive and profitable in the medical center; indeed, because of new and improved medical imaging equipment, Radiology was seeing and sharing many of the patients once seen mainly by Medicine, Surgery, and other departments.

Putman's appointment also challenged Anlyan's plans to "groom" Dr. Andrew Wallace to succeed him as chancellor for health affairs of Duke University. Anlyan had appointed Wallace CEO of Duke Hospital in 1981, at a time when Wallace was chief of the division of cardiology in the Department of Medicine. Wallace had also been appointed that year as the university's vice chancellor for health affairs, and he would remain in that position even after Brodie appointed Putman to it in 1985. Between 1986 and 1987, moreover, Brodie tried to move Anlyan out of the medical center by making Putman dean of the medical school—a position Anlyan had held in fact, if not in title, for the previous 20 years. And finally, Putman forged important personal and institutional links between the basic scientists at Duke and the drug, information, and biotechnology companies at Research Triangle Park—connections that Anlyan had tended to ignore. Putman soon became known as Duke's "ambassador" to the Research Triangle Park.[38]

Radiology's startling rise under Putman and Ravin occurred while the revolution in recombinant DNA was erupting at Genentech. Putman had been advised not to accept the radiology position when it was offered to him in 1977, as the word then had been that "radiology at Duke would be forever dwarfed and stifled by the lions of medicine and surgery." The department's first chairman, Dr. Robert Reeves, had certainly been dwarfed; he had remained a salaried employee of the hospital during his entire tenure as chief (1930–65), at a time when radiology was "entered in the financial record alongside medical illustration, the pharmacy, the library, the animal laboratory, physiotherapy, and the brace shop." Reeves had also been excluded from the medical school's executive committee, which included all of the department chairs. This meant that radiology lacked full stature as an academic department and thus that neither Reeves nor any of his staff had PDC privileges. As a result, the Department of Radiology "never accumulated separate funds adequate for development of the department." Reeves had also been powerless to stop the Departments of Surgery and Medicine from performing many of their own x-ray and other radiologic services. One of the several reforms attempted by Reeves's successor, Dr. Richard G. Lester, was that "radiologic services be restored to radiology."[39]

Putman inherited from his predecessor, Richard Lester, a department that had full status as an academic department and thus private practice privileges at the PDC. Putman also inherited a department that was expanding its outpatient services; that was interested in research; that had the latest technology at its disposal; and that had a tradition of working with Lincoln Hospital. According to the department's historians, "The first CT scanner in the South (third in the nation) was installed [at Duke] in 1974. A man of profound moral conviction, Lester also used his skills to help nurture the growth of an impoverished African-American hospital in the Durham community." Unfortunately, Lester also left Putman a department that was badly "balkanized by internecine sectional disputes. Section leaders reigned imperial. The file room had trouble tracking and controlling films. Clinicians grumbled about the service they were receiving." More to the point, Putman faced two closely related challenges at DUMC. One was Radiology's traditional place in the medical center's hierarchy. "Duke was among the very last of the major medical centers to abandon the old organizational model borrowed from Johns Hopkins that asserted the hegemony of the traditional clinical departments." Additionally, Putman faced the more specific challenge at which his predecessor had failed: to "achieve a rapprochement between radiologists and cardiologists over the tense battleground of angiography."[40]

Significantly, it was on the battleground of angiography that one encounters many of the forces that crossed the barrier between internal power struggles in Duke Medicine and the wider revolutions in genomics and health care. Angiography involves making x-ray pictures of blood vessels, generally arteries and usually coronary arteries, which helps explain why the radiologists and the cardiologists were at odds. They each wanted to control who looked at the heart, how they looked at it, and where they looked at it—all of which determined, in turn, who was paid for, and benefited from, not only the procedures but also the research they generated. This relationship was also becoming increasingly familiar to Radiology in its collaboration with both the clinical and basic science departments at DUMC. Advances in medical imaging equipment—from computerized tomography (CT) scanning and ultrasound to nuclear imaging and magnetic resonance imaging—were transforming the way diseases were diagnosed, investigated, and treated. New technologies and procedures were beginning to replace guesses about diagnosis while also eliminating dangerous and painful imaging tests. At the same time, however, the increasing demand for access to these expensive new advances was further fueling the already skyrocketing costs of medical care. The stakes were high for all concerned.

As for a rapprochement at DUMC, there wasn't one between Radiology and the division of cardiology. Their struggle was complicated by Anlyan's plans for Andrew Wallace and by several key scientists who wanted Duke to seize the opportunities being created by biotechnology and Bayh-Dole. Wallace had been named chief of the division of cardiology in 1969, two years after Eugene Stead had created the division within the Department of Medicine. To be sure, Stead and DUMC had groomed Wallace as much as Anlyan. Wallace had followed his M.D. degree at Duke with an internship, residency, and research fellowship there, before spending two years as an investigator at the National Heart Institute. Returning to Duke in 1964, Wallace had become chief resident in medicine under Stead, and in 1965 he had launched Duke's first cardiac care unit. Ten years later he started a heart disease prevention program called DUPAC (Duke University Preventive Approach to Cardiology), "and as an outgrowth of that," Anlyan later wrote, Wallace "was instrumental in establishing the Center for Living, a large, very successful program that helps people with cardiovascular diseases or at risk for heart disease to learn and follow healthy lifestyles." Thus, to the extent that there was any rapprochement at Duke, it represented Anlyan's efforts to reconcile some of the long-standing rivalries and differences between DUMC's giants, Medicine and Surgery, that went back to Hart, Hanes, Davison, and Stead. Surgeons had administered DUMC for the past 30 years, and Anlyan now intended to pass the baton to Andrew Wallace and the Department of Medicine.[41]

Putman carried no such personal or institutional loads, however, in pushing to have Radiology excel at teaching, research, and patient care. After taking undergraduate and medical degrees in his native Texas, Putman had interned in Iowa before returning to Texas for a residency in medicine. From there he had moved on to a residency in radiology at the University of California in San Francisco and then to the faculty at Yale Medical School, where, in addition to teaching radiology and internal medicine, he had been clinical director of diagnostic radiology at Yale-New Haven Hospital. His colleague there, Dr. Carl Ravin, joined him at Duke in 1978 and together they set about overhauling the department's filing system, eliminating the fiefdoms of imperious section heads, and permeating the hospital with radiologists. To the staff who objected, Putman responded with "a blunt, in-your-face directness that left little doubt about who was in charge. . . . Forty-seven members of the faculty resigned during the first five years of the Putman chairmanship, but the staff actually grew from 38 to 52 members." Putman and Ravin also made certain that "radiologists were everywhere present when films were reviewed and interpretations made. A radiologist was stationed in the emergency room around the clock." The two men also insisted "that the members of their staff be participants, not spectators; genuine practical physicians, not sterile academics. Within 5 years, the number of scientific papers published each year from the department rose from 18 to 190," and Radiology's PDC revenue rose, too.[42]

Putman first butted heads with Anlyan over space for CT scanning in the new North Division of Duke Hospital. According to the department's historians, "The original blueprint for Duke North provided no space for CT, but even as walls were being put up, Putman was having them torn down to accommodate three scanners." Later, Putman also challenged Duke Hospital CEO Andrew Wallace over the site for a new magnetic resonance device. When this "early high-field MR research unit was slated for construction in a distant part of Duke Forest, Putman insisted that the unit be grafted onto the hospital despite pervasive skepticism about the feasibility of imaging at high field." Indeed, by the early 1980s Putman and Ravin could not be ignored. They had taken "a foundering program and elevated it to peerage with the towering clinical departments at Duke and then into the highest echelons of academia."[43]

Putman's unusual upward mobility struck Bill Anlyan as part of a personal disagreement between Keith Brodie and Andrew Wallace. "I honestly felt that Andy Wallace was the best qualified person to succeed me as executive vice president and chancellor for health affairs at Duke University," Anlyan later wrote. "However, it became apparent that he and Keith Brodie, who was then the university president, did not get along. Looking into the matter subsequently, I gathered that when Andy was director of the hospital and Keith was chairman of psychiatry, Keith had appeared one day in Andy's office with some demand that Andy had denied. Apparently, Brodie never forgave him. I was not aware of that at the time."[44]

The Need for New Leadership

What Anlyan failed to see was the extent to which many at Duke considered him the problem. Keith Brodie explained, "Well, I think Terry Sanford really left the medical school alone. And under Bill Anlyan's leadership, he just let them build and build and get bigger and bigger and stronger, and it worked out. But when I went into the presidency, I began to see a plateau occur, and then I began to see some detriments: We lost major funding for our cancer center, and we were losing some really good scientists. So I spent a lot of time interviewing people and trying to get a handle on the cause of that. And it turned out at the end of the day that it was the person [Anlyan] who'd brought me to Duke in the first place that . . . needed new challenges. And so I had the chairman of the board of trustees meet separately with a number of the department chairmen in the medical center. He became convinced of that as well."[45] [Figure 8.6]

Brodie had also become convinced that Anlyan himself was incapable of promoting the concept of oneness at Duke. As chancellor Brodie had started to see the overall relationship between the medical center and the university. "I think the medical center, much like China, had tried to diminish any relationship between itself and the rest of the university," he explained. "There was really very little dialogue, and it was a great desire to be left alone, basically, that permeated the center."[46] What Brodie could not have seen, however, what he and most everyone else then at Duke had not experienced—indeed, what only Anlyan and those of his generation who had lived through it understood—was the extent to which the medical center's autonomy and economic power had been threatened by the postwar efforts of Willis Smith and Hollis Edens to impose their concept of oneness on Duke.

The most telling criticism of Anlyan, perhaps, was one shared by Brodie and many within Duke Medicine. Anlyan had failed to keep up with science. "I think there was a good amount of dissatisfaction first of all, within the medical center faculty with Dr. Anlyan's leadership," one close observer recalled. "I think that had a lot to do with the fact that Dr. Anlyan himself was not a scientist. He did not understand personally the direction or needs of biomedical science for the medical center. He was very, very dependent on the advice of a selected few. So, there were people, historically, who played a big role, like Dan Tosteson, Phil Handler, Tom Kinney, Bob Hill . . . Gene Stead. . . . I think that, when Kinney died, and when Handler went to the National Academy, and Dan Tosteson left for Chicago and then for Harvard, and Stead retired, . . . he was really robbed of his best advice." At the same time, many faculty also questioned Anlyan's priorities. "That, basically, it was just one building after another to be built, and that that was the major job of

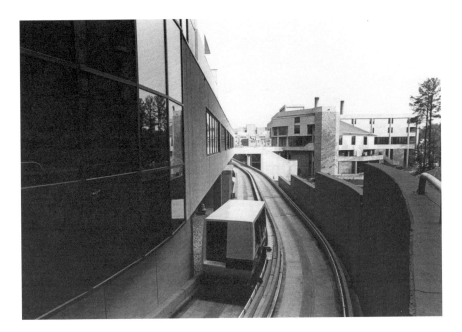

8.6 The PRT (personal rapid transit) system was designed to carry patients, faculty, staff, and visitors between the North and South Divisions of Duke Hospital. *Duke University Medical Center Archives.*

his administration was to build buildings. That's not fair, of course. But, that people and programs weren't nearly as intelligently managed."[47] [Figure 8.7]

Several of DUMC's best scientists were indeed looking for a leader who could make and manage wise connections between their own work and the exciting new world of genomics and business-biotech. One of those scientists was Dr. Dani Bolognesi, James B. Duke Professor of Surgery, whose research group was collaborating with Burroughs Wellcome on the anti-AIDS drug AZT. Three other members of the Department of Medicine were also keeping a close eye on the California biotech company Genentech and its new anticlotting drug, a tissue plasminogen activator (TPA) called Activase. Two of those three, Drs. Robert Lefkowitz and Robert M. Califf, were in Medicine's division of cardiology, while the third, Dr. Ralph Snyderman, was chief of the division of rheumatic-genetic disease in the Department of Medicine.

The biotech situation came to a head in February 1986, when Genentech announced that "the British Patent office had awarded the company a patent on its tissue plasminogen activator, used in treating heart attack and other blood-clot related diseases." According to the *New York Times*, "Genentech also said it would file suit in Britain against Burroughs Wellcome for patent infringement. Genentech already has been awarded patents in 10 other countries, not including America, for its tissue plasminogen activator, trademarked Activase, and the recombinant DNA technology used to make it." Burroughs Wellcome was already making TPA, and had recently announced that it was conducting clinical trials. Thus, when the British patent was awarded to Genentech, Wellcome filed suit to invalidate it. "Analysts said Activase, which has proved in tests to be twice as effective as existing anti-clotting agents, could account for as much as half of Genentech's revenues by the mid-1990s."[48]

More immediate and disruptive to Duke Medicine was President Brodie's 1986 appointment of Charles Putman as dean of Duke University's School of Medicine. The title was one that Anlyan had never relinquished; after becoming vice president for health affairs in 1969, he had transferred the "deanship responsibilities" to subordinates who held the titles "director of medical education," then "dean of medical and allied health education," and most recently "dean of undergraduate medical education." Brodie attached no qualifiers to Putman's title; the appointment, one insider recalled, was a blatant attempt by "Dr. Brodie to squeeze Dr. Anlyan out of the control of the medical center by appointing Dr. Putman to the position of dean."[49]

It was also in 1986 that Terry Sanford was elected to the United States Senate, Dr. Ernest Mario was named president and chief operating officer of Glaxo, Inc., at RTP, and Dr. Ralph Snyderman decided to leave Duke for Genentech in San Francisco. Sanford's victory was his last political hurrah; he would lose his reelection bid in 1992, and in 1998 he died and was buried in Duke Chapel. But Mario's relationship with Duke was just beginning. Riding the wave of Glaxo's profitable new antiulcer drug, Zantac, Mario, a pharmacist by training, became chief executive officer of Glaxo in 1988, and CEO of its parent company, Glaxo Holdings in 1989. He also became a trustee of Duke University in 1989, and is currently chairman of the board of the Duke University Health System.

Challenges for Research and Leaders

During Terry Sanford's final term as president of Duke, James Wyngaarden resigned as chair of the Department of Medicine to become director of the NIH. His absence from Duke, as well as his activities as director, affected DUMC's deepening leadership crisis. The kind of genetic research that he and his colleagues had been urging DUMC to invest in was now his mission at NIH. Wyngaarden was appointed to the position by President Ronald Reagan in 1982, and for the next seven years he fought to maintain NIH's political independence and funding against the ideological and fiscal onslaughts of the Reagan revolution.

In June of 1986, at a conference in London, one of Jim Wyngaarden's British colleagues asked the NIH director what he thought about the announce-

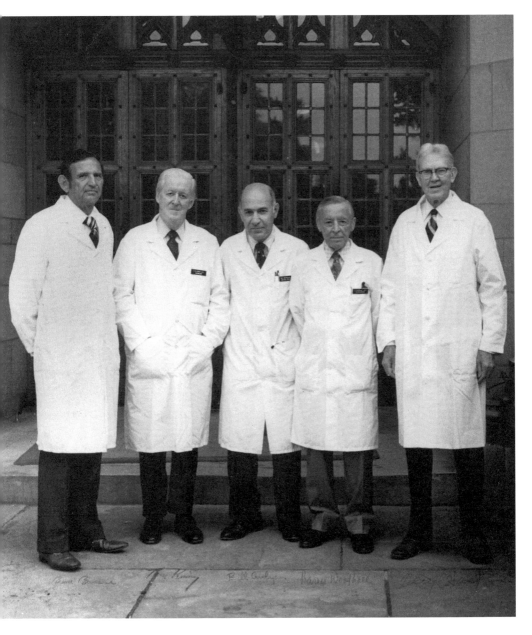

8.7 Left to right: Drs. Ewald W. Busse, Thomas D. Kinney, William G. Anlyan, Barnes
Woodhall, and J. Deryl Hart, ca. 1976. *Duke University Medical Center Archives.*

ment that the U.S. Department of Energy intended to commit $2 billion to launch a human genome sequencing project. Wyngaarden's reaction was "one of alarm at what appeared to be an attempt by DOE to usurp leadership of a major theme of biological research in which NIH had primogenitor seniority." Wyngaarden later reviewed that ancestral heritage. "Genetic research had been fundamental to the mission of the National Institutes of Health (NIH) since inception," he wrote. "NIH had supported programs in bacterial, phage, yeast, animal and human genetics since the 1950s. The deciphering of the genetic code by Marshall Nirenberg and his colleagues had brought NIH its first Nobel Prize in 1968. Identification and sequencing of structural genes of interest were common events in the intramural programs of almost all NIH institutes, and constituted major themes of extramural grants programs, especially those of the National Institute of General Medicine and Sciences (NIGMS). By 1986 there was a growing awareness of the possibility of sequencing entire human chromosomes, and a few editorials and several workshops had addressed the topic, including the formidable challenges involved."[50]

Frustrated by the constant struggle for funds, Wyngaarden planned to resign on November 1, 1988—just days before George Bush and Michael Dukakis squared off in the presidential elections. Wyngaarden felt "strongly that the position of NIH director should not turn over as soon as a new president takes office. After all," he said, "the job has never been a political one." So he delayed announcing his resignation from NIH until May of 1989. In explaining why he was stepping down, Wyngaarden said that there had been "no consistent science policy" during the Reagan years and that the budget process involved a situation where "the administration tries to get by with as little as it can, and then Congress repairs the damage to the greatest extent possible." He was able, however, to complete one other major project before he left office. "By that time the human genome project had started to come together," Wyngaarden said in May 1989, "the fraud and misconduct issue had heated up, and Vince DeVita resigned [as director of the National Cancer Institute] and I saw an opportunity to play a role in picking his successor."[51]

By the time Bush arrived at the White House, Vincent T. DeVita Jr. had been succeeded by AIDS researcher Samuel Broder, Congress had approved Wyngaarden's proposal for the new Office of Human Genome Research, and Wyngaarden had helped recruit Nobel laureate James Watson as associate director for Human Genome Research at NIH. Wyngaarden also later recalled that when the new secretary of the Department of Health and Human Services, Dr. Louis Sullivan, asked him if there was anything special he would like to see accomplished before he left NIH, Wyngaarden "cited the pending request for Center status for the Office of Human Genome Research. Secretary Sullivan approved the request on June 22; the Center became a reality on October 1, 1989 . . . and Jim Watson was appointed its first director." Congress finally appropriated $59.5 million for the new National Center for Human Genome Research.[52]

TO GENENTECH AND BACK

It was in the spring of 1986 that the Genentech corporation began aggressively recruiting the chief of Duke's division of rheumatology, Dr. Ralph Snyderman.[53] "At that time Genentech was a phenomenon," Snyderman later recalled. "It was the first major biotechnology firm. The impact of recombinant DNA technology in medicine was just becoming apparent. Cloning. Genentech was, it is hard to imagine what is was like, but I remember that the biggest and the best and the brightest scientists that I knew were there. . . . The research impact of that entity was so substantial, they were so far ahead of everybody else in the technology, and they had some of the best scientists in the country." Many other scientists, including Snyderman's friend, Dr. Robert Lefkowitz, feared Genentech's research prowess. "We ran together virtually every day. Bob had just gotten into molecular biology and wanted to clone a beta receptor. I remember one day on a run Bob almost swooned, he was so depressed because he had heard that Genentech was trying to clone a beta receptor. And, 'Oh my god, now, how in the world are we going to do it?' It really was a major threat, and I was so impressed by the power of Genentech."[54]

Things were going extremely well for Snyderman at Duke, however, when Genentech asked him to design a job he might consider taking. He had been appointed to the distinguished position of Frederic M. Hanes, M.D., Professor of Medicine at Duke. He had been given "almost a blank check" as a Howard Hughes medical investigator, his NIH grant had been renewed for five years, and also, he recalled, "I had broken out of the field of inflammation into the big time, so to speak, of the receptor G-protein biochemistry. . . . I was really in a foot race in opening up whole new areas of cell biology. And it was fun and it was exciting, and, there was no downside, everything seemed to be going real well."[55]

Still, Snyderman discussed the Genentech offer with his friend and running mate, Robert Lefkowitz. Both men were Howard Hughes investigators and both were involved in research on G-protein receptors (hormone and other intercellular signal receptors). These cell surface receptors are the largest class of receptors in the human body, and they are favorite target proteins for the development of new medicines. Signal molecules interact with these seven-membrane-spanning receptors to stimulate intracellular actions that result in tissue responses. The significance of these protein receptors was later explained by Lefkowitz, who by 2002 would be the most-cited scientist in the field of biochemistry. "There's no field of biology or medicine that's not

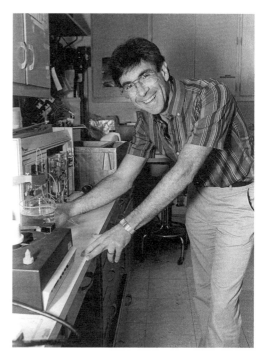

8.8 Dr. Robert J. Lefkowitz. *Duke University Medical Center Archives.*

impacted by them," he said. "We cloned the first of these receptors in 1986, the beta 2 adrenergic receptor, and in the years since then about 1,000 . . . receptors have been identified. They all share this structure in which the peptide chain runs across the plasma membrane back and forth seven times. By far this is the largest, most ubiquitous family of receptors that exist. And this family includes a huge diversity of receptors—virtually all sensory receptors, hundreds of smell receptors, dozens of taste receptors. . . . What's more, the drugs that target these receptors account for 60–70% of all the prescription drugs used in the world. Any antihistamines, for example. Anything that targets serotonin receptors. Opiates. And on and on."[56] [Figure 8.8]

Snyderman accepted the position of vice president for medical research and development at Genentech in October of 1986, and the following January began his official duties. [57] He was immediately thrown into the product pipeline for Activase—the clot-dissolving drug over which Genentech and Burroughs Wellcome were litigating. "The big blockbuster, the major blockbuster was going to be something called TPA, tissue plasminogen activator," Snyderman recalled. "The exciting thing about TPA is that it dissolved clots, it dissolved clots in coronary arteries, and there was a lot of animal data, and some clinical research had indicated that it would be the way to treat heart attacks. When I got there, or when I was negotiating for the position, which was in the fall of 1986, it was thought to be a done deal, that . . . it was pretty much approved and just needed to go through a few more regulatory turns, twists, and would be approved sometime in the early spring of 1987." But that didn't happen. "Lo and behold, on May 29th we got blown out of the water. It was disapproved," Snyderman stressed. "It was just awful. The streptokinase was approved, our competitor; TPA was disapproved."[58]

The setback transformed Snyderman as a leader and helped prepare him for many of the challenges that lay ahead. The catalyst, he recalled, was a confrontation with a colleague at Genentech. Snyderman remembered his colleague saying. "'Ralph, you may think that you are playing a big role in the approval of TPA, but you really are not leading,' He essentially told me . . . the difference between being a leader and being a participator and being an observer. . . . That was one of the biggest learning experiences I ever had."[59] Snyderman was so angry and inspired by the challenge that he demanded complete control of the TPA matter—something to which the company's president, G. Kirk Raab, agreed. And six months later, in November 1987, in one of the quickest reversals on record, the FDA approved TPA. "I did everything that I could," Snyderman said later. In addition to showing "all the data" to the FDA, he dealt with it in the same way he tries "to deal with everybody, and that's to be totally honest. Just really develop a relationship where people trust what I say."[60]

Early in 1988, Snyderman received a letter from Duke, from a member of the search committee, asking him if he wanted to be a candidate for the positions of dean of the medical school and chancellor for health affairs at Duke. The letter went unanswered by Snyderman, who was busy building what he later described as "appropriate relationships between industry and academic medicine." Snyderman explained: "I thought that if they were serious about me being a candidate, they knew me well enough that I didn't need to submit a CV or bibliography, so I didn't even bother to answer the letter, and was very slightly put off by it. That's the first I heard of it."[61]

REPERCUSSIONS IN DURHAM, RTP, AND CALIFORNIA

Back in Durham, Duke University was in administrative turmoil, much of it due to internal struggles of Duke Medicine. As Brodie pushed for more partnerships with corporate America, the university's Academic Council publicly challenged his leadership, questioning who was running Duke and how it was being run. Once again the banner of cross-campus, interdisciplinary studies was run up the pole, but this time the administration planned to unfurl it over a building designed specifically for that purpose: the Levine Science Research Center. The idea was to provide laboratory space for researchers from the medical school, the School of Engineering, the School of Forestry (later, the Environment), and the arts and sciences. Brodie explained: "And so we decided to bundle into one building with some shared research some very, very expensive equipment that no individual school could afford, but which as a collective group they could all chip in and use."[62]

Also evident in the building's plans were Brodie's efforts to realize in some measure the concept of oneness. "In my mind it was very, very important to have a central eating facility so these people could mingle and talk over meals. And so we tripled the size of the cafeteria." Anlyan, for his part, hoped the project "would assuage some of the anxieties" of the university faculty. But that didn't happen, at least not initially. According to Brodie, "the Academic Council was initially opposed, and we had to hold luncheons. . . . And pulling those people together, getting them to share first in the design concept of the building and then in the allocation of space in the building, was not the easiest thing in the world." What was more, the university "trustees were a little leery of it. It was a very, very costly building, $80 million."[63]

In the meantime, DUMC was having a terrible time putting its own house in order. Brodie's gambit with Charles Putman had proved disastrous; after a year as dean of the medical school, Putman had been replaced in 1987 by Dr. Doyle Graham. "One of the things that I had been really aware of was how Charles had been spit up and chewed up by the system in a very cruel way," Graham later mused. "I thought what happened to him was most unkind. I was reasonably convinced that that would probably also happen to me, but I wanted to do it so badly that I was willing to take the chance." Graham believed Bill Anlyan "was kind of in a pickle. He needed somebody to do this job. Not too many people were coming forward to volunteer." Graham also knew that Anlyan "wasn't going to redefine the dean's job and give over a lot of his power to me." And yet Graham stuck by Anlyan in a way that made things worse with Brodie. "Within a week of being in the dean's office," Graham recalled, "I was invited over for an interview by Keith Brodie who said to me something like 'Well, Charles and Andy Wallace called me regularly to discuss with me issues that are going on the medical center, and I would invite you to do the same.' I mean, basically inviting me into the same process that Charles had been in. My response to Keith was 'I negotiated this job with Bill Anlyan, I'm very satisfied with the negotiations that I went through. If I ever have anything to say to you about what's going on in the medical center, I will communicate to you through Bill Anlyan.' And I walked out."[64]

By then Charles Putman was focused on his duties as vice provost for research and development at Duke University, a position that increasingly meant strengthening Duke's ties to companies located in Research Triangle Park. This was not as simple as it sounds, however, for there was competition between corporate interests within the park, within Duke Medicine, and within the marketplace. There was DUMC's expanding AIDS work with Burroughs Wellcome, for example, and there were corresponding developments at Genentech. The collaboration with Burroughs Wellcome had progressed from early evaluation of AZT in the laboratory to using the drug in clinical trials and creating an HIV clinic for indigent patients at Duke. By the time the FDA licensed AZT for commercial distribution in 1987, Duke had also established an AIDS Treatment Evaluation Unit, the precursor of the university's AIDS Clinical Trials Group. By late 1988 researchers in the Duke unit had confirmed an independent study by Burroughs Wellcome showing that Retrovir, the brand name of its AZT drug, had greatly prolonged survival among some 5,000 AIDS sufferers.[65] As the *New York Times* reported that April, Retrovir was showing "promising results" for Burroughs Wellcome, even as Wellcome was "developing a blood-clotting drug that is expected to be ready to compete with TPA, made by Genentech Inc., probably in late 1989." Indeed, the *Times* reported, "Genentech . . . is also working on an AIDS virus-killer. Larger companies in the race to attack acquired immune deficiency syndrome include the Schering-Plough Corporation, the Bristol-Myers Company, Eli Lilly & Company and Hoffman LaRoche, Inc."[66]

By June of 1988 sales of Activase, Genentech's TPA drug, were at $100 million and expected to rise another $50–100 million by the year's end. Genentech also received a broad patent for TPA from the U.S. Patent Office that June and immediately filed suit, according to the *New York Times*, "against a team of companies that is closest to reaching the market with its own TPA drug." This team, the newspaper reported, "is composed of Burroughs Wellcome Inc. . . . and Genetics Institute Inc." But that was only one of the problems confronting Genentech. "Big Pharma" was betting big money on TPA, and Genentech, which was poised to become the first biotech company to transform into a major pharmaceutical firm, confronted numerous patent challenges and competitive research efforts throughout the world. Clinical trials were already under way in Italy, for example, where TPA was being compared with its vastly cheaper rival, streptokinase, for effectiveness in breaking up blood clots in heart attack victims. The results were due in 1990.[67]

It was in this context—of competition, litigation, and European trials—that Genentech halted production of TPA. In September of 1988 it decided it had enough TPA to meet demand for the foreseeable future.[68] By then Bill Anlyan was in the Allen administration building on the university campus. "Keith [Brodie] persuaded me that he seriously wanted me to be his chancellor, running the external affairs of the university," Anlyan wrote later. "I swallowed his bait hook, line, and sinker, until I got his proposed write-up of the job description of the chancellor's role, which was labeled 'chancellor for external affairs.'" Anlyan was wary of the label and "objected to this and said that my understanding when I said I would be willing to move from the Medical Center to the Allen Building was that I would be chancellor. [Philip] J. Baugh, vice chairman of the Board of Trustees and Alex McMahon, former chairman of the board, were doing the negotiating," Anlyan wrote, "and Keith Brodie finally agreed to my request. However, he did not tell me that he would not relinquish anything substantive when I moved to the Allen Building."[69]

It was now Robert Lefkowitz who made the crucial call to Snyderman at

Genentech. But Snyderman wasn't in. He was returning from a conference with the man who had first recruited him to Genentech, his good friend, Dave Martin. "We were driving back to San Francisco in my car, which was a Porsche 944T, a fun car to drive," Snyderman recalled. "We were having a great conversation talking about Genentech and all the exciting things we were going to do. We were getting ready to cross the Oakland Bay Bridge into San Francisco and going back to work at the end of an afternoon. I remember turning to Dave as we were driving, the vision of the Bay Bridge in front of me and the city beyond that, and telling Dave, 'You know, it's a remarkable thing I'm going to tell you. At this moment I feel as though I live in San Francisco, this is my city, I love it. This is the most beautiful place in the world.' We just kept on, drove back to Genentech. By that time it was 4:15 or 4:20 in the afternoon."

Snyderman found among his memos the phone message from Lefkowitz. "I remember calling up Bob. I was sitting in my office, and he said 'Ralph, I want you to get the time and the date, write it down on a slip of paper, because this phone call is going to change your life.' . . . Bob told me that I was at the top of the short list for Chancellor for Health Affairs, even though I hadn't been interested in the past, and the reason that they didn't consider me in the past is that I hadn't expressed any interest. Would I consider it now as the Institution really needed me, and they wanted me?" As soon as Snyderman said "'Bob, I would at least consider it at this time,' things moved very quickly from there. I was contacted formally by the Search Committee. I ended up having a meeting with a group from the Search Committee in New York at the apartment of [Duke trustee] Jerry Hudson. I don't remember everybody that was in the group, but it was a very memorable evening, because we spent maybe an hour and a half at Jerry Hudson's apartment then went to the 21 Club where we had a great meal, drank a lot of wine, and, by the end of the evening, were singing and toasting to Duke. I really felt reinvigorated in my love for the Institution."[70]

Snyderman had "never envisioned" returning to academic medicine, however, much less to Duke, and he was "extremely happy" at Genentech. "My time at Genentech was extremely important for my professional development as I became exposed to professions beyond those within academic medicine," Snyderman later noted. "I learned a tremendous amount about business, drive, initiative, organization and leadership. I also learned the meaning of having full responsibility for initiating and completing projects on which the institution depended for its survival. Had I not been amongst the senior leadership of Genentech, I would not have been interested in nor qualified for the position of Chancellor of Duke."[71]

In explaining his decision to accept the position, Snyderman later pointed to several factors. "First, subjectively and emotionally, this was an opportunity that was far too important for me to turn down given the fact that Duke was the place of my house staff medical training and my first academic position. Emotionally, it was a place that was treasured by my parents who both had died the previous year. Also," Snyderman continued, "my son Ted always wanted to go to Duke and was a Duke basketball crazy. He had planned to go to UC Berkeley, but certainly preferred to go to undergraduate school at Duke." The position also offered Snyderman a unique chance to reshape Duke Medicine. "The medical center was in a position for change, and change was inevitable," Snyderman recalled. "Of the 21 departments, 16 or more of their chairs were scheduled for retirement at the end of their five-year term. This meant that the new Chancellor would have the opportunity to rebuild the Medical Center."[72]

Snyderman believed he could use this opportunity to make a "real difference" in Duke Medicine. "I thought that this Medical Center had a reputation that it deserved, but in a sense, it was based on prior performance in that it needed to take the next very big jump, and a lot of it related to recruiting in outstanding chairs and a whole new group of faculty that were far more contemporary and had an opportunity to shape the future. I expressed to Keith Brodie and to the Search Committee that if I were to come back to Duke, this is what I would be excited about. It's not being a maintaining chancellor for health affairs, but reshaping the institution to be the leading or preeminent academic health center in the 21st century. That's what I came here to do. I think it fit in with Keith Brodie's desires for the chancellor of health affairs."[73]

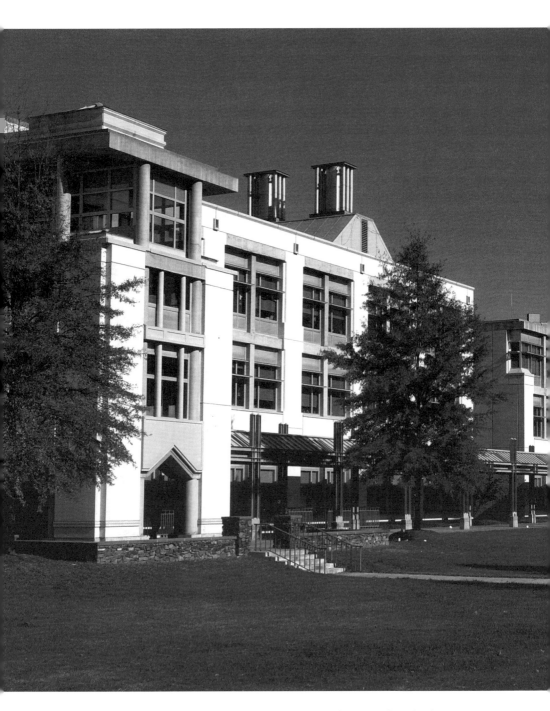

9.1 Levine Science Research Center. *Photograph by Butch Usery, Duke University Medical Center.*

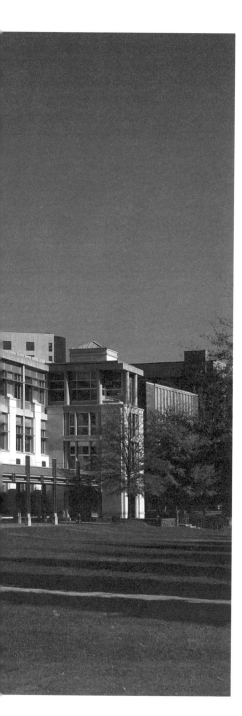

CHAPTER 9:

Duke Medicine and the Health Care Business, 1989–2004

Between 1989 and 2004 Ralph Snyderman and his colleagues developed a core academic business that helped Duke's medical center survive the revolution in managed health care. Keith Brodie assisted them, as did Brodie's successor, Nannerl O. Keohane, but both presidents also tried to keep the medical center "tail" from wagging the entire Duke Blue Devil. Keohane later explained. "I didn't come in with a strong priority to integrate the medical center more fully with the rest of the university. But very quickly, as I learned more about Duke . . . it became a very high priority for me to create a stronger sense of what we called *Big D*, all of Duke together. . . . The creation of the health system has been a new centrifugal force, however, which creates tensions within the medical enterprise as well as over against the university."[1]

Snyderman's Early Initiatives

Ralph Snyderman returned to Duke with several general goals in mind. One was to update the basic sciences at DUMC. Snyderman understood that the future of medicine would be based upon an understanding of how genes are structured, how they work, and what products they made. Snyderman wanted Duke Medicine to lead in the application of genomics to the human condition, and he wanted department heads who would lead their departments to unravel the important questions in biomedical research. He also wanted to prepare DUMC for changes in clinical care. Managed care was obviously coming, and rather than let it wash over DUMC and scavenge for pieces, Snyderman intended to prepare Duke Medicine for the changes ahead.

Snyderman's most immediate goal was to study the medical center and to have it study itself to begin planning for the future. Each week for his first several months on the job, the new chancellor did a 90-minute "walking around" visit designed to expose him "to a balanced collection of clinical, research, and education programs and services" at DUMC: "Finding out what's where and how things work. . . . Meeting people. . . . Finding out what's on peoples' minds." Snyderman considered this a "good, quick way . . . to find out how our employees perceive their work."[2] Snyderman also launched a major planning effort after taking office in July 1989. "Now that I have assumed the leadership role for the Medical Center," he wrote to the faculty and senior staff in the summer of 1989, "I have embarked on a series of departmental reviews that will enable me to identify the strengths, weaknesses and resource needs of the institution. This process will result in a plan to move us forward." Snyderman hoped to gain a "firm understanding" of what the faculty and staff had as their goals, and he combined formal visits to each department with the "walking around" visits mentioned above. He also held informal get-togethers at his home and had the director and chief planning officer of Duke Hospital, Duncan Yaggy, speak individually with many faculty and staff.[3]

By early August, Snyderman had the planning agenda set: "I have scheduled a retreat at the President's House on September 6 from 7:30AM to Noon," he wrote on August 3. "At that meeting, we will begin the discussion of academic and business plans for the next three years. My goal is to have clear and substantive statements of objectives and strategies and means of following progress for each unit by the end of December." The departmental statements would "then be collected and distributed for discussion at a retreat to be held after New Year's. At that time," he wrote to the department heads and staff, "we will have an opportunity to use the work that you have done to discuss our directions and our priorities, and to develop a plan for the future of the entire Medical Center."[4]

Snyderman's plans for Duke Medicine combined what was happening at Genentech with the personal and institutional goals that he and Brodie had discussed. And it was these plans that prevailed. In pursuing these goals, Snyderman relied on his experience both as a physician-scientist and as a biotech business liaison at Genentech. "Setting up models, testing them, learning from them, and improving them. That's what I did in research," he explained. And that's also what he did to some extent in leading the medical center, especially after 1993, when he confronted managed care and created the Duke University Health System. Snyderman and his advisers put together a complex, integrated-delivery health system that included a number of interrelated businesses, several of which proved unprofitable and were later sold.[5]

Snyderman considered it his "most important obligation" to focus on the academics of the institution, specifically, to build up and modernize the basic sciences. "They had not recruited an outside chair since 1968," Snyderman explained, "and had not played a leading role in the major emerging science of genetics." Between 1989 and 1992, Snyderman recalled, he "focused on bringing in the best scientists and making sure we had the right resources and the right programs to bridge disciplines." His first three major appointments were Dr. Dale Purves, a leading neurobiologist and a member of the National Academy of Sciences, as chairman of the Department of Neurobiology; Dr. Michael P. Sheetz as chairman of the Department of Cell Biology; and Dr. Anthony R. Means as chairman of the Department of Pharmacology. "The recruitment of these three chairs early in my tenure was indicative of the high priority I set for reforming the School of Medicine through the recruitment of outstanding chairs as the positions became open."[6]

Of less immediate concern to Snyderman were issues of institutional culture and the concept of university oneness. "When I returned to Duke, I did not envision making major changes in the overall governance of the Medical Center. The strong departmental structure had worked well for Duke's initial sixty years."[7] Yet Snyderman was also acutely aware that Duke Medicine "did not have an institutional way of governance, that the departments functioned quite independently, they were almost independent businesses." The new chancellor found the situation "almost like Somalia" when he returned. "We had independent warlords. . . . Some chairs were very powerful. . . . They were the power in running the Medical Center." In trying to convince these chiefs to become "a more coherent nation," as it were, to give up a little so that "everybody will get a heck of a lot more," Snyderman said, "I met tremendous suspicion from a few. Tremendous suspicion. Nevertheless, the key to the success of the Medical Center depended on an integrated planning and governance structure."[8]

Snyderman made it clear from the start that he was in charge and that planning for the "entire Medical Center" would take precedence over the traditional department-centered vision at Duke. One person who understood Snyderman's plans was Duncan Yaggy, the hospital's chief planning officer. Yaggy noted in a letter to Snyderman that Snyderman's staff would "carry the influence that cloaks a member of the chancellor's staff, but they will not exercise your authority. You will, and your authority will remain undivided. I start with that assumption because many other people make the opposite assumption: That you should delegate portions of your authority to individuals who will take charge of clinical programs, or education programs, or research programs, or space allocation, or money, or (fill in the blank). I think that that assumption is wrong and that acting on it would defeat the effort to make department chairmen and other unit heads truly accountable to you."[9]

Snyderman also applied to Duke Medicine his experience at Genentech as a businessman and liaison with universities. While Genentech applied management systems and philosophies to the entire company, DUMC did things "the Duke way"—which was pretty much the way each department chairman saw fit. As Snyderman described it, "One could think of the medical center as having consisted of, roughly, twenty-one fairly independent departments with faculty and divisions. It was almost like a shopping mall in which you have a whole bunch of businesses that are in the same place, same time but run their own operations. And when I came in here, the initial task was to look at these individual entities and try to make them the best that I could."[10]

THE GUSTO PROJECT

Proving particularly important for Duke Medicine were the kind of university-biotech alliances that Snyderman had supported in California. The first of these alliances was formed in 1990 and contributed significantly to both the demise of the medical center's traditional power structure and the foundation of a new one. Between 1990 and 1993, DUMC managed one of the largest heart attack studies ever conducted. The study compared the benefits and risks of streptokinase and tissue plasminogen activator (TPA) in treating heart attack victims at various times up to 30 days after the onset of their heart attack. The study, known as GUSTO (Global Utilization of Streptokinase and TPA for Occluded Arteries), began shortly after Genentech sold 60 percent of its stock in February 1990 to the large Swiss health-products company, Roche Holdings Ltd. Roche believed in TPA's ultimate success, and it paid $2.1 billion for the Genentech stock. Proceeds from the sale enabled Genentech to pour more than $40 million into the GUSTO trials.[11]

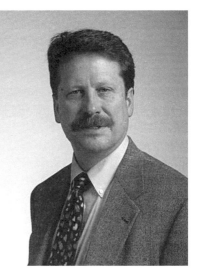

9.2 Dr. Robert M. Califf. *Duke University Medical Center.*

GUSTO involved Duke Medicine in the larger corporate wars then being waged by the world's biggest pharmaceutical companies. American physicians preferred TPA; European physicians preferred streptokinase; and clinical trials in Europe were favoring the cheaper streptokinase.[12] Genentech went to great lengths to assure that GUSTO's findings were above question. The company had no access to the data prior to publication, and it played no role in running the trials, which were conducted by an independent steering committee. Participating researchers could not own stock in Genentech, and they were also barred from acting as consultants to the company for at least a year after the final results were released. Dr. Eric J. Topol, a Duke-trained cardiologist at the Cleveland Clinic Foundation, directed the study and the Duke Databank for Cardiovascular Diseases, Eugene Stead's brainchild and the largest and longest running computerized cardiology databank in the world, served as clearinghouse for the data collected. Duke cardiologist Dr. Robert M. Califf collaborated closely with Topol on the trials, which included independent experts at academic medical centers in the United States and abroad. "We were very concerned that the European studies had missed the point," Califf later told the Raleigh *News & Observer.* He also stressed that it was not his goal "to compare the clot busters—it was to find out if a doctor can save more lives if he moves faster to open arteries after a heart attack."[13] [Figure 9.2]

The GUSTO trials involved more than 41,000 patients with confirmed heart attacks in 15 countries, including some 23,000 patients in the United States. The results were not what many had predicted. "Most experts expected the results to again show T.P.A. to be no better than its rival," the *New York Times* reported on May 1, 1993. "Confounding predictions, the trial showed a narrow but definable advantage for T.P.A. . . . The most successful strategy was the one in which the entire T.P.A. dosage was administered within 90 minutes, with most of the dose injected in a vein within the first hour."[14]

GUSTO fostered two important developments at Duke. It laid the foundation for one of DUMC's core academic businesses, the Duke Clinical Research Institute, and it also further aggravated the war over angiography. GUSTO not only demonstrated DUMC's ability to coordinate large-scale, multisite clinical trials throughout the world; it also provided Duke Medicine with the experience and infrastructure needed to conduct future megatrials—from site, data, and financial management to statistical analysis, technology, regulatory affairs, and personnel. Califf later lauded Snyderman's role in helping create the Duke Clinical Research Institute. "We benefited from Ralph Snyderman's leadership when he returned from Genentech," Califf said. "Because of his experience in a biotechnology firm, he understood that it takes a solid infrastructure to do clinical trials well, which most academic medical centers didn't—and don't—understand. Many still think you just go out onto the wards and treat a few patients. But Ralph had been functioning in a very regulated biotech community dealing with the FDA and he understood what we needed."[15]

GUSTO also exacerbated the angiography wars between the Departments of Radiology and Medicine at Duke. Not surprisingly, Califf, the cardiologist, was a key figure in that struggle. Califf had obtained both undergraduate and M.D. degrees from Duke before making the critical biotech connection in California as an intern and resident at the University of California, San Francisco. Returning to Duke in 1980, Califf served as a cardiology fellow in the Department of Medicine and became a certified specialist in both internal medicine and cardiovascular diseases and a fellow of the American College of Cardiology. More important, Califf directed the critical angiographic substudy of GUSTO. According to the Duke Clinical Research Institute, "The key finding of this 2431-patient GUSTO-I substudy was that blood flow to the heart muscle at 90 minutes mirrors outcomes at 30 days; that is, alteplase [generic TPA] resulted in both superior blood flow and superior outcomes compared with other therapies. This finding provided hard evidence that restoring blood flow to the heart muscle more quickly and completely corresponds directly with favorable outcomes."[16] The *New York Times* was even more to the point, noting in its May 1, 1993, story on GUSTO's results that "Dr. Robert M. Califf of Duke University, an important official in the study, said that angiogram X-rays had helped prove T.P.A.'s value conclusively."[17]

CHANGES IN DEPARTMENTAL STRUCTURE

Califf was not among the 200 physicians who signed a petition four days later, on May 5, calling for Snyderman's resignation. All of the signers were members of the Department of Medicine, and they were protesting Snyderman's decision not to reappoint their chairman, Dr. Joseph Greenfield Jr. Snyderman, in explaining his decision, denied that Greenfield, 61, had been forced out; it was simply a matter of the 10-year limit as chairman that Greenfield had agreed to in 1983. "There are a number of individuals in the department of medicine, primarily in the cardiology department, who are intensely loyal to Dr. Greenfield and who do not think he's been given the respect he deserves," Snyderman told reporters for the Raleigh *News & Observer*. The reporters, in asking physicians and others what they thought of Snyderman, found that "some see him as an ambitious, arrogant leader more interested in prestige than in the day-to-day operations of the medical center. Others view him as a visionary who is taking bold steps to prepare Duke Medical Center for upcoming changes in the health care system." One perceptive physician attributed the turmoil to the fact that "the nation's health care crisis has doctors on edge and they are just reacting to pressure."[18]

Snyderman received critical support from a number of important individuals at Duke. Yvonne Dunlap, a member of a minority advisory committee, told the *News & Observer* that Snyderman's opponents were at fault: "These are the people who are fighting so Duke doesn't have to change. . . . They are fighting to keep things exactly the same." Snyderman also received guarded praise from pediatrician Lois A. Pounds, head of DUMC's Advisory Committee on the Status of Women. "He has preliminarily delivered on what we have asked," she told the Raleigh newspaper, "and that's one step further than we've taken in the past." The chairman of Duke's board of trustees, Philip J. ("Jack") Baugh, pointed the journalists to a letter Snyderman had received in support of his actions. "He has a letter signed by the chairs of every one of those departments supporting his remaining. . . . I don't know how much more I need."[19]

Snyderman reviewed 11 chairmen for reappointment between 1989 and 1993, and Dr. Carl Ravin, chairman of Radiology, was one of only two reappointed. "Academic medical institutions are assessed in large part by the strengths of their departments," Snyderman later wrote, "with the reputations of the schools often being judged by the stature of their Departments of Medicine and Surgery in the clinical departments and Biochemistry and Microbiology/Genetics in the basic science departments." Among the nine chairmen not reappointed or who had their responsibilities altered were the chairman of Psychiatry, Bernard Carroll; the chairman of Biochemistry, Robert Hill; the chairman of Microbiology and Immunology, Wolfgang Joklik; and DUMC's two most powerful clinicians, Greenfield in Medicine and Dr. David Sabiston, who, at age 68, was ready to retire as chair of Surgery. In other words, Snyderman was changing the faculty in the way he had planned, and he was trying to complete the changes before Dr. Nannerl (Nan) Keohane succeeded Dr. Keith Brodie as president of Duke University in July of 1993.[20]

Snyderman fulfilled much of his mission in rejuvenating the basic sciences at DUMC, and he also oversaw the creation of several new departments. The early chair appointments of Purves, Sheets, and Means were the first of 25 eventually made by Snyderman. In 1991, a new department, the Department of Radiation Oncology, was created out of the divisions of nuclear medicine and radiation/oncology. The department's first chairman, Dr. Leonard R. Prosnitz, was nationally known for developing the use of alternative therapies to treat cancer and Hodgkin's lymphoma with various combinations of lumpectomy, radiation, and hyperthermia. Patient volumes doubled during Prosnitz's five years as chairman, while the number of faculty increased fivefold during his tenure. Prosnitz's successor, Dr. Edward C. Halperin, seized this momentum to expand the department to various locations in North Carolina and Virginia. He also oversaw construction of the new facilities for radiation oncology at Duke Hospital and at Raleigh Community Hospital.

It was also in 1991 that Duke's trustees approved five interdisciplinary research themes as part of Duke Medicine's strategic long-range plan. These research themes—genetics, immunology, neurosciences, structural biology, and signal transduction (the way cells, organs, and molecules communicate)—were identical to the expanded list of research themes articulated by Dr. James Wyngaarden and the other members of the advisory committee of the Howard Hughes Medical Institute in the late 1980s.[21] Implementation of the new research plans was followed by changes in personnel and departmental responsibilities. In 1993, Dr. Robert Hill was succeeded as chairman of the Biochemistry Department by Dr. Christian R. H. Raetz, an M.D.-Ph.D. who, as vice president for basic research at Merck Research Laboratories in New Jersey, had shepherded several drugs through the FDA, including the cholesterol-lowering medicine Zocor.[22] Although Wolfgang Joklik remained chairman of Microbiology, the Department of Microbiology and Immunology was reorganized between 1992 and 1994. Immunology was established as a separate department in 1993, and its first chairman, Thomas F. Tedder, Ph.D., is the current chair.[23]

By 1993 Joklik's Department of Microbiology had lost most of its genetics research to the new Department of Genetics, which was formed in 1991. Genetics' first chairman, Dr. Joseph R. Nevins, had received his Ph.D. in microbiology at Duke before studying the transcription of DNA into messenger RNA as both a fellow and a faculty member at Rockefeller University. Returning to Duke in 1987, Nevins, a Howard Hughes Investigator, became chairman of the new Department of Genetics in 1991 and continued as chair when the department was merged with the Department of Microbiology in 2002 to form the Department of Molecular Genetics and Microbiology.[24] At the same time, Dr. Brigid L. M. Hogan was appointed chair of the Department of Cell Biology. Hogan, a world leader in developmental biology and stem cell research, was the first woman to be appointed chair of a basic science department at Duke.[25]

Snyderman failed to dislodge Duke Medicine's top two powerbrokers, however, by the time Nan Keohane arrived as the university's new president in July 1993. He was forced to compromise. Greenfield was permitted to stay on in medicine until Sabiston's successor was appointed in surgery, and Snyderman himself had to negotiate a deal with the university's trustees: he agreed to a three-year reappointment rather than the standard five so that Keohane could have a hand in selecting her own senior management team.

The PDC and the Revolution of 1993

Snyderman's most difficult initial challenge was to integrate the PDC with the medical center in order to mobilize Duke Medicine for the rapidly changing clinical environment. Not only was the PDC the economic engine driving Duke's academic medical center, but the clinic's two major sources of fuel, the departments of Medicine and Surgery, were also, Snyderman later wrote, "a tremendous strength of the institution and a key to its lofty reputation. Dr. Sabiston was a pillar of the Medical Center and Academic Surgery for decades and led the development of the nation's strongest Department of Surgery. Nationally prominent leaders such as Drs. Stead and Wyngaarden built a top 5 Department of Medicine at Duke."[26]

Yet by the early 1990s it was also clear to Snyderman "that the structure which had sustained and benefited Duke for the initial 60 years was facing tremendous threat from the changing nature of clinical care and the movement of managed care into North Carolina." He explained: "This meant that departments such as Medicine, which relied so heavily on their clinical revenue to fund academic activities, were experiencing increasing pressure on their clinical margins. This led clinical departments within the Medical Center to compete with each other for clinical revenues. This was particularly troublesome between the Departments of Medicine and Radiology where a great deal of contention arose in the early 1990s in regard to the development of invasive intravascular intervention." By 1992, Snyderman was convinced that "there needed to be far greater collaboration, planning, and coordination so that the institution could approach the clinical 'marketplace' as a whole, focusing on the needs of the patient. A series of independent, competitive departments couldn't survive. The issue of shifting the balance of dominance from a small number of clinical departments to more cohesive institutional planning led to a great deal of angst between the Chancellor's office and the Department of Medicine."[27]

The major force that impeded Duke Medicine's shift to institutional planning was the PDC. Or, more specifically, it was the autonomy and power that the clinical chairmen derived from the PDC, especially the chairs of Medicine and Surgery, that had enabled Duke to flourish as a series of independent departments. The PDC is not actually part of Duke University and it never has been. It is the private practice plan of the attending senior faculty in Duke's school of medicine. Only in 1972, in fact, when faced with a legal challenge from the Internal Revenue Service, with the planning of Duke North, and with the construction of Durham Regional Hospital, had the PDC organized as a general partnership under the laws of North Carolina. And only then did it enter a "written agreement formalizing the terms under which the partnership would engage in medical practice through the use of Duke Hospital and other University facilities." A physician had to be on the school's faculty to be a member of the PDC and to practice there, and members of the PDC had priority on beds at Duke Hospital.[28]

Like almost everything else in Duke Medicine, the PDC was part of the great upheaval of 1993. Abandoning its general partnership structure, the practice became a limited liability partnership and adopted a revised operating agreement with the university. What it failed to do, however, at least initially, was to eliminate the administrative structure that provided Greenfield and Sabiston with much of their money and power. The PDC consisted of only two divisions, Medicine and Surgery, each of which had its own separate administrative structure and served as the umbrella for several specific departments. The two divisions handled all billing and collections for the departments within their respective division, and they also disbursed payments to those departments. Radiology, for example, was part of the surgical division of the PDC. The chiefs of the two PDC divisions, however, Greenfield and Sabiston, ran the practice as a dictatorship and not in partnership with the other departmental chairmen who sat on the PDC board. "Again, you look at the partnership meeting," the PDC's Paul Newman recalled, "and we're technically a partnership of physicians. You only had one meeting at the end of the year, as an annual meeting, and all they would talk about would be the retirement plan. And Dr. Sabiston was smart, and he would say, 'Any further business? And with none in front of us, Thank you very much for coming.' . . . Sabiston and Greenfield really ran the place. It wasn't a partnership of doctors."[29]

The restructuring of the PDC in 1993 was intended in part to make the practice more democratic, more of a true partnership, which also meant acknowledging the increasing power of the Department of Radiology. Indeed, the angiography wars and Radiology's rise to power were central to reform at the PDC. Newman, in explaining the restructuring, pointed to "some internal pressures of different cost allocations," and used a revealing example. "If a patient came in on surgical PDC and there was radiology done . . . there were two separate bills— . . . a bill for surgical PDC [with] . . . the radiology as part of it, and . . . then [one for] medical PDC. . . . [A]ll of that money [stayed in] the medical PDC bucket, and then we did transfers back and forth and allocations of cost." In other words, Radiology was filling the PDC's coffers but getting no voice, in turn, as to the disposition of the PDC's reserve funds controlled by Greenfield and Sabiston, which by 1993 amounted to almost $160 million.[30]

The structure of the PDC did not change until 1995, however, when, in the absence of Greenfield and Sabiston, the PDC amended its operating agreement to consolidate the business operations of the two divisions. Newman explained: "The chairmen looked at this and said, well, there's a lot of duplication; there's some efficiencies we can get out of one practice. We need to start—because of the advent of managed care coming in and competition, really, healthcare competition—we need to be more attractive. We need to put ourselves out as one to providers and not as a medical division and a surgical division; we need to gain efficiencies; we need to be more multidisciplinary in our care of medicine, so as we run the clinics and manage the clinics, you need to actually merge medicine and surgery physicians together around like services, so we can have a multidisciplinary approach and one-stop shopping for patients." The new structure also dispersed power and control at the PDC. "And it really has changed over the last, I'd say, ten years, really since Sabiston and Greenfield [stepped down] and—I think Ralph has been a part of it," Newman said of Snyderman in 2004, "but I would not sell the PDC chairmen out. I would say that [it was] their decision to come together as a group, to be one, to have a single voice, and it started with Chuck Hammond as the chairman of the PDC for four years and then the last six years it's been Carl Ravin. I think he certainly has been a proponent of that, but he also wants to show the physicians that they have a strong union and strong representation."[31]

The PDC and Duke Hospital had always funded much of Duke Medicine's core missions—of teaching, research, and clinical care—by charging 20 to 30 percent more than other hospitals and physician groups. Both Duke, DUMC, and its patients, moreover, had benefited immensely from this mutually reinforcing relationship. In the case of the PDC, for example, it was this 20–30 percent "margin" that, after deducting for PDC payments to the university and to other departmental and building funds, gave the medical and surgical divisions of the PDC the "reserve" funds that Greenfield and Sabiston distributed back to the medical school departments for unfunded research and teaching. As one close observer put it, the reserve funds gave Greenfield and Sabiston the power "to keep the faculty moving in the direction that you wanted them to move in"; moreover, "in the eyes of the leadership of the School of Medicine, the dean, the chancellor and ultimately the University (the people who knew what was going on in the University)," the PDC saved them from having to transfer money "to help support research and teaching" in the medical school. "There is a lot of money that flows out of the PDC over to the school, that ultimately flows back to the departments, that helps fund unfunded research and teaching."[32]

A CRISIS AT DUMC

By 1993, however, that cash flow was subsiding and DUMC was losing its margins in the face of cost-cutting HMOs and reduced federal funding. The situation was becoming particularly dire, as Snyderman noted, in the Department of Medicine, which was not only losing its margins but was also aggressively competing with the Department of Radiology for patients. Many patients previously seen and treated through the Department of Medicine were now being referred directly to Radiology by their primary care providers, the HMO "gatekeepers." It was at this point, Snyderman recalled, as Medicine and Radiology were "almost to the point of going to war with each other," that he decided that "this model of a free-standing shopping center, almost a flea market, was not going to work."[33]

That's also when Snyderman showed the spreadsheets to Duke's new president, Nannerl O. Keohane. Keohane had spent the previous 13 years as president of Wellesley College and had no experience dealing with a major academic medical center. "I knew it was complex," she later said. "I think maybe there were a number of warning signals on the horizon, but when I came, the general word on the street was 'The medical center is very healthy and one of the strongest parts of the university, so you will have plenty of time to learn about it. There are no crises facing you in that area.'" And she got that prognosis, she said, from both inside and outside observers alike. "But the reason I say this is to emphasize that, at least from my perspective, the pressures of managed care, especially in North Carolina, and the rapid transformation of health care was not something which was very visible in 1992. But by 1994, it had become extremely prominent, so that transition occurred while I was becoming president. I didn't come in with that foresight."[34]

It was therefore all the more surprising, Keohane recalled, when "six months later Ralph came in to my office and presented me with some spreadsheets that showed that unless we took some fairly specific action and some tough decisions, the lines were going to cross in the wrong direction and we were going to be facing some red ink. So the turmoil came relatively quickly after the fall of 1993." The situation grew much worse during the debate over Snyderman's reappointment, when many of the resentments reemerged that had first surfaced in May of that year over Snyderman's initial decision not to reappoint Joseph Greenfield. "There were a number of people who were supportive and a number of people who were critical of his work," Keohane later explained. "Basically I was asked to be involved in the decision about whether he would be asked to serve another term, and that was one of the first, most complex things on my plate when I came."[35] For Snyderman, personally, it was a "horrible time . . . when I went through my first review. . . . When there were scurrilous rumors about me that were patently untrue. . . . Having so many people in my own department, the Department of Medicine, sign a letter saying that I should not be renewed. That was very difficult."[36]

The question Keohane faced was whether to extend Snyderman's term to a full five-year term or have him step down in 1997 in accordance with the three-year agreement he had made with the trustees. The Raleigh *News & Observer* announced her decision in May of 1994. "On the recommendation of Keohane," the newspaper reported, "Duke's board of trustees last week extended Snyderman's appointment as chancellor for health affairs and dean of the medical school until June of 1999." The board's decision was bad news for Joseph Greenfield, however; as the newspaper reported, Greenfield had been allowed "to stay until another key position, that of chief of surgery, was filled. Duke recently made an appointment to that spot and a search for a new chief of medicine is next."[37]

Dr. Robert W. Anderson became the new chairman of Surgery at Duke in 1994, and over the next nine years, he facilitated the department's collaboration with both the hospital and the PDC to ensure that the faculty's private practice "was maximally efficient and effective and that its governance and other infrastructure systems were appropriately developed and fully realized."[38] Anderson was succeeded as chairman in 2003 by Dr. Danny O. Jacobs, an African American surgeon whose appointment followed close on the minority appointments of the first woman department chair, Brigid Hogan of the Department of Cell Biology, and the first African American department chair, Dr. Haywood Brown, who was appointed head of the Department of Obstetrics and Gynecology in 2002. In the meantime, Dr. Barton Haynes, a physician-scientist who specializes in human immunology and retroviral research, succeeded Joseph Greenfield as chairman of the Department of Medicine. Haynes had followed Snyderman as head of the division of rheumatic-genetic disease at Duke, and he would serve as Medicine's chair until 2002, when he stepped down to become the full-time director of the Duke Human Vaccine Institute. Haynes was succeeded as chairman in 2003 by the chief of cardiology at Duke, Dr. Pascal J. Goldschmidt.

Snyderman later reflected on the "important people" who supported him during the 1993–94 crisis, including David Sabiston and the other clinical chairmen (with the exception, of course, of Greenfield). "I will always want to recognize, extol, and give credit for my survival to the chairman of the board, Jack Baugh," Snyderman later stressed. "We talked a lot about what I was doing. He believed in me. He understood that this was an assault on an individual, who in a time of vulnerability was doing the right thing. And he understood that a heck of a lot of noise doesn't mean that an individual should be drummed out of office. . . . The board ultimately stood by me. Mary Semans stood with me. My family and other key people stood with me. And it was just enough to get through. And I didn't give up."[39]

The Duke Clinical Research Institute

Between 1994 and his second reappointment in 1999, Snyderman worked with his colleagues at Duke to manage managed care, to develop a core academic business at the medical center, and to shift Duke Medicine to an institutional form of planning and governance. Their approach combined a focus on biotech, Bayh-Dole, and large clinical trials with the aggressive acquisition of health and medical care businesses, hospitals, and private practices that in 1998 became part of the new Duke University Health System.

Their most successful effort, the Duke Clinical Research Institute (DCRI), was formed in 1996 and grew out of the Duke Databank for Cardiovascular Disease, a huge databank of computerized coronary angiography records started in the late 1960s. The more immediate origins of the DCRI, however, lay in Dr. Rob Califf's handling of GUSTO and its related studies. In 1992, for example, in association with several of the GUSTO principals, Califf published in the *Journal of the American College of Cardiology* an important article titled "Confronting the Issues of Patient Safety and Investigator Conflict of Interest in an International Clinical Trial on Myocardial Reperfusion." This was followed in 1993 by the publication of GUSTO's results, and in 1995 by the FDA's approval of a faster intravenous regimen for Activase, Genentech's TPA drug. Califf was named associate vice chancellor for clinical research at Duke in 1995, and in 1996, at the time DCRI was formed, he was named editor-in-chief of the *American Heart Journal*.[40]

"When I became chancellor," Snyderman recalled, "the cardiovascular database and cardiovascular research was well-developed." What Snyderman helped Califf do was move that research out of the Department of Medicine, where "it was flourishing but, as departments became more and more financially strapped," Snyderman explained, "it was really hemmed in, being a divisional function within a department. Recognizing the fact that clinical research was very important and should have an institutional face with the leadership of Rob Califf, who truly is a leader in clinical research nationally—we decided to institutionalize what had been cardiovascular research into a much broader institutional effort called DCRI. We backed it with a loan. We backed it with essentially a lot of promissory notes, and love and tenderness and appreciation, and the development of a business rigor, in which I give them all the credit. We played a facilitating role, and they grew it into this internationally prominent academic research organization."[41]

The DCRI built on GUSTO's excellent foundations with additional cardiovascular trials but quickly branched out into large clinical trials in psychiatry, genetics, neurology, rheumatology, and infectious diseases. "Soon, the same proven models were being applied to other therapeutic areas," the institute explains on its web site, "and the DCRI's extensive mentoring and fellowship programs ensured that the lessons learned were passed on to the next generation of scientists." One of those lessons was the difference between academic and commercial research. Dr. Robert L. Taber, director of DUMC's Office of Science and Technology, explained: "The thing about DCRI is it's academic—Rob [Califf] calls it an academic research organization, ARO." Taber noted that DCRI was in competition with clinical research organizations such as Quintiles and PAREXEL. "These people do clinical trials for industry," Taber stressed. "So if a drug company wants to do a trial with 5,000 patients, they go to these people, and they organize it for them. But they work for the company. And they do whatever the company tells them to do. When we work with a company, we get to publish everything we do. So if the trial ends up badly [from the commercial point of view], we get to publish it. We can also often use what we find for other purposes. We can analyze the data different ways. . . . [T]he Duke Clinical Research Institute does a hundred million dollars worth of business a year [and publishes] over 250 peer reviewed papers a year. So we get tremendous academic output."[42]

Nurturing DCRI was part of the larger approach that Snyderman and his colleagues developed to manage the revolution in managed care while also maintaining DUMC's traditional missions of excellence in research, teaching, and clinical care. "The nation is trying to define the role of academic medicine for the next century," Snyderman told a journalist in 1995, "and we want to be one of the institutions that provides that model." Which was not an outrageous ambition: DUMC had been rated among the top five medical centers in the United States for the previous three years.[43]

The Advent of Managed Care

Duke Medicine also found itself caught in what *Time* magazine called "a collision between money and medicine that is occurring in hospitals all over the country—nowhere more than in the elite academic medical centers that have always led the way in training the next generation of doctors, inventing the next generation of cures, and providing them to those who could least afford to pay. . . . All across the country, teaching hospitals are trying to figure out how to marry progress with profits, how to come up with the money that will let them continue to lead the world in death-defying discoveries, without going bankrupt in the process."[44] Indeed, by the late 1990s, financial failures had scarred the medical wings of Stanford and Georgetown universities. The University of Pennsylvania Health System was losing more than $100 million a year. Other universities, including Tulane, St. Louis, Indiana, and George Washington, were forced to sell their medical centers. And in 1998 the newly created Duke University Health System would inherit DUMC's own HMO, WellPath, which was losing $12 million a year.[45]

Running DUMC as a business was not something Snyderman eagerly embraced. "Because I still feel uncomfortable when I talk about the healthcare *business*," he recently explained. "I feel as though I am selling my heritage. My heritage was totally academic. I was a member of the Department of Medicine. I was the typical physician-scientist faculty member, and hence buried in my own activities. And to think of medicine as a business would be very offensive. . . . I still have trouble getting those words out."[46] But like it or not DUMC was a big business by the mid-1990s. With 8,000 employees, 1,000 faculty, and a budget of $700 million, it was one of the nation's 10 largest academic medical centers. It provided care for more than 35,000 inpatients and 550,000 outpatients each year. Its house staff included 855 residents and fellows who were enrolled in 60 training programs across all medical and surgical specialties. And by 1995 Duke's Medical Scientist Training Program had 230 biomedical science trainees—up from the 6 who first enrolled in the M.D.-Ph.D. program in 1966. DUMC also contained seven multidisciplinary centers of excellence—the Heart Center, Comprehensive Cancer Center, Eye Center, Stroke Center, Arthritis Center, Center for Digestive Health, and the Center for the Study of Aging and Human Development—where patients with complex illnesses are referred for diagnoses and treatment and "teams of clinicians and scientists approach health problems on multiple fronts, joining forces in both clinical care and research."[47]

One of the keys to operating DUMC as a successful business, of course, was to have its revenues exceed its expenses. But that seemed almost impossible for most academic medical centers in the 1990s. By the time the Clinton health plan failed in 1994, the majority of Americans with private insurance were enrolled in HMOs, and most of them were enrolled in for-profit HMOs that were competing with one another, that were eliminating what they saw as waste from the health care system, limiting choice of doctors and treatment, cutting costs by curbing tests and surgery, curtailing referrals to specialists, shortening and eliminating hospital stays, paying lower fees, promoting preventive medicine, and creating efficiencies wherever possible. Unfortunately for DUMC, its heavily specialized clinical care cost 25 to 30 percent more than market rates and that would not cut it under managed care. Specialists were becoming increasingly dependent on primary care physicians—the HMOs' gatekeepers—who referred patients only to specialists who had cut deals with the HMOs to be part of the referral network. Patients no longer paid their physicians directly and waited for insurance reimbursements to cover all or part of the costs; that system was all but gone. HMOs now paid primary care providers a capitation fee—a fixed amount per patient per year to cover all primary care expenses for that year. "It's the corporatization of health care," one market analyst said late in 1994. "And what's wrong with that?"[48]

Snyderman put together a leadership team that assumed managed care was coming to North Carolina and that Duke Medicine should control the process as much as possible. The team included William J. Donelan, a political scientist who holds a master's degree in management sciences from Duke's School of Business and who had worked with the PDC and Duke Hospital for almost two decades; Mark C. Rogers, M.D., a former associate dean at Johns Hopkins University who also holds a master's degree in business administration from Wharton; Mike Israel, an experienced hospital administrator who holds a master's degree in public health administration from Yale; and Robert Taber, Ph.D., a molecular biologist/entrepreneur recruited by Snyderman to make Bayh-Dole happen at Duke. If the team had one fleeting advantage in addressing managed care, it was DUMC's location. Managed care arrived in North Carolina later than it did in states with large urban populations. But by 1993 it was clearly in play, accounting for 6 to 7 percent of the state's health care market; 13 percent in the Research Triangle area; but only 3 percent of Duke Medicine's payroll mix.[49]

BENEFITS AND CHALLENGES FOR THE DUKE HEALTH SYSTEM

Snyderman and his colleagues moved quickly to cut costs and increase revenue. "We are taking the steps necessary to transform Duke University Medical Center into the Duke Health System," Mark Rogers announced in December 1993. "With health care reform moving so rapidly, we either have to make the changes ourselves or someone else will do it for us." Rogers made his remarks in connection with the announcement that Duke had formed a nonprofit subsidiary to develop a network of primary care providers in the Triangle and surrounding counties. The purpose of the subsidiary was to acquire existing medical practices and to affiliate DUMC with family practitioners, pediatricians, and obstetrician-gynecologists who would not only provide primary care but would also refer their patients to the specialists at Duke. The Raleigh *News & Observer* explained: "The current trend in health care reform, especially in North Carolina, puts high value on primary care doctors, funneling patients to the basic, less expensive care before allowing them to see specialists. Previously, most people decided which doctor they wanted to see, and the insurance company paid all or part of the bills. Insurance companies increasingly are insisting on the managed care scheme, not only because it saves money by forcing people to the less-expensive primary care doctor, but because it provides patients with preventive care that general practitioners are more apt to give."[50]

Much as the Clinical Research Institute would soon emerge from the Duke Databank for Cardiovascular Diseases, the new Duke University Affiliated Physicians, Inc. (DUAP), arose from Duke Medicine's existing clinical networks. DUAP grew out of the Affiliations and Outreach Program (1980), which was based, in turn, on decades of Duke's experience conducting referral clinics in outlying communities. Strengthening these existing connections became part of DUMC's strategy to create a network of primary care physicians and to link Duke's medical center to community physicians and hospitals. William Donelan helped shape that strategy. "Duke University Hospital—which was the mainstay of the clinical enterprise of Duke, along with the faculty practice, the Private Diagnostic Clinic—had broad referral networks and relationships across the Piedmont of North Carolina with hospitals and their medical staffs across a large number of communities in a geographic area that really ran from Greensboro to Greenville and from the Virginia border to the South Carolina border. One of the things that happens over time is those communities grow in population," Donelan explained. "Their ability to attract specialist physicians increases, and hospitals in those communities are desirous of expanding their own capabilities to more sophisticated services. So over time you begin to see a shrinkage in referrals from those areas."[51]

DUAP was created to keep the patients flowing to DUMC. "Duke generates $700 million in revenues from its clinical practice," Mark Rogers stressed in 1995. "Of that, we invest more than $70 million a year in cross-subsidization to support research and education. In a fully managed care environment, you wonder where that $70 million is going to come from. Then you begin to recognize the potential paralysis that threatens the academic medical centers."[52] DUAP acquired nine practices between 1994 and 1995. It opened two practice sites in neighboring Wake County, and it created a network of 17 offices and 65 physicians in 6 counties. DUMC also started sending its residents to the 230 annual community clinics in the medical center's Affiliations and Outreach Program. Training primary care physicians became critically important to DUMC, in fact, over the next several years. Although the numbers have slipped in recent years, by 1998 almost half of the 131 residents in the Department of Medicine were making primary care their specialty.[53]

Making it even more difficult for DUMC to prepare for managed care was that fact that Duke University had become the driving force behind Durham's economy. While the managed care team focused externally on fueling DUMC's clinical enterprise, it also implemented an internal Operations Improvement program designed to slash expenses and cut jobs. "Duke had become the major economic engine of Durham as industries closed down and went away," William Donelan noted. "The tobacco industry is largely gone from Durham now, and so we have a real stake in this community's health care service and so on, because our employees and their families make up an awful lot of the county population."[54]

Not surprisingly, the Operations Improvement program, which was announced in August 1994, raised fear and uncertainty in the local population. Between $50 million and $60 million in nonsalary expenses were targeted for cuts from the operating budget, while 1,500 jobs were scheduled to be eliminated by 1996. The fear of job loss was especially keen among Durham's black community. There was "a strong suspicion and belief that this would disproportionately disadvantage them," Snyderman recalled. "And there was minute oversight to make sure that people who were laid off were not disproportionately black."[55] By the fall of 1995, as a result of normal turnover and voluntary separation agreements, some 900 positions had been eliminated at DUMC— but only 10 employees, 4 of them managers, had been laid off. The estimated job loss was also revised downward, to between 1,000 and 1,300, as the $43 million saved from staff reductions was coupled with $59 million in nonsalary expenses cut from the hospital's operation budget for 1995–96.[56]

AN HMO AT DUKE

Even as they were cutting costs and creating primary care networks, the medical center leadership was partnering with Sanus Corporation Health Systems (the managed care division of New York Life Insurance Company) to link those feeder networks to a health maintenance organization of DUMC's own making. As Donelan described the larger plan, DUAP "created a geographically distributed array of access points to primary care physicians for our patients so that we would be in a position to contract with the insurers and have a complete enough network to provide services under this managed care form of insurance." At the same time, DUMC's leaders demanded as much control as possible in the HMO partnership with Sanus. "We also decided that it might be useful to understand managed care from the inside," Donelan explained. Managed care was a phenomenon "largely driven not by the medical profession but by the insurance industry," he stressed, and physicians throughout the country believed it was "beginning to affect their decision-making in a way that they were concerned about decisions being in the best interests of patients. There was not a lot of managed care form of health insurance in North Carolina, so we went through a process of concluding: 'Maybe we can influence the way this evolves if we're participating in a way other than just being a provider.'"[57]

New York Life gave DUMC a chance to try a new kind of HMO in North Carolina. "We found a partner who had a business strategy that was compatible with our objectives," Donelan said, "who shared our values, and who understood the role our institution would be playing in the future." Duke became part owner with Sanus of the new joint HMO venture, WellPath, which was approved by New York Life and Duke's board of trustees early in 1995.[58] Significantly, the WellPath agreement prompted one of the nation's largest HMOs, Kaiser Permanente, to drop Duke and Durham Regional Hospital from its list of preferred providers in favor of the UNC Hospitals at Chapel Hill. Likewise, Blue Cross and Blue Shield also suspended its long-time relationship with DUMC—a response that eliminated the majority of third-party payments to the PDC. "We were not happy when we were not in their network for a couple of years," the PDC's Paul Newman said, "and that was—once we got out of the old Duke Health Service and got into the relationship with WellPath, Blue Cross really said, 'We don't need you in our network.' And again it was . . . the notion that managed care was more competitive, and so they decided—I think it was a knee-jerk reaction—to not include us in their managed care network."[59]

WellPath and DUAP formed the core parts of a larger managed care model that Duke's leaders built and tested in North Carolina. This bigger model involved business strategies similar to those used by James B. Duke a century earlier in monopolizing the tobacco industry: vertical and horizontal integration. Creating a health care monopoly, however, was not what DUMC's leaders had in mind, on any level. What they designed was a health system that served as a delivery mechanism for the traditional clinical services provided by Duke Hospital and the PDC. "This had never been about some strategy to go statewide or go southeast regionwide and acquire more and more hospitals and more and more physician practices," Donelan recently stressed. "It was very focused strategically on some things that we felt we needed to do to build out from this very successful platform that had evolved over seven decades beginning with the creation of the medical school and Duke Hospital at the beginning of the thirties."[60]

Between 1995 and 1998 Duke's leaders pursued a strategy of "cradle-to-grave" integrated health delivery that led to the creation of the Duke University Health System. Rather quickly, however, they found themselves guided as much by chance and changing circumstances—by the need to move swiftly when opportunities arose—as by the models they brought to the task. By the time WellPath emerged, for example, HMOs had wrung much of the excess out the nation's health care system and many were beginning to lose money.

As the percentage of profitable HMOs dropped from 90 to 49 percent between 1994 and 1998, a wave of mergers and acquisitions arose—a trend that mirrored the larger business merger movement in the American economy, including the major for-profit hospital chains.

The 1993 merger of Columbia Healthcare, Inc., and HCA-Hospital Corporation, for example, had created the nation's largest investor-owned hospital chain, and the following year Columbia/HCA had acquired Healthcare Corporation, the nation's second largest hospital chain.[61] DUMC's leaders anticipated competition from Columbia/HCA and other large hospital chains, such as Tenet Healthcare and Health Management Associates, and especially from other HMOs. "As many as 75 HMOs may evolve in North Carolina over the next 5 to 10 years," Mark Rogers predicted in 1995. "They'll shrink down to 10 or 15, and ultimately there will be only 3 or 4 major providers of health care in the state. We expect to be one of them." What the DUMC team could not have foreseen, however, was the Balanced Budget Act of 1997, which reduced federal funding for hospitals and Medicare contributions. The act cost DUMC an estimated $200 million over the next five years.[62] One must look beyond campus, in fact, to the largest business merger movement in American history to understand fully the turmoil and complexity that accompanied the emergence of the Duke University Health System.

Divestment and Consolidation

Although the urge to merge began in the late 1980s, it exploded after the failure of the Clinton administration's health plan in 1994. And it soon transformed the corporate context from which Duke and DUMC had originally emerged. James B. Duke had monopolized the tobacco industry a century earlier, in the late 1890s, while playing a leading role in what was then the largest business merger movement in American history. Yet that earlier movement was dwarfed by comparison with the merger movement of the 1990s, which became the largest business merger movement in global history. Duke himself had gone global, of course, through control of the British American Tobacco Company, and he had also diversified his monopoly holdings beyond tobacco. He had cut a huge deal with the aluminum monopoly, Alcoa, involving water power properties in Canada, and he had gained control of one of the nation's largest chemical companies, American Cyanamid. He had also electrified the Carolina Piedmont through his Duke Power Company and had mandated use of the company's securities to fund his philanthropic interests through The Duke Endowment.

But that ensemble of Duke interests changed dramatically during the 1990s. The death of Doris Duke in October of 1993 made it possible for The Duke

Endowment to do something she had long opposed: sell a huge block of Duke Power stocks. The sale took place in the spring of 1994; the Endowment sold 16 million of its 26 million shares of Duke Power stock. In June of 1997, moreover, Duke Power merged with one of the nation's largest natural gas companies, PanEnergy of Houston, Texas, and became a subsidiary of the new Duke Energy Corporation. In the meantime, moreover, North Carolina continued to lose thousands of jobs in its traditional industries, tobacco, textiles, apparel, and furniture, and many of Duke's traditional state networks disappeared or diminished in importance. At the same time, new fortunes were being made in new industries, including telecommunications, information technologies, health care, and pharmaceuticals. And as new money shook hands with the old kind, new philanthropies emerged and a new wave of mergers and acquisitions occurred. The Duke Endowment dropped out of the top 10 wealthiest philanthropies in the United States, even as some of Duke's graduates gave generously to their alma mater in unprecedented amounts during the university's seven-year fundraising Campaign for Duke (1996–2003).[63]

Changes at American Cyanamid and in the RTP's largest drug companies—Glaxo, Burroughs Wellcome, and SmithKline Beecham—offer important examples of the economic and institutional changes in which the Duke University Health System emerged. Between 1937 and the early 1950s, Cyanamid's subsidiary, Lederle Laboratories, had played a major role at DUMC in facilitating the cancer and virus research of Dr. Joseph Beard and others. Indeed, Beard's collaboration with Lederle, first, on equine encephalomyelitis, and later, during World War II, on the flu virus, had given DUMC its earliest experience in balancing academic research with commercial opportunities. Although the Cyanamid networks had receded in importance at DUMC during the 1950s, they had resurfaced again briefly, in 1989, in connection with Davis & Geck, the surgical suture subsidiary of American Cyanamid. Working together with Duke's Department of Surgery, the Duke Graduate School, and Durham's largest black-owned business, the North Carolina Mutual Life Insurance Company, Davis & Geck joined Lederle in sponsoring the first meeting of the Society of Black American Surgeons.

Dr. David Sabiston hosted the meeting, which included a reception and banquet at the Washington Duke Inn on April 14, 1989. "Dr. John Hope Franklin, James B. Duke Professor Emeritus, addressed the gathering on 'The Vanishing Black Male,'" the society reported. "This outstanding address was appropriate and timely given what we now know of the status of the Black male in America." The society considered its first meeting "an unqualified success in achieving its goals of assembling and forming a national network of black academic surgeons. The information provided for the young surgeons

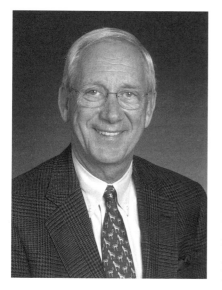

9.3 Dr. Ernest Mario. *Courtesy of Pharmaceutical Product Development, Inc.*

attending the meeting a broad perspective on the challenges and necessities for a successful career in academic surgery."[64]

Five years later, as consolidation swept the health care industry, American Home Products purchased American Cyanamid, only to sell it in July 2002, to BASF AG in Ludwigshafen, Germany.[65] Not part of that later deal, however, was Cyanamid's former subsidiary, Lederle-Praxis Biologics; it remained part of American Home Products, which in 2002 changed the name of the parent company to Wyeth.[66] Creating chaos closer nearby was the competition and consolidation of the British drug companies at Research Triangle Park. The career of Duke trustee Ernest Mario, who is currently chairman of the board of Duke University Health System, suggests some of the interconnected turmoil.

Mario was CEO of the world's second largest pharmaceutical company, London-based Glaxo Holdings, P.L.C., when he joined the Duke board of trustees in 1989, and before that he had held management positions at a number of pharmaceutical companies, including SmithKline, Squibb & Company, and Glaxo, Inc., at the Research Triangle Park. In 1990, moreover, just as the GUSTO trials were getting under way at DUMC, Mario, in his commencement address at Duke, garnered national attention for focusing "on the importance of ethical standards in business."[67] Mario left Glaxo three years later, after a dispute with its chairman, and in 1993 joined the new management team at Alza Corporation, the leading producer of skin patches for drug companies. Mario quickly became Alza's CEO, and in 1998 he also became the first chairman of the Duke University Health System. In 2001, Johnson & Johnson bought Alza for $10 billion, and in 2003, Mario, who was a trustee of Rockefeller University and chairman of the American Foundation for Pharmaceutical Education, became CEO and chairman of Reliant Pharmaceuticals.[68] [Figure 9.3]

In the meantime, Glaxo acquired Burroughs Wellcome (the Park subsidiary of the London-based Wellcome, P.L.C.) in a hostile takeover described by the *New York Times* in March of 1995 "as the second largest in any industry, behind the $30 billion merger between R. J. Reynolds and Nabisco in 1989."[69] Yet the financial community buzzed with even more excitement in 1998 when Glaxo Wellcome and SmithKline Beecham announced merger talks. "If the largest corporate marriage ever is completed in the next few weeks, as expected," the *Wall Street Journal* reported, "it will be the result of a profound revolution in human biology: the successful hunt for human genes. . . . The proposed deal is tentatively valued at between $65 billion and $70 billion, almost twice the size of the WorldCom Inc.'s planned takeover of MCI Communications."[70] Yet it took two more years before Glaxo Wellcome and SmithKline Beecham finally merged. The resulting company, GlaxoSmithKline, was the world's largest drug maker and represented the culmination of the British connection at Research Triangle Park.

Health Care Politics in Durham

It was in this rapidly changing context, then, that DUMC developed and launched its strategy for an integrated-delivery health care system. The process of horizontal integration—which involves acquiring and merging like or similar businesses—began with Durham Regional Hospital. "But the issue of Durham Regional really came up in a most interesting way," Snyderman recalled. The CEO at Regional, Richard Myers, called Snyderman in 1995 and told him that "Durham Regional is really facing tremendous financial problems. And we think we may need for you to help us out." Myers and his board continued to discuss the situation at Durham Regional, Snyderman explained, until "they made the decision that they could not make it on their own." "The considerations for us were capacity," William Donelan recalled. "Durham Regional was a four hundred-bed hospital running less than half full. It had operating rooms it wasn't using. Duke Hospital was chronically full and overfull in the Tuesday though Thursday period of the week, but under the State of North Carolina's certificate of need regulations, which controlled the supply of beds and operating rooms, there was no way we were going to get additional beds and operating rooms on this campus, on the Duke campus, while Durham Regional was running half empty, no matter who was in control of Durham Regional Hospital."[71]

The discussions that followed plunged Snyderman and his colleagues into the volatile local realities of race and health care politics. Durham Regional is a taxpayer-owned hospital run by a nonprofit corporation that answers to the Durham County Commissioners. According to Snyderman, after a year of exploratory talks "we came up with an agreement on the part of the Durham Regional board that Duke would take over the management, essentially run Durham Regional Hospital. And the financial agreement was that we would do it for a dollar a year. I mean, it would just be nominal because they were losing a whole bunch of money. That seemed to be all well and good until we hit the reality—you would think that this should have occurred earlier—that that deal needed to be approved by the county commissioners. When the county commissioners saw this, they indicated legally that they couldn't do this; it would have to be put up for bid. And at that time, there were aggressive acquisition strategies in the for-profit world. . . . [Companies] came in and aggressively bid for Durham Regional." The bidders included Duke and two large for-profits, Health Management Associates and Tenet Healthcare Corporation, as well as the state-owned, nonprofit UNC Hospitals. The "University of North Carolina, our buddies over in Chapel Hill, would have loved nothing more than to win this lease or contract from Durham to run Durham Regional Hospital," Snyderman remarked. "So they said they would manage Durham Regional Hospital—nice folks."[72]

UNC quickly dropped out of the bidding for Durham Regional, however, as Tenet and Health Management Associates "were very serious contenders and aggressive—they wanted it real bad," Snyderman said. "And I think the reason they wanted it real bad is that they felt that this was such a ripe area for getting some of the best and brightest Duke faculty to jump ship and go over to Durham Regional and to develop all these high-end services without any of the costs of doing business that we do. And what they did historically is very much limit the amount of charity care that they would do. . . . So we got into what amounted to a bidding war with them; and we felt, I think, for all the right reasons, that it would be a disaster for Durham Regional to be run by a for-profit." Snyderman focused in particular on Tenet, arguing that company's history suggested that it would turn Durham Regional "into a surgical hospital because that's where the money is. And we knew the distribution of healthcare economics, that Durham Regional primarily served Durham, which is not a high margin community for medical care, but that what they would try to do is skim as much as they could from Duke, shift as much of the indigent care as they could to Duke, and this would be a scenario for disaster for us as well as very poor care for the community."[73]

During hearings before the county commissioners, Durham's black community shared its concerns on the potential impact of a Duke-Regional alliance. One major concern was the future of the Lincoln Community Health Center, an affiliate of Durham Regional. Originally established in the early 1970s, as a prelude to the Watts-Lincoln hospital merger, the Lincoln Center received federal and county support as a primary care center for the poor. What would happen to it, many observers asked, under a Duke-Regional agreement? Another concern was raised by the chairwoman of the county commissioners, MaryAnn E. Black, an African American social worker. Black asked at one meeting what kind of "admitting privileges" Duke would grant

Lincoln's staff. "There was a perception that Duke was not as open to people having admitting privileges on their staff," Black told the Raleigh *News & Observer*. "Will Duke pick those physicians up?" she asked.[74]

Snyderman found his personal politicking in the black community both stressful and enlightening. At his first meeting with the Durham Committee on the Affairs of Black People, for example, he encountered "an incredible amount of hostility." Part of that anger was associated with the lingering uncertainty over the job cuts at DUMC; part of it was the kind of jobs African Americans held at DUMC; and part of it was the bitter legacy of racial and economic segregation. DUMC had always been "heavily oriented to the low-paying jobs for the African Americans with at times a feeling that there are a lot of dead ends in moving up the ladder," Snyderman said in 2004. "Now, obviously, we have done a tremendous amount to do everything we could to develop an upward mobility. But I think the perception certainly was there ten years ago that African Americans did a lot of service jobs here. Environmental services, nutrition, laundry, and not a whole bunch more." During his first years as chancellor, Snyderman recalled, Duke had been referred to as "the plantation. . . . And that was the perception on the part of the African-American community. And they were angry, distrustful."[75]

Particularly challenging for Snyderman was the story he heard from a black physician at one community meeting. "After the meeting he came up to me and he said, 'You don't recall me, but in 1977 you were head of the rheumatology division. And I came by as a fellow looking for a position on your program.'" As Snyderman described it, "I immediately thought, 'Boy, I hope we didn't turn this person down.' I said, 'How come you didn't come to Duke?' . . . He said, 'Well, you didn't realize it at the time—you were very, very nice to me, you wanted me to come. . . . But you took me around to see the clinics. And what was not apparent to you is that you were showing me a segregated delivery system.' Now, this was 1977," Snyderman explained. "This was probably . . . thirteen, fifteen years after Duke integrated. And what he meant by that is I took him to, at that time, the public clinic and the private clinic. The public clinic was almost entirely black. The private clinic was almost entirely white. I was blind to that. I mean, I saw it. It's what you call unintentional blindness. . . . I just did not perceive it the way he perceived it, which I think was more accurate than the way I perceived it."[76]

By 1997, Snyderman's work on Durham Regional had taught him a lot about "the local environment. And it was shocking to me," he recalled. "It wasn't just that I learned a whole bunch more, it was really shocking to me as to how divorced so much of the leadership of the medical center was with the community, the perceptions on the part of the community, the lack of understanding of each other. That was very striking." Snyderman also understood

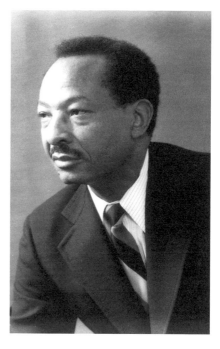

9.4 Dr. Charles Johnson. *Duke University Medical Center Archives.*

by then that the black community's political power was the key to any agreement between Duke and Durham Regional, and he worked closely with the university to strengthen its existing relationship with several local black leaders.[77]

One was Dr. Charles Johnson, Duke's first black faculty member. Johnson had arrived at DUMC in 1964, as a resident in Duke's collaborative medicine program with Lincoln Hospital, and he had worked at Lincoln for the next six years, building a practice and serving as director of the black hospital's medical servic-
es. Recruited to Duke in 1970, as a member of the faculty of the Department of Medicine, Johnson focused on health care issues for underserved minorities and also became a member of the medical school admission's committee. "By the time he retired in 1996," one source noted, "Duke had minority faculty and house staff in every clinical department, and more minority medical students than ever."[78] Duke awarded Johnson its highest award in 1997, the Medal for Distinguished Meritorious Service, and in September of that year, Johnson was named as a "special advisor" to Snyderman. His job was to recruit more black physicians to Duke and to serve "as a liaison between the community and the medical center."[79] [Figure 9.4]

Two months later, Snyderman named Dr. Jean Spaulding, a local black psychiatrist, as Duke's vice chancellor for health affairs. Her job description was similar to Johnson's: "to improve community relations and to help the university's medical center recruit and retain more women and minorities." Spaulding's appointment, like Johnson's, also represented nearly a century of effort by the Duke family and its allies to develop a new group of leaders in the South: men and women, black and white, local, state and regional. Spaulding was preceded, for example, by Durham's Harriett Amey, the black woman whose professional studies were supported by Doris Duke and her foundation officers, and who had broken the color line on Duke's staff in 1947 as a member of DUMC's Department of Social Services. Spaulding, as mentioned earlier, had married into one Durham's most prominent black families. She had been the

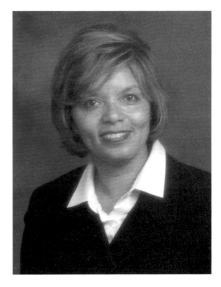

9.5 Dr. Jean G. Spaulding. *Duke University Medical Center*

first black woman to attend Duke's medical school and she had done her residency in psychiatry under Dr. Keith Brodie. By 1997 Spaulding was also a trustee of Duke University and divorced from her former husband, Kenneth Spaulding, the head of the Durham Committee on the Affairs of Black People. Spaulding, in addition to running her own psychiatric practice, was also doing a Saturday morning radio show with MaryAnn Black, chairwoman of the Durham County commissioners.[80] [Figure 9.5]

THE MERGER WITH DURHAM REGIONAL

Early in 1998 the negotiations with Durham Regional advanced quickly. The centerpiece of Duke's proposed "merger" included a 20-year lease to manage and operate Durham Regional for $3.5 million a year. The proposal also included $1.5 million in annual payments to the county for ambulance operations and $2.1 million a year for the Lincoln Community Health Center. Regional's doctors voted to support the proposal in March 1998, as did the hospital's governing board and the Durham Committee on the Affairs of Black People. The critical vote then came in April, when the Durham County commissioners voted 3–2 along racial lines to approve Duke's proposal. (The two white commissioners, both women, voted against it.) According to Joe Bowser, one of the African American commissioners, Duke had worked diligently and honestly to atone for its once haughty presumptions of power. "Duke University is not the old Duke of yesteryear," Bowser said. "There's a new group of people running Duke. I feel we can trust this group of people."[81]

For the commission's African American chairwoman, MaryAnn Black, the matter was both personal and practical. Black, a social worker with a master's degree from the University of North Carolina, had worked in the Community Child Guidance Clinic at Duke between 1973 and 1982. The clinic operates under the umbrella of DUMC's psychiatry department and is one of the medical center's oldest and most unusual links to the social welfare of the local community. Yet Black's main concern as chairwoman was to get Durham the best deal possible. And it certainly didn't look good for Duke at first, Black recalled, as "the votes were there to support Tenet. And I think, just time has

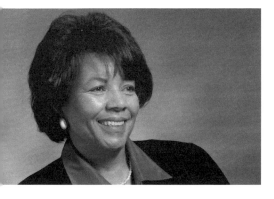

9.6 MaryAnn E. Black, chairwoman of Durham County Commission and later director of community affairs, Duke University Health System. *Duke University Medical Center.*

proven that Tenet was not the right group to go with." Black described her vote for the Duke proposal as both realistic and community based. "And I finally said, 'You know what? It may not be a perfect agreement, but there is one thing I know. I know where the Duke president's house is. And if I'm ninety years old and I've got to go knock on that door and say, 'Things are not going right,' I can do that. I don't know where the Tenet president lives. . . . And I'm glad that we made the decision not to go that route. So I think—and I think the county would have to look back and say that it was a good decision, although some of my colleagues would say, 'MaryAnn, you didn't get enough money, and this was not the right decision,' and blah, blah, blah. Before I left, I think I had a chance to say, 'It was the right decision, even if you don't believe it.'"[82] [Figure 9.6]

A Hospital Corporation

L ate in February 1998, Duke announced it was creating a new corporation, the Duke University Health System, that would begin operations in July. DUHS is a separate corporate entity from Duke University but it is controlled by the university's board of trustees and thus is a controlled affiliate corporation. Duke's trustees exercise control over the health system through the power to appoint DUHS's board of directors, and the chancellor for health affairs is, by virtue of that position, the CEO of the health system. The new corporation includes Duke Hospital and the affiliated businesses and clinical operations of the hospital, but it does not include DUMC's medical school and faculty, nor the PDC. DUHS's 30-member governing board has the power to make acquisitions and to handle all employee matters, from hiring and firing to pay and benefits, and between 13 and 17 of its board members must be university trustees or officers of Duke.[83]

Duke president Nan Keohane made it clear in announcing a diversified health system that the fate of the university and its medical center were closely intertwined. "The viability of the university as well as the medical center depends on the success of the medical center's clinical mission," Keohane said during the February announcement. This thought alarmed some faculty members, who rightfully raised the old fears of the tail wagging the dog. "Will the effect, intended or not, be that Duke becomes a diversified health system that operates a small university on the side?" one professor asked Keohane. No, Keohane responded; she considered "it highly unlikely that the health-care system will become a dominant corporate structure that skews the priorities of the rest of the university." What bothered her was the health system's potential to separate Duke Medicine even further from the university. Rather than help the university realize the concept of oneness—"the *Big D*, all of Duke together"—the health system might make the medical center more distant. "If that were to happen," she said, "the fruitful synergies that have historically characterized Duke—synergies of creativity, intellectual stimulation and mutual support both financial and administrative—would be lost."[84]

The new corporation, however, was focused on its mission. In May 1998, it purchased the 218-bed, for-profit Raleigh Community Hospital in nearby Raleigh for an estimated $175 million. The purchase was concluded quickly, without extended talks, after its overtures to Raleigh's two largest hospitals, Wake Med and Rex Hospital, had failed and after Raleigh Community's owner, Columbia/HCA, offered the hospital to Duke. "Wake County is fundamentally a physician strategy for us," William Donelan later noted, "it's a clinical program and physician strategy, it's not a hospital strategy. We didn't buy Raleigh Community because we wanted to have that particular hospital in Raleigh, but we needed a hospital in Raleigh through which we could offer and develop Duke clinical programs offered by Duke physicians; it's a distinction. . . . So Raleigh Community was an entrée into that marketplace."[85]

Duke continued to look for opportunities to expand horizontally, but the purchase of Raleigh Community Hospital marked the end of that strategy, at least for the time being. In the meantime, Snyderman and his colleagues also continued to implement their strategy for making DUHS a health system with integrated-delivery services from the cradle to the grave—that is, from prenatal care by DUAP physicians to hospital and home care services, nursing homes, and bereavement counseling. Specifically, Duke acquired a 50 percent interest in St. Joseph of the Pines, a long-term care organization, in January 1998, and then formally acquired Triangle Hospice, a facility for terminally ill patients. St. Joseph's 800 health care workers operated out of eight offices in central North Carolina, providing home care patients with a range of services from nursing and physical therapy to housekeeping. Duke also acquired full ownership later that year of Chartwell Southeast, a home drug-infusion company with which it had partnered since 1993. The new company, Duke Community Infusion Services, offered advanced mechanical devices for home care infusion of antibiotics, nutritional supplements, and medications, including chemotherapy and drug treatments for HIV/AIDS patients.[86]

And then there was the deal announced as imminent by the local press in October 1998: that Duke was on the verge of acquiring United Methodist Retirement Homes of Durham. "For Duke, the deal welds a new link in the health-care system it is building to serve patients from cradle to grave," the Raleigh *News & Observer* reported. "United Methodist offers options to retirees that range from separate cottages for people who don't need any care to beds for invalids. Those options fit well with the home health-care services offered by St. Joseph of the Pines, a Pinehurst non-profit that has a joint venture with Duke. Triangle Hospice, which has merged with Duke, offers services to the dying."[87]

DUMC *in the News*

By the fall of 1998, Snyderman had been reappointed to a third five-year term (1999–2004) as chancellor for health affairs and dean of the school of medicine and also to the new position of CEO of DUHS. Duke's health system then consisted of Duke Hospital and Clinics, Durham Regional Hospital, Raleigh Community Hospital, the DUAP regional network of primary care physicians, WellPath, Triangle Hospice, St. Joseph of the Pines, and Chartwell Southeast, with the acquisition of United Methodist Retirement Homes in the works.

Between 1994 and 1998, the number of employees associated with Duke's new ensemble of health interests almost doubled (from 8,000 to 14,000) as did the combined annual budgets of those interests (from $700 million to $1.3 billion). Snyderman quickly found it prudent, in fact, to give up his deanship. "Facts are," William Donelan later explained, "as the clinical environment became more complicated, and as the clinical enterprise became larger and more complicated, Ralph really had less time and attention to pay on being dean. And really driving the academic programs of the school. And before that became a problem—with substantial encouragement—decided that he should relinquish the deanship title himself and those responsibilities and recruit a dean for the medical school who would report to him but would take the day-to-day responsibility for the educational and research programs of the school of medicine and the clinical activities of the faculty." Dr. Edward W. Holmes Jr. served as the first dean under this new format (1999–2000) and he was followed by the current dean, Dr. R. Sanders ("Sandy") Williams.[88]

Duke's preemptive moves to protect its academic medical center drew the attention of UNC Hospitals and *Time* magazine. While UNC's medical leaders had expected the lease with Durham Regional, the deal for Raleigh Community Hospital—which supposedly went down in only 48 hours—"stunned" medical leaders in Chapel Hill. The deal drew an immediate response from

Dr. Jeffrey Houpt, the former Duke psychiatrist who was now dean of UNC's school of medicine. Houpt and his UNC colleagues had already responded to managed care in several ways, through purchasing physician practices, contracting with managed care insurers, creating an HMO with WakeMed, containing costs, and building a network of 400 affiliated physicians. What disturbed Houpt was the fact that UNC Hospitals was part of a big bureaucratic blob, a state-run behemoth that lacked the freedom and agility Duke had shown in acting quickly in Raleigh; without such nimbleness, Houpt feared, UNC Hospitals were doomed. "We're not talking about anything short of survival," Houpt said. "We prefer to retain our public status, but we have to get some of these things freed up or we won't be able to survive." In November 1998, the state legislature created the UNC Healthcare System with some of the latitude Houpt had requested.[89]

UNC created its health system less than a month after *Time* magazine published a 40-page cover story on the medical center at Duke, calling DUMC "one of the crown jewels of American medicine." A masked surgeon looks out intensely from the magazine's cover, his blue surgical uniform acting as a background for the title "A Week in the Life of a Hospital: On the Front Lines of the War Between Money and Medicine." The story uses Duke as an example of how America's academic medical centers were dealing with the challenges and opportunities presented by managed care, skyrocketing costs, dwindling federal funding, and widening inequities in care. In one of the story's many brief features, "An M.D. as CEO Redraws the Big Picture," *Time* noted that "what Snyderman is doing is not unique, but it is much talked about in medical circles. If it works, he's a genius. If it doesn't Duke could go the same route as the University of Minnesota, which sold its hospital, or the University of Pennsylvania, which reported a $40 million deficit this year."[90]

In another feature, "More Science . . . And Much More Money," *Time* briefly summarized the Duke Clinical Research Institute, the GUSTO studies with TPA and Genentech, and Rob Califf's assurance that the results of the institute's privately funded research "are published no matter what the outcome." Califf, *Time* explained, "has gathered a staff of 750 physicians, statisticians and computer jocks in a $44.8 million high-tech high-rise on the edge of the medical center. DCRI is currently coordinating 12 international studies, involving more than 1,500 clinical investigations in 35 countries. With net revenues projected this year to top $55 million (up from $30 million in '96), DCRI has the potential of becoming the largest single profit center at Duke."[91]

That kind of money, power, and publicity draws attention, of course, and in December 1998, representatives from the federal Office of Protection from Research Risks, which monitored all protocols involving research on humans, visited Duke and audited DUMC's Institutional Review Board records. The office identified 22 administrative deficiencies during its audit at Duke. Although DUMC responded in February with a plan for addressing those deficiencies, on May 10 the "OPRR notified us that they were suspending our Multiple Projects Assurance (MPA) immediately," Snyderman and Ed Holmes later wrote in *Science*. "(An institution submits an MPA document for approval by OPRR as an assurance of the institution's commitment to comply with the regulations of the DHHS [Department of Health and Human Services] for the protection of research subjects.) Without an MPA, DHHS-funded multiple trails cannot be conducted." The order shut down all government-funded trials at DUMC, and Snyderman and Holmes immediately instituted a self-imposed ban on all trials, even those being privately funded at DCRI.[92]

"We were the first, really big institution to have our research suspended," recalled Vicki Y. Saito, then associate vice chancellor of communications. "We thought that OPRR really wanted to use us as an example. And we believe that that was the case. Because there had been other reported incidents of problems involving patients, in which patients were actually harmed. And those never got to the national level. And yet, ours—in which no one was harmed—they were making a very big deal about it."[93]

Despite these reservations, Snyderman approached the problem as he had Genentech's initial failure to have TPA approved by the FDA. He formed a crisis team to deal openly, honestly, and immediately with the OPRR's concerns. Within days the team drafted a plan for corrective action and Snyderman, Ed Holmes, and several other team members took a chartered jet to Washington to meet with the OPRR. "That was absolutely brilliant because OPRR responded very favorably to that," Saito explained. "I think the fact that they had our two top leaders said to them . . . we were taking it seriously." The Duke group "met with the OPRR people who made some suggestions about needed changes for our Plan of Corrective Action," Saito continued. "They worked on those changes on the way back in this plane. And, by the time they got back here to the office, it was just a matter of a couple of hours they were able to incorporate those changes, and fax them up to Washington, and they accepted our plan. So, I mean, it was just—very quick."[94] To be sure, the OPRR reinstated Duke's MPA only four days after suspending it, and the following January, Snyderman and Holmes published an article in *Science* magazine on the matter. Their work, one source noted, provided one of the "opportunities for Duke to become a national model for improving human subject research."[95]

* * *

Successes with Long-Term Goals

Some people and programs fared better than others at Duke during the managed care crisis of the late 20th and early 21st centuries. The School of Nursing was reborn, and the university's successful seven-year Campaign for Duke (1996–2003) eventually raised more than $2.3 billion (including $706.4 million for the medical center). The face of Duke changed dramatically, in fact, as President Nan Keohane focused on student affairs, fundraising, and development, even as she expanded the minority and community outreach efforts of her predecessor Dr. Keith Brodie and launched an important study known as the Women's Initiative in 2003. [Figure 9.7]

The renaissance of Duke's nursing school reflected a combination of the managed care demand for primary care providers and the leadership of Mary T. Champagne, R.N., Ph.D. Snyderman recruited Champagne from UNC in 1991, at a time when Duke's undergraduate nursing program had been inactive for 10 years; only 5 faculty and 50 students remained in the graduate master's program. Champagne focused on creating "primary care, acute care, and tertiary care majors; nurse practitioner programs in acute care, pediatrics and geriatrics; and specialty programs in oncology, cardiovascular health, and nursing informatics." Champagne also helped establish the Nursing Research Center, a joint

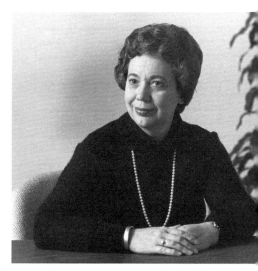

9.7 Ruby L. Wilson, dean of the School of Nursing, 1971–84. *Duke University Medical Center Archives.*

effort of Duke Hospital and the School of Nursing. And in 1996, in collaboration with Duke's Department of Community and Family Medicine, Champagne helped create the division of community health. During her 13-year tenure as dean, moreover, Champagne and her colleagues successfully mobilized significant funding from both NIH and private sources, and together with Keohane, Champagne secured an accelerated degree program, the bachelor of science in nursing, in 2002. The first graduates of the 18-month program received their diplomas in December 2003, and many immediately went to work for facilities in the Duke University Health System.[96]

By the time Champagne stepped down as its dean in July 2004, the School

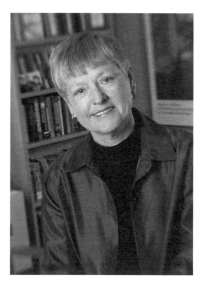

9.8 Mary T. Champagne, dean of the School of Nursing, 1991–2004. *Duke University Medical Center.*

of Nursing had 374 students, 38 faculty, and plans both to build a new building and to create a Ph.D. program in nursing. Snyderman, who also stepped down that July, praised Champagne for ushering in a "new era" at Duke's School of Nursing. "Her vision, her unflagging dedication, and her ability to rally people behind her have made all the difference in the progress the school has seen and the impact it will continue to make for years to come." Champagne also received great praise from Keohane, who joined Snyderman and the nursing dean in stepping down in July 2004. "Many students have benefited directly from Mary's efforts," Keohane said, "and thousands upon thousands of patients have benefited and will benefit. Her years will be remembered as transformational—a time of intelligent innovation that honored the best of Duke's traditions and history." In December of 2004, Duke's trustees approved both a new nursing building and the proposed Ph.D. program in nursing.[97] [Figure 9.8]

Snyderman's nursing initiative did represent the best of Duke's traditions and history. The Duke family and its philanthropies embraced the progressive spirit of educating and promoting women and African Americans, as well as white men, who would act as leaders and catalysts for change, whether in North Carolina, the South, or the world. Doris Duke maintained that commitment, as Mary Semans still does, and Duke Medicine, for most of its history and in concert with its traditional white patriarchy, has also pursued that commitment. It has pursued it in its work with Lincoln Hospital since the 1930s. It pursued it in recruiting black staff and nurses in the late 1940s and early 1950s. It pursued it during the sixties and seventies, through desegregation and recruitment of black faculty and students, and it remained committed to it throughout the 1980s and 1990s, during two decades of intense internal turmoil. Indeed, DUMC's traditional commitments were reinforced during the 1990s by the increasing democratization of American culture and by the simultaneous emergence of what might be called the feminization of health care. Managed care mangled up the traditional white male hierarchy of American medicine in many ways, giving women more power as both leaders and participants in a larger team of primary care providers, most of whom

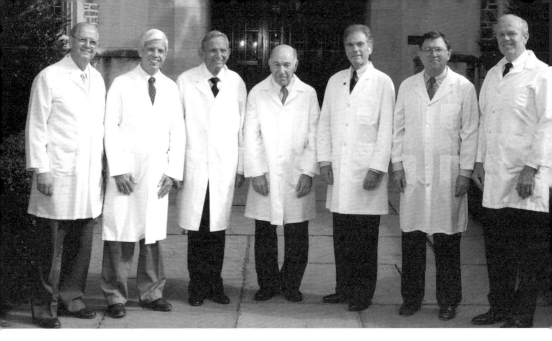

9.9 Several of the "deans" of Duke University School of Medicine. Left to right: Drs. Arthur C. Christakos, Dan G. Blazer, Ewald W. Busse, William G. Anlyan, Ralph Snyderman, Charles E. Putman, and Doyle G. Graham. *Duke University Medical Center Archives.*

are women. Almost half of the students accepted today to medical schools are women; at Duke they accounted for 48.5 percent of the entering class of 2004.[98]

Charles Putman's Legacy at DUMC

Although the patriarchy persists at Duke, it was diminished considerably through the synergy of Keohane's presidency with Snyderman's revolution in Duke Medicine and the fading feud between Bill Anlyan, Keith Brodie, and Charles Putman. Fittingly, it was the building envisioned as a great campus unifier, the Levine Science Research Center, that prompted Anlyan to move out of the Allen administration building and into another office off campus. According to Anlyan the LSRC was his first major assignment upon moving into the Allen Building as chancellor of Duke University in 1988. "When I became chancellor of the university," he recently wrote, "I was assigned to pull it all together."[99]

In 1989, however, Brodie tried again to put Anlyan and Putman together in the same building when he appointed Putman vice president for research and administration policy. This new nest proved no more nurturing, however, and in 1990 the situation reached a breaking point when Brodie appointed Putman

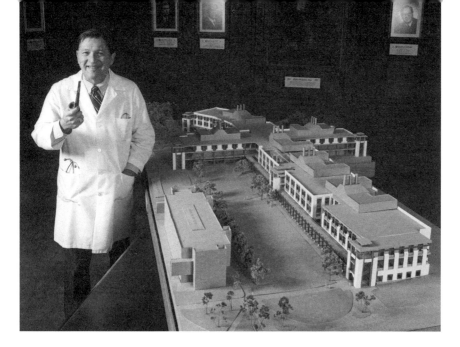

9.10 Dr. Charles E. Putman and a model of the Levine Science Research Center.
Photograph by Caroline Vaughan ©1991.

as executive vice president for administration, the university's senior financial officer. Anlyan, who together with Snyderman had developed the lead gift for the LSRC, became chancellor emeritus that year after accepting an invitation from Mary Semans to join The Duke Endowment. "Dr. Charles Putman, the former chairman of radiology, who was then coordinating research grants in the university, was asked to oversee the further development of the building," Anlyan later explained. "This was fine with me, because I was never good at details." The transition could not have been easier: "My staff and I moved our offices to the tenth floor of the First Union Building at Erwin Square, a new office building not far from the Medical Center."[100] [Figure 9.9]

Putman remained Duke's executive vice president of administration after Keohane assumed the presidency in 1993, and he was still the university's chief financial officer in 1994 when the new $80 million Levine Science Research Center opened. The following year Keohane appointed Putman to the new position of senior vice president for research administration and policy, and though he was considered in 1997 for the chancellorship of his alma mater, the University of Texas Medical School, Putman decided to withdraw his candidacy and remain at Duke. "This past year our faculty generated a record $275 million in externally sponsored projects," Keohane said in announcing Putman's decision to stay at Duke. "A good deal of credit for that accomplishment goes to Charles, who has worked closely with our deans and faculty to

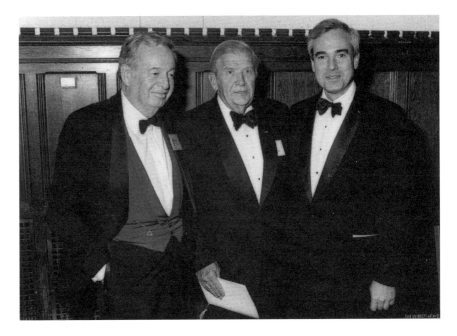

9.11 Dr. H. Keith H. Brodie with his immediate predecessors as president of Duke University, Douglas M. Knight, left, and Terry Sanford, middle. *Duke University Archives.*

ensure that we were aggressive in a very competitive environment in seeking support for our faculty's research interests. . . . Charles's knowledge of the important issues and relationships with research leaders in the Triangle, in North Carolina and in Washington, is particularly valuable to Duke, as is his thoughtful counsel on many different issues where his deep familiarity with Duke and the Medical Center make him a valuable repository of institutional memory."[101] [Figure 9.10]

In addition to his responsibilities at Duke, Putman was chairman of the board of the Microelectronics Center of North Carolina and a director and chairman of the North Carolina Biotechnology Center, both of which were located in Research Triangle Park. Putman was also a trustee of the Triangle Universities Center for Advanced Studies; a governor of the Research Triangle Institute; and a director of the North Carolina Alliance for Competitive Technologies. Twice, moreover, in 1992 and again in 1998, he received the state's Order of the Long Leaf Pine, and in 1994, as member of the Institute of Medicine, Putman chaired an institute committee that reviewed federal regulations governing the use of radioactive materials. Putman was also a principal investigator with the Howard Hughes Institute and an active and honored leader in the field of radiology, being the author or coauthor of some 200 published research reports and editor or coeditor of 9 textbooks.[102]

Putman's death from a heart attack on May 10, 1999, at the age of 57, was a blow to Duke and to his many friends and family. "No one loved Duke more nor was more dedicated to our university than Charles," Nan Keohane reflected. "Charles Putman was a dear friend and loyal colleague," Snyderman said. "I personally came to count on him as someone I could always turn to for advice, support and just plain good conversation." Mary Semans voiced sentiments shared by many of Putman's friends and colleagues. "We feel lost because we've lost a person who cared so much about Duke and for every single person there, regardless of where they worked, whether they were big or little, employee or staff. If someone were in trouble," Semans explained, "the first person who would come to mind to call was Charles. If he were out of state, he would call back. It's just simply terrible. There just isn't anybody like him."[103]

Putman's death hit Keith Brodie hardest of all. "He was my best friend, just a wonderful colleague, father and husband," Brodie told one local reporter. "Basically, it's just going to be impossible to replace him."[104] Brodie described the popular Putman as "sort of a renaissance man. He changed Duke in many wonderful ways. He left behind a top-ranking radiology department and an extraordinary science building that is without peer. As dean of the medical school, he substantially increased the admission of African American students, and then, as he moved on to become vice president for research, he dramatically increased research support for our faculty. And he was an ambassador for Duke in the Research Triangle and for Durham internationally. He was the consummate clinician, always available, helpful and effective. Duke has lost an extraordinary leader. We are all vastly diminished by his passing."[105]

Looking Back at Brodie's Presidency

Putman's passing certainly further diminished Brodie's own legacy at Duke. Many considered Brodie a sustaining president (1985–93) at best. Having inherited the best of Duke's progressive tradition, through Terry Sanford and Mary Semans, Brodie appeared unable to plot and pursue his own presidential journey. Amid angry faculty demands for increased power in the university's governance, Brodie facilitated the power of the marketplace in shaping Duke's future—and nowhere more so than at DUMC. But that was only part of Brodie's legacy as president. Keith Brodie hired Ralph Snyderman to be a transformational dean at DUMC and Snyderman was. Also, to the extent that Brodie had a hand in selecting Keohane as his successor, much as he himself had been selected by his own predecessor, Terry Sanford, Brodie recruited a transformational president to Duke. [Figure 9.11]

Brodie also returned to a severely diminished Psychiatry Department, where he taught a course in psychobiology until 2005. Managed care had reshaped DUMC's psychiatry department as much as the shifting fortunes of federal programs ever had. It moved the department from a combined focus on clinical care and research, with some 200 available inpatient beds, to a research-centered department with only 20 beds. Most of the department's residency training and service provision are done today at either the Veterans Hospital or the state mental hospital, as the number of beds for psychiatric patients has diminished rapidly across the state. Newman, the PDC administrator, offered one explanation for psychiatry's decline at Duke. "I think reimbursement was the main reason. One of the first things managed care companies and employers, as part of their plan design, really looked at curbing . . . was really around psychiatric services. . . . They would start with very rich benefits, and then cut it down to very minimal benefits right now. . . . If you go out to a private psychiatrist, they're not accepting insurance anymore. And so the economics have changed dramatically for psychiatric services."[106]

Paying for Excellence

The day Charles Putman died, May 10, 1999, was the same day that the OPRR suspended federally funded research trials at DUMC. Although the suspension was lifted in just four days, it portended changes in the Duke University Health System and the emergence of new models of health care based upon Snyderman's vision of the future of genomics.

THE SALE OF WELLPATH

Snyderman and his management team restructured the DUHS business model to focus on doing what Duke Medicine has always done best, provide outstanding medical care. This led them to abandon further acquisitions and to sell off pieces of the system that were not key to its operations and were unprofitable. In the spring of 1999, they broke off merger talks with the Methodist retirement homes, even as they were discussing the sale of WellPath, which was then the fifth largest HMO in North Carolina. Duke had assumed full ownership of WellPath in 1998, after New York Life sold its health insurance divisions to Aetna Life Insurance Company, and by the spring of 1999 WellPath had lost almost $12 million. Much of the loss was associated with the teachers and other state employees who made up a little more than half of WellPath's 111,000 members; they not only used their health benefits more than other individuals but they also paid less because of group rates. Indeed, Duke would lose another $12 million on WellPath by the summer of 2000. Worse still, Duke discovered in the fall of 1999 that Durham Regional had made auditing errors and had provided inaccurate financial information during the lease negotiations the previous year. The errors had already cost Duke $12 million in losses, and the projected losses for the fiscal year 1999–2000 were $15 million.[107]

Duke sold WellPath to Maryland's Coventry Health Plan late in 2000 for about $25 million. "By the time we sold WellPath . . . the bloom had kind of come off the rose of managed care," recalled William Donelan, the health system's chief operating officer. "The American people finally began to vote with their feet. They didn't like giving up their freedom of choice to access whatever physicians they wanted. Employers, after early success on the part of managed care insurance in reducing the rate of increase in health care costs, . . . had picked the low-hanging fruit, and further changes using that form were not really proving really effective, so employers became disenchanted. Their employees—patients—became disenchanted around the freedom of choice issues. And physicians never liked it, because they felt it really dictated practice decisions in ways that weren't always in the best interest of their patients." Snyderman described the sale of WellPath more simply. "No one was managing the care," he told one student journalist. "We learned that we did not want to be in the business of decreasing the amount of care that people had access to."[108]

THE INSTITUTE FOR GENOME SCIENCES AND RESEARCH

Snyderman's vision of the future of biomedical science drove another important initiative, the idea for an Institute for Genome Sciences and Policy, which emerged in connection with the beginning of the university's successful fundraising Campaign for Duke (1996–2003). "I was challenged," Snyderman later recalled, "as were other senior university leaders: What would be a transforming gift to Duke University? If somebody were to offer a gift of hundreds of millions of dollars, and you had to tell them how that would be transformational to Duke University, what would it be? Well, that got me thinking. And I couldn't help thinking that if it was transformational to Duke University, it ought to be transformational to the world. And that the most transformational event that seemed to be coming down the pike at the time, let's say '97, was the sequencing of the human genome, and from that the application of genomics to the human condition—very broadly speaking."[109] Although the science and technology already existed to do this, there were larger challenges. Snyderman explained: "It was clear that the technical aspects of implementing the genome revolution, while challenging, would be less so than resolving the socio-political-ethical issues it raised. Putting those two ideas together, I conceived of an institute that would bring together the health system, the school of medicine, biomedical research, law, ethics, and policy and have it be an overarching institution at Duke. I actually doodled all the structures interacting with each other on a napkin. It was like a daisy with the IGSP at the center and all other schools arrayed around it."[110]

In November 2000, Duke launched a series of events connected with the university's new $200 million Institute for Genome Sciences and Policy. The Institute was conceived as an on-campus network of five research centers that would offer integrated, interdisciplinary programs dedicated to advancing the genomics revolution and dealing with its implications for health and society. The director of the National Cancer Institute, Duke Medical School alumnus Dr. Richard D. Klausner, gave the keynote address and university president Nan Keohane moderated a round-table discussion on genetic testing. Snyderman, in discussing the public events, emphasized that, unlike genetic institutes at other universities, which emphasized either technology or the ethics of genetic research, Duke's new institute would provide a comprehensive approach. "We think we're doing it in very holistic way," Snyderman told a local reporter. "We don't see anybody doing it exactly like us."[111]

The Last Years under Snyderman

As Duke began to implement its plans for the institute, the university health system sold at a small loss its joint home health venture, St. Joseph of the Pines, and DUHS began to take on its present form: three hospitals, ambulatory surgery centers, primary and specialty care clinics, and four home care services offered by Duke Health Community Care (infusion, health, hospice, and bereavement). By the end of 2002, the Duke University Health System began to show sustainable economic growth. It continued to show excess margin through fiscal year 2003–4, when it made $55.5 million in net operating income, and in fiscal year 2004–5, when the figure was $90 million.[112] [Figure 9.12]

THE SANTILLAN CASE

On February 22, 2003, however, an event occurred that severely jolted the entire system: a seventeen-year-old illegal immigrant from Mexico, Jesica Santillan, died at Duke after a second heart-lung transplant failed to save her from a blood-type mismatch made during the first transplant at DUMC. The incident made national and international news, not only because it happened at Duke, but because of Santillan's immigrant status and the fact that, unlike the long waiting period most heart-lung recipients had to endure, her wait for a second set of organs was a matter of days. "All of us at Duke have agonized over the problems in Jesica's treatment and we have taken actions to ensure that nothing like this will ever happen again," said Duke Hospital CEO Dr. William J. Fulkerson Jr. "This has been a very tragic time and Jesica has

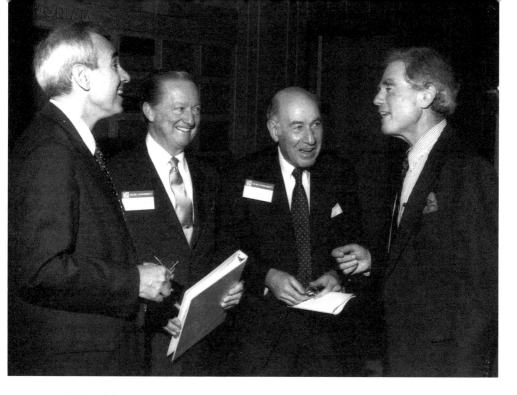

9.12 Left to right: Dr. H. Keith H. Brodie, Philip "Jack" Baugh, Dr. William G. Anlyan, and Dr. Ralph Snyderman. *Courtesy of Ralph Snyderman.*

had an enormous impact on all of us here. We are doing everything humanly possible to provide for all our patients, and we are committed to upholding the highest medical standards as we move forward."[113] The incident reminded everyone connected with Duke Medicine to remain vigilant about the most basic matters: careful medicine. Santillan's death proved especially tough for Snyderman, who, having helped transform Duke's academic medical center, was preparing to announce his retirement as chancellor at the end of his third term in June of 2004. "Everything surrounding it was incredibly painful," Snyderman later said of Santillan's death. "The event itself. The tragedy of this horrible mistake. The inevitability of this negative outcome. The skewering by the representatives of the family. The—what seemed to be—the unfairness of the press in how stories are played out. And just the difficulty. The pain in the institution, and seeing the institution brought down so low. That was horrible."[114]

SNYDERMAN'S LEGACY

Snyderman spent his final year as chancellor supporting several major initiatives: the IGSP, the Center for Integrative Medicine, and prospective health care. If one looks closely at the idea of integrative medicine it is possible to see the religious faith of James B. Duke, the psychosomatic approach of the Rockefeller Foundation, the alternative medicine pursued by Doris Duke, and the science-based, patient-centered focus present at DUMC since its creation. According to one source, integrative medicine "combines the best conventional and non-conventional approaches to medicine to treat the whole patient, not just the disease." And like the Institute for Genome Sciences and Policy, the Center for Integrative Medicine is interdisciplinary. "Specialists in obstetrics and gynecology, internal medicine, community and family medicine, psychiatry, and psychology see patients as a team. They then develop a personal health plan for patients that factors in healing-oriented medicine, nutrition, botanical medicine, meditation, spirituality, and other modalities." Snyderman, in describing his ideas for the center, points to the patient-physician combination of curing and caring. "That's what integrative medicine does," he said. "Its central feature is the patient's relationship to the physician and the health system and making that interaction more humane and effective." In November 2003, the Philanthropic Collaborative for Integrative Medicine in Minneapolis awarded Snyderman its first Bravewell Leadership Award for his "efforts to transform the culture of health care by establishing better methods of treating the whole person—mind, body, and spirit."[115]

What may prove to be Snyderman's most enduring contribution to health care is his work on another initiative: prospective health care. Prospective health care brings together the revolution in genomics with personalized medicine and the democratization of health care. According to Snyderman, the predictive tools that are becoming available—in science, technology, information, genomics, proteomics, and metabolomics—can alert individuals to their susceptibility of developing particular diseases and thus promote intervention at the earliest possible time in any given problem that a person develops. Put simply, "in addition to the usual modes of care, which is disease treatment," Snyderman says, "we're going to provide each willing individual with a personalized risk assessment to help them determine what it is that they could do to take better control of their own health and wellness and start developing plans for improving their own health. That's prospective care. How does it relate to integrative medicine? Once you give an individual a strategic plan for their own health, they become the captain of their health care team."[116]

Only time will tell if these new initiatives are as successful as Snyderman's efforts to save Duke's academic medical center. Snyderman stepped down in June 2004 as both chancellor for health affairs at Duke and the CEO of Duke University Health System. After spending the 2004–5 academic year as visiting professor at the University of California, San Francisco, he returned to Duke to work on prospective health care and a number of other ventures.

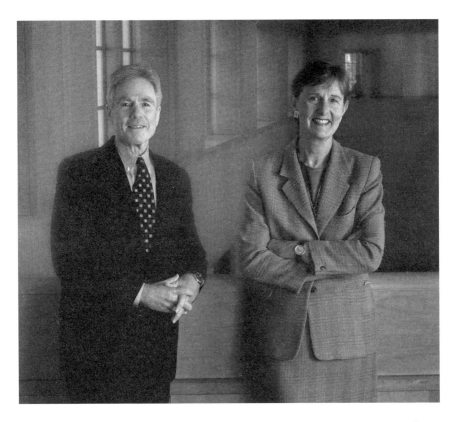

9.13 Dr. Ralph Snyderman, chancellor for health affairs, and Nannerl O. Keohane, president of Duke University, 2004. *Photograph by Chris Hildreth.*

Nan Keohane also stepped down as president of Duke in June 2004, and in the weeks before she departed, she reflected on Snyderman and his impact at Duke. "I share responsibility with Ralph and the board for having made the decision to build the large enterprise and then having made the decision gradually to dismantle parts of it," she said. "It's something that all of us did together. We made the wisest decisions we could at every stage, but I know that some of the critics of Ralph and of the health system may say . . . 'Look, they did all this stuff, and then they just had to undo it.' I think that's an unfair characterization. We didn't do as good a job in implementation at some stages as we might," she noted, "but all the decisions when we took them were the best ones we could have made at that point, given the enormously complicated evolution of health care in our country, in our region."[117]

"But the last thing I would say is even though there have been some organizational tensions between Ralph and me . . . I have a great deal of respect for Ralph's leadership. Fundamentally I think he's been a visionary leader who has done a lot to help the medical center and the health system understand their larger purposes and their reasons for being, and I think he will go down with that being increasingly clear after the dust clears on any particular leadership role." Finally, Keohane praised Snyderman's "sense of how important it is that the academic health center be sustained as an integrated unit so that patient care and education and research support each other powerfully, and his unyielding commitment to that principle, which a lot of other places abandoned, really served Duke well and made him a worthy successor of the people who saw that as our basic goal. He never lost sight of that goal even through the various organizational changes and structures. And his sense now of prospective medicine and how Duke should be engaged in that, his vision for the Institute for Genome Sciences and Policy, I mean, all those things are really major contributions."[118] [Figure 9.12]

Similar sentiments were expressed by the chairman of the Duke University Health System, Ernest Mario. "Ralph and I worked hand-in-glove during the formation of the DUHS," Mario recently wrote, "and we became not only business associates, but fast friends as well. The formation of DUHS which combined the Medical Center with Durham Regional and Raleigh Community was a bold initiative at the time. Several hospital management companies, including Tenet, were bidding against us for Durham Regional and Raleigh Community but fortunately we prevailed. It has been an interesting experience with the usual ups and downs. But today, I look back on our decisions and I am content that Ralph and I did what has turned out to be a good thing for patients in the Triangle area. It's not perfect," Mario conceded, "but given the scope of the adventure, on balance, I would do it again. Ralph carried the bulk of the responsibilities of course, so the success of DUHS is clearly his to claim."[119]

Snyderman himself recently wrote, in reflecting on his 15 years as chancellor, that "the change in thinking and practice from an independent departmental structure to an institutional organization was vital to the success and excellence of the Medical Center." The change enabled the university to act as an "integrated" institution, he explained, and thus to pursue "bold initiatives that positioned Duke as amongst the nation's leading medical centers. Indeed," Snyderman wrote in 2005, "during the last five years, Duke's reputation as an innovator and leader in academic medicine skyrocketed. The creation of the Duke Clinical Research Institute, the Duke Center for Integrative Medicine, the emphasis on translational research, and the Institute for Genome Sciences and Policy, and importantly, the Duke University Health System are all major institutional resources. This permitted entirely new approaches to health care delivery such as Prospective Care."[120]

As for what he regards as the most significant achievement of his chancellorship, Snyderman considers "the transition from a series of almost wholly independent departments to an institution built on coordinated strengths of departments, centers, and the PDC in integrated operation with medical center administration to be the greatest fundamental accomplishment." Today, Snyderman argues, "Duke is almost unique among American academic medical centers in its ability to act as a comprehensive entity. The institution can thus address big issues such as the development of better models of health care or create strategies to incorporate new technologies into more rational forms of care. This change in institutional form and function is hard to see on the surface but it permeates all of what Duke as a Medical Center and University is able to accomplish. Duke has thus created a new model for academic medicine and has found a new pathway for excellence. It can create wondrous benefits for society, and for this, I am extremely proud."[121]

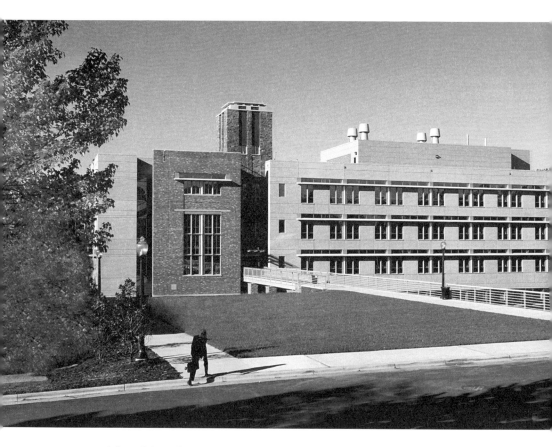

E.1 The Ralph Snyderman, M.D. Genome Sciences Research Building. *Photograph by Butch Usery, Duke University Medical Center.*

A Compassionate Global Business

On April 27, 2004, Duke president Nan Keohane stepped back from the podium as her successor-elect, Richard H. Brodhead, moved in to introduce Dr. Victor Dzau, M.D., as the next chancellor for heath affairs at Duke and the CEO of the Duke University Health System. After thanking the trustees for allowing him to participate in selecting Dzau, Brodhead turned to Dzau and said: "Victor, it will be an honor and a pleasure to be your colleague." [Figure E.1]

Two weeks earlier Keohane had received from the Duke trustees their "Final Report of the Ad Hoc Governance Committee for Duke University and Duke University Health System, Inc." The report offered what Keohane described as "a much-needed response to some of the lack of clarity in this hybrid structure" of the Duke University Health System. The health system "worked quite well in some ways but had some major shortcomings," Keohane explained, "and it was very difficult to fix them internally because there is a lot of potential tension involved. There's a lot of turf. There are a lot of people who have stakes in certain outcomes. So it became impossible to do it."[1]

Consequently, Keohane had called on the trustees for help—something she had tried to avoid while at Wellesley and at Duke. "They put together eighteen recommendations of things that needed to change," Keohane said of the trustees' report, "and from my perspective at least fifteen of them were spot on. Every one of those has been accepted, and that means that we leave this for Richard Brodhead and Victor Dzau as a much cleaner situation with a lot less murkiness about who's responsible for what and what role the president plays, what role the chancellor plays, what role the medical school plays, what role the health system plays. It's still a quasi-independent operation, but it reports indisputably to the president, which was never entirely clear. That created a lot of problems about who gets to make certain final decisions, who has responsibility. That was the first recommendation that was accepted, that that be made absolutely clear, and a lot of other things have followed from that: the way medical transfers are made in terms of the use of money, the role of the provost and the chancellor, the importance of the recognition of the nursing school."[2]

Dzau was aware of the trustees' recommendations when he was introduced to Duke, and he made it clear that he understood that Brodhead would be his boss. In noting their recent "wonderful encounters" together, Dzau said of Brodhead: "His warmth, sincerity, genuine interest in health care and intelligence truly impressed me. I told myself that I couldn't have found a better person to work for."[3]

If Brodhead came to Duke from Yale, as Keohane had come from Wellesley, lacking administrative experience with a major academic medical center, Dzau, 57, embodies much of what Ralph Snyderman laid the foundation for at DUMC. Dzau is a physician-scientist who emphasizes the importance of research to current and future health. As a cardiologist at Harvard and before that at Stanford, Dzau became familiar with managed care, genomics, and translational medicine both in Boston and in San Francisco and at two of the nation's largest, most prestigious academic medical centers. Dzau also brought with him to Duke his experience in creating two biotech companies and the expectation of soon seeing one of his own scientific discoveries "translated" into clinical practice.[4]

"In research I'm interested in the whole concept of *translation*," Dzau told a recent meeting of the university's Academic Council. "And I think you know that this is part of the emphasis of this institution. President Brodhead has certainly given great support to efforts to take basic knowledge and find how we can make it relevant in society. My work has to do with how do you take discoveries and make them applicable to man. One of the areas I work on—to do with the an inhibitor to transcription called decoy, DNA decoy—is now ready to be tried. So I keep my fingers crossed. It's one of those instances when you have physician-scientists advance to the point that an idea can actually become a therapy."[5]

Dzau also shares the progressive impulse at the heart of Duke Medicine's history. "I have come to Durham by way of Shanghai, Hong Kong, Montreal, San Francisco, and Boston," he recently said. "When I look at the diversity represented in the many faces of Duke, I realize that in addition to many people from this area, there are many others who, like me, have come from far and wide to be part of this great university."[6] Dzau likes to link this local diversity to his first major priority at Duke: the Global Health Initiative. To

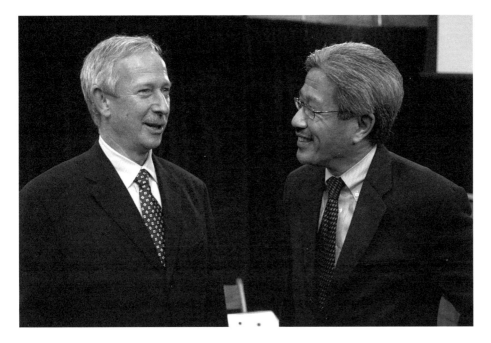

E.2 Richard H. Brodhead, ninth president of Duke University, and Dr. Victor J. Dzau, chancellor for health affairs, 2004. *Photograph by Jim Wallace Jr.*

Dzau "global" means everywhere at once, not something that is happening "out there," and the Global Health Initiative is aimed at addressing health disparities throughout the world. It includes "a think tank to inspire innovative ideas, a delivery arm to translate ideas into action, and an educational component to make sure that the leaders of the future are exposed to and trained in issues of global health." The initiative's importance is visceral to Dzau. "Five billion out of the six billion people of the world's population live in poverty and experience a disproportionate burden of disease and a shorter life expectancy because of poor environment, poor hygiene, poor access to health care and poor economics. I believe this inequity of health care is the defining issue of our time."[7]

Brodhead has supported Dzau's initiative from the start. As part of his inaugural speech in September 2004, the new president said, "In my dream, Duke would be the place where people from around the world come to learn and contribute to a growing understanding of our shared health future."[8] Brodhead also recently joined Dzau in celebrating the opening of the Walltown Neighborhood Clinic, one of two Durham clinics serving low-income patients as part the university's larger 12-neighborhood Duke-Durham Neighborhood Partnership. The clinic, which grew out of a collaboration between Duke and the grassroots Walltown Neighborhood Ministries, also received important financial support from The Duke Endowment. Dzau made it clear during the opening ceremonies, however, that the clinic was not imposed on the neighborhood by Duke. "We do not go around planting clinics like Johnny Appleseed," he said. "A community health center must emerge from the needs of the community, not from someone else's social engineering." Brodhead took a softer approach. "This is an example of what it means to be neighborly—everyone helping to do something together that they couldn't do by themselves," he said. "When health care can be made part of everyday life in the neighborhood, then progress can be made."[9]

One can only assume that James B. Duke and William Preston Few would have approved of what Brodhead and Dzau are doing. Few had sought an opportunity in 1921 "to create here in Durham a public health center for both white and colored people," and Duke, through the indenture he signed in 1924, had laid the foundation for that process. Indeed, the bold Durham entrepreneur would almost certainly have understood what Dzau meant when he said, "Health care may be a business but it's a compassionate business." And that's an excellent foundation on which to continue to build.

APPENDIX I: LIST OF DEPARTMENTS AND CHAIRS

Administration

CHANCELLOR FOR HEALTH AFFAIRS AND PRESIDENT AND CEO OF
   DUKE UNIVERSITY HEALTH SYSTEM
Position established in 1930 as the Dean of the School of Medicine
Name changed to Vice President for Health Affairs in 1969
Name changed to Chancellor for Health Affairs in 1983
Name changed to Chancellor for Health Affairs and Dean, School of
   Medicine in 1989
Name changed to Chancellor for Health Affairs, President and CEO of Duke
   University Health System, and Dean, School of Medicine in 1998
Wilburt C. Davison, 1927–60
Barnes Woodhall, 1960–64
William G. Anlyan, 1964–89
Ralph Snyderman, 1989–June 2004
Victor J. Dzau, July 2004–current

DEAN, SCHOOL OF MEDICINE
Position established in 1998

Edward W. Holmes Jr., 1999–2000
R. Sanders Williams, 2001–current

DEAN, SCHOOL OF NURSING

Bessie Baker, 1930–38
Margaret J. Pinkerton, 1939–46
Florence K. Wilson, 1946–54
Anne M. Jacobansky, 1955–68
M. Irene Brown, 1968–70
Anne M. Jacobansky (interim), 1970–71
Ruby L. Wilson, 1971–84
Rachel E. Booth, 1984–87

Dorothy J. Brundage (interim), 1987–91
Mary T. Champagne, 1991–2004
Catherine L. Gilliss, 2004–present

Clinical Sciences

DEPARTMENT OF ANESTHESIOLOGY
Established in 1950 as the Division of Anesthesiology in the Department of Surgery
Name changed to the Department of Anesthesiology in 1970

Chairs
Merel H. Harmel, 1970–83
W. David Watkins, 1983–90
Joseph G. Reves (interim), 1990–91, Chair, 1991–2001
Mark F. Newman, 2001–present

DEPARTMENT OF COMMUNITY AND FAMILY MEDICINE
Established in 1966 as the Department of Community Health Science
Name changed to the Department of Community and Family Medicine in 1979

Chairs
E. Harvey Estes Jr., 1966–85
George R. Parkerson Jr., 1985–94
J. Lloyd Michener, 1994–present

DEPARTMENT OF MEDICINE
Established in 1930

Chairs
Harold L. Amoss, 1930–33
Frederic M. Hanes, 1933–46
Eugene A. Stead Jr., 1947–67
James B. Wyngaarden, 1967–83
Joseph C. Greenfield Jr., 1983–95
Barton F. Haynes, 1995–2003
Harvey J. Cohen (interim), 2003
Pascal J. Goldschmidt, 2003–2006
Harvey J. Cohen (interim), 2006–present

DEPARTMENT OF PSYCHIATRY AND BEHAVIORAL SCIENCES
Established in 1940 as the Department of Neuropsychiatry
Name changed to the Department of Psychiatry in 1951
Name changed to the Department of Psychiatry and Behavioral Sciences in 1994

Chairs
Richard S. Lyman, 1940–51
Hans Lowenbach, 1951–53
Ewald W. Busse, 1953–74
H. Keith H. Brodie, 1974–82
Jeffrey L. Houpt (interim), 1982–83

Bernard J. Carroll, 1983–90
Dan G. Blazer (interim), 1990–92
Allen J. Frances, 1992–98
Ranga R. Krishnan, 1998–present

DEPARTMENT OF OBSTETRICS AND GYNECOLOGY
Established in 1930

Chairs
Robert A. Ross (acting), 1930–31
F. Bayard Carter, 1931–64
Roy T. Parker, 1964–80
Charles B. Hammond, 1980–2002
Haywood Brown, 2002–present

DEPARTMENT OF OPHTHALMOLOGY
Established in 1965

Chairs
Joseph A. C. Wadsworth II, 1965–78
Robert Machemer, 1978–91
W. Banks Anderson Jr. (interim), 1991–92
David L. Epstein, 1992–present

DEPARTMENT OF PEDIATRICS
Established in 1930

Chairs
Wilburt C. Davison, 1930–54
Jerome S. Harris, 1954–69
Samuel L. Katz, 1969–90
Michael M. Frank, 1990–2004
Dennis Clements (interim), 2004–2005
Joseph W. St. Geme III, 2005–present

DEPARTMENT OF RADIATION/ONCOLOGY
Established in 1991

Chairs
Leonard R. Prosnitz, 1991–96
Edward C. Halperin, 1996–2003
Leonard R. Prosnitz (interim), 2003–2004
Christopher G. Willett, 2004–present

DEPARTMENT OF RADIOLOGY
Established prior to 1936 as the Department of Roentgenology
Name changed to the Department of Radiology in 1940

Chairs
Robert J. Reeves, 1936–65
Richard G. Lester, 1965–77

Charles E. Putman, 1977–85
Carl E. Ravin, 1985–present

DEPARTMENT OF SURGERY
Established in 1930

Chairs
J. Deryl Hart, 1930–60
Clarence E. Gardner Jr., 1960–64
David C. Sabiston Jr., 1964–94
Robert W. Anderson, 1994–2003
Danny O. Jacobs, 2003–present

Basic Sciences

DEPARTMENT OF BIOLOGICAL ANTHROPOLOGY AND ANATOMY
Established in 1930 as the Department of Anatomy
Name changed to the Department of Biological Anthropology and Anatomy in 1988

Chairs
Francis H. Swett, 1930–43
Joseph E. Markee, 1943–66
J. David Robertson, 1966–88
Richard F. Kay, 1988–present

DEPARTMENT OF BIOCHEMISTRY
Established in 1930

Chairs
William A. Perlzweig, 1930–49
Philip Handler, 1950–69
Robert L. Hill, 1969–93
Christian R. H. Raetz, 1993–present

DEPARTMENT OF BIOSTATISTICS AND BIOINFORMATICS
Established in 2000

Chair
William E. Wilkinson (interim), 2000–present

DEPARTMENT OF CELL BIOLOGY
Established in 1988

Chairs
Harold P. Erickson (interim), 1988–90
Michael P. Sheetz, 1990–2000
Harold P. Erickson (interim), 2000–2002
Brigid L. M. Hogan, 2002–present

* * *

DEPARTMENT OF GENETICS

Established in 1994 when the Department of Micobiology and Immunology split

Merged with the Department of Microbiology and Immunology to form the Department of Molecular Genetics and Microbiology in 2002

Chair

Joseph R. Nevins, 1994–2002

DEPARTMENT OF IMMUNOLOGY

Established in 1992

Chair

Thomas F. Tedder, 1993–present

DEPARTMENT OF MICROBIOLOGY AND IMMUNOLOGY

Established as the Department of Bacteriology prior to 1936

Name changed to the Department of Bacteriology and Parasitology in 1938

Name changed to the Department of Bacteriology, Immunology, and Mycology in 1947

Name changed to the Department of Microbiology in 1952

Name changed to the Department of Microbiology and Immunology when combined with the Division of Immunology in 1964

Name changed to the Department of Microbiology in 1994 when the Department of Genetics was established

Merged with the Department of Genetics to form the Department of Molecular Genetics and Microbiology in 2002

Chairs

David T. Smith, 1936–58

Norman F. Conant, 1958–68

Wolfgang K. Joklik, 1968–94

Jack D. Keene (interim), 1994

Jack D. Keene, 1994–2002

DEPARTMENT OF MOLECULAR GENETICS AND MICROBIOLOGY

Established in 2002 with the merger of the Department of Genetics and Department of Microbiology and Immunology

Chairs

Joseph R. Nevins, 2002–2004

Thomas D. Petes, 2004–present

DEPARTMENT OF MOLECULAR CANCER BIOLOGY

Established in 1993

Merged with the Department of Pharmacology to form the Department of Pharmacology and Cancer Biology in 1995

Chairs

Robert M. Bell, 1993–95

Gordon G. Hammes (acting), 1995

DEPARTMENT OF NEUROBIOLOGY
Established in 1988

Chairs
William C. Hall (interim), 1988–90
Dale Purves, 1990–2002
James O. McNamara, 2002–present

DEPARTMENT OF PATHOLOGY
Established in 1930

Chairs
Wiley D. Forbus, 1930–60
Thomas D. Kinney, 1960–75
Robert D. Jennings, 1975–89
John D. Shelburne (interim), 1989–91
Salvatore V. Pizzo, 1991–present

DEPARTMENT OF PHARMACOLOGY
Established from the Department of Physiology and Pharmacology in 1977
Merged with the Department of Molecular Cancer Biology to form the Department
  of Pharmacology and Cancer Biology in 1995

Chairs
Norman Kirshner, 1977–88
Saul M. Schanberg (acting), 1988–91
Anthony R. Means, 1991–95

DEPARTMENT OF PHARMACOLOGY AND CANCER BIOLOGY
Established in 1995 as a result of the merger of the Department of Pharmacology
  and the Department of Molecular Cancer Biology

Chair
Anthony R. Means, 1995–present

DEPARTMENT OF PHYSIOLOGY
Established from the Department of Physiology and Pharmacology in 1977
Merged into the Department of Cell Biology as a division in 1988

Chairs
John V. Salzano (interim), 1975–77
Edward A. Johnson, 1977–88

DEPARTMENT OF PHYSIOLOGY AND PHARMACOLOGY
Established in 1930
Department was divided into two separate departments in 1975: the Department of
  Physiology and the Department of Pharmacology

Chairs
George S. Eadie, 1930–49
Frank G. Hall, 1949–61
Daniel C. Tosteson, 1961–75

APPENDIX 2: LIST OF FELLOWS AND HONOREES

Howard Hughes Medical Investigators

As of August 22, 2005

Vann Bennett
Joseph Heitman
Lawrence C. Katz
Robert J. Lefkowitz
Paul L. Modrich
Jonathan S. Stamler
Robin P. Wharton
John D. York

Howard Hughes Medical Institute Alumni

As of August 22, 2005

Stanley H. Appel, 1976–1977
Perry J. Blackshear, 1981–1997
Marc G. Caron, 1992–2004
George J. Cianciolo, 1979–1987
James R. Clapp, 1970–1973
Roberto Cotrufo, 1970–1972
Bryan R. Cullen, 1987–2004
Laura I. Davis, 1991–1996
Warner C. Greene, 1987–1991
John F. Griffith, 1970–1975
Edward W. Holmes Jr., 1974–1987
Robert H. Jones, 1975–1979
Nicholas M. Kredich, 1974–1989
Patrick A. McKee, 1977–1985

Joseph R. Nevins, 1986–2004
Keith L. Parker, 1986–1997
Sheldon R. Pinnell, 1973–1980
Allen D. Roses, 1977–1981
Wendell F. Rosse, 1976–1981
Ralph Snyderman, 1972–1987

National Academy of Science

Peter C. Agre
Irving T. Diamond
Irwin Fridovich
Gordon G. Hammes
Robert L. Hill
Brigid L. M. Hogan
Wolfgang K. Joklik
Robert J. Lefkowitz
Paul L. Modrich
Thomas D. Petes
Dale Purves
James B. Wyngaarden

National Institute of Medicine

As in June 9, 2005, Membership Directory

William G. Anlyan
Dan G. Blazer
H. Keith H. Brodie
Rebecca H. Buckley
Ewald W. Busse, *deceased*
Philip J. Cook
Victor J. Dzau

Joseph C. Greenfield
Charles B. Hammond
Barton F. Haynes
Robert L. Hill
Brigid L. M. Hogan
Danny O. Jacobs
Sherman A. James
Wolfgang K. Joklik
Samuel L. Katz
Robert J. Lefkowitz
Paul L. Modrich
Margaret Pericak-Vance
Dale Purves
David C. Sabiston Jr.
Debra A. Schwinn
Frank A. Sloan
Ralph Snyderman
Samuel A. Wells
Catherine M. Wilfert
R. Sanders Williams
Ruby L. Wilson
James B. Wyngaarden

American Association for the Advancement of Science Fellows

As of August 22, 2005

Rebecca H. Buckley
Joseph Heitman
Robert L. Hill
Lawrence C. Katz
Samuel L. Katz
Margaret L. Kirby
George L. Maddox
Paul L. Modrich
Miguel A. L. Nicolelis
Salvatore V. Pizzo
Leonard D. Spicer
Marilyn J. Telen
Samuel A. Wells
R. Sanders Williams

NOTES

NOTES TO FOREWORD

1. W. C. Davison, *The Duke University Medical Center (1892–1960): Reminiscences of W. C. Davison* (Durham: n.p., n.d.), 7.

2. Item 8, the will of James B. Duke, December 11, 1924.

3. The Duke Endowment Indenture of Trust, p. 13 (7th division).

4. William Osler, *Aphorisms: From His Bedside Teachings and Writings*, collected by Robert Bennett Bean, ed. William Bennett Bean (New York: Henry Schuman, Inc., 1950), 29.

5. Deryl Hart, *The First Forty Years at Duke in Surgery and the P.D.C.* (Durham: Duke University, 1971), 3.

6. Ibid., 3.

NOTES TO INTRODUCTION

1. E. C. Sage, memo to Dr. Flexner, January 21, 1921, folder 996, box 110 series 1, subseries 1, General Education Board Archives, RAC.

2. Few to Sage, February 15, 1921, in ibid.

3. *Lincoln Hospital, Thirty Eighth Annual Report* (Durham, 1939), 11.

4. The term "Duke Medicine" has been used throughout this history not only to refer with convenient brevity to the medical school and hospital at the time discussed but also to allude, in a way that is deliberately not bound to one particular point in time, to the growing and changing institution, its mission and enterprise, stretching into the future and back into the past.

5. Robert Durden, *Lasting Legacy to the Carolinas: The Duke Endowment, 1924–1994* (Durham: Duke University Press, 1998), 345.

6. Unless otherwise noted, the following is based upon Durden, *Lasting Legacy*, 1–28. The Duke indenture is reprinted on pages 335–348 of Durden's book.

7. Robert Durden, *Electrifying the Piedmont Carolinas: The Duke Power Company, 1904–1997* (Durham: Carolina Academic Press, 2001), 59.

8. Two percent is for retired Methodist ministers and their widows and orphans; 6 percent is for use in constructing rural Methodist churches; and 4 percent is for the maintenance and supervision of such churches.

9. It's not clear whether Duke left $10 million in cash or $10 million in preferred stock of Alcoa for construction of the medical center. The $6 million remaining after the center's construction, however, was in 6 percent preferred Alcoa stocks. See Durden, *Lasting Legacy*, 198; William G. Anylan, *Metamorphoses: Memoirs of a Life in Medicine* (Durham: Duke University Press, 2004), 144–145; and Davison, *The Duke University Medical Center (1892–1960)*, 18–19. For the history of Alcoa, see George David Smith, *From Monopoly to Competition: The Transformation of Alcoa, 1888–1986* (New York: Cambridge University Press, 1988).

10. For the litigation against Alcoa, see Smith, *From Monopoly to Competition*, passim.

11. Wilburt C. Davison, *The First Twenty Years: A History of Duke University Schools of Medicine, Nursing and Health Services and Duke Hospital, 1930–1950* (Durham: Duke University, 1952), 11.

12. Since 1946, Hill-Burton has provided over $6 billion in federal grants and loans to 6,800 health care facilities in more than 4,000 communities. In return for Hill-Burton funds, the facilities agree to provide free or reduced

charge medical services to those individuals who cannot pay. U.S. Department of Health and Human Services, Health Resources and Services Administration, "The Hill-Burton Free Care Program," http://www.hrsa.gov/osp /dfcr/ about/aboutdiv.htm [May 17, 2005]. On the Endowment's role as a template for Hill-Burton, see James F. Gifford Jr., *The Evolution of a Medical Center: A History of Medicine at Duke University to 1941* (Durham: Duke University Press, 1972), 174–175.

13. These matters are covered in detail in chapters 1–5 below.

14. For the research funded by Lederle and the RF see, Duke University, "Gift of Funds," Book 2, Duke University Archives. For a summary of Neurath's career, see his obituary in the *New York Times*, April 18, 2002. See *New York Times*, May 1, 1976, for a list of the physicians on the medical advisory board of the Howard Hughes Institute.

15. Nicole Kresge, Robert D. Simoni, and Robert L. Hill, "Blacktongue and Nicotinic Acid Metabolism: Philip Handler," *Journal of Biological Chemistry* 279 (November 26, 2004): 8–9. Robert Hill succeeded Handler as chairman of the Department of Biochemistry in 1969.

16. Davison, *The First Twenty Years*, 30.

17. Except where otherwise noted, the following discussion is based on Hart, *The First Forty Years*, 1–47.

18. Ibid., 11.

19. Private Diagnostic Clinic, "Description of PDC Organization," n.d. [ca. 2004–2005].

20. *Time*, April 27, 1931, 25

21. Keith Brodie and Leslie Banner, *Keeping an Open Door: Passages in a University Presidency* (Durham: Duke University Press, 1996), 7.

22. Ibid., 6.

NOTES TO CHAPTER 1

1. Rockefeller Archive Center, "Rockefeller Related Organizations: General Education Board," http://archive.rockefeller.edu/collections/rockorgs/geb.php [May 17, 2005].

2. James L. Leloudis, *Schooling the New South* (Chapel Hill: University of North Carolina Press, 1996), 151.

3. See the brief description of collections in the Rockefeller Archives Center, at http://archive.rockefeller.edu/collections/rf/#intl [May 17, 2005].

4. See Ferrell's obituary in the *New York Times*, February 20, 1965.

5. See W. S. Rankin to May McLelland, January 27, 1939, Watson Smith Rankin Papers, RBMSCL (first quotation); and James F. Gifford Jr., "Watson Smith Rankin and Standardization in Health Care: Hospitals, Philanthropy and Public Health, 1900–1950," unpublished manuscript, n.d., 5 (second quotation), DUMCA. For a biographical sketch of Rankin, see *National Cyclopedia of American Biography* (Clifton, N.J.: James T. White, 1975), 56:264–265.

6. Rankin, interview, 24.

7. Rankin to Davison, January 22, 1947, William Preston Few Papers, DUA.

8. Joseph S. Ross, "The Committee on the Costs of Medical Care and the History of Health Insurance in the United States," *Einstein Quarterly Journal of Biological Medicine* 19 (2002): 129–134.

9. *New York Times*, November 30, 1932.

10. Quoted in Ross, "The Committee on the Costs of Medical Care," 131.

11. Ibid.

12. Davison, *The First Twenty Years*, 58–59. For the statistics on DUMC, see Charles H. Frenzel, hospital report, May 18, 1959, in Wilburt C. Davison Papers, DUMCA.

13. Davison, *First Twenty Years*, 1–30, 46.

14. Jay M. Arena and John P. McGovern, eds., *Davison of Duke: His Reminiscences* (Durham: Duke University Medical Center, 1980), 147–148.

15. C. Rufus Rorem to Rankin, May 12, 1937, Rankin Papers, RBMSCL.

NOTES TO CHAPTER 2

1. See *New York Times*, March 27, 1933; January 13 and July 15, 1934; and June 27, 1935.

2. Beard to Alfred Blalock, February 8, 1937, Joseph Willis Beard Papers, DUMCA.

3. Peyton Rous to Beard, February 15, 1937, Beard Papers.

4. Joseph W. Beard, "Origin and Disposition of the Dorothy Beard Research Fund," 3, manuscript dated July 24, 1971, Beard Papers.

5. Bell to Davison, telegram, July 29, 1937; and Davison to Bell, July 29, 1937, Davison Papers.

6. *National Cyclopedia of American Biography* (New York: James T. White, 1965), 46:45–48; "New Attacks on Cancer Outlined by Bell at SCI Dinner" and "William Brown Bell" *Chemical and Engineering News* 27, no. 46 (November 14, 1949): 3351.

7. Frank Blair Hanson to W. P. Few, May 28,

1936, "Gift of Funds," 2:128-a, DUA (quotation); "David Tillerson Smith," *Aesculapian* (Duke University, 1980), special 50th anniversary issue, *1930–1980*. For the Smiths' research see *New York Times*, October 5, 1938. For their involvement with the Durham Monthly Meeting of Friends, see "History of Durham Meeting," http://durhammonthlymtg.home.mindspring.com/Handbook/DMMhistory.htm [May 17, 2005].

8. The best summary of Beard's career is R. McIntyre Bridges, "Dr. Joseph Willis Beard: A Mighty Man, 1902–1983," *North Carolina Medical Journal* 46, no. 5 (May 1985): 303–309.

9. *Lederle Veterinary Bulletin* 6, no. 4 (July–August 1937): 67.

10. *Lederle Veterinary Bulletin* 10, no. 1 (January–February 1941): 15.

11. Beard, "Origin and Disposition," 3, Beard Papers.

12. Marion B. Sulzberger, "Studies in Tobacco Hypersensitivity, I: A Comparison between Reactions to Nicotine and to Denicotinized Tobacco Extract," *Journal of Immunology* 24 (1933): 85–91.

13. Coca knew all of the immunologists with whom Beard worked at Rockefeller. Several of them, in fact, were officers and directors of the American Association of Immunologists. For information on Coca see University of Milwaukee–Wisconsin, Archives of the American Academy of Allergy, Asthma, and Immunology, http://www.uwm.edu/Library/arch/aaaai/president/coca.htm [May 17, 2005], and his obituary in the *New York Times*, December 13, 1959. The first issue of the *Lederle Veterinary Bulletin* appeared in April–May 1932.

14. Beard, "Origin and Disposition," 3.

15. For information on Wyckoff, see "Ralph W. G. Wyckoff, 1897–1994 — Obituary," *Acta Crystallographica* A51 (1995): 649–650; and his obituary in the *New York Times*, November 9, 1994. For Beard and Wyckoff's work together at Rockefeller, see Ralph W. G. Wyckoff to Coca, May 2, 1939; and Beard to Coca, May 18, 1939, both in the Peyton Rous Papers, American Philosophical Society.

16. *Lederle Veterinary Bulletin* 6, no. 3 (May–June 1937): 43. For the manufacture of sulfanilamide at the Calco Chemical Company, see Bell to Davison, October 9, 1937, Davison Papers.

17. For a list of Lederle's facilities, see *Lederle Veterinary Bulletin* 9, no. 4 (September–October 1940): 136.

18. Tony Travis, "Analysts in the Dye and Allied Industries: Calco Chemical Company and American Cyanamid, 1930–1960," paper presented at the Society for Alchemy and Chemistry, May 2002.

19. See Davis and Geck Company Records, Archives and Special Collections, Thomas J. Dodd Research Center, University of Connecticut Libraries, http://www.lib.uconn.edu/online/research/speclib/ACS/findaids/Davis-geck/biography.htm [May 17, 2005]. The company's film program continued until the 1980s as the Cliné Clinic Films Program.

20. Bell to Davison, August 6, 1937, Davison Papers. The letter is addressed to George Davison. Apparently, Bell addressed Davison as "George" in order to keep their correspondence as private as possible. See discussion below regarding the "secret" cancer research trials using an extract of aspergillus.

21. Ibid.

22. Davison to Bell, August 10, 1937, Davison Papers.

23. Davison to Bell, August 13, 1937, Davison Papers.

24. Bell to Davison, August 13, 1937, Davison Papers.

25. Ibid.

26. For references to the secrecy of the matter, see Bell to Davison, July 23, 1937, Davison Papers.

27. Leonard J. Ravenel to Beard, August 31, 1937, Davison Papers. Ravenel was one of the physicians administering the aspergillus treatment; Beard was the director of Lederle Laboratories.

28. For references to this meeting, see Bell to Davison, August 15, 1937; and Ravenel to Beard, August 31, 1937, both in Davison Papers.

29. Bell to Davison, August 15, 1937, Davison Papers.

30. Beard, "Origin and Disposition," 5.

31. Quoted in Arena and McGovern, *Davison of Duke*, 174. For Rankin's career, see *The National Cyclopedia of American Biography* (New York: James T. White, 1974), 56: 264–265; James F. Gifford Jr., "Watson Smith Rankin and Standardization in Health Care: Hospitals, Philanthropy and Public Health, 1900–1950," manuscript, n.d., James F. Gifford Jr. Papers, DUMCA. See Watson Smith Rankin, interview, 25, for McLeod's conversion to a nonprofit community hospital.

32. For information on Fred Rankin, see

his obituary in *New York Times*, May 23, 1954; Watson Smith Rankin to Fred Rankin, January 1, 1944, and Fred Rankin to W. S. Rankin, January 14, 1944, both in Rankin Papers, RBMSCL. For Fred Rankin's position on the AMA's council, see Council on Medical Education and Hospitals of the American Medical Association, *Survey of Medical Schools, 1934–1937* (Chicago: Privately printed, 1937).

33. See Perlzweig's memo in box 21, William Brown Bell Correspondence, Davison Papers. Reeves's response appears as a handwritten note on James McLeod to Davison, November 4, 1937, Davison Papers.

34. James McLeod to Davison, November 4, 1937, Davison Papers.

35. Bell to McLeod, September 17, 1937, Davison Papers.

36. See Davison's memo, September 22, 1937, Davison Papers.

37. Davison to Bell, October 12, 1937, Davison Papers.

38. Bell to Davison, October 9, 1937, Davison Papers.

39. Davison to Bell, October 12, 1937, Davison Papers.

40. *New York Times*, September 24, 1937, and October 8, 1937 (quotation).

41. For Rankin's stock holdings, see Rankin to C. D. Cooke Jr., May 16, 1938, Rankin Papers, RBMSCL. See Kenneth Towe, interview, for Inman's Cyanamid holdings. For B. N. Duke's Cyanamid holdings at the time of his death in 1929, see *New York Times*, June 11, 1935; for the Cyanamid holdings of his widow, Sarah P. Duke, see her obituary in the *New York Times*, July 1, 1937.

42. Altvater and Davison to Rankin, October 20, 1937, Davison Papers.

43. *New York Times*, December 12, 1936. The relationship between Duke's Department of Chemistry and Liggett & Myers is briefly mentioned in "Trial Transcript of Fred Darkis" (April 18, 1960), Bates: RC6000217-RC6000294, http://tobaccodocuments.org/ness/5281.html. Darkis worked as a chemist at Liggett & Myers between 1927 and 1932 before joining Duke's Department of Chemistry. He worked in the department from 1933 to 1947, when he returned to Liggett & Myers as research director of its new laboratory in Durham. See http://tobaccodocuments.org,"Purpose of Scientific Publication" (February 3, 1941), American Tobacco Company, for quote on the department's bright to-

bacco research; and J. Granville Myers to J. A. Crowe, September 4, 1934, http://tobaccodocuments.org for Gross's patents.

44. See *Time*, October 25, 1937; *New York Times*, October 4, 1937; and the "Scope and Content Note" for the Parapsychology Laboratory Records, 1893–1984, RBMSCL.

45. See Durden, *Lasting Legacy*, 335–348, for a copy of the indenture.

46. The disagreement over the Duke Power litigation is mentioned in Durden, *Electrifying the Piedmont Carolinas*, 145. For developments in the litigation in 1937, see *New York Times*, June 20, August 7, and October 26, 1937. For quotation, see Robert A. Lambert, officer's diary, July 16, 1934, RG 12.1, Rockefeller Foundation Archives, RAC.

47. See *New York Times*, June 29, 1937.

48. Michael Durham, *George Garland Allen: A Life to Be Honored* (Privately printed, 1983), 22.

49. Ibid.

50. Ibid.

51. See Introduction above.

52. Wilburt C. Davison, "Compulsory Health Insurance—Who Is Fooling Whom?" typed manuscript, Davison Papers, ca. 1948.

53. For the early history of DUMC, see Gifford, *The Evolution of a Medical Center*.

54. Quoted in William Buxton, "The Emergence of the Humanities Division Program in Communications, 1930–1936," *Rockefeller Archives Newsletter* (spring 1996), 3–4.

55. Quoted in ibid.

56. The best summary of the Rockefeller Foundation's psychosomatic program is Jack D. Pressman, "Human Understanding: Psychosomatic Medicine and the Mission of the Rockefeller Foundation," 189–208, in *Greater Than the Parts: Holism in Biomedicine, 1920–1950*, ed. Christopher Lawrence and George Weisz (New York: Oxford University Press, 1998). For a biography of Gregg by Davison's World War I buddy, see Wilder Penfield, *The Difficult Art of Giving: The Epic of Alan Gregg* (Boston: Little, Brown, 1967).

57. Pressman, "Human Understanding," 191.

58. See ibid., 196–197, for the Harvard Study. For specific information on the teaching of psychosomatic medicine at Harvard, see Theodore M. Brown, "The Historical and conceptual Foundations of the Rochester Biopsychosocial Model," Department of History, University of Rochester, Rochester,

New York (December 11, 2003), http://www. history.rochester.edu/history/fac/brown.htm. The major figures Brown mentions at Harvard—Drs. Soma Weiss, John Roman, and George Engle—were also colleagues there with Dr. Eugene Stead. See Galen S. Wagner, Bess Cebe, and Marvin P. Rozear, eds., *E. A. Stead, Jr., What This Patient Needs Is a Doctor* (Durham: Duke Hospital, 1981), 147–153.

59. Pressman, "Human Understanding," 201–202.

60. Mary Duke Biddle Trent Semans, interview, UNC-TV, 2003, http://www.unctv.org/biocon/msemans/prg03.html [May 17, 2005].

61. Seventeen of those were on the staff of the three state hospitals; seven worked in the state's four psychiatric institutions; three were in private practice; Crispell was the only one teaching.

62. "North Carolina Commission for the Study of the Insane and Mentally Defective, September 1, 1935–September 30, 1937," 4, folder 46, box 5, series 236A, RG 1.1, Rockefeller Foundation Archives, RAC.

63. Alan Gregg, officer's diary, June 4, 1936, RG 12.1, Rockefeller Foundation Archives, RAC.

64. "North Carolina Commission," 4.

65. Ibid.

66. Robert A. Lambert, memo, "September 1 to 12, 1937, Vacation in North Carolina with Dr. F. M. Hanes," folder 1112, box 126, series 200A, RG 1.2, Rockefeller Foundation Archives, RAC.

67. For Doris Duke's interest in and support for child guidance and dependent child care, see Watson Rankin to Marian Paschal, October 25, 1937, Davison Papers; and the correspondence in "Stern, William, Special Research Fund for European Scholars, 1933–1939," folder 1115, box 126, RG 1.2, Rockefeller Foundation Archives, RAC.

68. Social Service Division, Duke University Hospital, "Social Service Division, 1930–1940," pp. 2–3, DDCFA.

69. Davison to Dr. Marian Kenworthy (New York School of Social Work), April 18, 1944, Davison Papers.

70. See the division's annual reports in the DDCFA.

71. James E. Shepard to Paschal, September 18, 1937, DDCFA.

72. See the folder marked "North Carolina College in Durham," DDCFA.

73. *New York Times*, November 22, 1937.

74. Theodore M. Brown, "Friendship and Philanthropy: Henry Sigerist, Alan Gregg and the Rockefeller Foundation," in *Making Medical History: The Life and Times of Henry E. Sigerist*, ed. Elizabeth Fee and Theodore M. Brown (Baltimore: Johns Hopkins University Press, 1997), 290.

75. Clarence Gardner, October 30, 1964, "Testimonial Banquet at time of my retirement," Davison Papers.

76. Arena and McGovern, eds., *Davison of Duke*, 33.

77. Memo, April 28, 1931, "Visit of HAS and Jackson Davis," folder 997, box 110, series 1, subseries 1, General Education Board Archives, RAC.

78. Max Schiebel, "When I Was Younger: Looking Back at My Residency 65 Years Ago," *North Carolina Medical Journal* 60, no. 3 (May–June 1999): 132.

79. Gardner, "Testimonial Banquet," Davison Papers.

80. Anlyan, *Metamorphoses*, 33.

81. Robert A. Lambert, officer's diary, June 26, 1933, RG 12.1, Rockefeller Foundation Archives, RAC (first quotation); and Arena and McGovern, eds., *Davison of Duke*, 134 (second quotation).

82. Kevin Begos, quoting historian Robert Korstad, in "Selling a Solution: Group Founded by Hanes, Others Sent Sterilization in New Direction," from part 3 of "Against Their Will: North Carolina's Sterilization Program, Special Report," *Winston-Salem Journal*, n.d., http://extras.journalnow.com/againsttheirwill/parts/three/storybody1.html.

83. Hanes to Davison, February 16, 1937, Davison Papers.

84. Hanes to G. G. Allen, March 8, 1945, Frederic Moir Hanes Papers, DUMCA.

85. Hanes to Lambert, July 4, 1934, series 200A, Duke University (Kempner), RG 1.1, Rockefeller Foundation Archives, RAC.

86. See William S. Powell, ed., *Dictionary of North Carolina Biography*, 2:23–28.

87. Robert A. Lambert, officer's diary, October 13, 1933.

88. Hanes to Lambert, April 26, 1934, folder 1024, box 85, series 200, Walter Kempner, RG 1.1, Rockefeller Foundation Archives, RAC.

89. Deryl Hart, "The Responsibility of the Medical Profession to Medical Education: Contributions of the Geographic Full Time Staff to the Development of the Duke University School of Medicine and Suggestions for

the Assumption of More of the Cost of Medical Education by the Medical Profession as a Whole," *Annals of Surgery* 145 (May 1957): 601.

90. Hart, *The First Forty Years*, 9–10. The Hart quotes below are taken from this source.

91. This incident is discussed in Clarence Gardner and Ivan Brown, interview, December 7, 1991, DUMCA. For Agnes Hanes's obituary see *New York Times*, September 20, 1935.

92. Hanes to Hart, August 5, 1937, Davison Papers.

93. Ibid. (second quotation); and Hart, *The First Forty Years*, 10 (first quotation).

94. Hart, *The First Forty Years*, 12 (first quotation); and Hanes to Hart, August 5, 1937, Davison Papers (second quotation).

95. Hart, *The First Forty Years*, 12.

NOTES TO CHAPTER 3

1. Michael Kammen, *Mystic Chords of Memory: The Transformation of Tradition in American Culture* (New York: Alfred A. Knopf, 1991), 299–300.

2. See Durden, *Lasting Legacy*, 146.

3. W. S. Rankin to Davison, January 29, 1938, Davison Papers.

4. Lederle hired Wyckoff to work at Pearl River and purchased almost everything in his biophysics laboratory at the Rockefeller Institute in New York, including the ultracentrifuges and x-ray diffraction equipment Wyckoff had developed. See memo, December 23, 1937, "Used Equipment from Bio-Physics Laboratory Sold to Lederle Laboratories," in folder 2, RU-450 W972, Rockefeller University Archives, RAC. Likewise, Beard had staffed and equipped his laboratory at DUMC using the funds provided by Lederle and The Duke Endowment. For a description of work in Beard's laboratory, see Will C. Sealy, "The Hen's Egg versus the Horse's Brain: How Equine Encephalomyelitis Vaccine Established the Dorothy and Joseph Beard Foundation," manuscript in the Beard Papers, DUMCA, pp. 1–6. Sealy's piece was also published in *North Carolina Medical Journal* 47 (January 1986): 37–38.

5. Beard, "Dorothy Beard Research Fund," 6–7.

6. Ibid., 7.

7. Ibid., 9.

8. *Lederle Veterinary Bulletin* 6, no. 3 (May–June 1938). See also United States Patent Office, patent no. 2,204,064.

9. Beard, "Dorothy Beard Research Fund," 10.

10. Bell to Davison, June 22, 1938, Davison Papers.

11. Beard, "Dorothy Beard Research Fund," 8.

12. Hanes to Gregg, April 21, 1938, folder 114, box 126, series 200A, RG 1.2, Rockefeller Foundation Archives, RAC.

13. Davison to Gregg, April 22, 1938, Rockefeller Foundation Archives, RAC.

14. Ibid.

15. Hanes to Gregg, June 1, 1938, folder 114, box 126, series 200A, RG 1.2, Rockefeller Foundation Archives, RAC.

16. Hanes to Gregg, June 7, 1938, folder 114, box 126, series 200A, RG 1.2, Rockefeller Foundation Archives, RAC.

17. Gregg to Davison, June 13, 1938, Rockefeller Foundation Archives, RAC.

18. Gregg, officer's diary, June 21, 1938, RG 12.1, Rockefeller Foundation Archives, RAC.

19. Ibid.

20. *New York Times*, October 2, 1938.

21. "Duke University, The Duke Centennial Fund, 1838 Trinity College 1938," copy in folder 1001, box 111, series 1, subseries 1, pamphlets, General Education Board Archives, RAC.

22. Archie S. Woods to Davison, October 27, 1938, in "Gift of Funds," book 2, DUA.

23. *New York Times*, October 25, 1938.

24. Memo, September 27, 1935, folder 1023, box 85, series 200, subseries 200A, RG 1.1, Rockefeller Foundation Archives, RAC.

25. Davison to Lambert, April 18, 1936, Rockefeller Foundation Archives, RAC.

26. Davison, *First Twenty Years*, 40; W. Reece Berryhill, William B. Blythe, and Isaac H. Manning, *Medical Education at Chapel Hill: The First Hundred Years* (Chapel Hill: University of North Carolina School of Medicine, 1979), 38–41; and Lambert, officer's diary, May 5, 1936, folder 1023, box 85, series 200, subseries 200A, RG 1.1, Rockefeller Foundation Archives, RAC. For Brown's appointment at UNC, see Robert R. Korstad, *Dreaming of a Time: The School of Public Health, the University of North Carolina at Chapel Hill, 1939–1990* (Chapel Hill: School of Public Health, 1990).

27. Newbold first made his proposal in 1931. See N. C. Newbold to Jackson Davis, March 12, 1931, folder 997, box 110, series 1, subseries 1, General Education Board Archives, RAC. Apparently nothing more was said about the matter until 1934, when the GEB asked Newbold to resubmit his proposal. See Newbold to

Davis, February 22, 1934, General Education Board Archives, RAC.

28. Newbold to Davis, February 22, 1934, General Education Board Archives, RAC.

29. Ibid.

30. Ibid.

31. This account of Lincoln's reorganization is based on Gifford, *Evolution of a Medical Center*, 163–168.

32. Lincoln Hospital, *Thirty-Eighth Annual Report, 1938* (Durham, 1939), 21.

33. *New York Times*, January 8, 1939.

34. For the timing of Hanes's speech, see T. R. Waring Jr. to Hanes, October 23, 1938, in the Hanes Papers, DUMCA. A copy of the speech is with this letter.

35. *New York Times*, September 9, 1938 (quotation). See also Gifford, *Evolution of a Medical Center*, 174–175; Colin Gordon, *Dead on Arrival: The Politics of Health Care in Twentieth-Century America* (Princeton, N.J.: Princeton University Press, 2003), 17–18; and *New York Times*, October 7, 1937.

36. *Lederle Veterinary Bulletin* 8, no. 4 (September–October 1939): 63.

37. Beard, "Dorothy Beard Research Fund," 8.

38. Richard Shope to Beard, July 19, 1939, Beard Papers.

39. *Lederle Veterinary Bulletin* 8, no. 1 (January–February 1939): 19.

40. See Beard, "Dorothy Beard Research Fund," and "Gift of Funds," book 2, DUA.

41. Beard, "Dorothy Beard Research Fund," cover page. Beard reported that the fund was administered by Dr. Davison, Dr. Hart, and himself and that he was given "very great freedom with the Fund." See ibid., 11. For the Bell Building see Hart, *The First Forty Years*, 239.

42. See Albert Heinz to Treasurer of Duke University, July 7, 1938, "Gift of Funds," bk. 2, DUA, for Perlzweig's special project. For information on Neurath, see his obituaries in the *New York Times*, April 18, 2002, and the *Seattle Post-Intelligencer*, April 13, 2002.

43. See Albert Heinz to Duke University, August 10, 1939, "Gift of Funds," bk. 2, DUA.

44. Beard, "Dorothy Beard Research Fund," 11.

45. Beard to Arthur F. Coca, May 18, 1939 (first quotation); and George P. Berry to Coca, June 15, 1939 (second quotation), both in Peyton Rouse Collection, American Philosophical Society.

46. Beard to Coca, May 18, 1939, Peyton Rous Papers, American Philosophical Society.

47. George Packer Berry to Peyton Rous, July 15, 1939, Peyton Rous Collection, American Philosophical Society.

48. Thomas M. Rivers to Rous, July 19, 1939, Peyton Rous Collection, American Philosophical Society.

49. Memo, May 8, 1939, Davison Papers.

50. Rous to Coca, July 27, 1939, Peyton Rous Collection, American Philosophical Society.

51. Gifford, *Evolution of a Medical Center*, 89.

52. Gregg, officer's diary, December 13, 1938, folder 112, box 126, series 200A, RG 1.2, Rockefeller Foundation Archives, RAC.

53. See Hubert B. Haywood, "Mental Hygiene in North Carolina," *North Carolina Medical Journal* (March 1941): 139–142; and *Biennial Report of the North Carolina State Board of Charities and Public Welfare, July 1, 1938 to June 30, 1940* (Raleigh: Edwards and Broughton, 1940), 106.

54. Hanes to Lambert, January 10, 1939 (first quotation); and Hanes to Lambert, January 30, 1939 (second quotation), both in folder 112, box 126, series 200A, RG 1.2, Rockefeller Foundation Archives, RAC.

55. Hanes to Lambert, January 30, 1939, folder 112, box 126, series 200A, RG 1.2, Rockefeller Foundation Archives, RAC. Although Hanes wrote this letter requesting a fellowship for Graves, it accurately reflects his views on the kind of physician he wanted to head the new Department of Psychiatry.

56. Lambert to Hanes, January 23, 1939, folder 112, box 126, series 200A, RG 1.2, Rockefeller Foundation Archives, RAC.

57. Meyer's comments on Carroll are quoted in Lyman to Gregg, November 11, 1940, folder 112, box 126, series 200A, RG 1.2, Rockefeller Foundation Archives, RAC.

58. Robert S. Carroll, *Our Nervous Friends: Illustrating the Mastery of Nervousness* (New York: Macmillan, 1919).

59. Robert S. Carroll to Wendell Muncie, February 28, 1939, Highland Hospital Collection, Pack Memorial Library.

60. *National Cyclopedia of American Biography* (New York: James T. White, 1965), 47: 183–184.

61. Gregg, officer's diary, March 21, 1939, folder 112, box 126, series 200A, RG 1.2, Rockefeller Foundation Archives, RAC.

62. Carroll to Muncie, April 25, 1939, Highland Hospital Collection, Pack Memorial Library.

63. Hanes to Lambert, June 16, 1939, folder 112, box 126, series 200A, RG 1.2, Rockefeller Foundation Archives, RAC.

64. Hanes to Lambert, June 28, 1939, see "Excerpt from letter from Frederic M. Hanes to R. A. Lambert," folder 112, box 126, series 200A, RG 1.2, Rockefeller Foundation Archives, RAC.

65. Carroll to Muncie, August 2, 1939, Highland Hospital Collection, Pack Memorial Library. For information on Duke's lease with Highland Hospital, Inc., see the Highland Hospital Collection, Pack Memorial Library.

66. Carroll to Muncie, August 2, 1939, Highland Hospital Collection, Pack Memorial Library.

67. Lambert, officer's diary, October 12, 1939, folder 112, box 126, series 200A, RG 1.2, Rockefeller Foundation Archives, RAC.

68. Lambert to Davison and Hanes, Telegram, January 19, 1940, folder 112, box 126, series 200A, RG 1.2, Rockefeller Foundation Archives, RAC.

69. Wilburt C. Davison, "The First Ten Years of Duke University School of Medicine and Duke Hospital," *North Carolina Medical Journal* (October 1941): 527–532.

70. Charles Hampton Mauzy, "Cesarean Section: Its Incidence and Fetal Mortality in Some Cities in North Carolina," *North Carolina Medical Journal* (January 1942): 6.

71. "Annual Report of Social Service Department, Duke Hospital," July 1, 1941–June 15, 1942, 1–2, DDCFA.

72. Davison, "The First Ten Years," 530.

73. J. A. Long to Few, August 7, 1940, Few Papers, DUA.

74. Josiah W. Bailey to Watson Rankin, July 21, 1938, Rankin Papers, RBMSCL.

75. May McLelland to Rankin, January 24, 1939, Rankin Papers, RBMSCL.

76. For information on Stevens, see Davison, *The First Twenty Years*, 6, 283; and the *Aesculapian* (1980): 147. For the statistics on Duke University School of Medicine, see Davison, "The First Ten Years," 527–532.

77. See Davison, "The First Ten Years."

78. J. M. Van Hoy, *Aesculapian* (1980): 150; and K. D. Weeks, *Aesculapian* (1980): 153 (fourth quotation).

79. Earl A. O'Neill, *Aesculapian* (1980): 159.

80. Hanes to Davison, February 27, 1939, Davison Papers.

81. Lambert, officer's diary, May 9, 1939, box 34, RG 12.1, Rockefeller Foundation Archives, RAC.

82. See "School of Nursing," *Aesculapian* (1980): 351.

83. See ibid. (quotation); and Davison, *The First Twenty Years*, 61–66. For the two-year requirement, see Duke University, "Pictorial Bulletin of Information: Duke Hospital," March 1940, 6.

84. Dorothy Mary Smith, interview, March 26, 1979, p. 9.

85. Davison, *The First Twenty Years*, 8.

86. Few to Hanes, September 27, 1940, Davison Papers. Hanes's plan, in altered form, is mentioned in Hanes to George G. Allen, March 2, 1945, Hanes Papers, DUMCA.

87. Lyman to Gregg, November 8, 1940, RF, folder 112, box 126, series 200A, RG 1.2, Rockefeller Foundation Archives, RAC.

88. Gregg to Lyman, November 8, 1940, folder 112, box 126, series 200A, RG 1.2, Rockefeller Foundation Archives, RAC.

89. Hanes to Gregg, January 23, 1941, folder 113, box 126, series 200A, RG 1.2, Rockefeller Foundation Archives, RAC.

NOTES TO CHAPTER 4

1. See the "History" section of Fort Bragg's web site (December 2003), http://www.bragg.army.mil/history/HistoryPage/HistoryFortBragg/FortBragginthe1940s.htm.

2. See Dan Crozier, "History of the Commission on Epidemiological Survey," and William S. Jordan, "History of the Commission on Acute Respiratory Diseases, Commission on Air-Borne Infections, Commission on Meningococcal Meningitis, and Commission on Pneumonia," in *The Armed Forces Epidemiological Board: The Histories of the Commissions*, ed. Theodore E. Woodward (Washington, D.C.: Borden Institute, Office of the Surgeon General, Department of the Army, 1994). Electronic versions of the book can be found at Office of the Surgeon General, Office of Medical History, http://history.amedd.army.mil/booksdocs/historiesofcomsn/default.htm [May 18, 2005].

3. William S. Jordan, "History of the Commission on Acute Respiratory Diseases," 213. For DUMC's physicians on other commissions, see Davison, *The First Twenty Years*, 75.

4. See Jordan, "History of the Commission on Acute Respiratory Diseases," 10, for the commission's private funding. For research funding at DUMC during the war, see the entries for Lederle, Rockefeller, and Markle in Duke University, "Gift of Funds," bks. 2 and 3, DUA.

5. Hubert B. Haywood, "President's Address," *North Carolina Medical Journal* (June 1941): 277–278.

6. For information on Camp Butner, see GlobalSecurity.org, Military, "Camp Butner National Guard Training Center," http://www.globalsecurity.org/military/facility/camp-butner.htm [May 18, 2005]. Lynn K. Juckett, "Dad Goes to War" [May 18, 2005], http://www.thejucketts.com/ww2website/dadown-words.htm [May 18, 2005] (first quotation); and Jean Bradley Anderson, *Durham County* (Durham: Duke University Press, 1990), 383 (second quotation).

7. Ruth E. Barker, "Annual Report of the Social Service Department, July, 1940–July, 1941," DDCFA.

8. See University of Memphis, "The University of Memphis's First Distinguished Research Professor: W. Harry Feinstone," http://www.people.memphis.edu/research/cato1res.pdf [March 2004].

9. *New York Times*, August 17, 1941.

10. See W. Harry Feinstone to Alfred Blalock, December 9, 1942, Alfred Blalock Papers, DUMCA.

11. For DUMC's work with Cyanamid's sulfa drugs, see chapter 2 above and "Gifts through the Department of Medicine," June 27, 1939, in Duke University, "Gift of Funds," bk. 2, DUA.

12. Beard et al., "The Serological Diagnosis of Syphilis," *Science* (January 19, 1945).

13. See Davison, *The First Twenty Years*, 78–79; and "W. K. Kellogg Foundation," June 10, 1942, in "Gift of Funds," bk. 3, DUA.

14. Earl A. O'Neill, "Entering Class of 1938," *Aesculapian* (1980).

15. Davison, *The First Twenty Years*, 67–87.

16. Ibid., 67 (quotation). For the sizes of the different classes see the *Aesculapian* (1980): 163–175. Both the supplement to Duke's loan fund and the grant from Kellogg are discussed in "W. K. Kellogg Foundation," George Darling to Davison, April 20, 1942, and Davison to Darling, April 28, 1942, both in "Gift of Funds," bk. 3, DUA.

17. Lambert, officer's diary, February 18, 1942, RG 12.1, Rockefeller Foundation Archives, RAC.

18. Gregg to Davison, December 11, 1940, RG 12.1, Rockefeller Foundation Archives, RAC.

19. Davison to Lambert, April 2, 1943, Davison Papers.

20. Lambert, officer's diary, April 25, 1943, RG 12.1, Rockefeller Foundation Archives, RAC.

21. Lambert, officer's diary, April 22, 1942 (first quotation), and April 25 and 16, 1943 (second quotation), both in RG 12.1, Rockefeller Foundation Archives, RAC.

22. Lambert to Salvador Zubiran, January 21, 1943; and Davison to Lambert, January 25, 1943, both in Davison Papers, DUMCA.

23. Lambert to Davison, November 19, 1942 (first quotation); and Davison to Lambert, November 25, 1942 (second quotation), both in Davison Papers, DUMCA.

24. Andrew J. Warren to Davison, September 13, 1943; and Davison to Warren, September 21, 1943, both in Davison Papers, DUMCA.

25. Memo, May 29, 1929, folder 997, box 110, series 1, subseries 1, General Education Board Archives, RAC.

26. See "General Education Board" in "Gift of Funds," bk. 2, DUA. The economic projects were the "Economic Factors in the Utilization of Synthetic Fibres by Southern Textile Mills" and "The Potential Volume of Employment in Forest Industries of the South." The two forestry projects were "Optimum Size of a Sustained Forestry Enterprise—A Study of Land Use in Durham County" and "Studies of Markets for Forest Products in Central North Carolina."

27. Arena and McGovern, eds., *Davison of Duke*, 153–154.

28. The National Academies, "Advisory Committees to the Surgeons General of the War and Navy Departments and U.S. Public Health Service," http://www7.nationalacademies.org/archives/advcomsurgeons.html [May 18, 2005].

29. See *New York Times*, April 26, 1925, February 28, 1926 (quotation), and November 21, 1960.

30. Theodore E. Woodward, ed., *The Armed Forces Epidemiological Board: Its First Fifty Years* (Washington, D.C.: Borden Institute, Office of the Surgeon General, Department

of the Army, 1994), sec. 1, "The Commission System, 1940–1972."

31. Wilbur A. Sawyer to Davison, October 10, 1942, Davison Papers.

32. Quoted in Woodward, ed., *The Armed Forces Epidemiological Board*, 45.

33. Davison, *Davison of Duke*, 155.

34. Hanes to Davison, January 6, 1943, Davison Papers.

35. At some point Wise married W. Sterry Branning, who received his M.D. from Yale in 1939, two years after Wise received her M.D. there. Davison, *The First Twenty Years*, 208, lists Wise as a member of the house staff, a fellow and associate in medicine at DUMC between 1937 and 1947. He lists Branning as a member of the house staff and a fellow at Duke from 1939 to 1942 and 1945 to 1947, suggesting that Branning may have gone to and returned from New York with Wise.

36. Lambert, officer's diary, April 26, 1941 (first quotation), and April 25 and 26, 1943 (second quotation), both in RG 12.1, Rockefeller Foundation Archives, RAC.

37. Thomas J. Kennedy Jr., "James Augustine Shannon," National Academy of Sciences, *Biographical Memoirs* 75 (1998), http://www.nap.edu/readingroom/books/biomems/jshannon.html [May 18, 2005] (quotation). See Wise's article with Grace Kerby, "Cultivation of Brucella from the Blood," *Journal of Bacteriology* 46 (October 1943): 333–336. For Wise's work with Shannon at Welfare Island and later, see James A. Shannon with D. P. Earle Jr., B. B. Brodie, J. Taggart, R. W. Berliner, and resident staff of the Research Service, "The Pharmacological Basis for the Rational Use of Atabrine in the Treatment of Malaria," *Journal of Pharmacological Experimental Therapy* 81 (1944): 307–330. Wise is also listed with Shannon and several of the same authors on two of several studies published in the *Journal of Clinical Investigation* (1948).

38. Archie Woods to Davison, June 29, 1943, "Gift of Funds," bk. 2, DUA.

39. See Gordon N. Meiklejohn, "History of the Commission on Influenza," in Woodward, *Armed Forces Epidemiological Board*, 154.

40. See *Science*, December 31, 1943, 587–588.

41. Bell to Davison, March 6, 1944, "Gift of Funds," bk. 2, DUA.

42. Meiklejohn, "History of the Commission on Influenza," 156–157.

43. See note 40 above.

44. James F. Gifford Jr., "The Patients Made All the Discoveries: Walter Kempner and the Rice Diet Controversy," May 15, 1992, unpublished paper, Gifford Papers. See also Holmes Alexander and Joseph R. Slevin, "Mr. Welfare State Himself," *Collier's*, February 1, 1950, 15.

45. These developments are covered in detail in the chapters that follow.

46. Hanes to Davison, November 26, 1943 (emphasis in the original), Davison Papers.

47. See the correspondence between Davison and Hanes, November 1943, in Davison Papers.

48. Hanes to Gregg, December 15, 1943, folder 1294, box 106, series 200, subseries 200A, RG 1.1; and Lambert, officer's diary, November 5, 1943, RG 12.1, both in Rockefeller Foundation Archives, RAC.

49. Hanes to Davison, May 31, 1944, Hanes Papers.

50. R. McIntyre Bridges, "Dr. Joseph Willis Beard: A Mighty Man, 1902–1983," *North Carolina Medical Journal* (May 1985), afterword by Stead, 309.

51. Richard S. Lyman, "Report on Grant for Psychiatry at Duke University," October 11, 1947, folder 1114, box 126, series 200, subseries 200A, RG 1.2, Rockefeller Foundation Archives, RAC.

52. Robert S. Carroll to Frank Coxe, July 14, 1941, Highland Hospital Collection (quotation). For information on Suitt, see Davison, *First Twenty Years*, 285, and Suitt's December 1946 resume for the Veterans Administration in the Richard S. Lyman Papers, DUMCA. For Charman Carroll, see a copy of her obituary from the *Asheville Times Citizen*, April 1963, in the biography collection at Pack Memorial Library, and William S. Powell, *North Carolina Lives* (Hopkinsville, Ky.: Historical Record Association, 1962), 227.

53. Pressman, "Human Understanding," 196 (quotation). See chapters 2 and 3 above for a discussion of Gregg's funding of projects in psychiatry and psychosomatic medicine.

54. Lyman to Lambert, February 15, 1941, folder 1114, box 126, series 200, subseries 200A, RG 1.2, Rockefeller Foundation Archives, RAC.

55. Ruth A. Barker, "Annual Report of the Social Service Department, July 1940–July, 1941," 5, DDCFA.

56. Lyman to Lambert, February 25, 1941, folder 1113, box 126, series 200, subseries 200A,

RG 1.2, Rockefeller Foundation Archives, RAC.

57. Ibid.

58. Lyman, "Report on Grant for Psychiatry," 6.

59. Lyman to Lambert, February 25, 1941, folder 1113, box 126, series 200, subseries 200A, RG 1.2, Rockefeller Foundation Archives, RAC.

60. Lyman, "Notes on the Observation and Examination of Psychiatric Patients Including the Mental Status: Arranged for the Course for Student-Attendants, Duke Hospital, 1941," Durham, 1941.

61. Lambert, officer's diary, March 20, 1941, box 34, RG 12.1, Rockefeller Foundation Archives, RAC.

62. Ibid.

63. See "Robert Sproul Carroll," *National Cyclopedia of American Biography* (New York: James H. White, 1938), E:113–114.

64. See George A. Wright to Flowers, April 25, 1940, Highland Hospital Collection.

65. Lyman, "Report on Grant for Psychiatry," 2.

66. Lyman to Davison, March 24, 1942, folder 1113, box 126, series 200, subseries 200A, RG 1.2, Rockefeller Foundation Archives, RAC.

67. Ibid.

68. The chairman of the Morganton investigation, Judge Marshall T. Spears, was the brother-in-law of Duke president Robert Flowers; he was also a Durham attorney who taught part-time in Duke's School of Law. In addition, one of the strongest (and longest) letters Spears received on the matter came from Victor S. Bryant, the Durham attorney who had served with Hanes on the 1935 commission. Bryant made his one recommendation up front: "I would like to see your committee recommend in no uncertain terms the establishment of a unified department of mental hygiene in North Carolina supervised by one responsible head."

69. Quoted in "The Report of the State Hospital Investigation Board," *North Carolina Medical Journal* (September 1942): 506.

70. See *Durham Sun*, August 11, 1943; and Gregg to Davison, August 30, 1943, in Davison Papers.

71. Lambert, officer's diary, April 25 and 26, 1943, box 35, RG 12.1, Rockefeller Foundation Archives, RAC.

72. Memo, n.d. [with 1943 materials], "No laboratory courses . . . ," Lyman Papers.

73. Lambert, officer's diary, April 25 and 26, 1943, RG 12.1, box 35, Rockefeller Foundation Archives, RAC.

74. See Richard S. Lyman, "Report on Grant for Psychiatry," 3–4, folder 1114, box 126, series 200, subseries 200A, RG 1.2, Rockefeller Foundation Archives, RAC; and Lyman to Bettina S. Warburg, June 17, 1943, Lyman Papers.

75. Lambert, officer's diary, April 25 and 26, 1943, RG 12.1, box 35, Rockefeller Foundation Archives, RAC.

76. Ibid.

77. Katherine R. Lyman to Jeanette Hanford, July 10, 1945, Lyman Papers. Reference to Wiggins's work in Haiti is in Richard S. Lyman to State Department, May 31, 1943, Lyman Papers.

78. E. J. Wiggins and Lyman, "Manic Psychosis in a Negro: With Special Reference to the Role of the Psychogenic and Sociogenic Factors," *American Journal of Psychiatry*, 100 (July 1943–May 1944): 786–787. Lyman and Wiggins also emphasized that "a few patients are reluctant to let us make these photo and phonographic recordings. We have never overridden their wishes, and furthermore we have so far refused to make any recording without the knowledge of the patient."

79. Carroll to Rankin, April 10, 1943 (first quotation); and Rankin to Carroll, March 25, 1943 (second quotation), both in Highland Hospital Collection.

80. Carroll, memo, "Relating to Conference Held at Duke July 14, 1943," Highland Hospital Collection.

81. Lyman, "Report on Grant for Psychiatry," 3.

82. For a list of the recommendations, see "Recommendations (5/25/44)," Highland Hospital Collection.

83. Duke University Medical Center, "The 65th General Hospital in World War II," pamphlet, October 26, 2002, and "Duke Pays Tribute to Members of World War II Hospital Unit," *Dukemed news*, October 22, 2002.

84. Clarence Gardner, in Clarence Gardner and Ivan Brown, interview, December 7, 1991.

85. *New York Times*, August 22, 1954, July 25, 1956, and January 17, 1958.

86. See American Red Cross, "Charles Drew: Blood Pioneer" (July 24, 2004), http://

gso.redcross.org/info/CharlesDrew.htm [August 7, 2005].

87. See *New York Times*, April 9, 1943.

88. Arena and McGovern, eds., *Davison of Duke*, 156.

89. *New York Times*, October 2, 1944.

90. O'Connor to Davison, February 2, 1946, "Gift of Funds," bk. 3, DUA.

91. Arena and McGovern, eds., *Davison of Duke*, 160.

92. Calvin B. Hoover, interview, January 8, 1972.

93. Lambert, officer's diary, March 8–10, 1946, RG 12.1, Rockefeller Foundation Archives, RAC.

94. Howard E. Covington Jr., *Favored by Fortune: George W. Watts and the Hills of Durham* (Chapel Hill: University of North Carolina Press, 2004), 222, 227–231. For Huntingdon Gilchrist, see *New York Times*, July 21, 1927, and January 15, 1975.

95. See Davison, *First Twenty Years*, 29–30; and Arena and McGovern, eds., *Davison of Duke*, 168–169.

96. Hanes to Allen, March 2, 1945, Hanes Papers.

97. Ibid. (emphasis in original).

98. Allen to Hanes, March 5, 1945, Hanes Papers.

99. Hanes to Allen, March 8, 1945, Hanes Papers.

100. Carroll to Frank Coxe, February 28, 1945, Highland Hospital Collection.

101. Durden, *Electrifying the Piedmont*, 115; Smith, *From Monopoly to Competition*, 206–209; and Wallace C. Murchison, "Significance of the American Tobacco Company Case," *North Carolina Law Review* 139 (1947–48): 139–141.

102. Lambert, officer's diary, September 6–16, 1945, box 35, RG 12.1, Rockefeller Foundation Archives, RAC.

103. Ibid., March 8–10, 1946.

104. Ibid.

NOTES TO CHAPTER 5

1. See March 18, 1946, entry in Tappan Gregory's notes on his trip to Nuremberg with Smith, April 1946, in Willis Smith Papers, RBMSCL.

2. Jackson Davis, memo, October 23, 1946, box 110, series 1, subseries 1, General Education Board Archives, RAC.

3. Quoted in P. Preston Reynolds, "Hospitals and Civil Rights, 1945–1963: The Case of Simkins v. Moses H. Cone Memorial Hospital," *Annals of Internal Medicine* 126 (June 1, 1997): 898–906.

4. Rankin to Davison, June 1, 1946 (first quotation); and Davison to Rankin, June 4, 1946 (second quotation), Davison Papers, DUMCA.

5. Lambert, officer's diary, November 27, 1944, box 35, RG 12.1, Rockefeller Foundation Archives, RAC.

6. For the tradition at Emory, see Emory University Medical School, *Emory Medicine* (summer 1998), review of J. Willis Hurst, *The Quest for Excellence*, http://www.whsc.emory.edu/_pubs/em/1998summer/quest.html [May 19, 2005].

7. Lambert, officer's diary, June 19, 1946, box 35, RG 12.1, Rockefeller Foundation Archives, RAC.

8. For information on Stead's grant from the Life Insurance Medical Research Fund, see Francis R. Dieuaide to Stead, June 24, 1946, and Dieuaide to Davison, September 23, 1946, both in "Gift of Funds," bk. 3, DUA. For Stead's appointment to the cardiovascular section, see Gifford, "The Patients Made All the Discoveries." The National Institute of Health became the National Institutes of Health in 1948.

9. Lambert, officer's diary, August 9, 1946, in folder 1025, box 85, series 200, RG 1.1, Rockefeller Foundation Archives, RAC.

10. Ibid., September 1–12, 1946, box 35, RG 12.1, Rockefeller Foundation Archives, RAC.

11. Lyman, "Report on Grant for Psychiatry," folder 114, box 126, series 200, subseries 200A, RG 1.2, Rockefeller Foundation Archives, RAC.

12. *Durham Morning Herald*, March 12, 1947; Veterans Administration, "Neuropsychiatric Professional Opportunities in the Department of Medicine & Surgery of the Veterans Administration," n.p., May 1946, copy in Lyman Papers.

13. Lyman, "Report on Grant for Psychiatry," folder 114, box 126, series 200, subseries 200A, RG 1.2, Rockefeller Foundation Archives, RAC.

14. Maurice H. Greenhill to Lyman, April 26, 1946, Lyman Papers.

15. The Kirby Clinic became the Veterans Mental Hygiene Clinic, and the VA gave it the "assigned function" of administering *treatment* to veterans. But Lyman divided the building into two parts: "in one end of which Duke doctors gave 'N.P.' examinations which cost the VA $16 each, while in the other part

the VA used its own staff and the trainee doctors part-time to treat veterans." See *Greensboro Daily News*, July 11, 1948. This situation often led to double billing. While seeing veteran patients, for example, whose visits were billed to the VA, the Duke physicians who also received VA consulting fees were often teaching veteran residents who themselves regularly examined veterans and billed the VA for payment to Duke.

16. Davison, n.d., Davison Papers.

17. Katharine M. Banham, "The Early Days of the Department of Psychology (and Clinical Psychology)," Duke University, May 2, 1984, 7–8, Katharine M. Banham Papers, DUA.

18. *Durham Morning Herald*, March 12, 1947; "History of Durham Meeting," http://durhammonthlymtg.home.mindspring.com/Handbook/DMMhistory.htm; and Banham, "The Early Days," 2.

19. Banham, "The Early Days," 5.

20. Ibid. (second quotation); and Banham to Ruth Baker, February 19, 1991, in Banham Papers (first quotation).

21. Banham, "The Early Days," 13.

22. Ibid., 7 and 11; and Ewald W. Busse, "History of the Department of Psychiatry," unpublished manuscript, 83–84, DUMCA.

23. Florence Powdermaker to Gregg, December 20, 1946, folder 114, box 126, series 200, subseries 200A, RG 1.2, Rockefeller Foundation Archives, RAC.

24. Katharine M. Banham, "The Clinical Psychology Program at Duke University," n.d. [ca. 1947], Banham Papers.

25. Berryhill et al., *Medical Education at Chapel Hill*, 68–69.

26. Reynolds, "Hospitals and Civil Rights," 898–906.

27. Rankin to A. C. Bachmeyer, January 29, 1945, Rankin Papers.

28. Rankin, "Statement of W. S. Rankin, M.D., Member of the North Carolina Medical Care Commission, Opposing the Adoption of the Majority Report of the National Committee for the Medical School Survey," August 8, 1946, Davison Papers.

29. Davison to Don Elias, September 30, 1946, Davison Papers.

30. O. M. Mull to John Sanford Martin, October 29, 1946, John Sanford Martin Papers, RBMSCL, Duke University. For information on the Grayland Estate and Gordon Gray, see Donna S. Garrison, ed., *One Hundred Years of Medicine: The Legacy of Yesterday*

and the Promise of Tomorrow (Winston-Salem, N.C.: Wake Forest University Health Sciences Press, 2002), 29–34.

31. Hart, *The First Forty Years*, 28.

32. Jackson Davis, "Report on a Visit to Southern Institutions," February–March 1946, folder 998, box 110, series 1, subseries 1, General Education Board Archives, RAC. While Davis made no mention of where and with whom he visited at Duke, his usual contacts were Dr. Calvin Hoover in the Department of Economics, Dr. Paul Gross in the Department of Chemistry, and Dr. Taylor Cole in the Department of Political Science.

33. Ibid.

34. Unless otherwise noted, the following is based upon Lucy Morgan's transcript of the November 7, 1946, meeting at the North Carolina College in Durham. A copy of the transcript can be found in the "North Carolina College" folders in the DDCFA.

35. *Durham Morning Herald*, October 30, 1946.

36. See Lambert, officer's diary, November 1 and 2, 1946, box 35, RG 12.1, Rockefeller Foundation Archives, RAC.

37. Morgan, transcript.

38. See, for example, the Raleigh *News & Observer*, January 19, 1947. For additional information on the association, see the North Carolina Good Health Association Papers in the Southern Historical Collection, Manuscripts Department, University of North Carolina at Chapel Hill.

39. Excerpt from Lambert, officer's diary, December 13, 1946, in folder 1025, box 85, series 200, RG 1.1, Rockefeller Foundation Archives, RAC. (Emphasis in the original.)

40. Davison, *The First Twenty Years*, 3, 61.

41. Doris Duke to Davison, November 23, 1946 (first quotation); and Davison to Duke, November 25, 1946 (second quotation), both in Davison Papers.

42. See Byrnes's obituary in *New York Times*, October 11, 1959.

43. Department of Social Services, Duke University Hospital, "Annual Report of the Social Service Department, 1947," DDCFA.

44. Georgea T. Furst to Davison, January 14, 1947, DDCFA.

45. Berryhill et al., *Medical Education at Chapel Hill*, 72. These events are given additional treatment in chapter 6.

46. Elias to Smith, February 22, 1947, Willis Smith Papers.

47. Edwin L. Jones to Smith, February 22, 1947, Willis Smith Papers.

48. *New York Times*, December 18, 1946.

49. Raleigh *News & Observer*, March 11, 1947.

50. Quoted in Berryhill et al., *Medical Education at Chapel Hill*, 73.

51. Lambert, officer's diary, March 13, 1947, box 35, RG 12.1, Rockefeller Foundation Archives, RAC.

52. Lyman to Davison, March 26, 1947, Lyman Papers.

53. Unidentified newspaper clipping, April 15, 1947, Banham Papers, DUA.

54. See the undated newspaper clipping from the *Durham Morning Herald*, and Banham, "The Early Days," both in the Banham Papers, DUA.

55. Busse, manuscript, 54–55; *Durham Sun*, September 27, 1948.

56. Ruth Baker, "Annual Report of the Social Service Department, July, 1940–July, 1941," Department of Social Services, Duke Hospital, DDCFA; and Banham, "The Early Days," 6.

57. The quote is from Alex Rivera, "Duke University Hospital Takes the Lead in Integrated Training Programs," *Pittsburgh Courier*, December 13, 1952. For the integrated basketball game, see Scott Ellsworth, "The Secret Game: Defying the Color Line," *Duke Magazine* 82 (September–October 1996), 8–11, 40.

58. Unless otherwise noted the following is based upon an undated manuscript, ca. 1946–47, in the Lyman Papers.

59. Arena and McGovern, eds., *Davison of Duke*, 161.

60. Ibid., x.

61. Davison, *The First Twenty Years*, 6. Two of Davison's former pediatric residents at Duke, Grant Taylor and Jay Arena, spearheaded the portrait initiative. See Arena and McGovern, eds., *Davison of Duke*, 161. In 1947, Taylor was promoted from assistant to associate dean of Duke's School of Medicine, from assistant to associate professor of pediatrics, and from assistant professor of bacteriology to associate professor. Arena had been an associate professor of pediatrics since 1933.

62. Raleigh *News & Observer*, April 27, 1947. For the later fire, see *Durham Morning Herald*, May 13, 1947.

63. J. R. Smith to Willis Smith, May 26, 1947 (first quotation); and Calvin Hoover to Willis Smith, May 30, 1947 (second quotation), both in Willis Smith Papers.

64. Thomas M. Grant to Willis Smith, June 12, 1947, Willis Smith Papers.

65. Smith to Davison, July 19, 1946 (first quotation), and Davison to Smith, July 28, 1947 (second quotation), both in Willis Smith Papers. That the student in question was admitted is confirmed in *Aesculapian* (1980): 179, and Davison, *First Twenty Years*, 234, which also suggests that he dropped out of medical school in 1950.

66. George P. Harris to Smith, April 26, 1947, Willis Smith Papers.

67. M. Eugene Newsom to Smith, July 23, 1947, Willis Smith Papers.

68. Ibid.

69. Arena and McGovern, eds., *Davison of Duke*, 163.

70. George A. Burwell to Smith, January 5, 1948, Willis Smith Papers.

71. Oscar R. Ewing, interview, May 1, 1969, Harry S. Truman Library.

72. Wagner et al., *E. A. Stead, Jr.*, 158 (first quotation) and 169 (second quotation).

73. Gifford, "The Patients."

74. William K. Jackson to Smith, August 26, 1947; and Herman Horneman to Smith, September 2, 1946, both in Willis Smith Papers.

75. Dorothy Mary Smith, interview, March 26, 1979, p. 10.

76. Ibid.

77. Quoted in Alexander and Slevin, "Mr. Welfare State Himself," 15.

78. Ibid.

79. Lyman to Davison, September 29, 1947, Davison Papers.

80. Gregg to Powdermaker, December 31, 1946, folder 113, box 126, series 200A, RG 1.2, Rockefeller Foundation Archives, RAC.

81. See Lambert, officer's diary, October 13, 1947, box 35, RG 12.1, Rockefeller Foundation Archives, RAC.

82. George A. Burwell to Smith, January 5, 1948, Willis Smith Papers.

83. Raleigh *News & Observer*, February 7, 1948.

84. Durden, *The Launching of Duke University*, 486.

85. Davison, undated memo (ca. 1968), in Davison Papers.

86. *New York Times*, February 13, 1948.

87. *New York Times*, February 14 (first quotation) and February 15, 1948 (second quotation).

88. Oscar R. Ewing, interview, April 29, 1960, Harry S. Truman Library.

89. *New York Times*, March 12, 1948.

90. Smith to Clarence Cobb, March 15, 1948, Willis Smith Papers. For additional information on this matter, see Rebecca Merritt to Cobb, February 3, and Cobb to Merritt, February 5, 1948, in Willis Smith Papers.

91. H. E. Spence to Benjamin Few, March 12, 1948, included in Spence to Smith, March 15, 1948, both in Willis Smith Papers.

92. Smith to Davison, March 20, 1948, Willis Smith Papers.

93. Smith to Allen, March 26, 1948, Willis Smith Papers.

94. Lambert, officer's diary, May 1, 1948, box 35, RG 12.1, Rockefeller Foundation Archives, RAC.

95. Ibid.

96. Wagner et al., *Stead*, 160.

97. Lambert, officer's diary, May 1, 1948, box 35, RG 12.1, Rockefeller Foundation Archives, RAC.

98. Ibid.

99. Wagner et al., *Stead*, 162.

100. Department of Social Services, "Annual Report of the Social Service Department, Duke Hospital, 1947," 4, DDCFA.

101. Department of Social Services, "Annual Report of 1948," 1, DDCFA.

102. Wagner et al., *Stead*, 162.

103. Robert M. Gantt to Smith, May 31, 1948, Willis Smith Papers.

104. Copy of A. Brower to Davison, June 8, 1948, in Willis Smith Papers.

105. Davison to Furst, May 17, 1948 (second quotation); and Davison to Furst, June 28, 1948 (first quotation), both in DDCFA. See also Harold Bosley to Davison, May 12, 1948, in ibid.

106. *New York Times*, June 11, 1948. For Davison involvement with the study, see Davison to Furst, June 7, 1948, DDCFA.

107. Smith to J. H. Separk, July 2, 1948, Willis Smith Papers.

108. *Greensboro Daily News*, July 11, 1948.

109. *Durham Morning Herald*, October 24, 1948 (quotation). For Davison's trip to New York, see A. S. Brower to Smith, July 3, 1948, Smith Papers. The severity of the epidemic in North Carolina is suggested in *New York Times*, July 17, 1948.

110. Department of Social Services, "Annual Report of the Social Service Department, Duke Hospital, 1947," 6, DDCFA.

111. For the training program, see the *Pittsburgh Courier*, December 13, 1952.

112. Quoted in ibid., 493.

113. Memo, May 3, 1948, W. W. Brierly re interview with Walter M. Nielson, folder 998, box 110, series 1, subseries 1, General Education Board Archives, RAC.

114. Memo, October 4, 1948, Robert Calkins, interview with Alexander Sands, folder 998, box 110, series 1, subseries 1, General Education Board Archives, RAC.

115. Sands to Smith, October 5, 1948, Willis Smith Papers.

116. Bailey to Harry F. Byrd, September 13, 1948, James Hinton Pou Bailey Papers, RBMSCL, Duke University. For Smith's role in Truman's visit, see Jonathan Daniels to Smith, November 1, 1948, and Lamar Caudle to Smith, November 9, 1948, both in Willis Smith Papers.

117. Quoted in *New York Times*, October 20, 1948.

118. Smith to Harry S. Truman, November 3, 1948, telegram, Willis Smith Papers.

119. *Durham Morning Herald*, November 11, 1948.

120. Ibid., November 13, 1948. For Ewing's admission to the hospital, see ibid., November 12, 1948.

121. Edens to Taylor Cole, November 5, 1948, folder 998, box 110, series 1, subseries 1, General Education Board Archives, RAC.

122. Memo, Nov. 10, 1948, Calkins, interview with Sands, folder 998, box 110, series 1, subseries 1, General Education Board Archives, RAC.

123. Arena and McGovern, eds., *Davison of Duke*, 164. For Davison's support of Edens, see Durden, *The Launching of Duke University*, 495.

124. Mary Duke Biddle Trent to Smith, November 28, 1948, Willis Smith Papers.

125. A transcript of Thompson's broadcast can be found with Elias to Smith, April 8, 1949, in the Willis Smith Papers.

126. Bailey to Byrd, April 18, 1949, James Hinton Pou Bailey Papers.

NOTES TO CHAPTER 6

1. Except where otherwise noted, the narrative that follows is based upon Julian M. Pleasants and Augustus M. Burns, *Frank Porter Graham and the 1950 Senate Race in North Carolina* (Chapel Hill: University of North Carolina Press, 1990).

2. Maine Albright, interview, 1996. See also Walter E. Campbell, "Jesse Helms and Conservatism before 1972" (August 2002), paper in possession of author.

3. See Bailey's platform statement, February 4, 1950, in the James Hinton Pou Bailey Papers.

4. The other physician was Dr. Dwight H. Murray, who later served as president of the AMA in the mid-1950s. For Robins's feud with Ewing, see *New York Times*, May 6, 1950. For Bailey's activities on Smith's behalf, see the James Hinton Pou Bailey Papers.

5. William E. Leuchtenburg, interview by "Dr. Frank" documentary project, 1996.

6. Quoted in Covington and Ellis, *Terry Sanford*, 130.

7. Research Triangle Park, "About Us: Park History," http://www.rtp.org/index.cfm?fus eaction=page&filename=about_us_history. html [May 20, 2005].

8. Arena and McGovern, eds., *Davison of Duke*, 164.

9. Hart, *The First Forty Years*, 12 (first quotation) and 28 (second quotation).

10. Davison, memo, February 24, 1954, Davison Papers (first quotation); and Hart, *The First Forty Years*, 28 (second quotation).

11. Undated newspaper clipping included with H. W. Kendall to Smith, November 21, 1947, Willis Smith Papers.

12. Edward L. Fiske to Smith, August 10, 1948, Willis Smith Papers.

13. Smith to Charles E. Jordan, November 1, 1949, Willis Smith Papers.

14. Alexander and Slevin, "Mr. Welfare State Himself," 15.

15. *The Walter Kempner Foundation, Inc.* (Durham, N.C., 1950). The author would like to thank Dr. Barbara Newborg for making this pamphlet available. In addition to Edens and MacMillan, the incorporators included James L. Madden, Thomas B. Mullen, Donald M. Nelson, J. Robert Rubin, John H. Scatterty, and George P. Skouras.

16. Donna Hoel and Robert Howard, "Hypertension: Stalking the Silent Killer," *Postgraduate Medicine* 101 (February 1997): 116–124.

17. *New York Times*, August 29, 1948.

18. For the fund's Lasker Award, see *New York Times*, May 13, 1950. The grants to Handler, Bernheim, and Kempner can be found in "Gift of Funds," bk. 3., DUA.

19. *New York Times*, March 4, 1951.

20. Robert Calkins, memo, May 16, 1950, folder 999, box 110, series 1, subseries 1, General Education Board Archives, RAC.

21. Edwin L. Jones to Smith, February 22, 1947, Willis Smith Papers.

22. *New York Times*, December 26, 1951.

23. Ibid.

24. Ibid.

25. For information on the commission, see National Academy of Sciences, "Atomic Bomb Casualty Commission, 1945–1982," at http://www7.nationalacademies.org/archives/ ABCC_1945–1982.html. For Taylor's biography, see the collection description of his personal papers at the John P. McGovern Historical Collections & Research Center, Houston Academy of Medicine, Texas Medical Center Library in Houston, http://mcgovern.li brary.tmc.edu/text/collect/abcc/Taylor/intro. html#Bio. Davison mentions his visit to Japan in Arena and McGovern, *Davison of Duke*, 164. Handler's role in creating the Radiation Effects Research Foundation is mentioned in Frank W. Putnam, "The Atomic Bomb Casualty Commission in Retrospect," *Proceedings of the National Academy of Sciences* 94 (May 12, 1998): 5426–5431.

26. *New York Times*, May 27, 1950. For the grants to Duke between 1948 and 1956, see the annual *Bulletin of Duke University: Financial Report*.

27. For information on the Army Ordnance Research Office, see Peregrine White, "Office of Ordnance Research, U.S. Army: Semi-Annual Historical Summary 1 (1 July through 31 December 1951)"; and White, "A History of the Office of Ordnance Research/Army Research Office, 1951–1981," 1981, both in DUA.

28. *Durham Morning Herald*, June 30, 1949.

29. See Oak Ridge National Laboratory, "Swords to Plowshares: A Short History of Oak Ridge National Laboratory," http:// www.ornl.gov/info/swords/forties.html [May 20, 2005]. For Gross's election as president of the Oak Ridge Institute, see *Durham Morning Herald*, June 29, 1949.

30. Robert D. Calkins, memo, October 20, 1948, box 110, series 1, subseries 1, General Education Board Archives, RAC.

31. Davison, *The First Twenty Years*, 19–30. See Raleigh *News & Observer*, December 26, 1948, for the Atomic Energy Commission programs in physics at Duke. For information on Gross, see his biographical sketch in the web

pages of the Oak Ridge Associated Universities: http://www.orau.org/visitor/gross/.htm.

32. Davison, *The First Twenty Years*, 29–30.

33. Arena and McGovern, eds., *Davison of Duke*, 163.

34. For the ramjet rocket tests done at Topsail Island between 1947 and 1948, see National Park Service, "us Naval Ordnance Test Facilities, Topsail Island mps," http://www.cr.nps.gov/nr/travel/aviation/usn.htm. The connections between Duke's physics department and the Nike project were made through military contracts with Watson Laboratories in Red Bank, New Jersey. See Raleigh *News & Observer*, December 26, 1948; and Richard L. Weaver and James McAndrew, *The Roswell Report: Fact versus Fiction in the New Mexico Desert* (Department of the Air Force, Washington, D.C., 1995).

35. There are a number of web sites dealing with the Nike missile system. See, for example, Colonel Stephen P. Moeller, "Vigilant and Invincible," at http://www.fas.org/nuke/guide/usa/airdef/vigilant.htm. In 1954, the Nike Ajax missile system became the first guided, surface-to-air missile system in the world. Douglas Aircraft, the system's primary subcontractor, built more than 13,000 missiles at its plant in Santa Monica, California, and at the Army Ordnance Missile Plant in Charlotte. Deployment of the second Nike system, the Hercules, began in 1958, and by 1963, there were an estimated 134 Nike Hercules and 77 Ajax batteries defending the United States.

36. Edward D. Berkowitz and Mark J. Santangelo, *The Medical Follow-up Agency: The First Fifty Years, 1946–1996* (Washington, D.C.: National Academy Press, 1999), 2 (quotation).

37. Ibid., 1–21.

38. See ibid., 17, for Woodhall's follow-up study. For information on Woodhall, see Robert H. Wilkins, "Barnes Woodhall, M.D.: A Biographical Sketch," *Clinical Neurosurgery* 18 (1971): xvii–xx.

39. Quoted in Berkowitz and Santangelo, *The Medical Follow-up Agency*, 16. The other members of Davison's investigating committee were Dr. Michael DeBakey (then chairman of Surgery at Baylor), Dr. Allen O. Whipple (of Memorial Hospital in New York), and Herbert Marks (of the Metropolitan Life Insurance Company).

40. Arena and McGovern, eds., *Davison of Duke*, 42.

41. See Mary Duke Biddle Trent Semans,

"Josiah Charles Trent as a Collector," *Library Notes* (December 1956): 2–5.

42. Quoted in Gerald Oppenheimer's summary of his interview with Martin M. Cummings, June 23, 1987, National Library of Medicine, http://www. mlanet.org/about/history/m_cummings.html [May 20, 2005].

43. Martin M. Cummings, "Wilburt C. Davison and Medical Libraries," *American Journal of Diseases of Children* 124 (September 1972): 342.

44. Davison to Furst, January 3, 1951, DDCFA.

45. Lyman had expected the va to pay Scholz's salary, but that was impossible since Scholz was entering the country on a U.S. Army permit. Richard Lyman died in 1959 at the age of 68. See his biographical sketch in the *National Cyclopedia of American Biography* (New York: James T. White, 1965), 48:183–184. For the Scholz and Silver appointments, see Lyman to Forbus, June 17, 1950; for Lyman's resignation, see Lyman to Forbus, February 21, 1951, all in Lyman Papers. Robert Lambert first met with Scholz in 1937, during Scholz's trip to the United States, and Alan Gregg was close friends with Scholz's predecessor at the DFA in Munich, Walther Spielmeyer. See Cornelius Borck, "Mediating Philanthropy in Changing Political Circumstances: The Rockefeller Foundation's Funding for Brain Research in Germany, 1930–1950," http://archive.rockefeller.edu/publications/resrep/borck.pdf [May 20, 2005].

46. Lyman to Forbus, July 5, 1951 (first quotation), and Lyman to Davison, July 2, 1951 (second quotation), both in the Lyman Papers.

47. Greenhill and Sutherland are not among the staff listed by Busse as being part of the department upon his arrival. See Busse, "History of the Department of Psychiatry," 20. Greenhill helped established the Psychiatric Institute of the University of Maryland in 1954 before joining Albert Einstein College in 1957 and briefly serving the following year as director of New York City's Community Mental Health Board. See *New York Times*, January 22, 1981. Sutherland became chief of the division of psychiatric education of the Department of Mental Hygiene at Baltimore and was president of the Academy of Psychosomatic Medicine in 1960. See *New York Times*, October 16, 1960.

48. Busse, "History of the Department of Psychiatry," 64–67.

49. Paul Weindling, "Termination or Transformation: The Fate of The International Health Division as a Case Study in Foundation Decision-Making," *Research Reports* from the Rockefeller Archive Center, fall 2002.

50. For Rhine's grant, see folders 1109–1111, box 125, series 200A, RG 1.2, Rockefeller Foundation Archives, RAC. For the grant to Hanna, see "Gift of Funds," bk. 2, June 29, 1951, DUA.

51. Berryhill et al., *Medical Education at Chapel Hill*, 84.

52. Hart, *The First Forty Years*, 240–242.

53. P. Preston Reynolds, *Watts Hospital, 1895–1976* (Durham: Fund for the Advancement of Science and Mathematics Education in North Carolina, 1991), 55–56 (quotation). For information on UNC, see Berryhill et al., *Medical Education at Chapel Hill*, 91–96.

54. *North Carolina Medical Journal* (January 1950): 43 (quotation). See also Garrison, ed., *Wake Forest University*, 33.

55. *Bulletin of Duke University*, June 30, 1952, 6.

56. Ibid., June 30, 1956, 7.

57. George B. Webster to Smith, August 8, 1951, Willis Smith Papers.

58. Frank Daniels to Smith, August 8 (first quotation), and Smith to Webster, August 13, 1951 (second quotation), both in Willis Smith Papers.

59. See Preston Reynolds, manuscript, chap. 10, 34.

60. The "possibility of Mr. Gordon Gray being made head of the CIA" is discussed in a memo from the director of the Executive Secretariat to the undersecretary of state, March 8, 1949, National Archives and Records Administration, RG 59, Records of the Department of State, Records of the Executive Secretariat, NSC Files: lot 66 D 148, box 1555. A copy of the memorandum is at http://www.state.gov/www/about_state/history/intel/370_379.html.

61. See Jesse Helms to Smith, April 11, 1951, Willis Smith Papers.

62. Gray is quoted in Walter Spearman, "A University Examines Itself," *Journal of Higher Education* 25, no. 3 (March 1954): 122. For a summary of Gray's tenure at UNC, including the integration story, see William D. Snider, *Light on the Hill: A History of the University of North Carolina at Chapel Hill* (Chapel Hill:

University of North Carolina Press, 1992), 238–253. Duke's first black medical student, Del Meriwether, arrived in 1963 and received the M.D. in 1967. See the *Aesculapian* (1980): 204.

63. For Gray's work on the Psychological Strategy Board, see a copy of Gray to President Harry Truman, February 22, 1952, in the Edward Kidder Graham Papers, Manuscript Department, University of North Carolina at Greensboro. Gray resigned as director of the PSB in December, 1951, but continued to work with C. D. Jackson and others in the PSB's successor, the Operations Coordinating Board, which had its origins in the "cold war" board selected by Eisenhower in January of 1953. See *New York Times*, January 26, 1953. Jackson's appointment as a director of Independent Aid is mentioned in Furst to James Moseley, November 19, 1948, DDCFA. See *Time*, January 29, 1951, for Jackson's appointment as president of National Committee for a Free Europe.

64. *Durham Morning Herald*, December 2, 1951.

65. *New York Times*, November 30, 1951.

66. See *New York Times*, September 17, 1951, for the specific objectives of the commission, which included "An evaluation of the systems of payment for hospital care."

67. *Durham Morning Herald*, May 5, 1952.

68. Ibid., December 2, 1951.

69. *Pittsburgh Courier*, December 13, 1952.

70. Ibid.

71. Berkowitz and Santangelo, *The Medical Follow-up Agency*, 22.

72. Jesse Helms, interview, Helms Documentary Project (quotation). For the growing concern over Smith's reelection chances, see Bailey to Smith, May 8, 1953, in the James Hinton Pou Bailey Papers.

73. Raleigh *News & Observer*, July 2, 1953.

74. Durden, *Electrifying the Piedmont Carolinas*, 120.

75. Davison to Edens, February 24, 1954 (first quotation); and Davison, Stead, Hart, Busse, and Bayard Carter to Edens, October 13, 1954 (second quotation), both in the Davison Papers.

76. Leonard Goldner, interview, n.d. [2002?].

77. Dr. Charles Warren, memo, September 12–14, 1955, folder 923, box 101, RG 18.1, Commonwealth Fund Archives, RAC.

78. *Durham Morning Herald*, August 19, 1951.

79. Goldner, interview.

80. Ibid.

81. Hart, *The First Forty Years*, 81 (quotation). See also *Aesculapian* (1980): 76; and http://www.dukemednews.org/news/article.php?id=8368.

82. Harvey Estes, interview, April 28, 2004.

83. James B. Wyngaarden, "Remarks by James B. Wyngaarden at the Chief Residents Reunion, Department of Medicine," October 4, 2003, 2, copy in possession of author.

84. Ibid. For Wyngaarden's career prior to Duke, see Wyngaarden, interview by James F. Gifford Jr., April 9, 1982, DUMCA.

85. *Aesculapian* (1980): 261. Indeed, Stephen would resign when denied his request for full departmental status for the division of anesthesiology.

86. Hart, *The First Forty Years*, 28.

87. C. Warren, memo, September 15, 1955, folder 923, box 101, RG 18.1, Commonwealth Fund Archives, RAC.

88. Ibid.

89. Ibid.

90. J. C. Eberhart, memo, September 16, 1955, folder 923, box 101, RG 18.1, Commonwealth Fund Archives, RAC.

91. Ibid. Eberhart also noted, "Dean Davison mentioned to me that the Hospital is always crowded even though their average occupancy is 76 per cent."

92. Ibid.

93. Ibid.

94. Ibid.

95. See C. Warren, memo, September 15, 1955, folder 923, box 101, RG 18.1, Commonwealth Fund Archives, RAC.

96. Wyngaarden, interview, April 9, 1982.

97. Philip Handler and Eugene A. Stead Jr., "Historical Background," in James Gifford, ed., *Undergraduate Medical Education and the Elective System: Experience with the Duke Curriculum, 1966–75* (Durham: Duke University Press, 1978), 4.

98. Handler to Lester J. Evans, December 26, 1957, folder 923, box 101, RG 18.1, Commonwealth Fund Archives, RAC.

99. Gross to Evans, January 4, 1958, in ibid.

100. Handler to Evans, December 26, 1957, in ibid.

101. Dr. Heffron, memo, "The Duke University School of Medicine," November 22, 1957, folder 923, box 101, RG 18.1, Commonwealth Fund Archives, RAC (quotation). Information on funding for the RTP can be found in Philip

Handler to Malcolm P. Aldrich, May 17, 1961, in folder 924 of ibid.

102. Handler to Evans, December 26, 1956, folder 923, box 101, RG 18.1, Commonwealth Fund Archives, RAC.

103. Ibid.

104. Busse, interview, October 10, 2003, DUMCA.

105. Busse, "History of the Department of Psychiatry," 65.

106. Busse, interview, April 4, 2003, DUMCA.

107. Lester Evans, "Duke University School of Medicine—Experimental Training Program in the Basic Medical Sciences, Visit to School by Dr. Evans December 17–20, 1957," folder 923, box 101, RG 18.1, Commonwealth Fund Archives, RAC.

108. Busse, "History of the Department of Psychiatry," 67. Semans shared the bank note with Dillard Teer, see ibid., 68.

109. Duke Hospital *Intercom* (August 1957).

110. Busse, interview, April 4, 2003.

111. *New York Times*, August 4, 1957.

112. Duke Hospital *Intercom* (August 1957), 2.

113. Ibid., 1.

114. *New York Times*, August 4, 1957.

115. Hart, *The First Forty Years*, 52 and 243.

116. Ibid., 68–69.

117. Busse, interview, October 10, 2003.

118. Ibid.

119. Paul Gross to Preston L. Fowler (American Tobacco Company), June 13, 1951, in http://tobaccodocuments.org/atc/60334297.html (first and second quotation); and P. L. Fowler and H. R. Hanmer to Paul Hahn, May 16, 1931, http://tobaccodocuments.org/atc/60302252.html (third quotation), both in *Tobacco Documents Online*, http://tobaccodocuments.org/.

120. Memo, December 14, 1953, Tobacco Industry Meeting, http://tobaccodocuments.org/atc/0000291101, *Tobacco Documents Online*.

121. *New York Times*, December 23, 1953.

122. National Institute of Environmental Health Sciences, "Important Events in NIEHS History" (December 2003), http://www.nih.gov/about/almanac/1999/organization/niehs/history.html (quotation). See Gross to Walter Winchell (Damon Runyon Memorial Fund), April 9, 1953, http://tobaccodocuments.org/atc/60302340.html, *Tobacco Documents Online*, for the title of Gross's study. For Sanford and

Ewing's lobbying efforts, see *New York Times*, December 22, 1964.

123. For information on Kenneth C. Towe, see Towe, interview by Frank Rounds, February 27, March 17, 18, and 30, 1964, Duke Endowment Archives, RBMSCL.

124. See Henry Schuman, "The Josiah C. Trent Collection in the History of Medicine," *Bulletin of the Medical Library Association* 46 (July 1958): 354–355.

125. Unless otherwise noted, the following discussion is based upon Davison's correspondence in the DDCFA.

126. Davison to Van Theis, August 20, 1956, DDCFA.

127. Ibid., April 28, 1956.

128. Unless where otherwise noted, this section is based upon Davison's correspondence with Independent Aid and the Doris Duke Foundation between 1947 and 1972. See the DDCFA.

129. Davison to Van Theis, March 26, 1956 (first quotation); and Davison to May McFarland, April 11, 1958, both in DDCFA.

130. Van Theis to Davison, February 8, 1955, DDCFA.

131. Davison to Van Theis, December 28, 1956 (quotation), DDCFA. See also Van Theis to Davison, December 7, 1955; and McFarland to Davison, November 17, 1958, both in DDCFA.

132. Davison to Van Theis, October 14, 1955 (first quotation); Davison to Van Theis, January 24, 1955 (second quotation); and Davison to Van Theis, May 18, 1956 (third quotation), all in DDCFA.

133. Davison to James McCormick, October 8, 1964, Davison Papers.

134. *New York Times*, April 5, 1960.

135. Ibid., April 15, 1960.

136. Gross to Lindsley F. Kimball, May 31, 1960, folder 999, box 110, series 1, subseries 1, General Education Board Archives, RAC.

137. Ibid.

138. Arena and McGovern, eds., *Davison of Duke*, 176.

NOTES TO CHAPTER 7

1. Anlyan, *Metamorphoses*, 69.

2. Ibid., 52.

3. Daniel S. Greenberg, "The Politics of Science 2000," February 25, 2000, presentation at the meeting of the Philosophical Society of Washington, http://www.philsoc.org/2000Spring/2115minutes.html [May 21, 2005]

(quotation). For Sanford's leadership of the Humphrey campaign, see Covington and Ellis, *Terry Sanford*, 364–366. On Nixon's nomination for honorary doctorate degree at Duke see, William E. King, "Tabling Nixon," *Duke Dialogue* 12 (May 16, 1997): 15.

4. Quoted in *Duke Alumni Register*, May–June 1968.

5. William J. Rutter, interview, 1992.

6. *Medical Tribune*, July 6, 1970 (quotation). See *New York Times*, June 12, 1971, for a list of the Institute of Medicine's original members.

7. *New York Times*, November 3, 1977 (quotation). For Snyderman's career at Genentech, see Snyderman, interview, March 23, 1993, DUMCA.

8. For Wyngaarden's career, see Wyngaarden, interview, April 9, 1982, DUMCA, and *New York Times*, January 21, 1982. For Stetten's close relationship with Handler and Wyngaarden, see Dewitt Stetten, "How My Light Is Spent: The Memoirs of Dewitt Stetten, Jr." (spring 1983), http://history.nih.gov/articles/DeWittStettenMemoirs.pdf [May 21, 2005]. For general information on Stetten, see http://stills.nap.edu/html/biomems/dstetten.html.

9. Wyngaarden, interview, April 9, 1982, DUMCA.

10. Ibid.

11. Snyderman, interview, March 23, 1993, DUMCA.

12. Ibid.

13. Snyderman, interview, December 14, 1990 (second quotation), and April 23, 1994 (first quotation), DUMCA.

14. Snyderman, interview, December 14, 1990 (second quotation), and April 22, 1994 (first quotation), DUMCA.

15. Snyderman, interview, December 14, 1990, DUMCA.

16. Thelma Ingels, "An Experience in Learning," April 1957, folder 1516, box 167, series 200C, RG 1.2 (first and fourth quotations); Report, May 29, 1957, folder 1519, box 167, series 200C, RG 1.2 (third quotation); and Ingels to Virginia Arnold, March 13, 1961, folder 1520, box 167, series 200C, RG 1.2 (fifth quotation); all in Rockefeller Foundation Archives, RAC. The issue of accreditation is mentioned in Reginald D. Carter and Justine Strand, "Physician Assistants: A Young Profession Celebrates the 35th Anniversary of its Birth in North Carolina," *North Carolina Medical Journal* 61, no. 5 (September–October 2000): 279 (second quotation).

17. Pamela Preston Reynolds, unpublished manuscript, [no title], chap. 10, 24–28, copy in possession of author. The author would like to thank Ms. Reynolds for use of her manuscript.

18. For the evolution of the physician assistant idea, see Physician Assistant History Center, "Timeline," DUMCA, http://www.pahx.org/period07.html [May 21, 2005].

19. See Carter and Strand, "Physician Assistants," 249–256. See also Physician Assistant History Center, "Timeline," DUMCA, http://www.pahx.org/period07.html [May 21, 2005]; and Estes, interview, April 28, 2004, mentions the number of PA programs in the United States.

20. Melvin Berlin, interview, October 31, 2003, DUMCA.

21. East Carolina University, "The Brody School of Medicine," http://www.ecu.edu/med/bsom_about.htm (quotation) [August 15, 2005]. See also "Dr. Leo W. Jenkins, The Man Who Asked 'Why Not?'" ECU Medical Review 8, no. 3 (December 1985): 2–3.

22. Handler to Woodhall, memo, March 28, 1961, in Gifford Papers.

23. Ibid.

24. Thomas D. Kinney, Jane Elchlepp, and William D. Bradford, "Educational Activities Analysis of the Elective Curriculum," in Undergraduate Medical Education and the Elective System: Experience with the Duke Curriculum, 1966–1975, ed. James F. Gifford Jr. (Durham: Duke University Press, 1978). See ibid., 6–7, for Kinney, and for information on Tosteson, see Aesculapian (1980): 313.

25. Gifford, ed., Undergraduate Medical Education, ix–x.

26. Alfred Blalock to William G. Anlyan, January 17, 1964, Alfred Blalock Papers, DUMCA.

27. Ibid. For a summary of Sabiston's career, see the series of articles on him in Annals of Surgery 238 (December 2003).

28. Hart to Blalock, May 11, 1964, Blalock Papers, DUMCA.

29. Hart, The First Forty Years, 83.

30. Wyngaarden, interview, April 9, 1982.

31. Wyngaarden, "Jim Watson and the Human Genome Project," 6.

32. Wyngaarden, interview, April 9, 1982.

33. Ibid.

34. Aesculapian (1980): 124.

35. Duke Med Interactive, "The Medical Scientist Training Program," http://dukemed.duke.edu/Curriculum/index.cfm?method=MSTP [August 14, 2005].

36. Estes, interview, April 28, 2004.

37. Eugene Stead, "The Duke Plan," October 1969, folder 919, box 101, series 18.1, Commonwealth Fund Archives, RAC.

38. Ibid.

39. For the simultaneous formation of the two departments at Duke and UNC, see William W. McLendon, "Walter Reece Berryhill," chap. 10, 17–22, January 20, 2003, unpublished manuscript (copy in possession of author). The author would like to thank Dr. McLendon for use of this manuscript.

40. Estes, interview, April 28, 2004.

41. See Estes's summary of the department in Aesculapian (1980): 269–272.

42. Gifford, ed., Undergraduate Medical Education, x.

43. Anlyan, Metamorphoses, 127–133.

44. Booz, Allen & Hamilton, "Program and Implementation Recommendations," Long Range Plan for Physical Plant Development (New York: Booz, Allen & Hamilton, 1961), 1:78–80.

45. Ibid.

46. See Charlotte Observer, June 24, 1962; and the Aesculapian (1980): 204.

47. Anlyan, Metamorphoses, 133.

48. Between 1960 and the groundbreaking for the new hospital in 1975, the Duke Endowment trustees who occupied the foundation's three seats on the university's executive trustee committee were Thomas L. Perkins (1958–73), Benjamin Few (1960–65), Kenneth C. Towe (1960–63), Mary D. B. T. Semans (1971–81), and Amos R. Kearns (1948–62 and 1963–75). See Durden, Lasting Legacy to the Carolinas, 328–330.

49. James H. and Mary D. B. T. Semans, interview, January 20, 2004, DUMCA.

50. Reynolds, Watts Hospital, 64.

51. Ibid., 68.

52. See ibid., 57–88.

53. Berryhill et al., Medical Education at Chapel Hill, 165.

54. Anlyan, Metamorphoses, 134.

55. Ibid., 135.

56. William Donelan, interview, November 11, 2003, DUMCA.

57. See Reynolds manuscript, chap. 11, 8–11.

58. Donald L. Madison, "Durham's Exemplary Health Center—And Its Leader, Dr. Evelyn Schmidt," North Carolina Medical Journal

64, no. 4 (July–August 2003): 163. For information on Salber, see Duke University Medical Center, Department of Community and Family Medicine, "The Eva J. Salber Award for Projects in Community Medicine," http://communityhealth.mc.duke.edu/ED/Salber.htm [May 22, 2005]. During this period, between the resignation in 1969 of Knight as president of Duke, and the arrival of his successor, Terry Sanford, the university was led by three men: Marcus Hobbs, provost, Chuck Eustis, vice president for business and finance, and Dr. Barnes Woodhall, chancellor pro tem.

59. See "Curriculum Vitae, John Alexander McMahon,"http://faculty.fuqua.duke.edu/bio/mcmahonvita.pdf [May 22, 2005].

60. See ibid.

61. Covington and Ellis, *Terry Sanford*, 390.

62. Press release, draft, March 20, 1970, folder 920, box 101, RG 18.1, Commonwealth Fund Archives, RAC. For Sanford's study of the states, see Covington and Ellis, *Terry Sanford*, 352.

63. "Proposal for a Center for the Study of Health Policy at Duke University," n.a., n.d. [ca. 1972], folder 906, box 99, RG 18.1, Commonwealth Fund Archives, RAC. Other documents related to the center are located in folder 907 of ibid.

64. The AHA's "universal health insurance" plan is briefly summarized in *New York Times*, August 31, 1977.

65. Dr. Harvey Estes, lecture, November 9, 1978, DUMCA. Unless otherwise noted, the material that follows is taken from this lecture.

66. Estes, interview, April 28, 2004, DUMCA.

67. Wyngaarden to Edward C. Halperin, May 27, 2005, copy in possession of author.

68. Wyngaarden, interview, March 21, 2005.

69. Estes, interview, April 28, 2004.

70. For Stead's trainees, see Wagner et al., *E. A. Stead*, 231–232; for Wyngaarden's, see Wyngaarden to Halperin, May 27, 2005; and for Sabiston's, see W. Randolph Chitwood, "The Sabiston Heritage: Excellence in Surgical Education," *Annals of Surgery* 238 (December 2003): S4.

71. Quoted in Halperin to author, April 19, 2005.

72. See "The Walter Kempner Symposium," *Archives of Internal Medicine* 133 (May 1974): 751.

73. Wyngaarden to Sanford, June 13, 1972, copy in possession of author. The author would like to thank Dr. Barbara Newborg for bringing this letter to his attention. In the fall of 1972, Jim Wyngaarden reported allegations to Bill Anlyan that Kempner had been whipping one of his patients in Duke Hospital as part of an "aversive therapy" used to discipline certain patients on the rice diet. See Anlyan, *Metamorphoses*, 80. For Kempner's impact on Durham as a diet center, see Clancy Nolan, "Sin City," *Independent*, February 20, 2002; and Stephanie Saul, "Penny-Wise, Not Pound-Foolish," *New York Times*, May 19, 2005.

74. See Duke University Medical Center, "Interdisciplinary Research Training Program in AIDS," September 2001, 3–4, http://infectiousdisease.duke.edu/infectiousdiseases/images/AIDSBRO2000Research_Training.pdf [July 30, 2005].

75. Wyngaarden, interview, March 3, 2005.

76. For Beard's work in Florida, see David T. Kurtz and Philip Feigelson, "Multihormonal Induction of Hepatic α_{2u}-globulin mRNA as Measured by Hybridization to Complementary DNA," *Proceedings of the National Academy of Sciences* 74 (November 1, 1977): 4795; and Bridges, "Dr. Joseph Willis Beard," 308 (quotation).

77. Thomas F. Tedder and Jeffrey R. Dawson, "In Memoriam, D. Bernard Amos: April 16, 1923–May 15, 2003," *Journal of Immunology* 171 (2003): 6316–6317.

78. See Halperin to Campbell, April 19, 2005; *Aesculapian* (1980): 71; and Severe Combined Immunodeficiency, SCID.NET, http://www.scid.net/index.htm [July 30, 2005].

79. Duke University, Duke University Health System, dukechildren.org, "Dr. Samuel Katz, M.D., Receives 2003 Sabin Gold Medal," http://dukehealth1.org/childrens_services/press_release_katz.asp [July 30, 2005].

80. Anlyan, *Metamorphoses*, 75.

81. *Aesculapian* (1980): 289.

82. Ibid., 43.

83. See Cardiac Electrocphysiology Society, "Dr. Madison Spach," http://www.cardiaceps.org/annmeetings/spach2003.htm [August 1, 2005] (quotation); and Duke University Medical Center, Medical Alumni News (fall 2005), http://development.mc.duke.edu/medAlum/man/fa00/man1.html [August 1, 2005].

84. American Society for Cell Biology, "In Memory of J. David Robertson," http://www.

ascb.org/membership/obits/robertson95.htm [August 1, 2005].

85. Fridovich had taken his Ph.D. under Handler in the early 1950s and had joined the faculty of the Department of Biochemistry in 1958. See *Aesculapian* (1980): 72; and Society for Free Radical Biology and Medicine, November 1, 2003, http://www.sfrbm.org/tenth-annualDay1.html [August 1, 2005].

86. *Aesculapian* (1980): 293.

87. Ibid., 297. For information on Epstein, see Duke University, http://www.dukeye.org/doctors/epstein.html.

88. Ibid., 261. See also Duke University Medical Center, Department of Anesthesiology, "Chairpersons," http://simdot.org/alumni/chairpersons.htm [August 1, 2005].

89. *Aesculapian* (1980): 261.

90. Quoted in "Merel Harmel," *Duke Magazine* 89 (September–October 2003), archive ed., http://www.dukemagazine.duke.edu/dukemag/issues/091003/depface.html [August 1, 2005].

91. Chitwood, "The Sabiston Heritage," S10.

92. Ibid., S11.

93. For Brown's invention, see chapter 4 above. For Young's work, see Cardiothoracic Surgery Network, "Pioneer Surgeon W. Glenn Young Dies," April 4, 2005, http://www.ctsnet.org/announcements/announcement69.html [August 1, 2005].

94. Sealy, "The Hen's Egg," 2.

95. Andrew Wallace, "WPW at Duke—And Beyond," April 1, 2005, copy in possession of author.

96. Ibid.

97. Neurosurgery Online, Patrick J. Kelly, "Stereotactic Surgery: What Is Past Is Prologue," abstract, *Neurosurgery* 46 (January 2000): 16. Nashold introduced stereotactic surgery at Duke and became a collector of the method's instruments used worldwide; parts of his collection are on permanent display in the Duke University Medical Center Library. See Duke University Medical Center, "Guide to the Blaine Nashold Interview, 2004," http://archives.mc.duke.edu/ mcaoralnashold1_html [August 1, 2005].

98. *Aesculapian* (1980): 329.

99. Ibid., 285.

100. For Heyman, see Duke University Medical Center, "Albert Heyman," http://development.mc.duke.edu/medAlum/award_

heyman.htm [July 19, 2005]; for Roses, see Eliot Marshall, "Allen Roses: From 'Street Fighter' to Corporate Insider," *Science* 280 (May 1998): 1001–1004.

101. Wyngaarden, interview, March 3, 2005.

102. Ibid.

103. Ibid.

104. Estes, interview, April 28, 2004.

NOTES TO CHAPTER 8

1. Covington and Ellis, *Terry Sanford*, 423–432.

2. Snyderman, interview, April 22, 1994, DUMCA.

3. Ibid.

4. Busse, "History of the Department of Psychiatry," 68.

5. Ibid., 75.

6. Busse, interview, April 4, 2003.

7. Busse, "History of the Department of Psychiatry," 81–82.

8. Ibid.

9. Ibid.

10. For Brodie's activities at Stanford, see Busse, "History of the Psychiatry Department," 90; and Brodie, interview, June 17, 2004.

11. Busse, interview, October 10, 2003.

12. For Hamburg's career, see Carnegie Corporation of New York, "About Carnegie Corporation," http://www.carnegie.org/sub/about/hamburgd.html [May 22, 2005]; and Harvard University, John F. Kennedy School of Government, Belfer Center for Science and International Affairs, May 22, 2005, http://bcsia.ksg.harvard.edu/person.cfm?item_id=346&ln=full&program=CORE. For the Education Commission of the States, see Education Commission of the States, "About ECS," http://www.ecs.org/html/aboutECS/AwardsWinner.htm#Sanford [August 18, 2005]. Hamburg also served as president and then chairman of the board of the American Association for the Advancement of Science from 1984 to 1986.

13. Anlyan, *Metamorphoses*, 206–207.

14. Brodie, interview, October 10, 2003.

15. Ibid.

16. Ibid.

17. Ibid.

18. *Society for Executive Leadership in Academic Medicine* 3, no. 1 (January 2000): 9. For Spaulding's career prior to 1997, see Raleigh *News & Observer*, December 7, 1997.

19. Brodie, interview, June 17, 2004.

20. Ibid.

21. For Carroll, see Busse, "History of the Department of Psychiatry," 98.

22. Marcia Angell, "The Truth about the Drug Companies," *New York Review* 15, no. 12 (July 15, 2004): 54.

23. See Genentech, "Significant Scientific Milestones in Biotechnology," http://www.gene.com/gen/reserch/biotechnology/significant-milestones.jsp [May 23, 2005].

24. Information on the centers can be found at their respective web sites. For the Microelectronics Center of North Carolina, see the center's web site, http://www.mcnc.org [May 25, 2005]. For the North Carolina Biotechnology Center, see North Carolina Biotechnology Center, "The Biotechnology Center FAQ," http://www.ncbiotech.org/aboutus/center/faq.cfm [May 23, 2005].

25. Frank Maley, "Blood Work," *Business North Carolina* (July 2003), http://www.businessnc.com/archives/2003/07/trimeris.html. AZT was first synthesized in 1964.

26. Ibid.

27. See Research Triangle Park, "About Us: Park History," http://www.rtp.org/index.cfm?fuseaction=page&filename=about_us-history.html [May 23, 2005].

28. Angell, "The Truth about the Drug Companies."

29. See Durden, *Lasting Legacy*, 328, for Semans's office holding at The Duke Endowment and the university. See McMahon's resume for his information.

30. Estes, interview, April 28, 2004 (quotation). The changes in the PDC's organization are described in its "Description of PDC Organization," copy in possession of author.

31. Paul Newman, in Newman and Cecil Wallace, interview, November 30, 2004, DUMCA (first quotation), and Gordon, *Dead on Arrival*, 40 (second quotation).

32. Estes, interview, April 28, 2004.

33. Ibid.

34. Newman, in Newman and Wallace, interview, November 28, 2004.

35. Estes, interview, April 28, 2004.

36. Ibid.

37. Ibid.

38. For information on Putman, see Mark A. Kliewer and Carl E. Ravin, "A History of the Department of Radiology at Duke University Medical Center," *American Journal of Roentgenology* 165 (September 1995): 695–701;

and Duke University Medical Center, *Duke Med News* (May 11, 1999), "Dr. Charles E. Putnam [*sic*], Duke Senior Vice President, Dies at Age 57," http://dukemednews.duke.edu/news/article.php?id=395 [May 23, 2005]. Anlyan mentions "grooming" Andrew Wallace in *Metamorphoses*, 91. For Wallace, see *Aesculapian* (1980): 277; and "People," *Inside* (March 22, 2004), http://inside.duke.edu/section.php?section=people&IssueID=84.

39. Kliewer and Ravin, "History of Radiology at Duke," 696–698.

40. Ibid.

41. Anlyan, *Metamorphoses*, 91.

42. Kliewer and Ravin, "History of Radiology at Duke," 699 (quotation); and *Aesculapian* (1980): 321.

43. Kliewer and Ravin, *History of Radiology at Duke*, 699–700.

44. Anlyan, *Metamorphoses*, 92.

45. Brodie, interview, June 17, 2004.

46. Ibid.

47. Doyle Graham, interview, June 26, 1995, DUMCA.

48. *New York Times*, February 28, 1986.

49. Graham, interview, June 26, 1995.

50. James B. Wyngaarden, "Jim Watson and the Human Genome Project," 1, manuscript dated March 5, 2003, copy in possession of author.

51. Jeffrey Mervis, "Wyngaarden to Step Down as NIH Director," *Scientist* 3, no. 10 (May 15, 1989): 3.

52. Wyngaarden, "Jim Watson and the Human Genome Project."

53. See Snyderman, interview, March 23, 1993, DUMCA, for a discussion of his recruitment to Genentech.

54. Ibid.

55. Ibid.

56. Robert J. Lefkowitz, interview by Gary Taubes, *in-cites* (December 2002), http://in-cites.com/scientists/RobertJLefkowitz.html.

57. Snyderman, interview, March 23, 1993, DUMCA.

58. Ibid. For the FDA decision, see Food and Drug Administration, "Answers," http://www.fda.gov/bbs/topics/ANSWERS/ANSWER00310.html [August 20, 2005].

59. Snyderman, interview, March 23, 1993, DUMCA.

60. For a detailed discussion of TPA and its role in the early history of Genentech, see G. Kirk Raab, "CEO at Genentech, 1990–1995," an oral history conducted in 2002 by Glenn

E. Bugos, Regional Oral History Office, Bancroft Library, University of California, Berkeley, 2003 (first quotation); and Snyderman, interview, March 23, 1993 (second quotation).

61. Snyderman, interview, April 22, 1994, DUMCA.

62. Brodie, interview, June 17, 2004.

63. Ibid. (first and third quotations); and Anlyan, *Metamorphoses*, 146 (second quotation).

64. Graham, interview, June 26, 1995.

65. For the development of Duke's HIV clinics, see the profile of Dr. John A. Bartlett in "The Nexus," *Newsletter of the American Academy of HIV Medicine* (winter 2004), http://aahivm.org/new/nexus/WINTER04story_7.html. See *New York Times*, November 25, 1988, for Bartlett's comments on the Burroughs Wellcome Retrovir (zidovudine) study.

66. *New York Times*, April 1, 1988.

67. Ibid., June 22, 1988.

68. Raab, interview, "CEO at Genentech, 1990–1995," 24.

69. Anlyan, *Metamorphoses*, 206.

70. Snyderman, interview, April 22, 1994.

71. Snyderman to author, August 25, 2005, copy in possession of author.

72. Ibid.

73. Snyderman, interview, April 22, 1994.

NOTES TO CHAPTER 9

1. Nan Keohane, interview, May 26, 2004, DUMCA.

2. Snyderman to Andrew G. Wallace and Robert G. Winfree, July 21, 1989, Ralph Snyderman Papers, DUMCA.

3. Snyderman to Faculty and Senior Staff, August 16, 1989, Snyderman Papers.

4. Snyderman to Leonard R. Prosnitz, August 3, 1989, in ibid.

5. Snyderman, interview, March 6, 2003, DUMCA.

6. Snyderman to Campbell, August 25, 2005 (first and third quotation); and Snyderman, interview, March 6, 2003 (second quotation).

7. Snyderman to Campbell, August 24, 2005.

8. Snyderman, interview, April 22, 1994.

9. Duncan Yaggy to Snyderman, November 14, 1989, Snyderman Papers.

10. Snyderman, interview, March 6, 2003.

11. Raab, "CEO at Genentech," 21–27.

12. See *New York Times*, February 3, 1990, and April 4 and March 4, 1991.

13. Raleigh *News & Observer*, March 31, 1994.

14. *New York Times*, May 1, 1993.

15. Marsha A. Green, "The Future of Clinical Trials Delivered Today," *Inside* (January 26, 2004), http://inside.duke.edu/article.php?IssueID=80&ParentID=5796 [May 23, 2005].

16. Duke University Medical Center, Duke Clinical Research Institute, Research Activities, "Landmark Projects," http://www.dcri.duke.edu/research/landmarkproj.jsp [May 23, 2005].

17. *New York Times*, May 1, 1993.

18. Raleigh *News & Observer*, May 6, 1993.

19. Ibid., May 11, 1993.

20. Snyderman to Campbell, August 25, 2005.

21. *Inside* DUMC, June 28, 2004, 4. For the themes selected by the Howard Hughes Medical Institute, see Wyngaarden, interview, March 3, 2005.

22. See Duke University Medical Center, *dukehealth.org*, About Duke Health, "Christian Raetz," http://www.dukehealth.org/AboutDuke/Administration/DeptChairs/Biochemistry [May 23, 2005].

23. See *dukehealth.org*, "Thomas Tedder," February 7, 2005, http://www.dukehealth.org/AboutDuke/Administration/DeptChairs/Immunology [May 23, 2005].

24. Nevins stepped down as chairman of the Department of Molecular Genetics and Microbiology in 2004 to become director of genome technology at Duke's Institute for Genome Sciences and Policy. See dukehealth.org, "Joseph Nevins Named Director of IGSP Center for Genome Technology at Duke" (November 21, 2003), http://dukemednews.duke.edu/news/article.php?id=7218 [May 23, 2005].

25. See dukehealth.org, "Brigid Hogan to Head Cell Biology at Duke University Medical Center," http://dukemednews.duke.edu/news/article.php?id=5447 [May 23, 2005].

26. Snyderman to Campbell, August 25, 2005.

27. Ibid.

28. Private Diagnostic Clinic, "Description of PDC Organization," 2004–5 information packet (quotation). Busse, "History of the Department of Psychiatry," 53, mentions the PDC's legal question with the IRS.

29. Newman, in Wallace and Newman, interview, November 30, 2004.

30. Ibid.

31. Ibid.

32. Ibid.

33. Snyderman, interview, March 6, 2003.

34. Keohane, interview, May 26, 2004.

35. Ibid.

36. Snyderman, interview, February 23, 2004.

37. Raleigh *News & Observer*, May 13, 1994.

38. Duke University Medical Center, "Department of Surgery: Our History," http://dukehealth1.or/surgery/history.asp [August 21, 2005].

39. Snyderman, interview, February 23, 2004.

40. For the FDA's approval of the Activase infusion regimen, see *New York Times*, April 4, 1995. For information on Califf, see the DCRI timeline at http://www.dcri.duke.edu/who_we_are/timeline.swf [May 23, 2005].

41. Snyderman, interview, February 24, 2004.

42. Robert Taber, interview, August 25, 2004, DUMCA.

43. Hoechst Marion Roussel, Inc., *Hospital Management Profiles* (October 1995): 23.

44. Nancy Gibbs, "A Week in the Life of a Hospital," *Time* (October 12, 1998): 56.

45. *New York Times*, October 31, 1999. See also Mike Miller, "An Empire Contained," *Towerview* (March 2003): 8–13.

46. Snyderman, interview, February 24, 2004.

47. Roussel, Inc., *Hospital Management Profiles*, 12 (quotation) and 19. See Raleigh *News & Observer*, March 31, 1994, for patient numbers.

48. *New York Times*, December 18, 1994.

49. Roussel, Inc., *Hospital Management Profiles*, 10. Donelan was then vice chancellor for medical center administration and chief financial officer. Rogers was vice chancellor for health affairs at DUMC and CEO of Duke University Hospital and Health Network. Taber was associate vice chancellor for health affairs and director of the Office of Science and Technology.

50. Raleigh *News & Observer*, December 4, 1993.

51. Donelan, interview, May 26, 2004. See also Roussel, Inc., *Hospital Management Profiles*, 8–9.

52. Roussel, Inc., *Hospital Management Profiles*, 10.

53. Ibid., and Gibbs, "A Week in the Life of a Hospital," 76–77.

54. Donelan, interview, May 26, 2004, DUMCA.

55. Snyderman, interviews, December 16, 2003, and January 16, 2004.

56. Roussel, Inc., *Hospital Management Profiles*.

57. Donelan, interview, May 26, 2004.

58. Roussel, Inc., *Hospital Management Profiles*, 11.

59. Newman, in Newman and Wallace, interview, November 30, 2004.

60. Donelan, interview, May 26, 2004.

61. *New York Times*, October 3, 1993, and October 6, 1994.

62. Roussel, Inc., *Management Profiles*, 23 (quotation). For the change in profitability of HMOS, see Gibbs, "A Week in the Life of a Hospital," 57; for the impact on DUMC of the Balanced Budget Act of 1997, see Miller, "An Empire Contained," 10.

63. The indenture establishing The Duke Endowment required the unanimous consent of all the Endowment's trustees before any of the foundation's Duke Power stock was sold. See Durden, *Lasting Legacy to the Carolinas*, 311–324; and Durden, *Electrifying the Piedmont Carolinas*, ix and 239–260.

64. Society of Black Academic Surgeons, "History," http://www.sbas.net/history.htm [May 23, 2005].

65. *New York Times*, August 18, 1994.

66. American Home Products became Wyeth in 2002. See Wyeth, "About Wyeth," at http://www.wyeth.com/about/timeline.asp [May 23, 2005].

67. See Rutgers University, Ernest Mario School of Pharmacy, "Ernest & Mildred Mario Foundation pledges $5 million" (December 14, 2001), http://pharmacy.rutgers.edu/admin/new_name/ [May 23, 2005].

68. For a brief description of Mario's career, see Reliant Pharmaceuticals, Inc., Key Personnel (2004), http://www.reliantrx.com/corporate/key_personnel.html [May 23, 2005].

69. *New York Times*, March 8, 1995.

70. Elyse Tanouye and Robert Langreth, "Genetic Giant," *Wall Street Journal*, February 2, 1998.

71. Snyderman, interviews, December 16, 2003, and January 16, 2004, DUMCA (first quotation); and Donelan interview, May 26, 2004 (second quotation). Duke and Durham Regional had signed a letter of intent in December 1993, allowing the hospitals to "explore . . . collaboration for the future delivery of health care services." See Raleigh *News & Observer*, December 17, 1993.

72. Snyderman, interviews, December 16, 2003, and January 16, 2004, DUMCA.

73. Ibid.

74. Quoted in Raleigh *News & Observer*, February 4, 1997.

75. Snyderman, interviews, December 16, 2003, and January 16, 2004.

76. Ibid.

77. Ibid.

78. Duke University, "Medical Alumni Association Honors Nine," *Medical Alumni News* (October 27, 2000), http://www.dukenews.duke.edu/2000/10/medalumni027.html [May 23, 2005].

79. Raleigh *News & Observer*, November 11, 1997.

80. Ibid.

81. Raleigh *News & Observer*, April 7, 1998. Bowser is quoted in Raleigh *News & Observer*, June 23, 1998.

82. MaryAnn E. Black, interview, January 22, 2004, DUMCA.

83. Ibid.

84. Ibid.

85. Donelan, interview, November 11, 2003.

86. Raleigh *News & Observer*, June 8, 1993; January 17, September 16, and November 10, 1998.

87. Raleigh *News & Observer*, October 9 and November 3, 1998.

88. Donelan, interview, November 11, 2003.

89. Raleigh *News & Observer*, July 29, 1998, and November 10, 1998.

90. Gibbs, "A Week in the Life of a Hospital," 73.

91. Ibid., 68–69.

92. Ralph Snyderman and Edward W. Holmes, "Oversight Mechanisms for Clinical Research," *Science* 287 (January 2000): 595–597.

93. Vicki Y. Saito, interview by Walter E. Campbell, February 20, 2004, DUMCA.

94. Ibid.

95. *Inside*, June 28, 2004 (quotation). See Snyderman and Holmes, "Oversight Mechanisms for Clinical Research," 595–597.

96. "Farewell to a Transformational Dean," *DukeMed* (spring–summer 2004): 6–7, and "Nursing School's Future Home," *Dialogue*, December 10, 2004.

97. "Farewell to a Transformational Dean," 6–7 (quotations).

98. Duke admitted 217 women and 228 men to its medical school in 2004. See American Association of Medical Colleges, "FACTS—Applicants, Matriculants and Graduates," 2004, http://www.aamc.org/data/facts/2004/factsenrl.htm [May 23, 2005].

99. Anlyan, *Metamorphoses*, 147.

100. Ibid. (first quotation); ibid., 207 (second quotation).

101. Nannerl O. Keohane to Members of the Duke University Board of Trustees, memo, September 16, 1997, http://www.lib.duke.edu/archives/documents/reports-nok/RPT19970916.pdf [June 2004].

102. *DukeMed News*, May 11, 1999.

103. Ibid. (second quotation), and Raleigh *News & Observer*, May 12, 1999 (first and third quotations).

104. Ibid.

105. *DukeMed News*, May 11, 1999.

106. Newman, in Newman and Wallace, interview, November 30, 2004.

107. Raleigh *News & Observer*, June 18, 1999; June 3, 2000; and June 10, 2000.

108. Donelan, interview, May 26, 2004 (first quotation); and Miller, "An Empire Contained," 11 (second quotation).

109. Snyderman, interview, March 6, 2003.

110. Neil Chesanow, "Looking Back at Ralph Snyderman's 15 Years at the Helm," *DukeMed* (spring–summer 2004): 31.

111. Quoted in Raleigh *News & Observer*, November 20, 2000.

112. For the sale of St. Joseph of the Pines, see Raleigh *News & Observer*, June 14, 2002. For Duke Health Community Care, see dukehealth.org, Duke Health Community Care, http://dukehealth1.org/facilities_locations/dukehealthcommunitycare.asp [May 23, 2005.] See Raleigh *News & Observer*, May 23, 2002, and November 4, 2003, for DUHS's economic turnaround. DUHS's net operating income for 2003–4 is mentioned in Raleigh *News & Observer*, March 2, 2005.

113. See Duke University Medical Center, "Jesica Santillan Dies at Duke Hospital," *DukeMed News*, February 22, 2003.

114. Snyderman, interview, February 26, 2004.

115. Chesanow, "15 Years at the Helm," 31–32.

116. Snyderman, interviews, December 16, 2003, and January 16, 2004.

117. Keohane, interview, May 26, 2004.

118. Ibid.

119. Mario to Campbell, August 26, 2005.

120. Snyderman to Campbell, August 25, 2005.

121. Ibid.

NOTES TO EPILOGUE

1. Keohane, interview, May 26, 2004.

2. Ibid.

3. See http//:www.dukehealth.org/newchancellor/AboutNewChancellor/Introduction-

Ceremony/newchancellor_txt (quotation). This link is to a transcription of Dzau's presentation after being introduced by Brodhead and Keohane in April of 2004. See also "Statement by President-elect Richard H. Brodhead at the Introduction of Victor Dzau, M.D., as Duke University's New Chancellor for Health Affairs," April 30, 2004, http//:www.dukehealth.org/newchancellor/AboutNewChancellor/IntroductionCeremony/brodhead_txt.

4. For information on Dzau, see "The New Chancellor," *DukeMed* (spring–summer 2004).

5. Duke University *Dialogue*, January 28, 2005.

6. See note 3 above.

7. Duke University *Dialogue*, January 28, 2005.

8. Ibid.

9. *Inside*, February 28, 2005, 1, 8.

BIBLIOGRAPHY

Abbreviations

RAC   Rockefeller Archive Center
DUA   Duke University Archives
DUMCA   Duke University Medical Center Archives
RBMSCL Rare Book, Manuscript, and Special Collections Library
DDCFA   Doris Duke Charitable Foundation Archives

Manuscript Collections

ASHEVILLE, NORTH CAROLINA

Pack Memorial Library
      Highland Hospital Collection

CHAPEL HILL, NORTH CAROLINA

Southern Historical Collection, Louis Round Wilson Library, University
      of North Carolina
      North Carolina Good Health Association Papers
University Archives, Louis Round Wilson Library, University of North Carolina
      General Administration, Consolidated University Presidents' Office
      Records, Gordon Gray (1950–1955), Communications Center: General, 1950–1952

DURHAM, NORTH CAROLINA

Duke University Archives, William R. Perkins Library, Duke University
      Katherine M. Banham Papers
      William Preston Few Papers
Duke University Medical Center Archives
      Joseph Willis Beard Papers
      Alfred Blalock Papers
      Ewald W. Busse Papers
      Wilburt C. Davison Papers
      James F. Gifford Jr. Papers

Frederic Moir Hanes Papers
Richard S. Lyman Papers
David Sabiston Jr. Papers
Ralph Snyderman Papers
Rare Book, Manuscript, and Special Collections Library, Perkins Library,
    Duke University
    James H. "Pou" Bailey Papers
    John Sandford Martin Papers
    Watson Smith Rankin Papers
    Willis Smith Papers

GREENSBORO, NORTH CAROLINA

Special Collections, Walter Clinton Jackson Library, University of North Carolina
    at Greensboro
    Edward Kidder Graham Papers

PHILADELPHIA, PENNSYLVANIA

American Philosophical Society
    Peyton Rous Papers

POCANTICO HILLS, NORTH TARRYTOWN, NEW YORK

Commonwealth Fund Archives
General Education Board Archives
Rockefeller Foundation Archives
Rockefeller University Archives

SOMMERVILLE, NEW JERSEY

Doris Duke Charitable Foundation Archives

Government and University Documents

*Biennial Report of the North Carolina State Board of Charities and Public Welfare, July 1,
    1938 to June 30, 1940.* Raleigh: Edwards and Broughton, 1940.
Bulletin of Duke University: Financial Report
"Gift of Funds." Books 1–3. Duke University Archives.
Lincoln Hospital. *Thirty Eighth Annual Report*, 1938. Durham, 1939.
Private Diagnostic Clinic. "Description of PDC Organization." Durham: Duke
    University Medical Center, n.d. [ca. 2004–2005].

Directories and Biographical Dictionaries

National Cyclopedia of American Biography Vol. E. New York: James T. White, 1938.
National Cyclopedia of American Biography. Vol. 46. New York: James T. White, 1963.
National Cyclopedia of American Biography. Vol. 47. New York: James T. White, 1965.
National Cyclopedia of American Biography. Vol. 48. New York: James T. White, 1965.
National Cyclopedia of American Biography. Vol. 56. New York: James T. White, 1974.

Powell, William S., ed. *Dictionary of North Carolina Biography*. 6 vols. Chapel Hill: University of North Carolina Press, 1979–1996.
———. *North Carolina Lives*. Hopkinsville, Ky.: Historical Record Association, 1962.

Newspapers and Periodicals

Annals of Surgery, vol. 238 (December 2003)
Asheville Times Citizen
Charlotte Observer
Durham Morning Herald
Durham Sun
Greensboro Daily News
New York Times
News & Observer (Raleigh)
Pittsburgh Courier
Seattle Post-Intelligencer
Society for Executive Leadership in Academic Medicine 3, no. 1 (January 2000)
The Walter Kempner Foundation, Inc.
Winston-Salem Journal

Books, Articles, Pamphlets, and Addresses

Aesculapian. Special 50th anniversary issue: *1930–1980*. Durham: Duke University Medical Center, 1980.
Alexander, Holmes, and Joseph R. Slevin. "Mr. Welfare State Himself." *Collier's* (February 1, 1950): 13–15, 52–53.
American Medical Association. Council on Medical Education and Hospitals of the American Medical Association. *Survey of Medical Schools, 1934–1937*. Chicago: Privately printed, 1937.
Anderson, Jean Bradley. *Durham County: A History of Durham County, North Carolina*. Durham: Duke University Press, 1990.
Angell, Marcia. "The Truth about the Drug Companies." *New York Review* 15, no. 12 (July 15, 2004): 52–58.
Anlyan, William G. *Metamorphoses: Memoirs of a Life in Medicine*. Durham: Duke University Press, 2004.
Arena, Jay M., and John P. McGovern, eds. *Davison of Duke: His Reminiscences*. Durham: Duke University Medical Center, 1980.
Berkowitz, Edward D., and Mark J. Santangelo. *The Medical Follow-up Agency: The First Fifty Years, 1946–1996*. Washington, D.C.: National Academy Press, 1999.
Berryhill, W. Reece, William B. Blythe, and Isaac H. Manning. *Medical Education at Chapel Hill: The First Hundred Years*. Chapel Hill: University of North Carolina School of Medicine, 1979.
Booz, Allen & Hamilton. *Long-Range Plan for Physical Plant Development*. 3 vols. New York: Booz, Allen & Hamilton, 1961.
Bridges, R. McIntyre. "Dr. Joseph Willis Beard: A Mighty Man, 1902–1983." *North Carolina Medical Journal* 46, no. 5 (May 1985): 303–309.

Brodie, Keith, and Leslie Banner. *Keeping an Open Door: Passages in a University Presidency*. Durham: Duke University Press, 1996.

Brown, Theodore M. "Friendship and Philanthropy: Henry Sigerist, Alan Gregg and the Rockefeller Foundation." In *Making Medical History: The Life and Times of Henry E. Sigerist*, edited by Elizabeth Fee and Theodore M. Brown. Baltimore: Johns Hopkins University Press, 1997.

———. "The Historical and Conceptual Foundations of the Rochester Biopsychosocial Model." N.d. At http://www.history.rochester.edu/history/fac/brown.htm [December 11, 2003]. University of Rochester, Department of History, Rochester, New York.

Buxton, William. "The Emergence of the Humanities Division Program in Communications, 1930–1936." *Rockefeller Archives Newsletter* (spring 1996): 3–4.

Carroll, Robert S. *Our Nervous Friends: Illustrating the Mastery of Nervousness*. New York: Macmillan, 1919.

Carter, Reginald D., and Justine Strand. "Physician Assistants: A Young Profession Celebrates the 35th Anniversary of Its Birth in North Carolina." *North Carolina Medical Journal* 61, no. 5 (September–October 2000): 249–256.

Chesanow, Neil. "Looking Back at Ralph Snyderman's 15 Years at the Helm." *DukeMed* (spring–summer 2004): 31.

Covington, Howard E., Jr. *Favored by Fortune: George W. Watts and the Hills of Durham*. Chapel Hill: University of North Carolina Press, 2004.

Covington, Howard E., Jr., and Marion Ellis. *Terry Sanford: Politics, Progress, and Outrageous Ambition*. Durham: Duke University Press, 1999.

Cummings, Martin M. "Wilburt C. Davison and Medical Libraries." *American Journal of Diseases of Children* 124 (September 1972): 342.

Davison, Wilburt C. *The Duke University Medical Center (1892–1960): Reminiscences of W. C. Davison*. Durham: n.p., n.d.

———. "The First Ten Years of Duke University School of Medicine and Duke Hospital." *North Carolina Medical Journal* (October 1941): 527–532.

———. *The First Twenty Years: A History of Duke University Schools of Medicine, Nursing and Health Services and Duke Hospital, 1930–1950*. Durham: Duke University, 1952.

"Dr. Leo W. Jenkins, The Man Who Asked 'Why Not?'" ECU *Medical Review* 8, no. 3 (December 1985): 2–3.

Dorfman, Wilfred. "Psychophysiologic (Psychosomatic) Disorders: An Overview." In *International Encyclopedia of Psychiatry, Psychology, Psychoanalysis, & Neurology*, edited by Benjamin B. Wolman. New York: Aesculapius, 1977.

Durden, Robert. *Electrifying the Piedmont Carolinas: The Duke Power Company, 1904–1997*. Durham: Carolina Academic Press, 2001.

———. *Lasting Legacy to the Carolinas: The Duke Endowment, 1924–1994*. Durham: Duke University Press, 1998.

———. *The Launching of Duke University, 1924–1949*. Durham: Duke University Press, 1993.

Durham, Michael. *George Garland Allen: A Life to Be Honored*. Privately printed, 1983.

Ellsworth, Scott. "The Secret Game: Defying the Color Line." *Duke Magazine* 82 (September–October 1996): 8–11, 40.

Gibbs, Nancy. "A Week in the Life of a Hospital." *Time* (October 12, 1998): 56.

Gifford, James F., Jr. *The Evolution of a Medical Center: A History of Medicine at Duke University to 1941.* Durham: Duke University Press, 1972.

Gordon, Colin. *Dead on Arrival: The Politics of Health Care in Twentieth-Century America.* Princeton, N.J.: Princeton University Press, 2003.

Green, Marsha A. "The Future of Clinical Trials Delivered Today." *Inside*, January 26, 2004. At http://inside.duke.edu/article.php?IssueID=80&ParentID=5796 [May 23, 2005].

Handler, Philip, and Eugene A. Stead Jr. "Historical Background." In *Undergraduate Medical Education and the Elective System: Experience with the Duke Curriculum, 1966–75*, edited by James F. Gifford. Durham: Duke University Press, 1978.

Hart, J. Deryl. *The First Forty Years at Duke in Surgery and the P.D.C.* Durham: Duke University, 1971.

———. "The Responsibility of the Medical Profession to Medical Education: Contributions of the Geographic Full Time Staff to the Development of the Duke University School of Medicine and Suggestions for the Assumption of More of the Cost of Medical Education by the Medical Profession as a Whole." *Annals of Surgery* 145 (May 1957): 599–623.

Haywood, Hubert B. "Mental Hygiene in North Carolina." *North Carolina Medical Journal* (March 1941): 139–142.

———. "President's Address." *North Carolina Medical Journal* (June 1941): 277–278.

Hoechst Marion Roussel, Inc. *Hospital Management Profiles.* Norwalk, Conn.: Medical Age Publishing. October 1995.

Hoel, Donna, and Robert Howard. "Hypertension: Stalking the Silent Killer," *Postgraduate Medicine* 101 (February 1997): 116-121.

Kammen, Michael. *Mystic Chords of Memory: The Transformation of Tradition in American Culture.* New York: Alfred A. Knopf, 1991.

King, William E. "Tabling Nixon." *Duke Dialogue* 12 (May 16, 1997): 15.

Kinney, Thomas D., Jane Elchlepp, and William D. Bradford, "Educational Activities Analysis of the Elective Curriculum." In *Undergraduate Medical Education and the Elective System: Experience with the Duke Curriculum, 1966–1975*, edited by James F. Gifford Jr. Durham: Duke University Press, 1978.

Kliewer, Mark A., and Carl E. Ravin. "A History of the Department of Radiology at Duke University Medical Center." *American Journal of Roentgenology* 165 (September 1995): 695–701.

Korstad, Robert R. *Dreaming of a Time: The School of Public Health, the University of North Carolina at Chapel Hill, 1939–1990.* Chapel Hill: School of Public Health, University of North Carolina, 1990.

Korstad, Robert R., and James Leloudis. "Citizen Soldiers: The North Carolina Volunteers and the War on Poverty." In *Amateurs in Public Service: Volunteering, Service-Learning, and Community Service*, edited by Charles T. Clodfelter. Durham: Duke University School of Law, 1999.

Kresge, Nicole, Robert D. Simoni, and Robert L. Hill. "Blacktongue and Nicotinic Acid Metabolism: Philip Handler." *Journal of Biological Chemistry* 279 (November 26, 2004): 8–9.

Madison, Donald L. "Durham's Exemplary Health Center—And Its Leader, Dr. Evelyn Schmidt." *North Carolina Medical Journal* 64, no. 4 (July–August 2003): 163.

Mauzy, Charles Hampton. "Cesarean Section: Its Incidence and Fetal Mortality in Some Cities in North Carolina." *North Carolina Medical Journal* (January 1942): 6.

Mervis, Jeffrey. "Wyngaarden to Step Down as NIH Director." *Scientist* 3, no. 10 (May 15, 1989): 3.

Miller, Mike. "An Empire Contained." *Towerview* (March 2003): 8–13.

Murchison, Wallace C. "Significance of the American Tobacco Company Case." *North Carolina Law Review* 139 (1947–48): 139–141.

One Hundred Years of Medicine: The Legacy of Yesterday and the Promise of Tomorrow, edited by Donna S. Garrison. Winston-Salem, N.C.: Wake Forest University Health Sciences Press, 2002.

Penfield, Wilder. *The Difficult Art of Giving: The Epic of Alan Gregg*. Boston: Little, Brown, 1967.

Pleasants Julian M., and Augustus M. Burns. *Frank Porter Graham and the 1950 Senate Race in North Carolina*. Chapel Hill: University of North Carolina Press, 1990.

Pressman, Jack D. "Human Understanding: Psychosomatic Medicine and the Mission of the Rockefeller Foundation." In *Greater Than the Parts: Holism in Biomedicine, 1920–1950*, edited by Christopher Lawrence and George Weisz. New York: Oxford University Press, 1998.

Private Diagnostic Clinic. "Description of PDC Organization," n.d. [ca. 2005].

Putnam, Frank W. "The Atomic Bomb Casualty Commission in Retrospect." *Proceedings of the National Academy of Sciences* 94 (May 12, 1998): 5426–5431.

"Ralph W. G. Wyckoff, 1897–1994–Obituary," *Acta Crystallographica* A51 (1995): 649–650.

Reynolds, P. Preston. "Hospitals and Civil Rights, 1945–1963: The Case of *Simkins v. Moses H. Cone Memorial Hospital*." *Annals of Internal Medicine* 126 (June 1, 1997): 898–906.

———. *Watts Hospital, 1895–1976*. Durham: Fund for the Advancement of Science and Mathematics Education in North Carolina, 1991.

Rivera, Alex. "Duke University Hospital Takes the Lead in Integrated Training Programs." *Pittsburgh Courier*. December 13, 1952.

Ross, Joseph S. "The Committee on the Costs of Medical Care and the History of Health Insurance in the United States." *Einstein Quarterly Journal of Biological Medicine* 19, no. 31 (2002): 129–134.

Schiebel, Max. "When I Was Younger: Looking Back at My Residency 65 Years Ago." *North Carolina Medical Journal* 60, no. 3 (May-June 1999): 132.

Sealy, Will C. "The Hen's Egg versus the Horse's Brain: How Equine Encephalomyelitis Vaccine Established the Dorothy and Joseph Beard Foundation." *North Carolina Medical Journal* 47 (January 1986): 37–38.

Shannon, James A., D. P. Earle Jr., B. B. Brodie, J. Taggart, R. W. Berliner, and resident staff of the Research Service. "The Pharmacological Basis for the Rational Use of Atabrine in the Treatment of Malaria." *Journal of Pharmacological Experimental Therapy* 81 (1944): 307–330.

Smith, George David. *From Monopoly to Competition: The Transformation of Alcoa, 1888–1986.* New York: Cambridge University Press, 1988.

Snider, William D. *Light on the Hill: A History of the University of North Carolina at Chapel Hill.* Chapel Hill: University of North Carolina Press, 1992.

Snyderman, Ralph, and Edward W. Holmes. "Oversight Mechanisms for Clinical Research." *Science* 287 (January 2000): 595–597.

Spearman, Walter. "A University Examines Itself." *Journal of Higher Education* 25, no. 3 (March 1954): 122.

Sulzberger, Marion B. "Studies in Tobacco Hypersensitivity, I. A Comparison between Reactions to Nicotine and to Denicotinized Tobacco Extract." *Journal of Immunology* 24 (1933): 85–91.

Tanouye, Elyse, and Robert Langreth. "Genetic Giant." *Wall Street Journal* (February 2, 1998).

Travis, Tony. "Analysts in the Dye and Allied Industries: Calco Chemical Company and American Cyanamid, 1930–1960." Paper presented at the Society for Alchemy and Chemistry, May 2002, Sutton, England.

Wagner, Galen S., Bess Cebe, and Marvin P. Rozear, eds. *E. A. Stead, Jr., What This Patient Needs Is a Doctor.* Durham: Duke University Hospital, 1981.

Weaver, Richard L., and James McAndrew. *The Rosewell Report: Fact versus Fiction in the New Mexico Desert.* Washington, D.C.: Department of the Air Force, 1995.

Weindling, Paul. "Termination or Transformation: The Fate of The International Health Division as a Case Study in Foundation Decision-Making." *Research Reports from the Rockefeller Archive Center* (fall 2002).

Wiggins E. J., and R. S. Lyman. "Manic Psychosis in a Negro: With Special Reference to the Role of the Psychogenic and Sociogenic Factors." *American Journal of Psychiatry* 100 (July 1943–May 1944): 786–787.

Wilkins, Robert H. "Barnes Woodhall, M.D.: A Biographical Sketch." *Clinical Neurology* 18 (1971): xvii–xx.

"William Brown Bell." *Chemical and Engineering News* 27, no. 46 (November 14, 1949): 3351.

Woodward, Theodore E. *The Armed Forces Epidemiological Board: Its First Fifty Years.* Washington D.C.: Borden Institute, Office of the Surgeon General, Department of the Army, 1994.

———. ed. *The Armed Forces Epidemiological Board: The Histories of the Commissions.* Washington D.C.: Borden Institute, Office of the Surgeon General, Department of the Army, 1994.

Interviews

Albright, Maine. Interview by "Dr. Frank." Documentary project. Chapel Hill, North Carolina, 1996. John Wilson Productions, Inc.

Berlin, Melvin. Interview by Walter E. Campbell. Durham, N.C., October 31, 2003. DUMCA.

Brodie, H. Keith H. Interview by Jessica Roseberry. Durham, N.C., June 17, 2004. DUMCA.

Busse, Ewald W. Interview by Walter E. Campbell. Durham, N.C., April 4, 2003. DUMCA.

Busse, Ewald W. Interview by Jessica Roseberry. Durham, N.C., October 10, 2003. DUMCA.

Cummings, Martin M. Interview by Gerald Oppenheimer. Washington, D.C., June 23, 1987. National Library of Medicine http://www.mlanet.org/about/history/m_cummings.html [May 23, 2005].

Donelan, William J. Interview by Jessica Roseberry. Durham, N.C., November 11, 2003. DUMCA.

Estes, E. Harvey, Jr. Interview by Jessica Roseberry. Durham, N.C., April 28, 2004. DUMCA.

Ewing, Oscar R. Interview by J. R. Fuchs. Chapel Hill, N.C., May 1, 1969. Harry S. Truman Library.

Gardner, Clarence E., and Ivan W. Brown Jr. Interview by James F. Gifford Jr. Orange City, Florida, December 7, 1991. DUMCA.

Goldner, J. Leonard. Interview by William Richardson, [ca. 2002]. DUMCA.

Graham, Doyle G. Interview by James F. Gifford Jr. Durham, N.C., June 26, 1995. DUMCA.

Helms, Jesse. Interview by Helms Documentary Project. Raleigh, N.C., [n.d.]. John Wilson Productions, Inc.

Hoover, Calvin B. Interview by B. U. Ratchford. Durham, N.C., January 8, 1972. Department of Economics, Duke University.

Lefkowitz, Robert J. Interview by Gary Taubes. December 2002. *in-cites*. At http://in-citex.com/scientists/RobertJLefkowitz.html [May 23, 2005].

Leuchtenburg, William E. Interview by "Dr. Frank" documentary project. Chapel Hill, 1996. John Wilson Productions, Inc.

Newman, Paul R., and Cecil Wallace. Interview by Walter E. Campbell. Durham, N.C., November 30, 2004. DUMCA.

Raab, G. Kirk. "CEO at Genentech, 1990–1995." Oral history conducted in 2002 by Glenn E. Bugos. Regional Oral History Office, Bancroft Library, University of California, Berkeley, 2003.

Rankin, Watson Smith. Interview by Wiley D. Forbus. January 11, 1965. DUMCA.

Rutter, William J. Interview by Sally Smith Hughes. 1992. Program in the History of the Biological Sciences and Biotechnology, University of California at San Francisco. At http://texts.cdlib.org/dynaxml/servlet/BookView?source=oac/oh/rutter/rutter.xml&style=oac/xsl/dynaxml/dynaxml.xsl&query=Rutter [May 23, 2005].

Saito, Vicki Y. Interview by Walter E. Campbell. Durham, N.C., February 20, 2004. DUMCA.

Semans, James H., and Mary D. B. T. Semans. Interview by Jessica Roseberry. Durham, N.C., January 20, 2004. DUMCA.

Semans, Mary Duke Biddle Trent. Interview by North Carolina Public Television. Research Triangle Park. At http://www.unctv.org/biocon/msemans/prg03.html [December 15, 2004].

Smith, Dorothy Mary. Interview with Stephen Kerber. Gainesville, Florida, March 26, 1979. University of Florida Health Center, University of Florida, Gainesville, Florida.

Snyderman, Ralph. Interviews by James F. Gifford Jr. Durham, N.C., December 14, 1990; March 23, 1993; and April 22 and 23, 1994. DUMCA.

———. Interviews by Walter E. Campbell. Durham, N.C., March 6, 2003; December 16, 2003; and January 6, 2004. DUMCA.

Taber, Robert L. Interview by Jessica Roseberry. Durham, N.C., August 25, 2004, DUMCA.

Towe, Kenneth C. Interview by Frank Rounds. New York, February 27; March 17, 18, and 30, 1964. Duke University, RBMSC.

Wyngaarden, James B. Interview by James F. Gifford Jr. Durham, N.C., April 9, 1982. DUMCA.

Wyngaarden, James B. Interview by Jessica Roseberry. Durham, N.C., March 3, 2005. DUMCA.

Web sites

Note: bracketed dates indicate the date web site URL was accessed.

Alza Corporation. "ALZA and SmithKline Beecham Sign International Commercialization Agreement for Nicoderm." November 17, 1997. At http://www.prnewswire.com/cgi-bin/stories.pl?ACCT=105&STORY=/www/story/11-17-97/361214 [May 23, 2005].

American Association of Medical Colleges. "FACTS—Applicants, Matriculants and Graduates." At http://www.aamc.org/data/facts/2004/factsenrl.htm [May 23, 2005].

Borck, Cornelius. "Mediating Philanthropy in Changing Political Circumstances: The Rockefeller Foundation's Funding for Brain Research in Germany, 1930–1950." Rockefeller Archive Center Research Reports Online, 2001. At http://archive.rockefeller.edu/publications/resrep/borck.pdf [May 24, 2005].

California Health Institute. "ALZA CEO elected chairman of Biomedical Industry Group." January 18, 1999. At http://www.chi.org/home/article.php?aid=7104 [May 23, 2005].

"Davis and Geck Company Records." Archives and Special Collections, Thomas J. Dodd Research Center, University of Connecticut. At http://www.lib.uconn.edu/online/research/speclib/ASC/findaids/Davisgeck/biography.htm [May 17, 2005].

Department of Energy. "DOE Openness: Human Radiation Experiments: Roadmap to the Project. Chapter 5: The Manhattan District Experiments." At http://

www.eh.doe.gov/ohre/roadmap/achre/chap5_2.html [May 20, 2005].

Duke University, Fuqua School of Business. "Curriculum Vitae, John Alexander McMahon." At http://faculty.fuqua.duke.edu/bio/mcmahonvita.pdf [May 23, 2005].

Duke University Medical Center. "Dr. Charles E. Putman, Duke Senior Vice President, Dies at Age 57." *DukeMed News*, May 11, 1999. At http://dukemednews. duke.edu/news/article.php?id=395 [May 23, 2005].

———. "Genomic-Based Prospective Medicine Collaboration." *dukehealth.org*, May 29, 2003. At http://dukemednews.org/news/article.php?id=6605 [May 23, 2005].

———. "Joseph Nevins Named Director of IGSP Center for Genome Technology at Duke." *dukehealth.org*, November 21, 2003. At http://dukemednews.duke.edu/ news/article.php?id=7218 [May 23, 2005].

———. "The Eva J. Salber Award for Projects in Community Medicine." At http:// communityhealth.mc.duke.edu/ED/Salber.htm [May 23, 2005].

———. "Thomas Tedder." *dukehealth.org*, February 7, 2005. At http://www.duke-health.org /AboutDuke/Administration/DeptChairs/Immunology [May 23, 2005].

Durham Monthly Meeting of Friends. "History of Durham Meeting." At http://dur-hammonthlymtg.home.mindspring.com/Handbook/DMMhistory.htm [May 17, 2005].

Emory University Medical School. Review of J. Willis Hurst, *The Quest for Excellence. Emory Medicine* (summer 1998). At http://www.whsc.emory.edu/_pubs/em/ 1998summer/quest.html [May 19, 2005].

Genentech. "Significant Scientific Milestones in Biotechnology." At http://www. gene.com /gen/reserch/biotechnology/significant-milestones.jsp [May 23, 2005].

Greenberg, Daniel S. "The Politics of Science 2000." February 25, 2000. Presentation at the meeting of the Philosophical Society of Washington. At http://www. philsoc.org/ 2000Spring/2115minutes.html [May 21, 2005].

Juckett, Lynn K. "Dad Goes to War." At http://www.thejucketts.com/ww2website /dadownwords.htm [May 18, 2005].

Kennedy, Thomas J., Jr. "James Augustine Shannon." National Academy of Sciences, *Biographical Memoirs* 75 (1998). At http://www.nap.edu/readingroom/books/ biomems/jshannon.html [May 18, 2005].

Microelectronics Center of North Carolina. May 23, 2005. At http://www.mcnc.org/.

Moeller, Stephen P. "Vigilant and Invincible." At http://www.fas.org/nuke/guide/ usa/airdef/vigilant.htm [May 20, 2005].

National Academy of Sciences. "Advisory Committees to the Surgeons General of the War and Navy Departments and U.S. Public Health Service." At http:// www7.national academies.org/archives/advcomsurgeons.html [May 18, 2005].

———. "Atomic Bomb Casualty Commission, 1945–1982." At http://www7.nation-alacademies.org/archives/ABCC_1945–1982.html [May 23, 2005].

National Archives and Records Administration. RG 59, Records of the Department of State, Records of the Executive Secretariat, NSC Files: Lott 66 D 148, Box 1555. Memorandum from the Director of the Executive Secretariat to the Under Secretary of State, March 8, 1949. At http://www.state.gov/www/about_state/ history/intel/370_379.html [May 23, 2005].

National Institute of Environmental Health Sciences. "Important Events in NIEHS History." 1999. At http://www.nih.gov/about/almanac/1999/organization/ niehs/history.html [November 1, 2004].

National Park Service. "US Naval Ordnance Test Facilities, Topsail Island MPS." At http://www.cr.nps.gov/nr/travel/aviation/usn.htm [May 20, 2005].

Newsletter of the American Academy of HIV Medicine. "The Nexus." Winter 2004. At http://aahivm.org/new/nexus/WINTER04story_7.html [May 23, 2005].

North Carolina Biotechnology Center. "The Biotechnology Center FAQ." At http:// www.ncbiotech.org/aboutus/center/faq.cfm [May 23, 2005].

Oak Ridge National Laboratory. "Swords to Plowshares: A Short History of Oak Ridge National Laboratory." At http://www.ornl.gov/info/swords/forties.html [May 20, 2005].

Research Triangle Park. "About Us: Park History." At http://www.rtp.org/index. cfm?fuseaction=page&filename=about_us-history.html [May 23, 2005].

Rutgers University, Ernest Mario School of Pharmacy. "Ernest & Mildred Mario Foundation pledges $5 million." December, 14, 2001. At http://pharmacy.rutgers.edu/admini/newname/ [May 23, 2005].

Stetten, Dewitt. "How My Light Is Spent: The Memoirs of Dewitt Stetten Jr." Spring 1983. http://history.nih.gov/history/DeWittStettenMemoirs.pdf. At http://stills.nap.edu/html/biomems/dstetten.html [May 21, 2005].

Tobacco Documents Online. At http://tobaccodocuments.org/.

United States Department of Health and Human Services, Health Resources and Services Administration. "The Hill-Burton Free Care Program." At http:// www.hrsa.gov/osp/dfcr/about/aboutdiv.htm [May 17, 2005].

United States Military, Army, Fort Bragg. "History." At http://www.bragg.army.mil/ history/HistoryPage/HistoryFortBragg/FortBraggin the1940s.htm [December 2003].

University of Milwaukee–Wisconsin, Archives of the American Academy of Allergy, Asthma, and Immunology. At http://www.uwm.edu/Library/arch/aaaai/president/coca.htm [May 17, 2005].

Unpublished Manuscripts

Campbell, Walter E. "Jesse Helms and Conservatism before 1972." August 2002. Copy in possession of author.

Gifford, James F., Jr. "Watson Smith Rankin and Standardization in Health Care: Hospitals, Philanthropy and Public Health, 1900–1950." Undated manuscript, James Gifford papers DUMCA.

McLendon, William W. "Walter Reece Berryhill." Chapter 10. January 20, 2003. Copy in possession of author.

Reynolds, Pamela Preston. Unpublished manuscript, [no title]. Copy in possession of author.

Wyngaarden, James. "Jim Watson and the Human Genome Project." March 4, 2003. Copy in possession of author.

———. "Remarks by James B. Wyngaarden at the Chief Residents Reunion." Duke University Medical Center, Department of Medicine, October 4, 2003. Copy in possession of author.

INDEX

Academic Council (Duke University), 341
Adams, Donald K., 140, 155–156
Adler, Alexandra, 134–135, 145
Advisory Committtee on the Status of Women, 353
Aeromedical Laboratory (U. S. Army), 98
Aetna Life Insurance Company, 386–387
African Americans
  care at DUMC for, 91–94, 284–286
  as Duke Hospital patients, 282
  institutions in Durham for, 76–77
  mental illness among, 135–136, 185–186, 417n.78
  morbidity and mortality statistics in North Carolina for, 72
  photos at Duke Hospital of, 75, 91, 175
  venereal disease prevalence among, 103
AIDS Clinical Trials Group, 342–343
AIDS research, Duke participation in, 324, 335, 342–343
AIDS Treatment Evaluation Unit, 342
Alderman, Sidney, 148, 190
Alexander, Leo, 132, 134, 137–138, 145
Alex H. Sands Jr. Medical Sciences Building, 281
Allen, George G., 29, 41–42, 45–47
  as Duke Endowment trustee, 53–54, 110, 142–143, 177, 182, 186–190
  photos, 21, 46
allergy research at DUMC, 297, 302
Aluminum Company of America (Alcoa), 5, 367, 407n.9
  antitrust suit involving, 45–46, 55, 144, 182
Aluminum Ltd., 46
Alyea, Edwin P., 41
Alza Corporation, 369
Alzheimer's disease, DUMC research on, 309
American Association of Immunologists, 34, 409n.13
American Bankers Association, 60
American Bar Association, 149
American Cancer Society, 213
American Cyanamid, 7, 29–30, 66, 109–110, 367
  aerosol research at Duke and, 253–254
  American Home Products purchase of, 369
  cancer research and, 40–41
  economic and institutional changes in, 368

  electron microscope from, 82
  equine encephalitis vaccine development and, 31–37, 66–68
  intelligence operations and, 140–141
  stock holdings of, 41–42
  sulfa drug development by, 104–105
  virology research initiatives and, 117–119
American Home Products, 369
American Hospital Association (AHA)
  Commission on Financing of Hospital Care and, 231
  Committee on Hospital Service, 27
  DUMC and, 289, 291–292
American Journal of Digestive Diseases and Nutrition, 38
American Journal of Psychiatry, 135–136
American Medical Association (AMA)
  Committee on the Costs of Medical Care, 22–23
  Council on Medical Education and Hospitals, 39
  kidney research rejected by, 120
  national health policy opposed by, 77–78
  political contributions from, 208
American Pediatric Society, 194
American Psychiatric Association, 50, 321
American Public Health Association, 214
American Red Cross, 138–139
American Tobacco Company, 13, 47–48, 57, 144, 218, 252–253
American Veterinary Medical Association, 80
Amey, Charles C., 52–53
Amey, Clementine, 168
Amey, Harriett, 168, 175, 197, 373
Amos, D. Bernard, 296–297, 298, 302–303
Amoss, Harold L., 57
Anderson, Robert W., 359
Angell, Marcia, 325
angiography, DUMC program for, 331–333
Anlyan, William G.
  appointment to DUMC, 264–265
  Brodie and, 317, 321–322, 330–333, 341–343, 382–385
  building expansion campaign and, 281, 283
  family medicine at Duke and, 326–330
  leadership style of, 334–336

photos, *265, 339, 382, 389*
racial integration at Duke and, 285–288
research programs and, 305–306
Surgery Dept. at DUMC and, 275–276
virology research and, 303
Anna M. Hanes Research Fund, 59, 115, 117, 123
anti-Semitism at DUMC, 184
Arena, Jay M., *298*, 303–304, 420n.61
Armed Forces Epidemiological Board, 218
Army Medical Library, 223–224
Army Ordnance Missile Plant, 221
Army School of Malariology, 114
Army Specialized Training Program, 106, 117, 121
Arnold, Virginia, 270
arrhythmia surgery, DUMC advancements in, 307–308
Asheville Christian Academy, 315
Asheville Times Citizen, 157
Aspergillus, Duke research on, 38–41, 63
Association of Collegiate Schools of Nursing, 95
asthma research at DUMC, 297, 302
Atomic Bomb Casualty Commission, 142, 217–219, 224
Atomic Energy Commission (AEC), 8, 43, 142, 216–223, 258
Atrabine antimalarial drug, development of, 115–116
Avery, Osvald T., 31

Bailey, James Hinton Pou, 189, 199, 203, 207–208
Bailey, Josiah W., 91–92, 171, 189, 199
Baker, Bessie, 95
Baker, Lenox D., 177, 237–238
Baker, Roger D., 41
Banham, Katharine M., 155–156, 173
Baptist State Convention of North Carolina, 57
Barker, Ruth (Elizabeth), 104
Barnard, Chester, 226
Barnes, Bowling, 35–36
Barnes, Robert H., 248
Baugh, Philip J. ("Jack"), 353, 389
Bayh, Birch (Sen.), 322–325
Bayh-Dole Act. *See* University and Small Patent Procedures Act
Beard, Dorothy, 32, 68, 119
Beard, Joseph W., 7–9, 62, 368
controversy over research methods of, 79–83
encephalitis vaccine research, 30–37, 39, 51, 63, 66–68, 412n.4
on military commissions, 103
patent application by, 67–68
photos, *31, 68*
viral research programs of, 117–119, 121, 127–128, 255, 295–297, *298*, 302–303
behavioral science at Duke, 248–252
Bell, William B., 119, 127
cancer research projects and, 38, 40–41
capital expansion campaigns and, 41–42
death of, 255
Duke Endowment and, 45, 53–54, 62, 110
encephalitis vaccine research and, 30, 32, 66–68
photo, *21*
Bell Research Building, 81, 126–128, 143, 220, 227, *312*
Berlin, Melvin, 272–273
Bernheim, Frederick, 213–214
Biddle, Anthony J. Drexel Jr., *21*, 49

Biddle, Mary Duke, 10, 21, 49–50, 71. *See also* Semans, Mary Duke Biddle Trent; Trent, Mary Duke Biddle
Billig, Otto, 134
Black, MaryAnn E., 371, 374–375
Blalock, Alfred, 7, 30–31, 275–276, 306–307
Blazer, Dan G., *382*
Blood Transfusion Betterment Association, 138–139
blood transfusions, Duke procedures for, 137–139
Blue Cross and Blue Shield of North Carolina, 60, 232, 289–290, 366
Blue Cross Associations, 26–27
Board for Investigation and Control of Influenza and Other Epidemic Diseases, 102–105, 118
Boineau, John P., 308
Bolognesi, Dani P., 296, *298*, 324, 335
Booz, Allen & Hamilton, 282–283
Bosley, Harold A., 194
Bowman Gray School of Medicine (UNC), 123, 158–160, 172, 228–229
regional cooperation with DUMC, 286–288
Bowser, Joe, 374
Branning, W. Sterry, 416n.35
British American Tobacco Company, 367
Broder, Samuel, 337
Brodhead, Richard H., 16, 395–398
Brodie, H. Keith H., 9–10, 15–16, 264, 380
Anlyan and, 330–336, 382
as Duke President, 313–322, 341–345, 347, 385–386
early career of, 316–322
photos, *318–319, 384, 389*
Private Diagnostic Clinic and, 325–330
Putman and, 385
Broughton, Melville (Gov.), 133, 199, 202
Brower, Alfred S., 180–181, 194–195
Brown, Harold W., 74
Brown, Haywood, 359
Brown, Ivan W. Jr., 138, *298*, 307–308
brucellosis, Duke research on, 115–116
Bruton, John F., 149
Bryant, Victor S., 50, 417n.68
Bryson, Edwin C., 136
Bryson, T. D. (Judge), 183
Buckley, Rebecca H., *298*, 302
Bugher, John, 271
Burkholder, Charles I., *21*
Burney, Leroy, 250–251, 323
Burroughs Wellcome Company, 323–325, 335–336, 340–343, 369
Burwell, George A., 182, 186
Bush, George H. W. (President), 272
business opportunities, Duke Medicine's involvement in, 11–16
Busse, Ewald W. ("Bud"), 9, 225, 248–252, 314–317, 423n.47
photos, *249, 339, 382*
Busse Building, 251

Calco Chemical Company, 35–36, 41
Califf, Robert M., 335, 351–352, 360, 378–379
Calkins, Robert, 198, 201–202, 214–215
Callaway, J. Lamar, 103, 105
Campaign for Duke, 368, 379–380, 387–388
Camp Butner (Durham), 103–104
cancer research

Duke Medicine's involvement in, 38–41, 63, 281
  radioactive fallout and, 221–223
  smoking risks and, 216–223
  Veterans Administration and, 239–240
capital expansion, for Duke research programs,
  41–42
Cargill, Walter H., 190
Carnegie Foundation, 22–23, 272, 290, 317
Carroll, Bernard J., 321–322, 353
Carroll, R. Charman, 129–130, 188, 315
Carroll, Robert S., 129–130, 132, 136, 143–144, 152
  as Highland Hospital director, 87–89, 184, 188
  photo, 99
Carter, F. Bayard, 94, 298, 305
Center for Integrative Medicine, 389–393
Center for the Study of Aging and Human
  Development, 250
Center for the Study of Health Policy, 291
Central Intelligence Agency (CIA), 140–141
Champagne, Mary T., 380–381
charity, DUMC and principles of, 11–12
charity cases, statistics at DUMC on, 90–91
Charles D. Barney & Company, 60
Chartwell Southeast, 376
Cherhavy, Irene, 225
Cherry, R. Gregg, 171–172, 199
China
  Duke connections in, 140
  Lyman's work in, 185
Christakos, Arthur C., 382
Ciba Pharmaceutical Products, 73
Citizens for Humphrey-Muskie Committee,
  265–266
Civil Rights Act of 1964, 274–275, 290–291
Civitan Building, 282, 315
Clark, James H., 233
Clinical Associates Program (NIH), 268
clinical psychology, Duke-VA collaboration on,
  155–157
Clinton, Bill (President), 367
Cobb, Clarence H., 188
Cobb, Stanley, 129–130
Coca, Arthur F., 34, 38, 82, 138–139, 409n.13
Cocke, Norman A., 21, 236, 283
Cohen, Louis D., 140, 156
Cohen, Sanford, 248
Cole, R. Taylor, 200–201
Collier's magazine, 212
Columbia Healthcare, Inc., 367
Columbia University, School of Tropical
  Medicine, 113
Colwell, Ernest C., 193, 198
commercial aspects of medicine, avoidance at
  Duke of, 111
Commission on Acute Respiratory Diseases,
  102–103, 117–118
Commission on Epidemiological Survey, 102, 116
Commission on Financing of Hospital Care, 27,
  231
Commission on Influenza, 102–103, 117–119
Commission on Tropical Diseases, 102, 113–114
"Committee of 50," 317
Committee of Four Hundred, 77–78
Committee of Veterans Medical Problems, 223
Committee on the Costs of Medical Care, 22–23,
  26–27, 229, 231
Committee to Study Watts Hospital Proposal, 288

Commmonwealth Fund, Community Health
  Sciences funding at DUMC by, 291
Commonwealth Fund, 8–9, 103, 112, 118, 281
  behavioral science research funding and,
    249–252
  Center for the Study of Health Policy fund-
    ing, 291
  DUMC assessment by, 242–245
  physician assistant program funding, 272
  Research Training Program and, 245–248, 258
Community Chest (Durham), 173
Community Health Organization Committee,
  229
Conant, Norman F., 103, 298, 302
Congress on Medical Education and Licensure,
  106–107
conscientious objectors, at DUMC, 134, 134–135
Cooper, Beatrice, 192–193
Cooper, George M., 162, 165, 168
Coordinating Office on Information, 140
Coppridge, William M., 164
Cornell, Beaumont S., 38
Council, C. T., 117
Coventry Health Plan, 387
Cox, Jonathan E., 21
Cox, Nola Mae, 135
Crick, Francis, 8
Crispell, Raymond S., 49–50, 132, 411n.61
Cromwell, James H. R., 46, 53–54, 166
Cummings, Martin M., 223–224

Dai, Bingham, 134, 136, 140
Damon Runyon Memorial Fund, 218–219, 252–
  253, 255
Daniels, Frank, 229
Daniels, Josephus, 13
Dann, William J., 73, 116–117
Darby, William J., 116
Darkis, Fred, 410n.43
Davey Compressor Company, 170
Davidson College, 5
Davis, Graham L., 26–27, 231
Davis, Jackson, 149, 161, 419n.32
Davis, James E., 285
Davis, Michael M., 25–26
Davis & Geck, 36–37, 368
Davison, Wilburt C. ("Dave"), 6, 9, 12, 22, 26–27
  American Red Cross and, 139–140
  Atomic Bomb Casualty Commission and, 142
  blood transfusion research and, 139
  budgeting controversy of, 144–145, 209
  candidacy for Duke presidency, 176–178, 186–
    190, 209, 253
  on charity cases at DUMC, 90
  committees controlled by, 166
  Commonwealth Fund assessment of, 243–245
  corporate partnerships and, 29, 32, 36
  critique of Edens by, 210
  as dean of DUMC, xiii–xiv
  death of, 286
  dissolution of Neuropsychiatry Department
    and, 224–227
  Doris Duke and, 55, 166–168, 194, 256–258
  Duke cancer projects and, 38–41, 66
  Duke Endowment and, 53–54, 101, 186–190
  Duke Hospital expansion project and, 231,
    236–237

Duke University Trustees and, 169–170
DUMC building expansion and, 283–284
equine encephalitis research and, 67–68, 81
financial support for medical students and,
    106–107
general practitioner training supported by, 294
gerontology research and, 250
Hanes and, 57–63
Hill-Burton Act and, 150
Hospital Care Association and, 290
Kempner and, 120, 152, 181–186, 212–214
Latin American medical students at Duke and,
    108–109, 112–113
leadership of Medical School, 121–128, 264–265,
    280–281
Lincoln Hospital and, 76–77
Medical Follow-up Agency and, 234–235
medical library program and, 223–224
North Carolina College for Negroes and,
    162–165
photos, 17, 26, 68, 99, 141, 283
political tensions involving, 147, 149, 165–168
portrait of, 177, 181, 420n.61
Private Diagnostic Clinic and, 54–55, 241–242
psychiatric medicine and, 50, 52–53, 69–71, 89,
    101–102, 133, 136–137, 152–153
public health and preventive medicine research
    and, 73–74
racial integration efforts of, 284–285
on radioisotope research, 220–221
retirement of, 261, 294
School of Nursing and, 95
Smith and, 170–172, 188–190, 236
staffing and financial issues facing, 144–145
Stead and, 151–152, 190–193
tropical disease research and, 113–116
UNC medical school expansion oposed by, 159
viral research programs and, 118–119
Davison Building, 28–29
Dean, Gordon, 220
DeBakey, Michael E., 222, 423n.39
Dees, Susan C., 297, 298, 302
De Jong, Herman H., 134, 136, 145
Democratic Party
    Duke involvement in, 170–172, 206–209,
        263–266
    Gray's involvement in, 230
Dent, Sara, 298, 306
DeVita, Vincent T. Jr., 337
Dewey, Thomas, 199
Diggs, Edward O., 230
Dingle, John H., 118
Dole, Elizabeth, 323
Dole, Robert (Sen.), 322–325
Donelan, William J., 288, 363–366, 370, 377,
    432n.49
Doris Duke Foundation, 29, 45, 55, 256–258
Dorothy Beard Research Fund, 12, 68, 80–81, 118,
    127, 413n.41
Downstate Medical College, 270–271
Drew, Charles R., 138–139, 186
Dublin, Louis, 222
Duke, Arden, 166
Duke, Benjamin N. ("Ben"), 2, 71
    African American community and, 284
    Flowers and, 177
Duke, Doris, 10, 14, 45–46, 215, 373

black colleges supported by, 52–53
Davison and, 55, 166–168, 194, 256–258
death of, 367–368
DUMC building expansion and, 281, 284
photos, 141, 283
psychiatry research supported by, 51–54
Duke, James Buchanan ("Buck"), xiii, 1–2, 367
    African American community and, 284
    Alcoa stockholdings of, 46
    American Cyanamid controlled by, 76
    corporate interests of, 4
    death of, 38
    Duke Endowment Indenture and, 4–5, 44–45,
        161
    DUMC creatiion and, 13, 19
    goals of, 54
    Rockefeller and, 47–48
Duke, Nanaline H., 45
Duke, Washington, 284
Duke Clinical Research Institute, 14–15, 351–352,
    360–361, 378
Duke Community Infusion Services, 376
Duke Comprehensive Cancer Center, 240, 281
Duke Council on Gerontology, 250
Duke Databank for Cardiovascular Diseases, 351,
    360
Duke-Durham Neighborhood Partnership,
    397–398
Duke Endowment
    Bell Building construction funding by, 81
    building expansion at Duke funded by, 281–283
    Busse Building funded by, 251
    charitable tradition of, 11–12
    Commission on Financing of Hospital Care
        and, 231
    community hospital system funding and, 79
    corporate ties in, 44–47
    creation of, xiii, 2
    curriculum reforms funded by, 275
    Davison and, 53–54, 121, 176–177
    Duke family tensions with, 53–54
    Duke Hospital expansion supported by, 242,
        286–288
    DUMC funding from, 4–6, 9–10, 13, 19, 55, 109–
        110, 180–181, 241–242, 281, 407n.8
    Durham Child Guidance Clinic funding, 250
    economic challenges facing, 144–145
    general practitioner training support from,
        294–295
    health care reform and, 24–25
    health insurance plans and, 26–27
    Highland Hospital and, 132, 136–137
    Hospital and Orphans Section, 21–22, 38
    Hospital Savings Association and, 289–290
    indenture requirements of, 44
    Lincoln Hospital African American residency
        program and, 272
    Lincoln Hospital and, 76–77
    medical library funding, 223–224
    mission of, 4, 6, 8, 44–47
    neighborhood clinics supported by, 397–398
    photo of trustees, 21, 283
    Physics Building funding by, 198
    political tensions within, 12–14, 149
    Private Diagnostic Clinic and, 84–85, 160–161
    racial integration initiatives funded by, 285–286
    Republican connections in, 235

research mission of, 29, 126–128
Smith's relations with, 209–212, 236–237
stock sales by, 367–368, 432n.63
trustees of, 7, 21, 45–46, 169–170, 215, 236, 283, 427n.48
Wake Forest funding from, 148
during World War II, 101
Duke Energy Corporation, 368
Duke Eye Center, 282
Duke family, 4
African American relations with, 284–286
black colleges supported by, 52–53, 381
Duke Medicine's relations with, 47–54
DUMC funding by, 9–10
Hanes's relations with, 60
stockholdings of, 42
Duke Farms, 46
Duke Health Community Care, 388
Duke Hospital
African American patients at, 75
black nurses training program at, 197–198
Blood Bank photo, 137
community clinic, 195
Doris Duke Foundation funding for, 256
expansion of, 59, 282, 286–288
financial problems at, 228–229, 232
funding requests from, 42
integration at, 174–176, 282–286
medical school faculty photo, 24
Medical Social Service Division at, 52
Out-patient clinic photo, 233
pediatric medicine at, 194–195
photos, i–iii, xv, 24, 75, 91, 94, 167, 175, 195, 197, 201, 286–287, 312–313
portable x-ray equipment, 167
Private Diagnostic Clinic and, 14–16
Syphilis Clinic at, 104
Duke Hospital Blood Bank, 137
Duke Human Vaccine Institute, 359
Duke Medical Alumni Association, 55
Duke Out-Patient Clinic, 24–25, 233
Duke Power Company, 4–5, 13, 30, 367
American Cyanamid shareholdings of, 42
antitrust litigation and, 55
Duke Endowment and, 44–47, 144, 236, 367–368
Duke Rehabilitation Clinic, 137, 153–154
Duke Southern Power Systems, 4
Duke University
administrative turmoil at, 341–345
Brodie as president of, 313–322
centennial celebration (1938), 65, 71–79
charitable tradition of, 11–12
Chemistry Department of, 42–44, 252–255, 410n.43
corporate connections of, 42–44
curriculum changes at, 273–275, 281
Department of Psychology at, 155–157
Department of Social Services at, 10, 14, 168, 175, 197, 256
DUMC building expansion funding, 281
DUMC integration with, 4, 14–16, 314–322
Edwin L. Jones Basic Cancer Research Building, 141–142
founding of, 2–3
genetics research funding by, 8
Long Range Planning Committee, 215

map of, 154
photo of campus, 64–65
Physics Department at, 198, 201–202, 220–223
racial integration of, 230–231, 282, 424n.62
Research Training Program funding, 258
state's relations with, 12–14
trustees of, 46, 178–179
West Campus quadrangle photo, 18–19
Duke University Affiliated Physicians, Inc. (DUAP), 364–367
Duke University Health System (DUHS), 3, 16, 286
as corporate entity, 375–377
creation of, 366–367
Durham Regional merger with, 374–375
economic and institutional changes in, 368–370
managed care issues and, 362–365
Mario as chairman of, 369
media coverage of, 378–379
sale of Wellpath and, 386–387
Santillan case, 388–389
Duke University Law School, 235
Duke University Medical Center (DUMC)
administrative turmoil at, 341–345
Bell Building constructed at, 81
biomedical research at, 295–297, 302–306
Brodie's leadership of, 314–322
building expansion at, 281–284
business operations of, 10–12
cancer research at, 38–41
charity caseload at, 90
Commonwealth Fund assessment of, 242–245
construction funding for, 227–229
Coronary Care Unit, 308
corporate partnership with, 29–63
curriculum changes at, 93–94, 273–275
daily hospital census at, 90
Davison's leadership of, 177–178
definition of, 407n.4
departmental restructuring at, 352–355
Department of Anesthesiology, 305–309
Department of Biochemistry at, 265, 304–305, 353–354
Department of Community Health Sciences, 278–280, 289, 291, 325, 329–330
Department of Medicine at, 277–279, 331–333, 352–355
Department of Microbiology and Immunology, 297, 302–306, 354–355
Department of Molecular Genetics and Microbiology, 354–355
Department of Neuropsychiatry, 97–98, 98, 101–102, 128–131, 148, 151–154, 172–174, 221, 224–227
Department of Obstetrics and Gynecology, 305
Department of Ophthalmology, 305–306
Department of Pediatrics, 297, 302, 315
Department of Psychiatry, 9–10, 15, 248–252, 314–322, 385–386
Department of Radiation Oncology, 353–354
Department of Radiology, 330–333, 352–353, 356–360
Department of Social Services, 197
Department of Surgery at, 263–264, 275–277, 306–309, 355–357
double billing controversy with VA and, 193, 196
Duke University and, 4, 14–16
emergence of, 2

expansion vs. consolidation at, 123–125
faculty changes at, 93–94
financial issues at, 143–145, 180–181, 358–360
financial support for students at, 106–109
general practitioners vs. physician-scientists at,
 293–295
government-sponsored research and, 30–32
grant programs of, 81–83
GUSTO Project at, 350–352
health care reform and, 24–25, 24–26
Hill-Burton funding for, 27
HMO formed at, 365–367
inpatient/outpatient statistics at, 122
integration with Duke University, 314–322
legacy of, 3–6
library reading room photo, 160
local network of, 289–291
major projects of 1930s, 20–22
map of, 154
medical libraries at, 223–224, 282
medical students at, 105–106
military relations with, 102–105, 216–223,
 241–242
mission of, 4–8
national health policy debate and, 77–78
opens in 1930, 19
Operations Improvement program, 364–365
outpatient clinic, 233
photos, i–iii, iv, 43, 122, 262–263, 318–319
physician assistant program, 272–273
polio clinic at, 196–198
politics and, 121–133, 202–203
postwar expansion of, 142–143, 147–203
poverty, race, and reform programs, 71–79
prewar years at, 90–100
Private Diagnostic Clinic as core business for,
 83–85
psychiatric research at, 49–54, 69–71, 85–89
public health research of, 8, 20, 73–79
public-private partnerships at, 105, 117–119
quality of care issues at, 91–94
racial integration of, 233–234, 283
racial politics at, 174–176
as regional research center, 214–223
reputation and influence of, 280–288
research programs at, 66–68, 110, 252–255
Rockefeller Foundation ties with, 47–54
salary issues at, 125–126, 151–152
Smith's influence on, 205–206, 208–212
Snyderman as chancellor of, 344–345, 347–355
social services at, 51–54
staffing issues at, 131–133, 143–145
state's relations with, 12–14
survey commissioned by, 157–168
venereal disease programs at, 104–105
during World War II, 101–145
World War II and, 105–109
Duke University Preventive Approach to
 Cardiology, 332
Duke University School of Medicine
 admissions policies at, 178–180, 210–211
 curriculum changes at, 273–275, 305
 Davison Building photo, 28–29
 Osler ivy ceremony, xiii, 17
 photos, i–iii, xv, 1, 24, 43, 179, 382
 regional cooperation with, 286–288

Duke University School of Nursing, 379–381
 cadet nurses photo, 100–101
 expansion of, 105, 142–143
 Hanes Annex photo, 100–101, 146–147
 Master of Science program, 271–273
 in prewar years, 90, 95–100
 staff and student photos, 25, 167
Duke-Veterans Administration Hospital Stroke
 Center, 309
Dulles, Allen W., 141
Dulles, John Foster, 226
Dunlap, Yvonne, 353
Durham, North Carolina
 Lincoln Hospital and, 76
 racial politics in, 174–176
 syphilis prevalence in, 103–105
Durham Chamber of Commerce, 285
Durham Child Guidance Clinic, 173–174, 226–227,
 249–250
Durham Committee on Negro Affairs, 288–289
Durham Committee on the Affairs of Black
 People, 372, 374
Durham County General Hospital, 3, 286, 291–
 292, 320, 327
Durham Hospital Association, 26
Durham Regional Hospital, 3, 370–375, 386–387
Durham Social Planning Council, 173
Durham Sun, 133
Dzau, Victor J., 16, 395–398

East Carolina University, 273, 286
Eberhart, John, 242–245
Edens, A. Hollis, 12, 111, 198–202, 205–206
 dissolution of Neuropsychiatry Dept. and,
 226–227
 Duke Endowment relations with, 236
 Duke Hospital expansion project and, 236–237,
 242
 DUMC regional research program and, 214–216,
 218–223
 photos, 220, 232
 Private Diagnostic Clinic criticized by, 241–242
 resignation of, 258, 260
 Smith and, 210–212, 235–236
 statewide health care planning and, 228–230
 tobacco industry and, 253
Edwin L. Jones Basic Cancer Research Building,
 281
Edwin A. Morris Building, 281
Eichner, Ludwig, 270–271
Eichorn, A. A., 34–35
Eisenhower, Dwight (President), 206, 233–234,
 252
Elias, Don S., 157–159, 169–170, 181, 203
Eli Lilly and Company, 323
Elizabeth P. Hanes House for Nurses, 227
Enders, John, 302
Engel, Frank L., 191, 269
Epstein, David L., 306
equine encephalomyelitis vaccine
 development of, 7, 30–37, 46, 66–68
 success and controversy surrounding, 79–83
Estes, E. Harvey Jr., 240, 288–289, 291–293, 295
 family medicine programs and, 279–280, 310–
 311, 326–330
 photo, 292
Eustis, Chuck, 427–428n.58

Evans, Lester, 248–249, 252
Ewing, Helen D., 213
Ewing, Oscar Ross
  health care reform and, 199–200
  Kempner and, 181–188, 212, 234
  NIH Environmental Health Sciences Center
    and, 325
  photo, 183
  political activities of, 206, 208–209, 323
  research programs at Duke and, 255
Extra-Sensory Perception, 44
extra-sensory perception, Duke research on, 44

Fair Employment Practices Commission, 206–207
Falk, Isadore, 23
family medicine
  DUMC programs for, 273, 310–311
  Private Diagnostic Clinic and, 325–330
Family Medicine Center (Durham County
  General Hospital), founding of, 280, 310–311
Family Medicine Program (DUMC), 289
Farrar, Judith, 201
Farrar, Mildred P., 201
Farrar & Rinehart, 44
federal funding, Duke Medicine and, 157–158
Federal Reserve Bank, 60
Federal Security Administration, 181–182, 187–188,
  206, 209, 228, 234
Feinstone, W. Harry, 104–105
Ferrell, John Atkinson, 20–22, 48, 116, 233
Few, Benjamin F., 189, 253, 427n.48
  photo, 283
Few, William Preston, xiii–xiv, 1–2, 55, 74–75, 97,
  253, 284
*First Forty Years at Duke in Surgery and the P.D.C.,
  The*, 62
Fishbein, Morris, 72, 77
Fitzgerald, Zelda Sayre, 87, 188
Fleishman, Joel, 291
Fletcher, A. J., 207
Flexner, Abraham, 1–2, 11, 48, 111, 191, 210
Flowers, Robert L., 21, 155, 162, 417n.68
  Duke Endowment and, 53–54, 170
  photos, 21, 99
  psychiatric research and, 97
  research programs and, 119
  retirement as Duke president, 177
  staffing and financial issues and, 143
  VA double-billing controversy and, 196, 226
Forbus, Wiley D., 6, 93, 102–102, 117, 192, 274, 298
Ford Foundation, 290
foreign medical students, wartime admission of,
  107–109
Fort Bragg, Duke Medicine activities at, 102–105
Fortune magazine, 231
Fosdick, Raymond, 226
Fowler, John A., 248–249
Frank, Michael M., 302
Fridovich, Irwin, 298, 304, 428n.85
Fulkerson, William J. Jr., 388–389
Furman University, 5
Furst, Georgea T., 169
Fuseon (AIDS drug), 324

Gallagher, Harold J., 183
Gallo, Robert C., 324

Gardner, Clarence E. Jr. (Lt. Col.), 56, 137–138,
  264, 273, 298
Gardner, John W., 290–291
Gardner, O. Max, 171–172
Genentech, 323, 331, 335–336, 338, 340–345,
  349–350
general practitioners, Duke policies concerning,
  279–280, 293–295
genetics research
  DUMC and, 310
  human genome sequencing project, 337
Georgia Workers Education Service, 194
Gilchrist, Huntingdon, 140–141
Gildea, Edwin, 88
Glaxo Holdings, P.L.C., 324, 336, 369
GlaxoSmithKline, 370
Glaxo Wellcome, 369–370
Global Health Initiative, 397–398
Goldner, J. Leonard, 237–238
Goldschmidt, Pascal J., 359
Graham, Doyle G., 342, 382
Graham, Frank Porter, 148, 202, 206–208, 219,
  230
Graves, Robert W., 86–89, 102, 413n.55
Gray, Gordon, 160, 205–206, 209, 229–233, 255,
  424n.63
  photo, 232
Great Society programs, Duke involvement in,
  273, 279–280
Green, Estelle Markin, 173–174
Greenfield, Joseph C. Jr., 326–327, 352–359
Greenhill, Maurice H., 129–130, 136–137, 153–155,
  173–174, 196
  dissolution of Neuropsychiatry Department
    and, 225, 423n.47
  photo, 130
  Stead and, 192
Greensboro Daily News, 196
Gregg, Alan, 9–10, 57, 98, 107
  American Red Cross and, 139
  Lyman and, 185–186
  psychiatric medicine and, 69–71, 85–88, 133,
    156–172
  Rockefeller Foundation work of, 48–51, 54, 109,
    111, 128, 226
  salary policies at DUMC and, 125–126, 191
Gregory, Tappan, 148
Grimson, Keith S., 296, 299
Gros, François, 277
Gross, Paul M., 142, 214–216, 218–219, 419n.32
  curriculum reform and, 273
  gerontology research and, 250
  photo, 220
  Research Training Program and, 42–43, 206,
    242, 246–248, 252
  resignation of, 258–261
  Smith and, 210–212, 235–236
  tobacco research and, 252–255
group medical insurance, Duke Medicine's involvement in, 26–27
Guaranty Trust, 47
GUSTO (Global Utilization of Streptokinase and
  TPA for Occluded Arteries) Project at DUMC,
  350–352, 360–361, 378

Hackel, Donald B., 295, 299
Halperin, Edward C., 354

Halsted, William S., 56
Hamblen, Edwin C., *299*, 305
Hamburg, David A., 316–317, 323, 429n.12
Hammond, Charles B., *299*, 305
Handler, Philip, 8–9, 206, 213–214, 218–220
    curriculum reform and, 273–274
    gerontology research and, 250
    at National Academy of Sciences, 266–268, 304
    photos, *267, 299*
    political activism of, 265–266
    Research Training Program and, 241–242, 245–248, 255, 258, 265
Hanes, Agnes Michel, 62, 227
Hanes, Betty (Elizabeth) P., 51
Hanes, Frederic M., 9–10, 12, 29, 49–51
    conflict with Hart, 61–63, 145
    Davison and, 121–128
    death of, 145, 148
    expansion of DUMC and, 123–125
    kidney research supported by, 120
    Life Insurance Medcial Research Fund and, 213
    malarial research and, 114–115
    national health policy debate and, 78–79
    neurology research of, 309
    photos, *57, 99*
    postwar expansion of DUMC and, 142–145
    Private Diagnostic Clinic and, 54, 57–61, 85
    psychiatry research and, 51, 69–71, 85–89, 101, 172
    salary policies at DUMC and, 125–126
    as School of Medicine faculty member, 93–94
    School of Nursing and, 96–97
Hanes, John Wesley Jr., 60
Hanes, P. Frank, 236
Hanes, Pleasant Huber, 60
Hanes, Robert March, 60
Hanes Annex, photo of, 146–147
Hanna, Frank A., 227
Hansen-Pruss, Oscar C., 297, *299*
Harmel, Merel H., 241, *299*, 306–307
Harris, Jerome S., 219, 274, *299*, 303
Hart, J. Deryl, 7, 11, 29, 32, 37
    conflict with Hanes, 61–63, 145
    Davison as dean and, xiv
    Department of Psychiatry and, 251–252
    Department of Surgery and, 276–277
    Duke Endowment and, 160–161
    Duke Hospital expansion project and, 237, 242
    equine encephalitis research and, 81
    expansion of DUMC and, 123–125, 127–128, 149
    photos, *37, 56, 264, 339*
    as president of Duke, 215, 258–261, 263
    Private Diagnostic Clinic and, 54, 56–57, 61–63, 85, 123, 210, 243–244
    salary policies at DUMC and, 125–126
    as School of Medicine faculty member, 93–94
Harvard University
    Commission on Epidemiological Survey and, 102
    encephalitis research at, 68
    psychiatry research at, 49
Haymaker, Webb, 222
Haynes, Barton J., 296, *299*, 359
Haywood, Hubert B. Jr., 103
HCA-Hospital Corporation, 367
health and hospital insurance, evolution of, 26–27
health care reform

Duke Medicine's involvement in, 19–27, 71–79, 199–200, 227–229
    Durham politics and, 370–375
health maintenance organizations (HMOs), 362–363, 365–367
Health Management Associates, 367, 371
Health Planning Council for Central North Carolina, 229, 285–286, 289
Heartt, Philip, *283*
Helms, Jesse, 207–208
Henricksen, G. R., 136
Heyman, Albert, *299*, 309
Hickam, John B., 191
Hicks, John M. W., 57
Highland Hospital
    DUMC psychiatric facility at, 86–89, 97, 101–102
    fire at, 188
    photo, *84*
    sale of proposed, 185–186, 315–316
    staffing and financial issues at, 130–133, 136–137, 143–145, 151–153
Hill, George Watts, 26, 140, 285, 290
Hill, Robert L., *299*, 304, 326, 353–354
Hill, Thomas F., *283*
Hill-Burton Act. *See* Hospital Survey and Construction Act
Hobbs, Marcus E., 218, 427–428n.58
Hoey, Clyde (Gov.), 51, 70, 86
Hoffman-LaRoche, 324
Hogan, Brigid L. M., 354, 359
Hohman, Leslie B., 154–155, 196, 224–225
Holmes, Edward W. Jr., *299*, 309, 377, 379
hookworm eradication program, DUMC's involvement in, 20–22, 48
Hoover, Calvin Bryce, 140–141, 178–179, 187, 194, 419n.32
Horack, H. Claude, 182–183
Horneman, Herman, 183
Hospital Administration: A Career, 26
Hospital Care Association, 26, 232, 290
Hospitalized Veterans Service of the Musicians Emergency Fund, 257
Hospital Savings Association of North Carolina, 26, 60, 232, 289
Hospital Survey and Construction Act (Hill-Burton Act), 6, 13–14, 27, 407n.12
    expansion of DUMC and, 147–148
    impact on Duke Medicine, 150–158, 209
    North Carolina College for Negroes and, 162–165
    Smith's influence with, 228–229
Houpt, Jeffrey L., 321–322, 377–378
Howard Hughes Medical Institute, Duke medical investigators at, 8, 269, 275, 338, 384
Howard University Medical School, 163
Hughes, Hubbard & Ewing, 182
human testing, Duke cancer research and issue of, 40–41
Humphrey, Hubert, 265–266
Hunt, Jim (Gov.), 317

IBM, at Research Triangle Park, 325
immunology research at DUMC, 295–297, 302–306
Independent Aid, Inc., 52–53, 55, 166–169, 194, 224, 231, 256–258
Ingles, Thelma, 270–272

Inman, Walker P., 42
Institute for Genome Sciences and Policy, 387–390
Institute of Government, 289
Institute of Inter-American Affairs, 112
Institute of Medicine, 267, 292–293
Institute of Nuclear Studies, 142
Institute of Policy Studies and Public Affairs, 291
insurance industry, DUMC and, 213–214
integrative medicine at Duke, 389–393
Intercom (Duke Hospital newpaper), 250
International Association of Insurance Counsel, 213
"Isolation and Characterization of Influenza Virus B (Lee Strain)," 118
Israel, Michael, 363

J. A. Jones Construction Company, 141, 166
Jackson, C. D., 231
Jackson, Robert A. (Justice), 148
Jackson, William K., 183–184
Jacobs, Danny O., 359
James B. Duke (Liberty ship), 166
Jenkins, Leo W., 273
Jenkins, W. M., 173
John and Mary R. Markle Foundation, 20, 73, 103, 114, 116–119, 246–248, 258
Johns Hopkins School of Medicine, 6–7, 20, 22, 88–89
    Davison's attendance at, 55
    Duke's connections to, 112–113, 275–276
    Hanes at, 58
    Hart's attendance at, 56
Johnson, Amos N., 329
Johnson, Charles, 373
Johnson, Charlie, 186, 199
Johnson, Lyndon Baines (President), 252, 264, 273, 323
Johnson, Mary Elizabeth, 56–57
Johnson C. Smith University, 5
Johnson & Johnson, 369
Joklik, Wolfgang K., *300*, 302–303, 326, 353–354
Jones, Edwin L. Sr., 141, 170, 215
    curriculum reform and, 273
Jones, Nell Cooke, 197–198
Jones, Robert R. Jr., 41
Jordan, Charles E., 211
Josiah Macy Jr. Foundation, 9, 272
Journal of Clinical Investigation, 116
Journal of Immunology, 34
Journal of Parapsychology, 44
Journal of the American College of Cardiology, 360
Journal of the American Medical Association (JAMA), 23, 72, 216, 218
Journal of the History of Medicine and Allied Sciences, 223
Joyner, George William, *xiii*
Junior League of Durham, 173–176

Kammen, Michael, 65–66
Katz, Samuel L., *300*, 302
Kearns, Amos R., 427n.48
Keeping an Open Door: Passages in University Presidency, 15
Kelley, William H., 309–310
Kempner, Robert, 149
Kempner, Walter, 59, 124, 127, 144, 149, 165, 197

Davison and, 152, 181–186, 188, 191
    hypertension research of, 119–121, 295–296
    photos, *120, 300*
    rice diet research, 212–214, 234, 428n.73
Kendall, Henry, 210–211
Kennedy, John F. (President), 252, 263, 315
Kennedy, Robert F., 49
Keohane, Nannerl O., 16
    Brodie and, 347
    DUMC department restructuring and, 353–355
    financial crisis at DUMC and, 358–360
    hospital acquisitions and, 375–376
    Institute for Genome Sciences and Policy and, 388
    photo, *391*
    Putman and, 383–385
    retirement of, 390–392, 395
    School of Nursing and, 380–381
    Snyderman and, 353, 391–393
Kerby, Grace, 116
kidney disease, Duke research programs on, 119–121, 182–185, 191, 295–296
Killian, James R. Jr., 198
Kinney, Thomas D., 274–275, *339*
Kirby Clinic, 154–157, 196
Kirksville College of Osteopathic Medicine, 257
Klausner, Richard D., 388
Knight, Douglas M., 263–264, 290, 384, 427–428n.58
Kohn, Henry I., 108
Korean War
    DUMC activities during, 216–223
    veterans at Duke from, 238–239

La Barre, Maurine Boie, 173–174
La Barre, Weston, 173–174
LaGuardia, Fiorello H., 167
Lambert, Robert A., 51–54, 58, 86–89
    dissolution of Neuropsychiatry Dept. and, 226
    Hanes's relations with, 60–61, 144–145
    on Latin American medical students, 108–109
    photo, *60*
    psychiatric medicine and, 133–135, 172–173
    research staffing issues and, 131
    Rockefeller Foundation work of, 109
    on School of Nursing, 95
    Stead and, 151–152, 165–166, 190–193
    tropical disease research by, 113, 115
Lassiter, Robert, 60
Latin American medical students, wartime admission to DUMC, 108–109, 112
Lederle Fellowship in Biochemistry, 81
Lederle Laboratories, 7–8, 368
    blood bank and transfusion research, 138–139
    cancer research at, 38–41
    equine encephalitis vaccine development and, 32–37, 51–52, 67–68, 79–83, 412n.4
    military commission partnerships with, 103
    nutrition research at, 116
    pellagra research and, 73
    sulfadiazine development by, 105
    viral research at, 117–119
Lee, William S., *21*
Lefkowitz, Robert J., 296, *300*, 335, 338, 340–341, 344
Lemkin, Raphael, 148–149

Lester, Richard G., 331
Leuchtenburg, William E., 208
Levine Science Research Center (LSRC), 341,
  346–347, 382–383
Lewin & Company, 329
Life Insurance Medical Research Fund, 152,
  213–214
Life Sciences Research Laboratories, 297
Liggett & Myers Tobacco Company, 42, 144, 177,
  252–253, 259–260, 410n.43
Lincoln Community Health Center, 3, 289, 371, 375
Lincoln Hospital
  African American residency program at, 272
  becomes Lincoln Health Center, 3
  Doris Duke Foundation support for, 256–257
  Duke family support of, 284–286
  Duke Medicine and, 71–72, 76
  early building, xviii
  evolution of, 76–77, 164
  expansion of, 228, 286, 288–289
  Flowers as trustee for, 177
  founding of, 2
  Medical and Dental Advisory Committee, 289
  School of Nursing at, 284
  segregation of, 174–176
  social work at, 135
Liversedge, Lawrence, 108
Llewellyn, Charles E., 248
Lordeaux, Stan, 94
Lowenbach, Hans, 130–131, 134, 224
lung cancer, research on smoking and, 216–223,
  259–261
Lyman, Katherine Ham, 174
Lyman, Richard S., 10, 87–89, 97–98, 143, 145
  anti-segregation efforts of, 174–176
  dissolution of Neuropsychiatry Department
    and, 224–227
  Highland Hospital and, 185–186, 315–316
  Kirby Clinic and, 152, 154–158, 418n.15
  Neuropsychiatry Department and, 128–137,
    172–174, 423n.45
  OSS career of, 137, 140, 156
  photos, 87, 99
  VA work of, 193, 196

MacDonald, Aleta Morris, 167
MacDonald, Byrnes, 167
Machemer, Robert, 300, 305–306
MacMillan, John H. Jr., 212–213
malaria, Duke research on, 114–115
managed care, DUMC and, 361–365, 379–381
Manhattan Project, 141, 215
Manning, Isaac H. Jr., 26
Mario, Ernest, 336, 369, 392
Markee, Joseph E., 238, 300, 304
Markle Scholars-in-Medicine program, 116–117
Marks, Herbert, 423n.39
Marshall, Edward C., 21
Marshall I. Pickens Building, 282
Martin, David, 344
Martin, Samuel P. III, 244–245
Mason, Max, 48
Matas, Rudolph, 97
Matte-Blanco, Ignacio, 132, 134
Matthews, Thomas, 324
Mayo, Charles, 39

McBryde, Angus M. Jr., 41
McCallister, Frank, 194
McCarran, Patrick (Sen.), 230
McCarthy, Joseph (Sen.), 230
McCloy, John, 226
McCord, Joe M., 300, 304
McCuiston, Fred, 198
McGovern, John P., 17
McHugh, Gelolo, 156
McLean, I. William Jr., 118
McLelland, May, 92
McLendon, L. P. (Maj.), 169–170, 233
McLeod Infirmary, 38–41, 63, 66
McMahon, John Alexander, 285, 289–292, 326
Means, Anthony R., 349, 353
Medical Alumni Association, 90, 92–93, 178–179
Medical Care for the American People, 23
medical education
  racial integration and, 175–176
  World War II impact on, 105–109, 121–123
Medical Follow-up Agency, 221–223, 226, 234–235
medical library at Duke, 223–224
  Seeley G. Mudd Building for, 282
Medical Scientist Training Program, 8–9, 278–
  279, 362
Medicare/Medicaid program
  creation of, 273–275, 279
  funding cuts in, 314, 327
Meharry Medical College, 163, 224
mental health care
  Duke Department of Neuropsychiatry and,
    97–99, 101–102, 128–131, 148, 151–154, 172–174
  Duke Department of Psychiatry and, 9–10, 15,
    248–252
  Duke Medicine's initiatives in, 49–54, 251–252
Mental Retardation Facilities and Community
  Mental Health Centers Construction Act of
  1963, 314–315
Meriwether, W. Delano, 282, 424n.62
Metabolic Basis of Inherited Diseases, The, 270
Methodist Church, Duke ties with, 177, 235–236,
  258–261
Meyer, Adolph, 49, 87–88, 97–98, 99
Microelectronics Center of North Carolina, 323,
  384
Milam, Daniel F., 103, 116
Milbank Memorial Fund, 231
military research, Duke Medicine's involvement
  in, 102–105, 216–223, 241–242
Morelock, Isabelle, 257
Morelock, Josephine, 257
Morgan, Lucy Shields, 162–163
Morgan Guaranty Trust, 47
Morris, Lewis Gouverneur, 167
Muncie, Wendell S., 86–89
Murray, Dwight H., 422n.4
Myers, Jack D., 190–191
Myers, Richard, 370

Nanaline H. Duke Medical Sciences Building, 281
Nashold, Blaine S. Jr., 300, 308, 429n.97
National Academy of Sciences, 266–268
National Cancer Act of 1971, 281
National Cancer Institute, 39, 184, 240, 297, 305
  DUMC grants from, 82, 128, 142
National Committee for Mental Hygiene, 86

National Committee for the Medical School
  Survey, 157–168
National Conference on the Costs of Medical
  Care, 23
National Environmental Health Sciences Center,
  255
National Foundation for Infantile Paralysis, 139,
  196, 231, 238
National Health Council, 184
National Health Insurance plan, 199–202,
  206–208
national health policy, debate at Duke concern-
  ing, 77–79
National Institute of General Medicine and
  Sciences, 337
National Institutes of Health (NIH)
  Cardiovascular Section, 152
  Duke gerontology research funded by, 251
  Duke Medicine and, 4, 7–10, 30–32, 79, 82, 128,
    209, 266–268
  DUMC building expansion funding from, 281
  Environmental Health Sciences Center, 325
  funding cuts at, 314
  kidney research grants from, 121, 182–185, 191,
    295–296
  racial integration of, 290–291
  research mission of Duke Medicine and, 7,
    294–295
  Research Training Program and, 246–247, 258
  wartime origins of, 113
National League of Nursing, 271
National Library of Medicine, 224
National Mental Health Act, 153
National Research Council, 112–118, 139, 217
  Committee on Veterans Medical Problems,
    221–222
  Division of Medical Sciences at, 235
National Venereal Disease Control Act of 1938, 104
Nature, 8
Navy V-12(S) Programs, 106, 121
Neurath, Hans, 8–9, 81
Nevins, Joseph R., 354–355, 431n.24
Newbold, Nathan Carter, 74–77, 162, 412–413n.27
New England Journal of Medicine, 294
New Frontiers of the Mind, 44
Newman, Paul R., 328, 356–357, 366
Newsom, Eugene, 181
New York Hospital for Tuberculosis, 32
New York Life Insurance Company, 365–367,
  386–387
Nielsen, Walter M., 36–37, 170, 219
Nike Ajax missile system, 218, 221, 423n.35
Nirenberg, Marshall, 337
Nixon, Richard M. (President), 233, 292, 294, 323
  anticancer campaign of, 252
  racial integration policies of, 281
  ties to Duke, 235, 265–266, 313
  Veterans Administration policies of, 239–240
North Carolina
  African American morbidity and mortality rates
    in, 72
  DUMC's relations with, 12–14
  health care reform in, 19–27
  mental health legislation in, 50, 132–133, 417n.68
North Carolina Association of Launderers and
  Cleaners, 228

North Carolina Baptist Hospital, 123, 228
North Carolina Biotechnology Center, 323, 384
North Carolina Board of Charities and Public
  Welfare, 86
North Carolina Cerebral Palsy Hospital, 3
North Carolina College for Negroes, 52–53, 76–77,
  135, 162–165
  anti-segregation drives and, 175–176
  Duke family funding for, 284–285
  Flowers as trustee for, 177
  integrated basketball with Duke, 175
  Medical School established at, 172
North Carolina Department of Agriculture, 252
North Carolina Department of Instruction,
  Division of Cooperation in Education and Race
  Relations, 75
North Carolina Good Health Association, 164–
  165, 211–212
North Carolina Hospital and Medical Care
  Commission, 124–125
North Carolina Hospital for Cerebral Palsy, 177
North Carolina Hospital Study Committee, 205–
  206, 232–233
North Carolina Medical Care Commission, 12–13,
  20, 150, 157, 160–161
  Duke Hospital expansion supported by, 242
  Duke Medicine's cooperation with, 205–206
  Durham Child Guidance Clinic funding, 250
  location at DUMC, 315
  Medical Training for Negroes Committee, 163
  political issues and, 165–166, 169–170, 172
  Smith and, 209–212
  statewide health care planning and, 227–229
North Carolina Medical Journal, 119–120, 223
North Carolina Medical Society, 11–12, 26–27
North Carolina Memorial Hospital, 227–228
North Carolina Regional Medical Program, 289
North Carolina State Board of Health, 20, 39, 116
  venereal disease research on, 103–105
North Carolina State Sanitorium, 77
Nursing Research Center, 380
nutrition research
  Duke initiatives in, 7–8, 73, 116–117
  kidney disease and, 119–120

Oak Ridge Institute of Nuclear Studies, 142, 215,
  219–221
Oak Ridge power plant, 141–142
occupational therapy, psychiatric medicine and, 87
O'Connor, Basil, 139, 196
Odum, Howard W., 74–75, 209
Office for Coordination of Commercial and
  Cultural Relations between the American
  Republics, 112
Office of Coordinator of Inter-American Affairs,
  112
Office of Human Genome Research, 337
Office of Protection from Research Risks, audit of
  DUMC, 378–379, 386
Office of Scientific Research and Development,
  113, 118
Office of Strategic Services (OSS), DUMC and, 137,
  140–142, 156
oneness concept, Brodie's advancement of, 313–
  322, 334, 341–345, 347–349
Orgain, Edward S., 295–296, 300

Osler, William (Sir), xiii–xiv, 54
Our Nervous Friends, 87
Outpatient Clinic at Duke, 122–123

parapsychology research, Duke involvement in, 44, 226–227
Parker, John J. (Judge), 149
Parker, Roy T., *300*, 305
Parker, Walter C., *21*
Parkerson, George R. Jr., 330
Parran, Thomas Jr., 6, 23, 39, 79, 104, 139
    controversy over Kempner and, 182, 184–185, 187–188, 212
Paschal, Marian, 52–53, 167–169
Paullin, James E., 152
Pavlov, Ivan, 88
Peace College, 92
Peck, Elizabeth, 58
Peking Union Medical College, 87–88
pellagra, Duke research on, 7, 32–33, 73, 116
Penrod, Kenneth E., 243–245
Peripheral Nerve Injuries: Principles of Diagnosis, 222
Perkins, Thomas L., *283*, 427n.48
Perkins, William R., 41–42
Perlzweig, William A., 8, 40, 81, 93, 117
Perry, Jessie, 92
personal rapid transit (PRT) system, *335*
Peters, John Punnett, 72, 77
physician assistant program at Duke, 272–273, 278–280, 304–306
physician-scientists, training of, 7–9, 279–280, 283–285
Pickens, Marshall I., *283*
Pickett, Clarence, 167
Pickrell, Kenneth L., 105
Pinkerton, Margaret I., 95
Pittsburgh Courier, 233
Plasma for Britain Project, 138–139
politics
    Duke Endowment trustees' involvement in, 169–172, 186–187
    Duke faculty and staff involvement in, 202–203, 206–207, 234–235, 263–266
    health care in Durham and, 370–375
    statewide health care planning and, 227–229
Porter, F. Ross, 232
Pounds, Lois A., 353
poverty, Duke's reform initiatives concerning, 71–79
Powdermaker, Florence, 156
preventive medicine, DUMC initiatives in, 73–79, 118
Preventive Medicine Service, 118
primary care physicians, DUMC policies for, 291–293
Principles of Biochemistry, 268
Pritchard, Otto E., 259
Private Diagnostic Clinic (PDC), 4
    Bell Building construction funding by, 81
    building fund of, 281–283
    business success of, 241–242
    as commercial operation, 12–14
    construction funding by, 227–228
    as core business of Duke Medicine, 83–85
    Department of Neuropsychiatry and, 102, 151–152
    Department of Psychiatry funded by, 251–252, 315
    Duke Endowment and, 84–85, 160–161
    Duke Hospital expansion supported by, 242
    evolution of, 10–12, 14–16
    expansion of, 110, 149, 205–206
    family medicine and, 325–330
    health care reform and, 24–26
    integration with Duke Medicine, 355–357
    Kempner's success at, 183–184
    leadership of, 54–63
    medical and surgical divisions in, 29
    photos, *96*, *204–205*
    political ascendancy of, 121–128
    radiology privileges at, 331–333
    referral clinics of, 237–238
    Smith's influence on, 188–189, 210–212
    space and expansion concerns of, 61–63
    tensions with DUMC, 241–242
private practice, DUMC's reluctance concerning, 111, 191, 210
Prosnitz, Leonard R., 354
Psychiatric Institutes of America, 316
psychiatry
    at Duke University Medical Center, 49–54, 69–71, 85–89, 151–154
    in North Carolina, 133–137, 417n.68
Psychological Strategy Board, 230–231
Psychological Warfare Center, 231
psychosomatic medicine, Duke Medicine's research on, 49–54, 192–193, 244–245, 389–390
Public Mental Health Act, 173
public-private partnerships at DUMC, 105, 117–119, 127–128, 139–140, 206
Puerto Rico School of Tropical Medicine, 102
Purdue University, 323
Purves, Dale, 349, 353
Putman, Charles E., 330–333, 336, 342, 382–385

R. J. Reynolds Tobacco Company, 46, 143–144, 236, 251
Raab, G. Kirk, 341
racial politics
    building expansion at DUMC and, 281–286
    dissolution of Neuropsychiatry Dept. and, 225–226
    at Duke Medicine, 174–176
    in Duke research staffing, 131–133
    DUMC and, 13–14, 71–79, 197–198
    Durham health care and, 370–375
    health care reform and, 19–27
    integration at DUMC and, 233–234
    integration of Duke University and, 230–231, 424n.62
    Lyman's involvement in, 136–137, 417n.78
    North Carolina College for Negroes and, 162–165
    in postwar North Carolina, 206
    quality of care at Duke and, 91–94
Radiation Effects Research Foundation, 218
radioactivity and cancer, Duke research on, 221–223
Radio Corporation of America (RCA), 30, 82
radioisotope research at Duke, 142, 219–223, 240–241
radiology at DUMC, 330–333

Raetz, Christian R. H., 354
Raleigh Community Hospital, 376
Raleigh *News & Observer*, 13, 56–57, 186, 353, 359, 363–364
Ralph Snyderman, M.D., Genome Sciences Research Building, *394–395*
Rankin, Fred, 39
    Lincoln Hospital and, 76–77
    on McLeod Infirmary projecty, 66
Rankin, R. Grady, *283*
Rankin, Watson Smith, 6, 20–22
    American Cyanamid shareholdings of, 42
    Committee on the Costs of Medical Care and, 22–23, 26–27, 231
    Duke Endowment duties of, xiii, 21–22, 38–39, 150, 169–170, 182
    DUMC building expansion and, 283–284
    expansion of UNC Medical School and, 158–159
    legacy at DUMC of, 281
    Medical School Survey and, 157–158
    North Carolina College for Negroes and, 164–165
    photos, *21, 283*
    quality of care issues and, 92
Rapid Treatment Center for venereal disease, 104–105
Ravenel, Leonard J., 409n.27
Ravin, Carl E., 330, 333, 353
Reaction to Injury, 93
Read, Florence, 151
Reagan, Ronald (President), 268, 314, 322, 327, 336–337
recombinant DNA research, impact on DUMC of, 322–325, 330–331
Reeves, Robert J., 40, 331
Regional Center for Research on Aging, 250
Reliant Pharmaceuticals, 369
Reminiscences, 176–177
Republican Party, Duke involvement in, 208, 233–234
research programs at Duke
    building and facilities for, 126–128
    corporate funding, 29–63
    as Duke Medicine mission, 7–9
    Hanes's commitment to, 59–61
    interdisciplinary focus of, 252–255, 305–306, 341–345, 354–355
    on kidney disease, 119–120
    military projects, 216–223
    nutrition research programs, 7–8, 73, 116–117
    regional research center, 214–223
    risks and rewards of, 66–68
    staffing demands for, 131–133
    on tropical diseases, 102, 113–116
    viral research, 30–32, 117–119
    wartime expansion of, 110, 112–120
Research Training Program (RTP), 206, 241–242, 245–248, 265, 305
    founding of, 8–9, 43, 258
    interdisciplinary curriculum of, 252–255, 305, 341–345
    photo, *259*
    Wyngaarden as director of, 268, 277–279, 294
Research Triangle Institute, 326, 384
Research Triangle Metropolitan Health Planning Group, 229, 285

Research Triangle Park, 209
    biotechnology at, 323–325
    British drug companies in, 369
    DUMC ties with, 330–333, 342–345
    National Environmental Health Sciences Center at, 255
    Research Training Program and, 247–248
Retrovir drug development, 343
Reuther, Walter, 199–200
Rex Hospital (Raleigh), 228, 376
Reynolds, R. J., 46
Reynolds, William N., 46, 177
Rhine, Joseph B., 44, 226–227
rice diet, development of, 119–120, 211–214, 296
Rich, William, 163–164, 232, 256–257
Rivera, Alex, 233–234
Robertson, J. David, *300*, 304
Robins, R. B., 208
Robinson, Walter Smith O'Brien, *283*
Rockefeller, John D., 19, 47–48
Rockefeller Foundation, 4
    Bell Building construction funding by, 81
    Commission on Financing of Hospital Care and, 231
    Committee on the Costs of Medical Care and, 22–23
    Community Health Sciences funding at DUMC by, 291
    Division of Medical Sciences and Public Health, 226
    Duke Power and, 45
    DUMC funding by, 7–8, 19, 47–54, 109–112, 281
    foreign medical student program of, 107–109
    formation of, 48
    General Education Board, 1–4, 11, 19, 29, 48, 55, 74–76, 110–111, 131–133, 214, 252
    International Health Board, 19–20, 48
    International Health Division, 20, 109, 113–116, 118, 127
    Lambert's tenure with, 60–61
    Latin American fellowships program, 112
    military commission funding by, 103–105
    Neuropsychiatry Dept. funding by, 112, 128–131, 226
    North Carolina College for Negroes and, 163–165
    nutrition research funding by, 73, 116–117
    physician assistant program funding, 272–273
    physics funding at Duke from, 201–202
    psychiatric research funding by, 9–10, 49–51, 69, 85–89
    race relations research funded by, 74–79
    reorganization of, 48–49
    research funding from, 29–32, 131–133
    School of Nursing funding by, 271–272
    Spelman Fund, 29
    Stead's resignation from Duke and, 192–193
    tropical disease research funding by, 113–116
    VA-Duke collaborations and, 156–157
    wartime funding programs of, 107–109
Rockefeller Institute for Medical Research, 30–32, 34–35, 41, 48, 82, 115
Rockefeller Sanitary Commission for the Eradication of Hookworm Disease, 19–22, 48
Rodnick, Eliot H., 250
Rogers, Mark C., 363–364, 432n.49

Roosevelt, Eleanor, 217
Roosevelt, Franklin Delano (President), 23, 32, 39, 45, 65, 213
Rorem, C. Rufus, 27, 231
Rosenau, Milton J., 74
Rosenwald Fund, 27, 77
Roses, Allen D., *300*, 309
Rous, Peyton, 7, 31, 83
Royall, Kenneth, 230
Ruffin, Julian M., 103
rural medicine, DUMC programs for, 273, 279–280
Rusk, Dean, 226
Sabiston, David C. Jr., 7, 359
  biomedical research programs and, 295
  Department of Surgery at Duke and, 264, 275–277, 306–308, 326
  general practitioner training opposed by, 328
  photos, *276, 301*
  physician-assistant program and, 273
  Private Development Clinic and, 356–357
  retirement of, 327, 353
  Society of Black American Surgeons and, 368
Sage, E. C., 1–2
St. Joseph of the Pines, 376, 388
Saito, Vicki Y., 379
salary issues at DUMC, 125–126
Salber, Eva, 289
Sands, Alexander H. Jr., *21*, 149, 177, 186–188, 193–194, 198, 201–202
Sanford, Terry (Gov.), 208, 255, 427–428n.58
  Brodie and, 319–320, 385
  building expansion at Duke and, 286–287, 289–290
  elected senator, 336
  NIH Environmental Health Sciences Center and, 325
  Nixon library controversy and, 313
  photos, *321, 384*
  political activities of, 263–266, 314
Santillan, Jesica, case of, 388–389
Sanus Corporation Health Systems, 365
Sarah P. Duke Gardens, 58
Sawyer, Wilbur A., 113–114
Schmitt, Miss, 130
Scholz, Willibald, 224, 423n.45
Science magazine, 31, 118
scientific research at Duke, 245–248
  physician-scientist concept and, 279–280, 293–295
  Research Training Program and, 247–248
Scientists and Engineers for Humphrey, 266
Scott, W. Kerr, 186, 199, 202, 233
Scudder, Atala, 55
Scudder, Townsend, 55
Sealy, Will Camp, *301*, 307–308
Searle Center, 282, 292
Securities and Exchange Commission, 60
Seeley G. Mudd Building, 282
Selective Training and Service Act, 102
Semans, James H., 255, 285, 290
Semans, Mary Duke Biddle Trent, 427n.48
  Brodie and, 319–320, 385
  building expansion campaign and, 280–281, 283–286, 290
  Duke Endowment and, 250
  as Duke Endowment chair, 326
  expansion of Duke Hospital and, 288

  photos, *17, 283*
  progressive politics of, 314
  Putman and, 382–385
  research programs and, 255
Shadow on the Land, 104
Shannon, James A., 115–116, 247, 267–268
Sharp, D. Gordon, 119, *254*
Sheetz, Michael P., 349, 353
Shepard, James E., 53, 77, 162–164, 169
Shingleton, William W., 239, 281, *301*
Shope, Richard, 7
Silver, Georga A. III, 224
Silverman, Albert J., 248
Sinclair Oil Company, 167
65th General Hospital, 97–100, 102, 137–139
  photo, *138*
Smith, David T., 32–37, 40–41, 62, 302–303
  Commission on Epidemiological Survey and, 102–103
  nutrition research by, 7, 73, 116–117
  photos, *33, 301*
Smith, Susan Gower, 32
Smith, Willis, 12, 147–149, 170–172, 178–181
  curriculum reform and, 273
  Davison's presidential candidacy at Duke and, 186–190, 193–196, 198–199
  death of, 206, 235
  election to Senate of, 206–208, 230, 235
  influence on Duke Medicine of, 205–206, 208–212, 252
  military research projects and, 216–223
  national health insurance proposals and, 199–200, 203
  photo, *183, 207*
  regional research center project of, 214–223
  rice diet research funding and, 212–214
  statewide health care planning and, 227–229
smoking, Duke research on, 216–223, 252–255, 259–261
Snyderman, Ralph, 14–15, 314, 335–336
  Brodie and, 316, 385–386
  chancellorship of DUMC, 344–345, 347–355, 377
  Duke Clinical Research Institute, 360–361
  Duke University Health System and, 376–377
  family medicine and, 325–327
  financial problems at DUMC and, 358–363
  Genentech and, 338, 340–341, 344
  GUSTO Project and, 351–352
  immunology research and, 296
  Institute for Genome Sciences and Policy, 387–388
  integration of PDC and, 355–357
  legacy of, 389–393
  photos, *301, 382, 389, 391*
  Putman and, 385
  racial politics and Durham health care and, 370–375
  research audit and, 378–379
  Stead and, 268–271
social services, at Duke Medicine, 51–54, 74–79
Society of Black American Surgeons, 368
Southeastern Regional Trophoblastic Center, 305
Southern Conference for Human Welfare, 206
Spach, Madison S., *301*, 303–304, 308
Spaulding, Asa, 320
Spaulding, C. C., 77
Spaulding, Elna, 320

Spaulding, Jean G., 320, 373–374
Spaulding, Kenneth, 374
Spears, Marshall T. (Judge), 417n.68
spectrophotometry
  research applications of, 35–36
  Rockefeller Foundation funding for, 112
Sponer, Hertha, 112
Sprunt, Douglas H., 103, 117
Stamford Laboratories, 35–37, 40
Standard Oil Company, 45–46, 48
Stanford University, 102, 316
Stanley, Wendell, 119
Stead, Eugene A. Jr., 10, 49, 109, 128, 147, 165–166
  cardiology research of, 332, 351
  as Department of Medicine chair, 277–279
  Duke Hospital expansion project and, 237
  gerontology research and, 250
  initiatives at DUMC of, 270–273
  Kempner and, 182–183
  Life Insurance Medical Research Fund and, 213
  National Institutes of Health and, 267–268
  photos, 190, 271
  physician assistant program and, 295, 329
  psychiatric medicine at Duke and, 151–152, 174
  public health policies and, 279–280
  Research Training Program and, 246, 265
  resignation of, 190–193
Stephen, C. Ronald, 240–241, 306, 425n.85
Stetten, DeWitt, 268
Stevens, Joseph B., 92–93
Steward, Bob, 149
Stotesbury, Edward, 46
Strode, George K., 115
Suitt, R. Burke, 129
sulfanilamide, research involving, 35, 41
Sullivan, Louis, 272, 337
Surgical Instrument Shop, 237
Sutherland, George F., 225, 423n.47
Swanson, Louis E., 232
syphilis, Duke research on, 103–105, 174
Syphilis Clinic (Duke Hospital), 104, 174

Taber, Robert L., 361, 363, 432n.49
Taylor, A. R., 119
Taylor, H. Grant, 173, 217–218, 420n.61
Tedder, Thomas F., 354
Teer, Dillard, 250
Ten Broeck, Carl, 82–83
Tenet Healthcare, 367, 371
10th Special Forces Group, 231
Textbook of Bacteriology, 303
Thayer, William S., xiii
Thompson, Bob, 202–203
Time magazine, 15, 44, 361–362, 378–379
Tisdale, Wright, 182
tissue plasminogen activator, Duke research on, 335–336, 343, 350–352
tobacco industry, Duke research programs and, 216–223, 252–255, 259–261
Topol, Eric J., 351
Tosteson, Daniel C., 274
Toth, Cynthia A. (Cindy), 306
Towe, Kenneth C., 255, 283, 427n.48
Treadwell, Henry Lee ("Buddy"), 329
Trent, Josiah Charles, 71, 202, 223
Trent, Mary Duke Biddle, 10, 14, 71, 201–202, 232, 255. See also Semans, Mary Duke Biddle Trent

Triangle Hospice, 376
Triangle Universities Center for Advanced Studies, 384
Trimeris company, 324
Trinity College (Duke University predecessor), 1–2, 43, 60, 110, 149, 171, 177
tropical disease research, Duke involvement in, 102, 113–116
Truman, Harry S. (President), 153, 181–182, 187, 199, 206–208, 217, 230
Turner, J. Clyde, 57
Twentieth Century Fund, 22

U.S. Bureau of Animal Industry, 35
Umstead, William B., 171, 199
Undergraduate Medical Education and the Elective System: Experience with the Duke Curriculum, 281
United Fund, 173
United Methodist Retirement Home of Durham, 376–377
United States Department of Health, Education and Welfare, 206, 234–235
United States Office of Economic Opportunity, 289
United States Public Health Service, 4, 127–128, 184–185
  Duke gerontology center funding, 250
  grant to Neuropsychiatry Dept. at Duke, 173–174
  integration initiatives funded by, 286
  Latin American fellowships program, 112
  partnerships with DUMC, 206, 209, 213
  venereal disease programs of, 104–105
United States Supreme Court, 207
University and Small Patent Procedures Act, 311, 322–325
University of North Carolina (UNC), 13–14, 27
  Division of Education and Research in Community Medical Care, 280
  Duke partnership with, 111
  Durham Regional Hospital and, 371
  expansion of medical school at, 124, 148, 157–159, 169–170, 172–174, 205–206, 210, 226, 286
  Gray as president of, 229–233
  health system created by, 377–378
  psychiatric center at, 227
  race relations and public health programs, 71, 74–79
  School of Public Health, 116
  School of Public Welfare at, 73–74
  social services division at, 52

vaccine development, Duke initiatives in, 118, 296–297, 302–306
Vanderbilt University, 1–2, 7
Van Theis, Sophie, 167
venereal disease, military research on, 103–105
Veterans Administration
  budget review of, 234–235
  double-billing controversy with DUMC, 193, 196
  Duke collaboration with, 155–157, 238–241, 418–419n.15
  Durham Hospital of, 3, 9, 102, 228
  Lyman's work with, 185–186, 193
  Mental Hygiene Clinic, 155
  photo of hospital, 239
  research programs at, 142, 216–223

Veterans Resident Training Program, 153
Veterinary Bulletin, 33–34, 67, 79–80
veterinary research, Duke involvement in, 30–37
virology research at DUMC, 30–32, 117–119, 295–297, 302–306
vitamin deficiency research at Duke, 116–117

W. K. Kellogg Foundation, 103, 105–106, 118, 231, 281
Wachovia Bank and Trust Company, 60
Wade, Wallace, 44
Wadsworth, Josph A. C. II, *301*, 305
Wake Forest College, 13, 20, 27
    Bowman Gray medical school at, 77, 123–124, 148, 209, 229–233
    move to Winston-Salem, 159–160
Wake Med Hospital, 376, 378
Walker, Charlotte (Frisch), 134
Wallace, Andrew G., *301*, 308, 326, 330, 332–333
Walltown Neighborhood Clinic, 397–398
Walltown Neighborhood Ministries, 397–398
Walter Kempner Foundation, Inc., 212–214
Wannamaker, William H., *141*, 170, 187
War on Poverty programs, 274–275
Warren, Charles, 242–245
Warren, James V., 191, 240
Watson, James, 8, 277, 337
Watts, Charles DeWitt, 289
Watts, George Washington, 1–2, 285
Watts Hospital
    closing of, 3, 286
    early building, xviii
    expansion of, 228, 288
    founding of, 1–2, 140
    physician-patient ratios at, 72
    racial integration of, 285–286
    segregation at, 174–175, 284–285
Weed, Lewis H., 112–115, 139
Weiss, Soma, 151
Welch, William H., xiii
WellPath, Duke agreement with, 366–367, 386–387
Westinghouse "Sterilamp," use at Duke Medicine of, 37
Wheeler, John, 285, 288–289
Whipple, Allen O., 423n.39
Whitaker, Paul, 211
Whitehorn, John, 222

Wiggins, Ethel J., 135–136, 417n.78
Wilkins, Robert H., *301*, 308–309
Williams, R. Sanders ("Sandy"), 377
Wilson, Florence K., 166
Wilson, Ruby L., 380
Wilson Times, 210
Wise, Nancy Bowman, 115–116, 416n.35
women at DUMC
    admission in wartime of, 107–109
    feminization of health care and, 381
    Hanes's attitudes concerning, 115–116
Women's Initiative, 380
Woodhall, Barnes, 86, 199–200, 221–223, 246, 423n.38
    building expansion at DUMC and, 283
    curriculum reform and, 274
    as dean of DUMC, 261, 264–265, 281
    gerontology research and, 250
    photos, *222*, *339*
    racial integration of Duke Hospital and, 282, 285–286
    retirement of, 326
Woods, Archie S., 114, 117
World War II, Duke Medicine during, 101–145
Wyckoff, Ralph W. G., 30–32, 35–37, 67–68, 82–83, 139, 297, 412n.4
Wyngaarden, James B., 8–9, 240, 246
    curriculum reforms and, 273
    as director of NIH, 326, 336–337
    Howard Hughes Medical Institute and, 354
    on immunology research, 296
    on Kempner's research, 296, 428n.73
    legacy of, 309–310
    photos, *269*, *301*
    as Research Training Program director, 258, 277–279, 293–294, 316
    Stead and, 267–269

Yaggy, Duncan, 350
Young, W. Glenn Jr., *301*, 307–308

Z. Smith Reynolds Foundation, 250
Zenith Radio Corporation, 44
Zinsser, Hans, 303
Zinsser Microbiology, 303
Zuidema, George D., 276